FAMILY HEALTH CARE NURSING

Theory, Practice, and Research

SECOND EDITION

SHIRLEY MAY HARMON HANSON
RN, PMHNP, PhD, FAAN, CFLE, LMFT
Professor, Oregon Health Sciences University
School of Nursing, Portland, Oregon

F.A. DAVIS PUBLISHERS
Philadelphia, Pennsylvania

F. A. Davis Company
1915 Arch Street
Philadelphia, PA 19103

Printed in the United States of America

Last digit indicates print number: 10 9 8 7 6 5 4 3 2 1

Acquisitions Editor: Joanne P. DaCunha, RN, MSN
Cover Design: Louis J. Forgione

Library of Congress Cataloging-in-Publication Data
First Edition co editor was Sheryl Thalman Boyd
Family health care nursing : theory, practice, and research / [edited by] Shirley May Harmon Hanson.—[2nd ed.]
p. ; cm.
Includes bibliographical references and index.
ISBN 0-8036-0598-6
1. Family nursing. 2. Family—Health and hygiene. 3. Sick—Family relationships. 4. Child health services. I. Hanson, Shirley M. H., 1938–
[DNLM: 1. Nursing Care. 2. Child Health Services. 3. Family Practice. 4. Health Promotion. 5. Nursing Process.
WY 100 F198 2000]
RT120.F34 F35 2000
610.73—dc21 00-031483

FAMILY HEALTH CARE NURSING:

Theory, Practice, and Research

To my sisters, Marjorie, Peggy, and Kathleen, who have stood steadfast beside me all of my life, but especially during the difficult times

To my children, Derek and Gwen, and their families, who continue to give me reason to celebrate family

To my God who created families to love, protect and care for each other

SHIRLEY MAY HARMON HANSON

ACKNOWLEDGEMENTS

There are many significant people to acknowledge for their direct or indirect contribution to the **second** edition of *Family Health Care Nursing.*. First, I would like to acknowledge Sheryl T. Boyd who was co-editor and contributed to the **first** edition which was published in 1996. Second, I am thankful to the twenty-four contributors who wrote for this **second** edition. Without their cooperation, hard work, and commitment to family nursing, this edition would never have come to fruition. Third, I would like to acknowledge the assistance and support received from my editors at FA Davis—Joanne DaCunha the Nursing Acquisitions Editor, and Diane Blodgett, the Developmental Editor. They helped to smooth the wrinkles in the long arduous process of giving birth to this edition of the book. Fourth, thanks to all the blind reviewers who read chapters in process and helped us make this book better and more user friendly. Fifth, several of us received special editorial assistance from Elizabeth Tornquist, a person who has dedicated much of her life to making nurses look good when they write. Sixth, a special thank you to Barbara Bodine, my staff assistant in getting this book put together. Every person who has ever published books, knows that books do not happen without a dedicated and loyal secretary and Barbara performed her duties par excellence! I am indebted to Barbara and only hope she is still available when the **third** edition rolls around. Finally, my sisters participated by going through family archives to select pictures that liven up the book. Thank you Marjorie and Peggy for your love and devotion to me and our family.

FOREWORD

This book represents an important contribution to advancing the integration of theory, practice, and research for nursing care of families. The first edition was published in 1996. This second edition, written especially for the new millennium, updates the information and demonstrates the significance of family social and health policy with family health care nursing. The authors retain the clinical focus of the book to guide the learners through a systematic review of the knowledge derived from family sciences, family therapy, and family nursing—all of which form the foundations for the theory, practice, research and social policies important in family health care nursing. The first half of the book addresses theoretical foundations for family nursing, and the second half of the book describes how nurses can and should practice with families in a variety of clinical settings. The book guides students in learning to apply theory to practice and provides examples of how this is done. Examples of assessments and interventions with families are significant contributions of the book.

Editor Hanson has enlisted many of the highly qualified family nurses across the country to describe their varying approaches to the nursing care of families. This variety reinforces that there is no one person, theory, or approach that works for all families and situations. Family nursing is broad and those who call themselves family nurses often exercise their skills within clinical specialties across the age continuum and settings such as acute care and primary health care. Because of this integration of family focused nursing across age and practice settings, family nursing is seen by some as an emerging specialty while others see this integration as evidence that family nursing is established. The authors of this book make it clear that family can and should be the focus for all health care.

Contributions to advance the state of the science and clinical practice of families and their family members occur through several approaches: textbooks written for clinicians, scientific conferences, scholarly journals, research, research critiques, and synthesis reviews of the literature. Some of these approaches are described briefly in an effort to place this textbook within the broader scientific advances of family nursing. What is evident in each example of the approaches cited below is that to advance practice knowledge, the work must be deliberate, extend over time, and be research based. Those involved must be willing to systematically critique their own work and that of other scholars. Efforts such as this book, where the authors critiqued and revised their own previous successful edition, is one important approach to advance the knowledge of families and family health care. In this second edition, Hanson and the other authors have not only updated the text but they have conducted careful analysis to assure the currency and relevancy of the text.

Another major approach that has contributed to family nursing science is the initiation of the scholarly journal, the *Journal of Family Nursing*. This journal, edited by Dr. Janice Bell of the University of Calgary, provides an ongoing forum for peer reviewed cutting edge articles pertaining to family nursing education, practice, and research. In less than a decade, it is recognized for its significant contributions to the science and practice of family nursing. Another means of moving family nursing science forward has been through the mechanism of scientific conferences. The International Family Nursing Conference held every three years around the world is an example of this kind of commitment to the advancement of family nursing. The first conference was in Calgary, Alberta Canada in 1988, and followed in Portland, Oregon (1991); Montreal, Canada (1994); Valdavia Chile (1997); and in

Chicago in 2000. The publications derived from the first and second meetings solidified the contributions of the family nursing scholars attending these meetings and demonstrate the growing breadth and depth of our knowledge of family health care (Bell, Watson & Wright, 1990; Feetham, Meister, Bell & Gilliss, 1993).

Other approaches to advancing family nursing science are the reviews and synthesis of nursing research. An example of this synthesis is the landmark book *Handbook of Clinical Nursing Research* edited by Hinshaw, Feetham & Shaver(1999) . In Feetham's (1999) synthesis of the state of the science of nursing research of families in this handbook, she described three common themes and gaps: the continuing need for family theory development in nursing research, the need for increased progress in intervention research, and the increased need for the integration of research and practice.

Family Health Care Nursing: Theory, Practice, and Research is an example of the integration that Feetham stated was needed. Of significance is how the authors of this text continually draw on research and the state of the science reviews for their integration. Textbooks such as this can bridge the gap of the translation of research to practice as well as the gap from practice knowledge to research. Research and practice are interactive and this is one of the themes apparent in this textbook.

Strengths of nursing research in general and nursing research of families in particular are evident in this text including the diversity in the populations studied with a focus on vulnerable or at-risk groups. Another contribution of the text is that the chapters include the developmental perspective of families, and the interdependence of issues of practice and policy in the health care of families. Another important message in this text is the recognition of the varying family forms in society. The authors acknowledge that there is not a better or dominant family form. The authors document that the traditional family of two parents and two children, espoused since the 1950s, does not exist as the dominant structure in society (Coontz, 1992). Inherent in the authors' discussions is that achieving family functions is the marker of all families and not one particular family form or structure. The underlying message is that society is acknowledging the varying family forms as evidenced in our changing social policy rather than the fact that family structure and functions are changing.

Nursing practice and research can inform health and social policy. Nursing research that translates best practices into public policy addressing access, quality and cost is essential to the health of families. The authors demonstrate the integration of family exemplars with distinct social policies. For example, Gebbie and Gebbie (2000) note that families live within social policies that have evolved in or been legally created by the culture and government surrounding them. These policies have an impact on who can be considered family, how parenting is supported, caregiving for dependents, access to health services and basic economic welfare. Understanding this interdependence between policy, families and nursing is central to providing the best care. Through their exemplars the authors reinforce that many of those for whom we care are not in a position to actively advocate for changes and for themselves. They describe the roles and actions for nursing to advocate for families and family members.

This book is reflective of nursing in general in that there is limited attention to the significance of the discoveries in technology and science. For example, there is an imperative that all health professionals must have genetic literacy to interpret the burgeoning knowledge of gene function from the Human Genome Project (Collins, 1999; Hayflick & Eiff, 1998). The genetic discoveries are changing our understanding of the mechanisms, diagnosis, treatment and prevention of disease. What little research is reported on the psychosocial issues from the new genetic and technological knowledge, essentially none is conducted in the context of family (Feetham, 1999; Rolland, 1999). While specific exemplars and content would have been a strength, the frameworks and strong clinical perspectives of the authors of this text enable the readers to translate the family context to the burgeoning knowledge in technology and science. This book makes an excellent contribution to the next generation of family nurses that includes researchers, practitioners, theoreticians, educators and policy makers who have health and families as their focus. The editor and the contributing authors display a high level of scholarship in guiding this new generation to provide family health care nursing in the 21st century. The authors provide direction to students, faculty and practicing clinicians for the integration of family to practice, research, and health and social policy.

Suzanne L. Feetham, PhD, RN, FAAN
Professor, Harriet Werley Research Chair
College of Nursing, University of Illinois at Chicago

REFERENCES

Bell, J., Watson, W.L. & Wright. L.M. (Eds.) (1990), *The Cutting Edge of Family Nursing*. Calgary: Calgary Press.

Collins F. S. (1999) Shattuck Lecture—Medical and societal consequences of the Human Genome Project. New Engl J Med. 411, 28–37.

Coontz, S. (1992) *The Way We Never Were: American Families and the Nostalgia Trap*. New York: Basic Books.

Feetham, S. L. (1999). Families and the genetic revolution: Implications for primary health care, education, and research. *Families, Systems and Health* 17:1, 27–44.

Feetham, S.L. (1999) Section Overview Families in health, illness and life transitions. In A.S. Hinshaw, S. Feetham, J. Shaver (Eds) *Handbook of Clinical Nursing Research*. Thousand Oaks, CA: Sage Publications. 199–200.

Feetham, S.L, Meister, S.B., Bell, J.M., & Gilliss, C. L. Eds. (1993) *The Nursing of Families: Theory, Research, Education, Practice*. Newbury Park, CA: Sage Publications.

Hayflick S. J., Eiff M. P. (1998) Role of primary care providers in the delivery of genetics services. *Community Genetics* 1:18–22.

Hinshaw, A. S., Feetham, S., Shaver, J.L.F. (Eds) (1999) *Handbook of Clinical Nursing Research*. Thousand Oaks, CA: Sage Publications. Page xvi.

Rolland, J. S. (1999). Families and genetic fate: A millennial challenge. *Families, Systems & Health: The Journal of Collaborative Family Health Care* 17:1, 123–127.

PREFACE

Family health care nursing has arrived! We in the health care professions, particularly nursing, have been preaching for the last ten years or so about the importance of the interaction that exists among individuals, families and their health status. We have become acutely aware of the therapeutic triangle that exists between individuals, families, and the health care team. Much has evolved in family nursing since the early thinkers and writers started twenty years ago and we are now in the second and even third generation of family nursing scholars. We all stand on the shoulders of our earlier family nurses including Florence Nightingale. I am grateful for the exchange of ideas and what I learn from the work of other contemporary family nursing scholars: Kathryn Barnard, Janice Bell, Perri Bomar, Marion Broome, Carol Danielson, Suzanne Feetham, Marilyn Friedman, Marie-Luise Friedemann, Catherine Gillis, Brenda Hamel-Bissell, Mary Ann Johnson, Kathleen Knafl, Maureen Leahey, Judy Malone, Marilyn McCubbin, Karen Pridham, Wendy Watson, Patricia Winstead-Fry, Lorraine Wright, Beth Vaughan-Cole, B. Lee Walker, just to name some and hope I have not forgotten others.

This first edition of this book came out in 1996 and was extremely well received. In fact, it is being translated right now in Japan. The second edition of *Family Health Care Nursing* prepared for the new millennium is completely rewritten resulting in a new, refined and expanded edition. There were 16 chapters in the first edition and 17 chapters in the second edition. Some people who wrote for the first edition dropped away for a variety of reasons, but most stayed on with the project. A few mentors turned their chapter revisions over to next generation mentees. There are three brand new chapters in this edition: Chapter 2 (Theoretical Foundations for Family Nursing, Chapter 3 (Research in Families and Family Nursing), and Chapter 16 (Families, Nursing and Social Policy). All in all, this edition is a new and improved model.

The purpose of this book is to provide a foundation in the concepts of family health care nursing, to learn how these concepts and theories are practiced in the traditional specialities within the nursing profession, and to see how these concepts play out in the social policy arena or predict the future of family nursing and families. It is my belief that family nursing is no longer just another evolving specialty in nursing, but rather family nursing is THE umbrella under which all specialties could/should/do practice nursing. For example, childrearing family nursing draws on different theories and research than gerontological family nursing, but they are both "family nursing". To be able to practice family nursing, it appears to be a matter of whether nurses have been educated in a family nursing paradigm as part of their formal undergraduate/graduate education or are self taught by experience. I believe this book forwards the art and science of family nursing into the new millenium. It does this by integrating the theory, practice and research (TPR) of family nursing; it accomplishes this by integrating the TPR of nursing scholarship with the TPR of family social science and family therapy. This book makes the cognitive connection between assessment and intervention strategies. The book was created to be a comprehensive textbook to be used by student nurses and practitioners at all levels. I realized there is a deficit of literature in family nursing, when I was teaching both undergraduate and graduate family nursing core courses. It was through teaching and practicing family nursing myself, that my own ideas continued to form and I asked and answered some questions about the nature of family nursing. What is it that nurses need to know about family health care nursing and how can this be applied in a variety of health care settings by different levels of practitioners? It was through teaching graduate students that I realized that many students do not receive any family nursing foundation through their original associate, diploma, or baccalaureate programs. They were being exposed to these ideas the first time during their masters or doctoral program. This book is appropriate for both undergraduate and graduate students who need a foundation in family health care nursing. Every nurse practitioner program today should include an advanced course in family nursing and this book would serve as a resource. This text is also suitable for registered nurses already practicing but who want to learn more about family health care nursing, or as a general reference text for all practicing nurses.

Family Health Care Nursing is organized so that it can be used in its entirety from cover to cover for a course in family nursing. Another alternative approach for the use of this text is to first teach Section I pertaining to the Foundations of Nursing Care of Families early in the nursing curricula, and then expose students to the individual specialty chapters in Section II related to Family Nursing Practice while these same students are going through the various clinical rotations in their curricula. Section III on Families, Nursing, Social Policy and Futures could be addressed during the latter part of the senior year. The third alternative use is to use this book as a reference text or as an adjunct to other textbooks that address specific specialties such as: maternity, pediatrics, geriatrics, or community health. There is something in this book for all levels of students and there is something in this book for all levels and specialties of practicing nurses.

Concerning the contributors for this textbook, great efforts were made to garner the best talent available in family nursing from across the country, nurses who were sound theoreticians, practitioners, researchers, and yes teachers! This was no small feat and it was compounded by some of the usual problems that editors experience—people drop out for one reason or the other, new co-authors are added, or manuscripts are late and I had to nag. On a whole, I found nurse authors responsible. articulate, and committed. I found this second edition of the book easier to develop four years after the first edition because of the electronic age technology and because I had an excellent working team. I believe that nurses are growing in their sophistication in scholarly publication efforts and that no one person has the knowledge and skills to single author a textbook in todays world. Textbooks of this kind are always group efforts. Congratulations to these contributors for their tenacity in this two-year process and for their commitment to families and nursing!

The book is divided into three sections. **Unit I addresses the Foundations of Nursing Care of Families.** There are nine chapters in this section. **Chapter 1, Family Health Care Nursing: An Introduction** was written by Shirley Hanson (the editor of this textbook) from Oregon Health Sciences University School of Nursing (Portland) . This chapter lays a foundation by giving an overall introduction to family health care nursing. Family, family health and family nursing are defined and the reasons for learning about family nursing are discussed. Next the author talks about the history of family nursing, approaches to family nursing, variables influencing family nursing, family nursing roles and obstacles influencing family nursing practice. There is a section on the history of families in America, functions and demographics of families, and concepts for family health care.

Chapter 2, Theoretical Foundations for Family Nursing, a brand new chapter for this book, was developed by Shirley Hanson, Oregon Health Sciences University School of Nursing, and Joanna Kaakinen from University of Portland School of Nursing. This chapter addresses what is theory, the functions of theory, and the criteria for evaluating theory. Selected theories from family social science, family therapy, and nursing science that help frame research and practice in family nursing are summarized and integrated approaches to family nursing are described. This chapter would also fit nicely with a course in nursing research. This chapter also lays the foundation for the theory discussion within each of the practice chapters in Section II of this book.

Chapter 3, Research in Families and Family Nursing, is another new chapter developed especially for this edition. It was authored by Gail Houck and Sheila Kodadek, both from Oregon Health Sciences Univeristy School of Nursing. This chapter addresses methods used to identify and validate family theory. Research methods and issues particular to family research are addressed in order to enhance the reader's ability to evaluate research on families for use in nursing practice. This chapter discusses the central issue of family as a "unit of analysis" and describes how resolution of this issue impacts the nature of research questions asked. This chapter would also fit nicely with a course in nursing research. There are examples of nursing research where some of these methods and issues are discussed.

Chapter 4, Family Structure, Function & Process was written by Naomi Ballard, Professor Emeritus from Oregon Health Sciences University School of Nursing. She summarizes basic core issues pertaining to families in America. Her sociological bent shows through as she discusses family structure, family function and family process and how these concepts relate to health care of families. Her discussion of family process includes an overview of familial roles and the effects of communication, power, and decision making upon the enactment of these roles. This chapter is important as a basic foundation in understanding families.

Eleanor Ferguson-Marshalleck and J. Kim Miller from California State University, Department of Nursing (Los Angeles) wrote **Chapter 5, Socio-cultural Influences on Family Health.** This chapter discusses and explicates some of the complex socio-cultural influences on family health. It defines key concepts of culture and ethnicity, social class and family health and discusses the growth in cultural diversity and the disparity between social classes in the United States. The chapter also examines the extent to which health beliefs and practice as well as family values/communication/power/ roles/coping styles influence family health. An exploration of social class structure as a decisive factor in family health is included. Implications for family nursing practice are suggested.

Chapter 6, Factors influencing Family Functioning and the Health of Family Members, was developed by Marcia Van Riper from the College of Nursing at Ohio State University in Columbus. Van Riper examines the relationship between family systems and health relationships and how these health factors influence family functioning and the health of individual family members. Both factors within the family and outside the family are addressed. In addition, the Resiliency Model of Family Stress, Adjustment and Adaptation is presented as well as Rolland's work on how illness characteristics and illness time phases influence family recovery from chronic illness.

Beverly Ross, Professor Emeritus from Indiana University School of Nursing wrote **Chapter 7, Nursing Process and Family Health Care.** Ross first summarizes the systematic steps of the nursing process and then shows how these ideas fit the paradigm for family nursing. In addition, she reviews two classification systems (NANDA diagnostic framework and the Omaha classification system) and describes and uses them to define family health problems and concerns. Families involvement in each step of the nursing process is emphasized. A case study is presented using the cyclic and dynamic family nursing process.

The editor of this book Shirley Hanson from Oregon Health Sciences School of Nursing wrote **Chapter 8, Family Assessment and Intervention,** was written by Shirley Hanson. She expands on the concept of assessment as the first and essential ingredient to provide comprehensive family health care. She differentiates between assessment and measurement and then presents three different family nursing assessment models that can be used by clinicians in the field. These models are followed by a case example that demonstrate the varying level and scope of information derived from using the various models and instruments, including a sample family genogram and ecomap.

Chapter 9, Family Health Promotion—is presented by Perri Bomar and Pammela Baker-Word from University of North Carolina School of Nursing at Wilmington. This chapter provides an overview of the history of health promotion and its historical relevance to family nursing in the United States. Models of both family health and family health promotion are presented. Bomar points out that the nursing process is used as an approach to empower families to achieve optimum wellness and includes such activities as assessment, contracting, health teaching, and anticipatory guidance. Finally the implications for practice, education, family policy and research are discussed in relation to family health promotion.

Unit II of this book addresses Family Nursing Practice and consists of 6 chapters focused on the practice of family nursing in six major clinical areas. **Chapter 10** was written by Louise Martell, University of Washington School of Nursing and is entitled **Family Nursing with Childbearing Families.** This chapter includes a brief history of family nursing, use of theory to guide childbearing family nursing process, health promotion, threats to health, and implications for education, research and policy. Emphasis is on health promotion in relation to developmental tasks of childbearing families. A case study of a family experiencing preterm birth is used to illustrate the impact of threat to health on childbearing families. Throughout the chapter, nursing interventions with childbearing families are emphasized. The chapter concludes with implications for education, research and policy development.

Chapter 11, Family Child Health Nursing, was co-authored by Vivian Gedaly-Duff and Marsha Heims, both from Oregon Health Sciences University

School of Nursing. This chapter describes the practice of family child health nursing. It begins by examining the history of family centered care and then describes the Family Interaction Model, using examples to illustrate the connection between theory and practice. Application of this interactional model to four areas of practice is examined: health promotion, acute illness, chronic illness, and life-threatening illness. In addition, practice, education, research and health care policy relevant to family child health nursing care are reviewed.

Chapter 12 was created by Nancy Trygar Artinian from Wayne State University College of Nursing and is titled **Family-Focused Medical-Surgical Nursing.** The purpose of this chapter is to describe factors and issues for nurses to consider as they plan care for families in medical-surgical settings. Included is a review of the stressors that families often face during hospitalization and the discussion of the use of the therapeutic quadrangle to analyze family needs during an illness episode. This chapter examines caring for families before, during and after acute/chronic illness and during the terminal illness experience. It also reviews broad categories of family nursing interventions during phases of illness. Included are a discussion of theoretical models and a case example is highlighted.

Chapter 13 is co-penned by Helene Moriarty from Philadelphia Veterans Affairs Medical Center and Margaret Shepard from Temple University Department of Nursing(Philadelphia). This chapter is called **Family Mental Health Nursing.** The authors provide a historical overview of trends in family mental health nursing relating conceptual models to the practice of family mental health nursing. The focus is on health promotion, and acute and chronic mental illness with appropriate case studies to demonstrate the issues. Strategies are identified that assist nurses in creating a healthy environment for families within any health care setting. Implications of the family approach to mental health nursing for practice, education, research and health policy conclude the chapter.

Beverly Richards and Mary LuAnne Lilly from Indiana University School of Nursing wrote **Chapter 14, Gerontological Family Nursing.** The purpose of this chapter is to describe the nature, scope and goals of gerontological family nursing and to discuss the demographic and social trends that influence the dynamics and structure of the contemporary older family.

Then the authors describe normative and non-normative events that challenge older families functioning and care giving. This is followed by a demonstration of the use of the Family Life Cycle Model and the Resiliency Model of Family Stress. Following intervention strategies are implications for future research and social policy.

Families and Public Health Nursing in the Community, was coauthored by Debra Anderson (University of Kentucky School of Nursing), Cecelia Capuzzi (Oregon Health Sciences University School of Nursing) and Diane Hatton (University of San Diego School of Nursing). **Chapter 15** describes how the principles and practice of family nursing and community/public health nursing are integrated into family-centered community nursing. It includes a discussion of the historical roots of the care of families in community settings, theoretical perspectives, and concepts basic to care of families such as health promotion, disease prevention, and nursing interventions in acute and chronic illness. Implications for family community health nursing practice, education, research, and social policy are reviewed.

Unit III focuses on Families, Nursing, Social Policy and Futures. Chapter 16 is titled **Families, Nursing and Social Policy** and it is a new chapter written especially for this book. It is completed by a mother/daughter team: Kristine Gebbie from Columbia University School of Nursing, and Eileen Gebbie, who is a doctoral student in the Department of Sociology from the University of Illinois. This chapter discusses some of the dominate ways in which public social policy affect families, particularly family health. Included are policies affecting the ability to parent or provide care for family members, gain access to needed services, and provide for family welfare. The goal is to illustrate the variety of lived family experiences by social structure and review important legal and social policies regarding family in order to facilitate the highest quality of nursing care and health care policy.

The last chapter of the book, **Chapter 17,** was authored by the editor Shirley Hanson (Oregon Health Sciences University School of Nursing) and is entitled **Families and Family Nursing in the New Millennium.** It summarizes general patterns of changing families, future demographics of American families and glimpses of world demographic trends. Also it discusses the future of family nursing theory, practice, research, education, and social policy. It concludes with other factors influencing family nursing such as religion, sexuality, health care technology and health care reform. This chapter brings closure to the book.

As editor of this book and author of some of the

chapters, I am glad this nearly two year project is finished. I encourage anyone to write me with your critiques, your counterpoints and your ideas that could be included in the next edition of this textbook. This book was not meant to be a template but rather a catalyst to move the art and science of family nursing forward.

I can be contacted at:

Shirley May Harmon Hanson
Oregon Health Sciences University
School of Nursing
3181 SW Sam Jackson Park Road
Portland, Oregon 97201-3098
Voicemail: 503-494-3869
Fax: 503-494-3878
E-mail: hansons@ohsu.edu

CONTRIBUTORS

Debra Gay Anderson, RNC, PhD
Associate Professor
University of Kentucky
College of Nursing
Lexington, Kentucky

Nancy Trygar Artinian, RN, PhD
Associate Professor
Wayne State University
College of Nursing
Detroit, Michigan

Cecelia Capuzzi, RN, PhD
Professor
Oregon Health Sciences University
School of Nursing
Portland, Oregon

Pammela Baker-Word, RN, MSN, FNP
University of North Carolina-Wilmington
School of Nursing
Wilmington, North Carolina

Naomi R. Ballard, RN, MA, MS
Associate Professor Emeritus
Oregon Health Sciences University
School of Nursing
Portland, Oregon

Perri J. Bomar, RN, PhD
Associate Dean and Professor
University of North Carolina-Wilmington
School of Nursing
Wilmington, North Carolina

Eleanor Ferguson-Marshalleck, RN, MPH, PhD
Professor and Associate Chair
School of Nursing
California State University, Los Angeles

Eileen Gebbie, MA
Teaching Assistant and Teaching Fellow
University of Illinois
Department of Sociology
Urbana, Illinois

Kristine M. Gebbie, DrPH, RN
Elizabeth Standish Gill Associate Professor of Nursing
Director, Center for Health Policy
Columbia University School of Nursing
New York, New York

Vivian Gedaly-Duff, RN, DNSc
Associate Professor
Oregon Health Sciences University
School of Nursing
Portland, Oregon

Shirley May Harmon Hanson, RN, PMHNP, PhD, FAAN, CFLE, LMFT
Professor
Oregon Health Sciences University
School of Nursing
Portland, Oregon

Diane Hatton, RN, CS, DNSc
Associate Professor
University of San Diego
Hahn School of Nursing and Health Science
San Diego, California

Marsha L. Heims, RN, EdD
Associate Professor
Oregon Health Sciences University
School of Nursing
Portland, Oregon

Gail M. Houck, RN, PhD
Associate Professor
Oregon Health Sciences University
School of Nursing
Portland, Oregon

Joanna Rowe Kaakinen, RN, PhD
Associate Professor
University of Portland
School of Nursing
Portland, Oregon

Sheila M. Kodadek, Ph.D., RN
Professor
Oregon Health Sciences University
School of Nursing
Portland, Oregon

Mary LuAnne Lilly, RN, PhD, Fellow
Indiana University School of Nursing
Indianapolis, Indiana

Louise Martell, RN, PhD
Associate Professor
University of Washington
School of Nursing
Seattle, Washington

Jung Kim Miller, RN, PhD
Professor
California State University
Associate Director, The Roybal Institute for Applied Technology
Los Angeles, California

Helene J. Moriarty, PhD, RN, CS
Nurse Researcher
Philadelphia Veterans Affairs Medical Center
Philadelphia, Pennsylvania

Beverly S. Richards, RN, DNS
Associate Professor
Indiana University School of Nursing
Adjunct Associate Professor and-Family Care Coordinator
Alzheimer's Disease Center
Indiana University School of Medicine
Indianapolis, Indiana

Beverly J. Ross, RN, MANEd, MSEd
Assistant Professor Emeritus
Indiana University
School of Nursing
Indianapolis, Indiana

Margaret P. Shepard, RN, PhD
Assistant Professor
Director of Graduate Studies in Nursing
Temple University
Department of Nursing
Philadelphia, Pennsylvania

Marsha Van Riper, RN, PhD
Assistant Professor
College of Nursing,
The Ohio State University
Columbus, Ohio

CONSULTANTS

Teri Aronowitz, RN-CS, MSN, FNP
Doctoral Student
University Rochester
School of Nursing
Rochester, New York

Ellen G. Christian, MS, RN-C
Professor
Institutional Nursing
University of Massachusetts
North Dartmouth, Massachusetts

Ruth P. Cox, PhD, LMFT, CRNP, ARNP
Assistant Professor, Graduate Studies
University of Alabama
School of Nursing
Birmingham, Alabama

Susan B. Fowler, RN, MS, PhD(c), CCRN, CNRN, CS
Reseaarch Assistant and Instructor
Robert Wood Johnson University Hospital
New Brunswick, New Jersey

JoAnn K. Gottlieb, ARNP, CS, MS
Assistant Professor
Barry University
North Miami, Florida

June Andrews Horowitz, PhD,RN, CS, FAAN
Associate Professor
Boston College
School of Nursing
Chestnut Hill, Massachusetts

Melinda Jenkins, RN, PhD
Assistant Professor of Primary Care
Director, FNP Program
University of Pennsylvania
School of Nursing
Philadelphia, Pennsylvania

Patricia S. Jones, RN, PhD, FAAN
Professor
Loma Linda University
School of Nursing
Loma Linda, California

Heather J. McKnight, RN, MSN
Course Coordinator, Undergraduate Pediatrics
University of Pennsylvania
School of Nursing
Philadelphia, Pennsylvania

Lynette Leeseberg Stamler, RN, PhD
Associate Professor
University of Windsor
School of Nursing
Windsor, Ontario, Canada

Nancy Symmes, RN, BSN, MAEd(c)
Faculty
College of New Caledonia
Prince George, British Columbia, Canada

Elizabeth S. Tiechler, RN-C, FNP, MSN, PhD(c)
Senior Instructor
University of Colorado Health Sciences Center
Denver, Colorado

CONTENTS

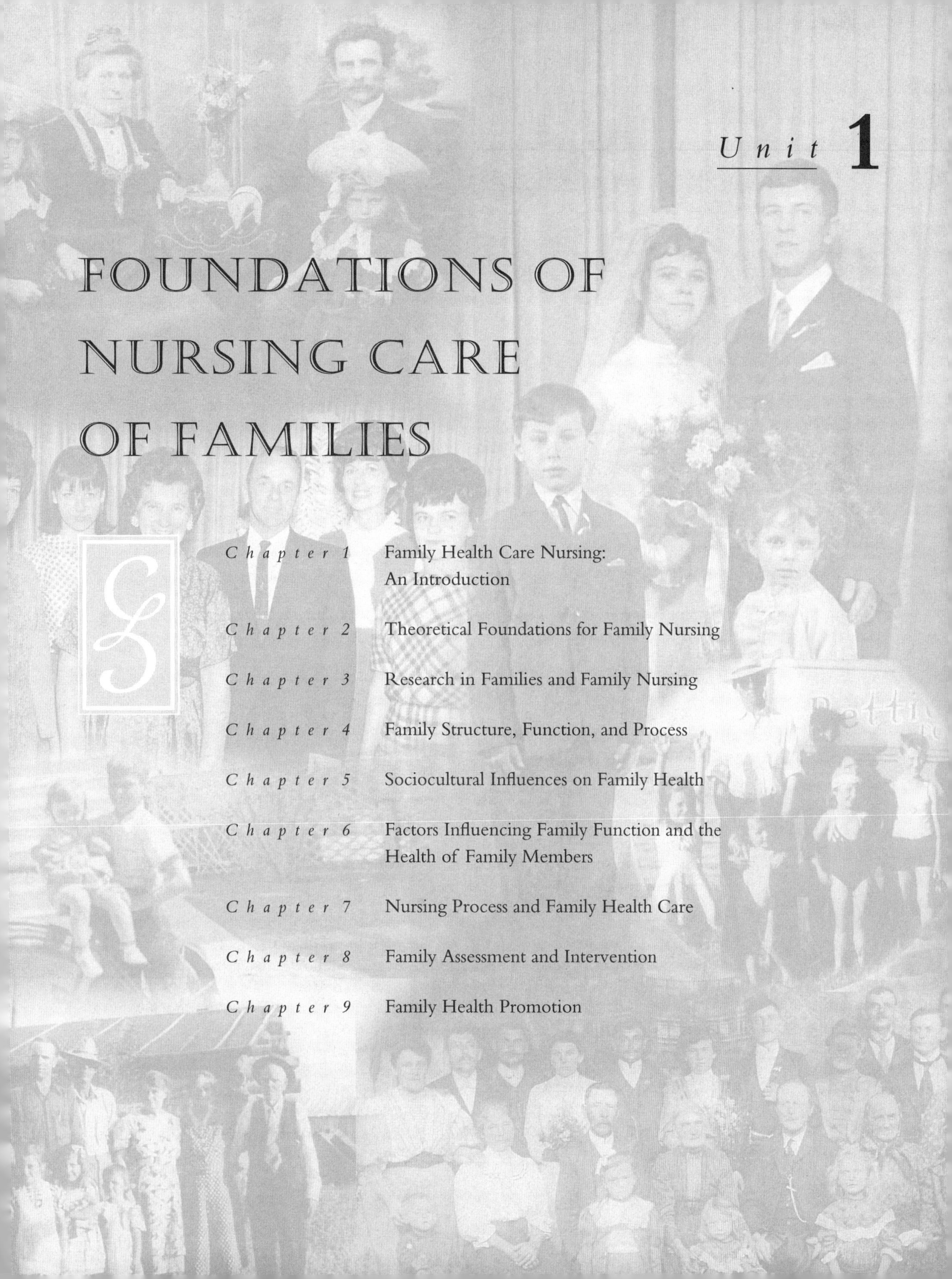

Unit **1**

FOUNDATIONS OF NURSING CARE OF FAMILIES

Focus On

FAMILY HEALTH CARE NURSING: AN INTRODUCTION

Welcome to *Family Health Care Nursing*. Family nursing is more than an emerging specialty; it is a new way of thinking about families and nursing. Family nursing is a lens through which we view the nursing care of families. It is important that this lens becomes clear and that the concepts are incorporated into your development as a beginning or advanced nurse.

Chapter 1 introduces you to one of the most important clients in nursing practice today: the human family. Traditionally, the focus of most nursing education is on the practice of nursing with individual clients. In this chapter, you will get to know the family client, one of the many aggregate clients you will encounter in professional nursing practice. It is anticipated that readers bring to this study of families a background in natural and social sciences as well as in the humanities, all of which will assist readers to understand the complex client that we call "the family."

All of us learn about families by being a member of one. Therefore, some of us tend to view ourselves as experts about families on the basis of this narrow egocentric viewpoint, and we question the need for focused study about families and nursing. You may have assumed that nursing practice is uniform for individuals or families with similar nursing diagnoses. Let us recall that nursing is an interpersonal profession; just as a nurse's personal characteristics affect individual client relationships, so too a nurse's experience and assumptions from his or her own family influence that nurse's interactions with client families. For this reason, it is essential to make a systematic study of the many kinds of families and how nurses can work with this important basic unit of society in the health care system.

The chapter begins with a broad overview of families, family health, and family nursing, all of which brings us to the full spectrum of family nursing. This big picture includes a summary of the history of family nursing and how nursing has arrived at its present status. The chapter proceeds with a discussion of concepts for family health care, including the family health and illness cycle, levels of family care, the therapeutic triangle, and when to gather the family in health care settings.

Finally, the chapter examines the history, the functions (past and present), and the demographics of American families. In summary, the purpose of this chapter is to immerse you in the subject of families and nursing and give you a foundation to begin your journey—a journey that will change your personal and professional opinions on how you think about and work with families. I hope you enjoy the discoveries you make as you learn about challenging new insights in the chapters to come.

Chapter 1

FAMILY HEALTH CARE NURSING: AN INTRODUCTION

Shirley May Harmon Hanson, RN, PhD

OUTLINE

OBJECTIVES

On completion of this chapter, the reader will be able to:

- Explain why it is important to have a family focus in nursing.
- Define family, family health, and family health care nursing.
- Describe the changing demographics of American families and the implications of these changes for the future of family nursing.
- Describe the interactions between families and the health-to-illness continuum.
- Compare and contrast the four different views of families.
- Summarize the history of the modern family and family nursing.
- Differentiate between family theory, family therapy, and family nursing.
- Know the roles of the various health professionals involved in family health care, particularly the role of the family nurse.

INTRODUCTION TO FAMILY HEALTH CARE NURSING

Family health care nursing is emerging as an art and a science. Much nursing talent and effort during the last 10 years has been used to move the specialty to where it is today. Family health nursing has evolved to the point of the following achievements: (1) a number of textbooks focus on the emerging theory, practice, and research; (2) articles written by nurses are published in an array of scientific journals; (3) family nursing scholars are celebrated all over the world, particularly in the United States and Canada; (4) there is unquestioned inclusion of family content in both undergraduate and graduate nursing curricula; (5) national and international family nursing conferences are being held; and finally, (6) a new journal, called the *Journal of Family Nursing,* was born. Box 1–1 lists journals that explore themes related to families and nursing. Although the specialty has come a long way, efforts continue to: (1) conceptualize and classify the phenomena of interest in family nursing, (2) build a science that is cumulative rather than isolated, and (3) develop theories drawing from clinical practice that explain nursing and family interaction in health and illness (Gilliss, 1990, p. v).

WHY TEACH NURSES ABOUT FAMILY NURSING?

Why teach nurses about families, when many people believe they are "experts in the family," having had personal experiences with their own families? Based on this limited experience, family members make assumptions and judgments about their own and other families with whom they work. However, when nurses operate from only their own experience, they have an egocentric view of families. Individual socialization, culture, and value systems effect the way nurses work with families. The overall goal of this book is to enhance your knowledge and skills that pertain to the theory, practice, and research important for the nursing of families.

Why is a family focus important for nursing? The research literature generally concludes that: (1) health and illness behaviors are learned within the context of family (Pratt, 1987); (2) family units are affected when one or more members experience health problems, and families are a significant factor in the state of health and well-being of individuals (Gilliss, 1993); (3) families affect the health of individual members, and each individual member's health events and health practices affect the family as a whole (Doherty, 1985; Doherty & Campbell, 1988); (4) health care effectiveness is improved when emphasis is placed on the family, rather than just on the individual (Gilliss & Davis, 1993); and (5) promotion, maintenance, and restoration of the health of families is important to the survival of society (Anderson & Tomlinson, 1992).

There is also a growing recognition that health crises are critical events in the life of a family, which make them a population at risk. Families at risk are vulnerable to deterioration in mental and physical health and family function. Families at risk have an opportunity to increase their adaptive capacity and mental health during a crisis, and nurses can provide supportive interventions during these critical events.

The centrality of the family in health care delivery is emphasized by the futuristic policy statement of the American Nurses Association (ANA, 1995; ANA, 1996), as well as legal definitions of nursing in many states that mandate nurses to provide family care. Although families have been recipients of nursing care for many years, recent challenges to the individual paradigm of nursing now include the family as the unit of care or the family as the context of care. This paradigm shift is affecting the development of family theory, practice, research, and education.

What is the Family?

Family is a word that conjures up different images for every individual and group, and the word has evolved in its meaning over time. Definitions focus on different aspects according to the paradigm of the respective discipline, for example:

- Legal: relationships through blood ties, adoption, guardianship, or marriage
- Biological: genetic biological networks among people
- Sociological: groups of people living together
- Psychological: groups with strong emotional ties

The U.S. Bureau of the Census has used the same definition for years: the family is a group of two or more persons related by blood, marriage, or adoption who are residing together. Therefore, early family social science theorists (Burgess & Locke, 1953) adopted the following definition in their writing:

> The family is a group of persons united by ties of marriage, blood, or adoption, constituting a

Box 1-1

JOURNALS RELATED TO FAMILIES AND FAMILY NURSING

American Journal of Family Therapy
Community and Family Health
Family and Child Mental Health Journal
Journal of the Jewish Board of Family and Children's Services
Families in Society: The Journal of Contemporary Human Services
Family and Community Behavior
Family and Community Health
Family Behavior
Family Health
Family Medicine
Family Planning Digest
Family Planning Perspectives
Family Planning/Population Reporter
Family Process
Family Relations (previous title: Family Coordinator)
Family Science Review
Family Studies Review Yearbook
Family Systems Medicine
Family Therapy Collections
Family Therapy Networker
Family Therapy News
Health and Social Work
Health Care for Women International
Inventory of Marriage and Family Literature
Journal of Adolescent Research
Journal of Child and Family Nursing
Journal of Comparative Family Studies
Journal of Divorce
Journal of Family History
Journal of Family Issues
Journal of Family Nursing
Journal of Family Practice
Journal of Family Psychology
Journal of Marital and Family Therapy
Journal of Marriage and The Family
Marriage and Family Review
Maternal-Child Health
Merrill-Palmer Quarterly of Behavior and Development
Social Forces
Social Problems
Social Work
Social Work and Health Care
Sociology of Health & Illness
The Family Journal: Counseling and Therapy for Couples and Families
Women and Health
Women and Health Care
Youth and Society

> single household; interacting and communicating with each other in their respective social roles of husband and wife, mother and father, son and daughter, brother and sister; and creating and maintaining a common culture (pp. 7–8).

The definitions of early family nursing scholars also followed these trends.

It was not until the 1980s that the broader definitions of family moved beyond traditional blood, marriage, or legal constrictions. In 1985, one of the first family nursing departments in the country adopted this definition:

> The family is a social system composed of two or more persons who coexist within the context of some expectations of reciprocal affection, mutual responsibility, and temporary duration. The family is characterized by commitment, mutual decision making, and shared goals (Department of Family Nursing, Oregon Health Sciences University, 1985).

The definition for family adopted by this textbook is:

> **Family refers to two or more individuals who depend on one another for emotional, physical, and economical support. The members of the family are self-defined.**

Nurses working with families should ask clients who they consider as their family and then include those persons in health care planning. The family may range from traditional notions of the family, for example, the nuclear and extended family, to such "post-modern" family structures as single-parent, step, extended, and same-gender families. In a study reported by Ford (1994), people were asked about their perceptions of what "family" is. Ford found that for young college students the definition of family was shifting to include a greater variety of possibilities, such as cohabitating couples without children, same-gender partners, and certain extended groups. Females in her study were more likely than males to consider various alternative scenarios as families. She concluded that there will be even more alternative family forms in the future and that professionals must explore their own perceptions and definitions of families to enhance their work with alternative family structures.

What is Family Health?

What is meant by the term family health? Health has been described as a state or process of the whole person in interaction with the environment in which the family represents a significant factor of the environmental matrix (Anderson and Tomlinson, 1992).

Despite the focus on family health within nursing, the construct of family health lacks consensus and precision. Anderson and Tomlinson (1992) said, "the analysis of family health must include simultaneously both health and illness and the individual and the collective." There is growing evidence that the stress of a member's serious illness exerts a powerful influence on family function and health, and that families' behavior patterns can, in turn, influence individual health (Campbell, 1987).

The World Health Organization has always defined health as a state of complete physical, mental, and social well-being and not merely the absence of disease and infirmity: this definition could apply to individuals as well as families. The term "family health" is often used interchangeably with the terms family functioning, healthy families, or familial health. To some, family health is actually the composite of individual family members' physical health, because it is impossible to make a single statement about the whole family's physical health. The term "healthy" family versus "unhealthy" or "dysfunctional" family is often used to connote negative mental status and not physical health per se, so a healthy family is one that is functioning well in society, and this may or may not have much to do with physical health. Years ago, McEwan (1987) concluded that family health refers to the comparative health status of individuals within the family and that familial health is an evaluative description of functions and structures of the family, with dual focus on both health of individual members and health of the family as a whole. Pender (1996) supported the notion that health and illness are qualitatively different and should be considered separate but related phenomena. The definition adopted by this textbook is:

> **. . . Family health is a dynamic changing relative state of well-being which includes the biological, psychological, spiritual, sociological, and culture factors of the family system.**

This approach, which combines the biological, psychological, social, cultural, and spiritual aspects of life, refers to individual members as well as the whole family unit. An individual's health (on the wellness-to-illness continuum) affects the entire family's function and, in turn, the family's function affects each individual's health. Thus, assessment of family health involves simultaneous assessment of individual family members and the whole family system. Family health nursing includes health promotion as well as treatment of chronic and acute illness.

Healthy Families

Terms used to refer to healthy families or family strengths have varied throughout time in the literature. Otto (1963) was the first scholar to develop psychosocial criteria for assessing family strengths that emphasized the need to focus on positive family attributes instead of the pathological approach that accentuates family weaknesses. Pratt (1976) introduced the idea of the "energized family" as one whose structure encourages and supports persons to develop their capacities for full functioning and independent action, thus contributing to family health. Stinnett, Chesser, and DeFrain (1979) researched characteristics of family strengths. Curran's research (1983, 1985) investigated not only family stressors but also traits of healthy families incorporating moral and task focus into traditional family functioning (Box 1–2, Traits of Healthy Families).

What is Family Health Care Nursing?

The specialty area of family health care nursing has been emerging over the last decade. It has become a specific focus of practice that cuts across the various other specialty areas of nursing, although as a distinct specialty, it is still in its early youth. There is still some disagreement as to how it is distinctive from other specialties that might involve families, such as maternal-child health nursing, community health nursing, and mental health nursing. For the purpose of this book, family health care nursing is defined as:

> . . . the process of providing for the health care needs of families that are within the scope of nursing practice. Family nursing can be aimed at the family as context, the family as a whole, the family as a system or the family as a component of society.

One conceptual framework for family nursing is depicted in Figure 1–1. This framework shows how the concepts of the individual, the family, nursing, and society intersect with one another. Family nursing takes into consideration all four approaches to viewing families and, at the same time, cuts across the individual,

Box 1–2 TRAITS OF HEALTHY FAMILIES

- Communicates and listens
- Fosters table time and conversation
- Affirms and supports each member
- Teaches respect for others
- Develops a sense of trust
- Has a sense of play and humor
- Has a balance of interaction among members
- Shares leisure time
- Exhibits a sense of shared responsibility
- Teaches a sense of right and wrong
- Abounds in rituals and traditions
- Shares a religious core
- Respects the privacy of each member
- Values service to others
- Admits to problems and seeks help

Source: Curran, D. (1983). *Traits of a healthy family*. Minneapolis: Winston Press (Harper & Row).

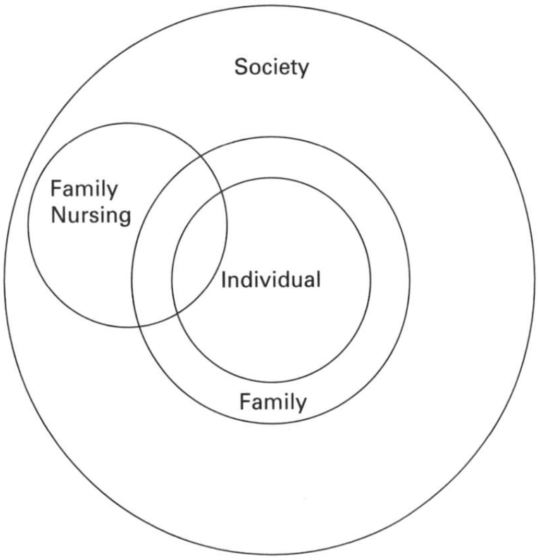

FIGURE 1–1
Family nursing conceptual framework.

family, and community for the purpose of promoting, maintaining, and restoring the health of families important to societal survival. Figure 1–2 contains a model for viewing family nursing theory, where family nursing is seen conceptually as the confluence of theories and strategies from nursing, family therapy, and family social science. Over time, family nursing continues to incorporate more ideas from family therapy and family social science into the practice of family nursing as a result of more nurses having pursued advanced preparation in those disciplines.

Some family nursing scholars have differentiated among the varying levels of knowledge and skill family nurses need for a generalist versus specialist practice and have defined the role of advanced academic preparation for different levels of practice. Wright and Leahey (1984, pp. 7–9) proposed that nurses receive a generalist or basic level of knowledge and skill in family nursing during their undergraduate work, and advanced specialization in family nursing or family therapy at the graduate level. They proposed differences between the generalist family nurse and the specialist family nurse. In summary, they recognized that advanced specialists in family nursing have a much narrower focus than generalists and that family assessment is an important skill for nurses who practice with families. Building on previous work, Bomar (1996) developed five different levels of family nursing practice using the novice to expert paradigm (see Table 1–1).

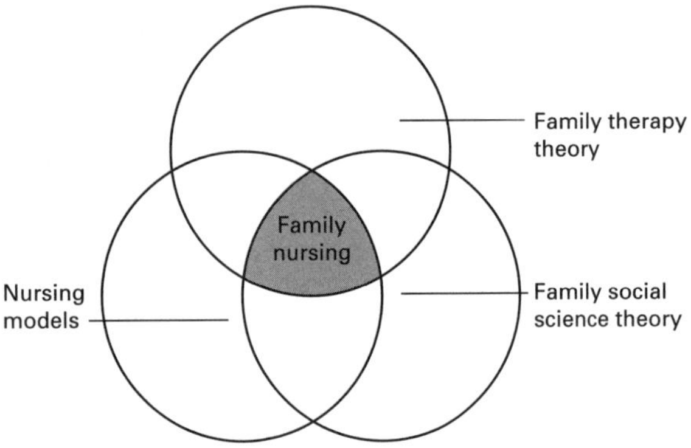

FIGURE 1–2
Family nursing practice.

Nature of Interventions in Family Nursing

Gilliss, Roberts, Highley, and Martinson (1989, pp. 71–72) identified 10 characteristic or distinctive features of family nursing, emphasizing the multivariate nature of the relationship between family health and the health of individual members. In describing the nature of interventions in family nursing, they determined:

1. Family care is concerned with the experience of the family over time. It is considerate of both the history and the future of the family group.
2. Family nursing is considerate of the community and cultural context of the group. The family is encouraged to receive from and give to community resources.
3. Family nursing is considerate of the relationships between and among family members and recognizes that, in some instances, all individual members and the family group will not achieve maximum health simultaneously.
4. Family nursing is directed at families whose members are both healthy and ill. Family health is not indexed by the degree of individual health or illness.
5. Family nursing is often offered in settings in which individuals present with physiologic or psychological problems. Along with being competent in treatment of individual health problems, family nurses must recognize the reciprocity between individual family members' health and collective health within the family.

TABLE 1–1
Levels of Family Nursing Practice

Level of Practice	Generalist/Specialist	Education	Client
Expert	Advanced Specialist	Doctoral degree	All levels Family nursing theory development Family nursing research
Proficient	Advanced Specialist	Master's degree with added experience	All levels Beginning family nursing research
Competent	Beginning Specialist	Master's degree	Individual in the family context Interpersonal family nursing Family unit Family aggregates
Advanced beginner	Generalist	Bachelor's degree with experience	Individual in the family context Interpersonal family nursing (family systems nursing) Family unit
Novice	Generalist	Bachelor's degree	Individual in the family context

Source: Bomar, P.J. (Ed.) (1996). *Nurses and Family Health Promotion: Concepts, Assessment, and Interventions,* ed. 2. Philadelphia: W. B. Saunders, (p. 17).

6. The family system is influenced by any change in its members; therefore, when caring for individuals in health and illness, the nurse must elect whether or not to attend to the family. Both individual and collective health are intertwined and will be influenced by any nursing care given.
7. Family nursing requires that the nurse manipulate the environment to increase the likelihood of family interaction; however, the absence of family members does not preclude the nurse from offering family care.
8. The family nurse recognizes that which person in a family is the most symptomatic may change over time; this means that the focus of the nurse's attention will also change over time.
9. Family nursing focuses on the strengths of individual family members and the family group to promote their mutual support and growth as it is possible.
10. Family nurses must define with the family which persons constitute the family and where they will place their therapeutic energies.

These are the distinctive characteristics of family nursing that continuously reappear in the care and study of families in nursing, regardless of the theoretical model in use.

Approaches to Family Nursing

Nursing literature defines the different approaches to care inherent in family nursing. This chapter presents four different views, perspectives, or approaches to family nursing practice, research, and education: (1) family as the context for individual development, (2) family as a client, (3) family as a system, and (4) family as a component of society. Figure 1–3 shows the approaches to family nursing. Each approach has its roots in different specialties within the nursing profession: maternal-child nursing, primary care nursing, psychiatric or mental health nursing, and community health nursing (Hanson & Boyd, 1996; Berkey & Hanson, 1991). All of these specialty orientations have contributed to the emerging field of family nursing. All four approaches have legitimate implications for nursing assessment and intervention. The approach that nurses use is determined by many factors, including the health care setting, family circumstances, and nurse resources. Figure 1–4 depicts these four views through

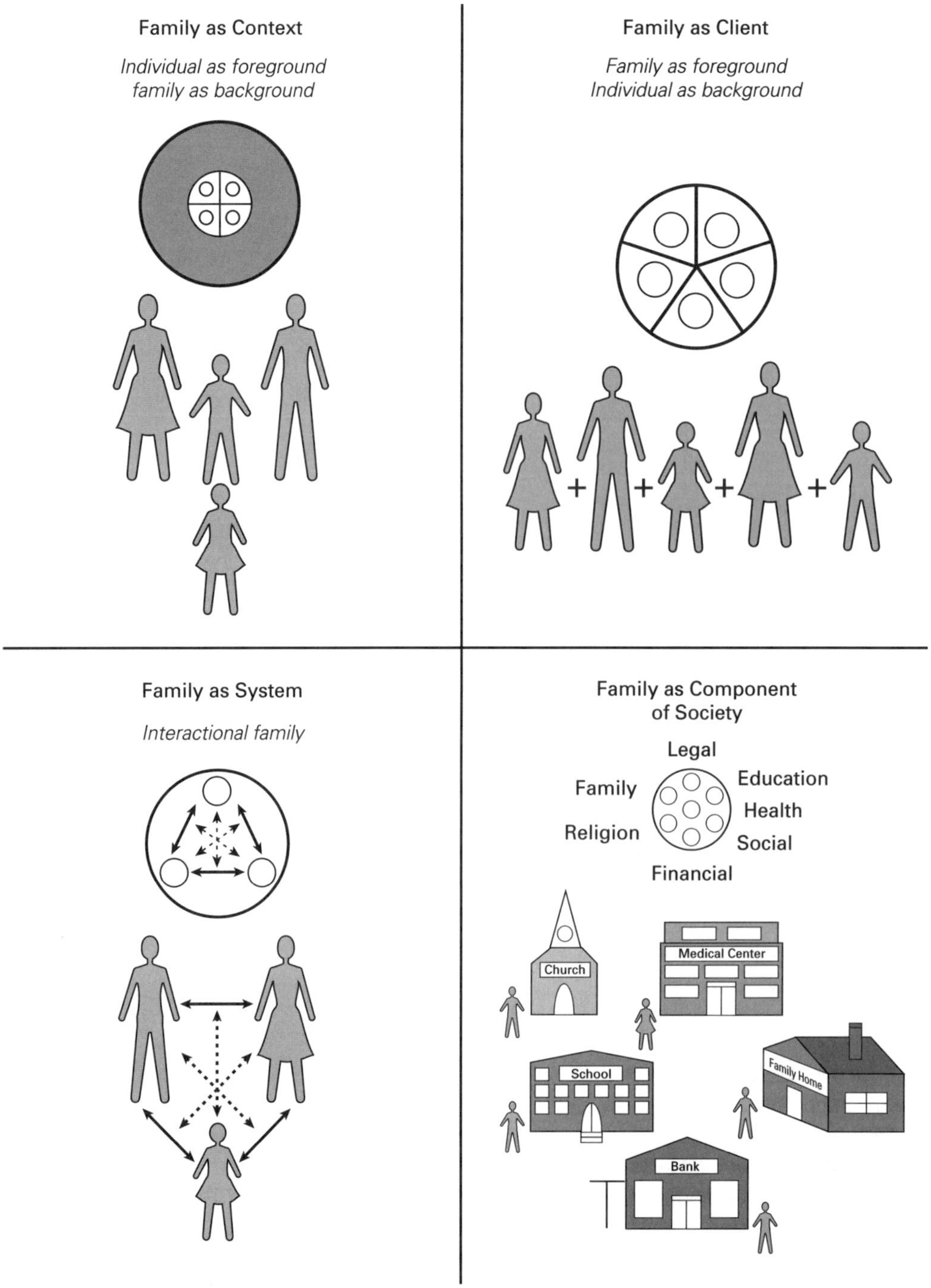

FIGURE 1–3
Approaches to family nursing.

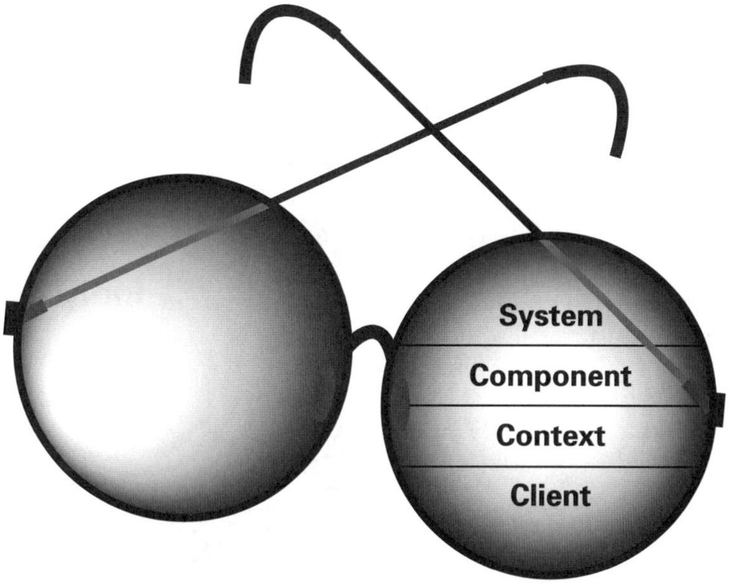

FIGURE 1–4
Four views of family through a lens.

one lens. It is important to keep all four perspectives in mind when working with any given family.

The first approach to family nursing care focuses on the assessment and care of an individual client in which *the family is the context.* This is the traditional nursing focus, in which the individual is foreground and the family is background. The family serves as context for the individual as either a resource or a stressor to their health and illness. Most existing nursing theories or models were originally conceptualized using the individual as a focus. Alternate labels for this approach are "family-centered" or "family-focused." This approach is rooted in the specialty of maternal-child nursing and underlies the philosophy of many maternity and pediatric health care settings. A nurse using this focus might ask an individual client: "How has your diagnosis of juvenile diabetes affected your family?" or "Will your nightly need for medication be a problem for your family?"

The second approach to family nursing care centers on the assessment of all individual family members; *the family as client* is the focus of care. In this approach, the family is in the foreground and individuals are in the background. The family is seen as the sum of individual family members, and the focus is concentrated on each individual. Each person is assessed, and health care is provided for all family members. However, the family unit is not necessarily the primary consideration in providing care. Medicine's primary care movement provided the impetus for this approach to family care and, more recently, the responsibility for this approach was assumed by family nurse practitioners. This approach is typically seen in family health care settings in the community in which family practice physicians or family nurse practitioners eventually provide care to all family members. From this perspective, a nurse might ask a family member who has just become ill: "Tell me about what has been going on with your own health and, while you are here, tell me about how your sister is getting along with her recent diagnosis of juvenile diabetes." It is worth noting that some family nursing theorists combine the family as client with the family as system, but for the sake of this discussion, they are viewed differently.

The third approach to care focuses on *the family as a system.* The focus is on the family as client, and the family is viewed as an interactional system in which the whole is more than the sum of its parts. That is, the interactions between family members become the target for nursing interventions that result from the nursing assessment. The family nursing system approach focuses on the individual and family simultaneously. The emphasis is on the interactions between family members; for example, the direct interactions between the parental dyad or the indirect interaction between the parental dyad and the child (see Fig. 1–3). The more children there are in a family, the more complex these interactions become.

The family system is imbedded in a larger community system. The systems approach always implies that when something happens to one part of the system, the other parts of the system are affected. So, if one family member becomes ill, it affects all other members of the family. Questions that nurses ask in a system approach may be: "What has changed between you and your spouse since your child was diagnosed with juvenile diabetes?" or "How has the diagnosis of juvenile diabetes affected the ways in which your family is functioning and getting along with each other?" This interactional model had its start with the specialty of psychiatric and mental health nursing.

The fourth approach to care views *the family as a component of society,* in which the family is viewed as one of many institutions in society, similar to the health, educational, religious, or economic institutions. The family is a basic or primary unit of society, as are all the other units, and they are all a part of the larger system of society (Figure 1–5). The family as a whole interacts with other institutions to receive, exchange, or give communication and services. Family social science first used this approach in its study of families in society. The approach uses a structural functional and exchange theory point of view. Community health nursing has drawn many of its tenants from this perspective as it focuses on the interface between families and community agencies.

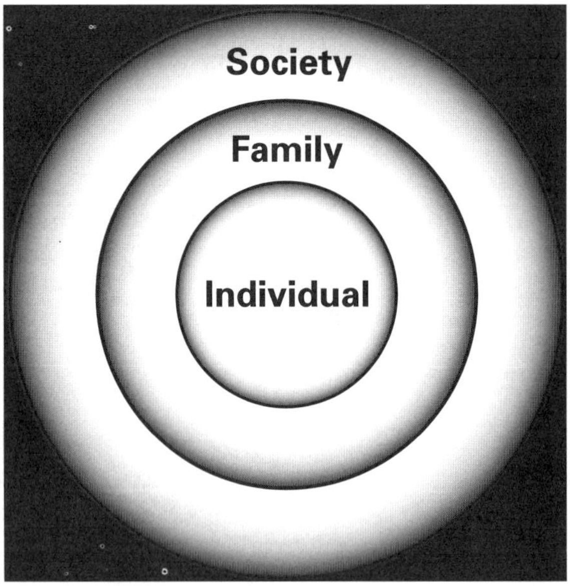

FIGURE 1–5
Family as primary group in society.

Variables Influencing Family Health Care Nursing

The evolution of family health care nursing has been influenced by many variables that are derived from both historical and present events within society and the profession of nursing, such as nursing theory, practice, education, and research; knowledge derived from family social sciences and health care sciences; national and state health care policies; changing health care behavior and attitudes; and national and international political events. A detailed discussion of some of these areas are contained elsewhere in this text (see Chap. 16). Also, Bomar (1989, 1996) discussed a few of these areas in her book on family health promotion.

Figure 1–6 shows a sample of the many variables that influence contemporary family health nursing, making the point that the status of family nursing is dependent on what is occurring in the wider society. A recent example of this point is that health practices and policy changes are under way because of the recognition that current costs of health care are escalating and, at the same time, greater numbers of people are underinsured or uninsured and have lost access to health care. The goal of this health care reform is to make access and treatment available for all at an affordable cost. That will require a major shift in priorities, funding, and services. A major movement toward health promotion and family care in the community will greatly affect the evolution of family nursing.

Family Nursing Roles

The roles of family health care nurses are evolving along with the field. Figure 1–7 shows the many roles that nurses can assume with families as the focus. This figure was constructed from some of the first family nursing literature that appeared and is a composite of what various scholars believe to be the role of the nurse today (Bomar, 1996; Friedman, 1998; Hanson and Boyd, 1996b). Each health care setting may affect the role that the nurse plays with families.

1. Health teacher. The family nurse teaches about family wellness, illness, relations, and parenting,

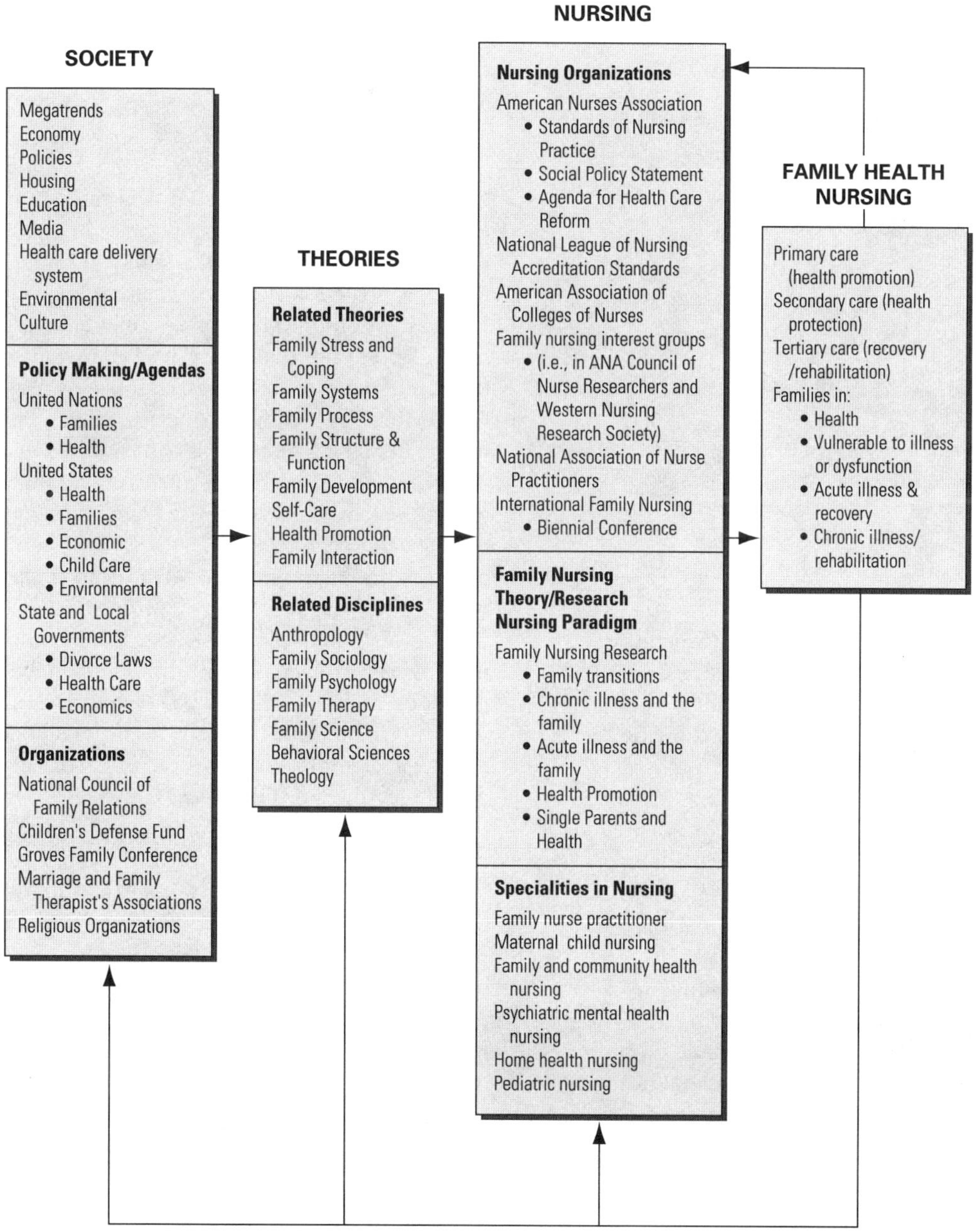

FIGURE 1–6
Variables influencing contemporary family health nursing. (From Bomar, PJ: *Nursing and Family Health Promotion: Concepts, Assessment, and Interventions.* 2nd Edition. W. B. Saunders, Philadelphia, 1996, with permission.)

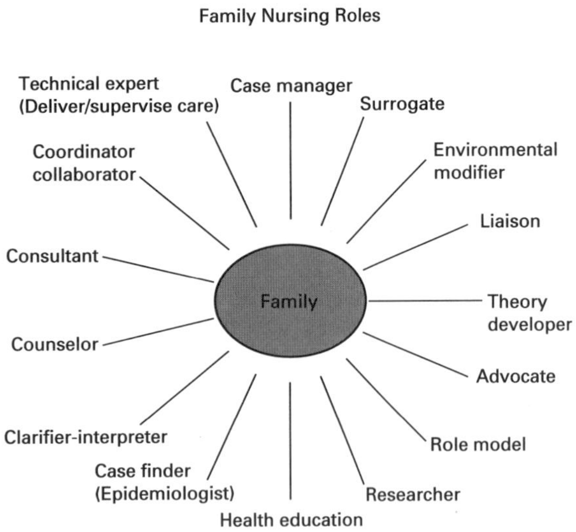

FIGURE 1–7
Family nursing roles. (Data from Leavitt [1982], Bomar [1989], Friedman [1992], and Hanson [1991].)

to name a few. The teacher-educator function is ongoing in all settings in both formal and informal ways. Examples include teaching new parents how to care for their infant and giving instruction about diabetes to a newly diagnosed adolescent boy and his family members.

2. Coordinator, collaborator, and liaison. The family nurse coordinates the care that families may receive, collaborating with the family in the planning of this care. For example, if a family member has been in a traumatic accident, the nurse would be a key person in helping families to access resources—from inpatient care, outpatient care, home health care, and social services to rehabilitation. The nurse may serve as the liaison among these services.
3. Deliverer and supervisor of care and technical expert. The family nurse either delivers or supervises the care that families receive in various settings. To do this, the nurse must be a technical expert both in terms of knowledge and skill. For example, the nurse may be the person going into the family home on a daily basis to consult with the family and help take care of a child on a respirator.
4. Family advocate. The family nurse advocates for families with whom they work; that is, the nurse empowers family members to speak with their own voice or the nurse speaks out for the family. An example is the nurse who is advocating for family safety by supporting legislation that requires wearing seat belts in motor vehicles.
5. Consultant. The family nurse serves as a consultant to families whenever asked or whenever necessary. In some instances, he or she consults with agencies to facilitate family-centered care. For example, a clinical nurse specialist in a hospital may be asked to assist the family in finding the appropriate long-term care setting for their sick grandmother. The nurse comes into the family system by request for a short period of time and for a specific purpose.
6. Counselor. The family nurse plays a therapeutic role in helping individuals and families solve problems or change behavior. An example from the mental health arena is a family that requires help with coping with a long-term chronic condition, such as when a family member has been diagnosed with schizophrenia.
7. Case-finder and epidemiologist. The family nurse gets involved in case-finding and becomes a tracker of disease. For example, consider the situation in which a family member has been recently diagnosed with a sexually transmitted disease. The nurse would engage in sleuthing out the sources of the transmission and in helping to get other sexual contacts in for treatment. Screening of families and subsequent referral may be a part of this role.
8. Environmental modifier. The family nurse consults with families and other health care professionals to modify the environment. For example, if a man with paraplegia is about to be discharged from the hospital to home, the nurse assists the family in modifying the home environment so that the patient can move around in a wheelchair and engage in self-care.
9. Clarifier and interpreter. The family nurse clarifies and interprets data to families in all settings. For example, if a child in the family has a complex disease, such as leukemia, the nurse clarifies and interprets information pertaining to diagnosis, treatment, and prognosis of the condition to parents and extended family members.
10. Surrogate. The family nurse serves as a surrogate by substituting for another person. For

example, the nurse may stand in temporarily as a loving parent to an adolescent who is giving birth to a child by herself in the labor and delivery room.

11. Researcher. The family nurse should identify practice problems and find the best solution for dealing with these problems through the process of scientific investigation. An example might be collaborating with a colleague to find a better intervention for helping families cope with incontinent elders living in the home.
12. Role model. The family nurse is continually serving as a role model to other people through his or her activities. A school nurse who demonstrates the right kind of health in personal self-care serves as a role model to parents and children alike.
13. Case manager. Although case manager is a temporary name for this role, it involves coordination and collaboration between a family and the health care system. The case manager has been formally empowered to be in charge of a case. For example, a family nurse working with seniors in the community may become assigned to be the case manager for a patient with Alzheimer's disease.

What are Some Obstacles to Family Nursing Practice?

The question arises: why has family nursing only been practiced in recent history? A number of reasons exist.

First, there is a vast amount of literature on the family, but there was little on the family in nursing curricula until the past decade. The majority of practicing nurses have not had exposure to family concepts during their undergraduate education and continue to practice using the individualist paradigm.

Second, there has been a lack of good comprehensive family assessment models, instruments, and strategies in nursing. More scholars are developing ideas and material in this arena; the chapter on family assessment and intervention presents three of the better known models.

Third, many students and nurses believe that the study of family and family nursing is just common sense and does not belong formally in nursing curricula, either in theory or practice. Learning about subjects that have personal familiarity can be of help or hindrance to learners, and most undergraduate nursing students are more attracted to learning about pathology than wellness.

Fourth, nursing has strong historical ties with the medical model. The medical model has traditionally focused on the individual as client, not the family. At best, family has been viewed in context, and many times, families were considered a nuisance in health care settings—an obstacle to overcome in providing care to the individual.

Fifth, the traditional charting system in health care has been oriented to the individual. For example, Subjective, Objective, Assessment, Plan (SOAP) focuses on the physical care of the individual and does not lend itself easily to a whole family or lots of members of families.

Sixth, the medical and nursing diagnostic systems used in health care are disease-centered, and diseases are focused on individuals. The International Classification of Disease (ICD) (AMA, 1997), *the Diagnostic and Statistical Manual of Mental Disorders* (DSM-IV) (APA, 1994), North American Nursing Diagnosis Association (NANDA) (Gordon, 1994; NANDA, 1998), and *The Omaha System: Application for Community Health Nursing* (Martin & Scheet, 1992) have only some diagnostic codes that take the whole family into consideration. Nurses select their diagnosis from these existing manuals, which because they include few choices for family diagnosis, also do not help in determining the family intervention.

Seventh, most insurance carriers require that there be one identified patient with a diagnostic code drawn from an individual disease perspective. Thus, even if health care providers are intervening with entire families, this requires the provider to choose one person in the family group as the identified patient and to give that person a physical or mental diagnosis, even though the client is the whole family. There is a need for better family diagnostic codes that are accepted by vendors as legitimate reasons for reimbursement.

Finally, the eighth obstacle to increased family care has been the established hours during which health care systems provide services. Traditionally, this has been during the day, when family members cannot accompany each other to seek care and become acquainted with the health care provider. Increasingly, this is changing because urgent care centers and other outpatient settings are incorporating evening and weekend hours into their schedules, making it possible for family members to come in together. These obstacles to family-focused nursing practice are slowly changing;

nurses can continue to lobby for changes that are more conducive to caring for the family as a whole.

History of Family Nursing

Family health nursing has roots in society from prehistoric times. The historical role of women has been inextricably interwoven with the family, for it was the responsibility of women to care for family members who fell ill and to seek herbs or remedies for the illness. In addition, by housekeeping, women made efforts to provide clean and safe environments for the maintenance of health and wellness (Bomar, 1996; Ham and Chamings, 1983; Whall, 1993).

During the Nightingale era, the historical development of families and nursing became more explicit. Florence Nightingale influenced both the establishment of district nursing of the sick and poor and the work of "health missionaries" through "health-at-home" teaching. She believed that cleanliness in the home could eradicate high infant mortality and morbidity. She encouraged family members of the fighting troops to come into the hospitals during the Crimean War to take care of their loved ones. Nightingale supported helping women and children toward good health by promoting both nurse midwifery and home-based health services. In 1876, in a document entitled *Training Nurses for the Sick Poor,* Nightingale encouraged nurses to serve in nursing both sick and healthy families in the home environment. She appears to have given both home-health nurses and maternal-child nurses the mandate to carry out nursing practice with the whole family as the unit of service (Nightingale, 1949, p. 32).

In colonial America, women continued the centuries-old traditions of women who nurtured and sustained the wellness of their families and cared for the ill. During the Revolutionary War, women called "camp followers" provided nursing care. These untrained nurses performed many functions for the troops.

During the Civil War (1861 to 1865), nursing of the wounded solders became more organized. Women formed Ladies Aid Societies, groups who met regularly to sew, prepare food and medicines, and gather other items needed by the soldiers. Dorothea Dix was named the Superintendent of Women Nurses of the U.S. Army. Hundreds of women received a month's training to prepare them for military nursing work.

During the industrial revolution of the late 18th century, family members began to work outside the home. Immigrants, in particular, were in need of income, so they went to work for the early hospitals. This was the real beginning of public health and school nursing. The nurses involved in the beginning of the labor movement were concerned with the health of workers, immigrants, and their families. Concepts of maternal child and family care were incorporated into basic curriculums of nursing schools.

Maternity nursing, nurse midwifery, and community nursing historically focused on the quality of family health. Margaret Sanger fought for family planning. Mary Breckenridge formed the famous Frontier Nursing Service (midwifery) to provide training nurses to meet health needs of mountain families.

There was a concerted expansion of public health nursing during the Depression to work with families. However, before and during World War II, nursing became more focused on the individual, and care became centered in institutional and hospital settings, where it remained until recently.

Since the 1950s at least 19 disciplines have studied the family and, through research, have produced family assessment techniques, conceptual frameworks, theories, and other family material. Recently, this interdisciplinary work has become known as "family social science." Family social science has greatly influenced family nursing in the U.S. because of the National Council of Family Relations and their large number of family publications. Many family nurses have become active in this organization. In addition, many nurses are now receiving advanced degrees in family social science departments around the country.

Nursing theorists started in the 1960s to systematize nursing practice. Scholars began to articulate the philosophy and goals of nursing care. Initially, theorists were concerned only with individuals, but gradually, individuals became viewed as part of a larger social system. In the 1960s, the nurse practitioner movement began espousing the family as a primary unit of care in their practice.

In the 1970s, only one theorist included families as part of the assessment in her system for nursing practice. Other theorists developed models which did not speak specifically to families but families could be the identified client in some of these theories (Orem, 1995; Roy, 1999; Neuman, 1995).

During the 1980s, the refocusing on families as a unit of care was evident in America. Small numbers of people from throughout the country gathered together at their personal expense to discuss and share family nursing concepts (for example, Wingspread in Racine, Wisconsin). Family nurses started defining the scope of practice, family concepts, and how to teach this information to the next generation of nurses. Family nursing is both old and new—long traditions and new definitions. Family nursing is still in the stage of youth, a state of becoming. Table 1–2 provides a composite of historical factors contributing to the development of family health as a focus in nursing.

State of the Art and Science of Family Nursing Practice, Research, and Education

Family Nursing Practice

Family nursing practice is in the process of being defined and developed. Many nurses call themselves "family nurses," but can they truly practice family nursing without the whole family being present? According to Friedemann (1995) family nursing can be practiced at three levels: (a) the individual level, with the family seen as the context of the individual; (b) the interpersonal level, with the family consisting of dyads, triads, and larger units; and (c) the system level, in which the family is a system with its own structural and functional components and interacts with environmental systems and its own subsystems. A family nurse who practices on one of the higher levels also includes the levels below (Friedemann, 1995).

The goal for practice on the *individual level* is physical health and personal well-being of family members; interpersonal change and system change are by-products. Family nursing at the *interpersonal level* has as its main goal mutual understanding and support of the family members. Personal change is anticipated and the interaction between personal and interpersonal factors is understood and included in the nursing care plan. Advanced practitioners anticipate system change so that harmful situations are avoided. The goal for nurses who practice at the *system level* is change in the family system as a whole and increased harmony between system and subsystems, as well as between system and environment. Changes at all system levels are carefully predicted, monitored, and corrected, if the need arises.

Friedemann (1995) says family nursing can and should be practiced at all three levels by all nurses. Nurse generalists are equipped to care for relatively well-functioning families at the individual level and the interpersonal level. Family systems nursing and advanced interpersonal nursing of families with dysfunctions are reserved for advanced nursing specialties that have knowledge and skills in family theory and practice.

Nursing practice at the systems level is focused on family health and strengths, is holistic in character, and requires knowledge of complex interactions of a multitude of family factors at all systems levels. The reciprocal relationship between health problems and family functioning is well-known to clinicians and theoreticians and is well-documented. Health problems influence family perceptions and behaviors; likewise family perceptions and behaviors influence health outcomes.

Wright and Leahey (1993) name the system level "family systems nursing," which is defined by them as focusing on the whole family as a unit of care. There is simultaneous concentration on both the individual and the family; it is inclusive rather than exclusive. The focus is always on the interaction and reciprocity of the family. Family systems nursing is the integration of nursing, systems, cybernetics, and family therapy theories. Wright and Leahey hypothesize that the future trend in family nursing will be towards increased diversity in clinical practice with families and that more nurses will be involved with families in health care, no matter what type of practice settings nurses choose. Families will be invited in more often for interviews and more intervention will take place at a systems level. Finally, more one-way mirrors will be used in health care settings to enhance interdisciplinary collaboration and practice.

A survey was reported concerning family nurses and their practices (Kirschling and associates, 1994). After four regional continuing education workshops on family nursing, 201 nurses responded to a survey in which they were asked to relate "successes" in family-centered nursing interventions. Using a qualitative approach, five themes were identified as successful outcomes, with commensurate examples of changes in family behavior as a result of family nursing intervention:

1. Families were able to seek help or identify a problem as demonstrated by calling the nurse when experiencing stressors in family members' lives.
2. Families and family members behaved differently as a result of family nursing interventions, such as encouraging an asthmatic client's family member to stop smoking to provide a smoke-free environment for their child.
3. Family members experienced a change of feel-

TABLE 1–2
Factors Contributing to the Development of Family Health as a Focus in Nursing

Time Period	Events
Pre–Nightingale era	Revolutionary War "camp followers" were an example of family health focus before Florence Nightingale's influence.
Mid-1800s	Nightingale influences district nurses and health missionaries to maintain clean environment for patient's homes and families.
	Family members provide for soldiers' needs during Civil War through Ladies Aid Societies and Women's Central Association for Relief.
Late 1880s	Industrial Revolution and immigration influence focus of public health nursing on prevention of illness, health education, and care of the sick for both families and communities.
	Lillian Wald establishes Henry Street Visiting Nurse Service (1893).
	Focus on family during childbearing by maternal-child nurses and midwives.
Early 1900s	School nursing established in New York City (1903).
	First White House Conference on Children occurs (1909).
	Red Cross Town and Country Nursing Service was founded (1912).
	Margaret Sanger opens first birth control clinic (1916).
	Family planning and quality care become available for families.
	Mary Breckinridge forms Frontier Nursing Service (1925).
	Nurses are assigned to families.
	Red Cross Public Health Nursing Service meets rural health needs after stock market crash (1929).
	Federal Emergency Relief Act passed (1933).
	Social Security Act passed (1935).
	Psychiatry and mental health disciplines begin family therapy focus (late 1930s).
1960s	Concept of family as a unit of care is introduced into basic nursing curriculum.
	National League for Nursing (NLN) requires emphasis on families and communities in nursing curriculum
	Family-centered approach in maternal-child nursing and midwifery programs is begun.
	Nurse-practitioner movement—programs to provide primary care to children are begun (1965).
	Shift from public health nursing to community health nursing occurs.
	Family studies and research produce family theories.
1970s	Changing health care system focuses on maintaining health and returning emphasis to family health.
	Development and refinement of nursing conceptual models that consider the family as a unit of analysis or care occur (e.g., King, Newman, Orem, Rogers, and Roy).
	Many specialties focus on the family (e.g., hospice, oncology, geriatrics, school health, psychiatry, mental health, occupational health, and home health).
	Master's and doctoral programs focus on the family (e.g., family health nursing, community health nursing, psychiatry, mental health, and family counseling and therapy).
	ANA Standards of Nursing Practice are implemented (1973).
	Surgeon General's Report (1979).
1980s	ANA Social Policy Statement (1980)
	White House Conference on Families
	Greater emphasis is put on health from very young to very old.
	Increasing emphasis is placed on obesity, stress, chemical dependency, and parenting skills.
	Graduate level specialization is begun with emphasis on primary care outside of acute care settings, health teaching, and client self-care.
	Use of wellness and nursing models in providing care increases.
	Promoting Health/Preventing Disease: Objectives for the Nation (1980) is released by U.S. Department of Health and Human Services.

Continued on the following page

TABLE 1–2 (*continued*)
Factors Contributing to the Development of Family Health as a Focus in Nursing

Time Period	Events
	Family science develops as a discipline. Family nursing research increases. National Center for Nursing Research is founded, with a Health Promotion and Prevention Research section. First International Family Nursing Conference occurs (1988).
1990s	*Healthy People 2000: National Health Promotion and Disease Prevention Objectives* (1990) is released by U.S. Department of Health and Human Services. Nursing's Agenda for Health Care Reform is developed (ANA, 1991). Family leave legislation is passed (1991). *Journal of Family Nursing* is born (1995).

Source: Bomar, P.J. (Ed.). (1996). *Nurses and Family Health Promotion: Concepts, Assessment, and Interventions*, ed. 2. Philadelphia: W. B. Saunders, (p. 8).

ings as a result of such family nursing interventions as helping them feel satisfied with their ability to solve their own problems.

4. Family members increased their knowledge of health terminology, family process, and the beliefs and understanding of other family members as a result of family nursing interventions, such as helping them learn to care for their high-risk infant at home.
5. Family and individual development continued in spite of illness as a result of family nursing interventions that assisted families to allow children to lead normal (versus protected) lives, even when they had a chronic illness such as diabetes.

In summary, nurses who considered themselves to be practicing family nursing described family nursing interventions that involved families and family members, including assessment and intervention as well as support, education, and exploration of feelings, as common occurrences (see Chap. 10 through Chap. 15). Vaughn-Cole and colleagues' (1998) book on *Family Nursing Practice* is a valuable new resource on this topic.

Family Nursing Research

Although families have been growing in importance in family nursing practice, they have been neglected in nursing research. Most nursing research has focused on the individual; the culture of individualism supersedes commitment to social groups. Recently nursing has awakened to the connection between family dynamics and health and illness. Research pertaining to family and mental health is further advanced than family and physical health (Campbell, 1987).

Studies on the family's effect on physical health of family members have predominantly been from a social and epidemiologic view. For example, family interactions have been examined in studies of diabetes and hypertension. Poor diabetic control and hypertension have been associated with unresolved marital conflicts. Marital status has been shown to influence the overall mortality and morbidity of cardiovascular disease. Recent studies have shown that patients respond more to their family's response to illness than to the disease or condition itself.

There are some summaries available on family nursing research and some of the inherent methodologic problems. See the work by Murphy (1986); Feetham (1990); Moriarty (1990); Broome, Knafl, Pridham, and Feetham (1998); and Gilliss and Davis (1993) on this topic. Wright and Leahey (1993) discussed three major implications for future nursing research:

1. Family assessment techniques must be further developed.
2. Research on the reciprocal relationship between family functioning and the course and treatment of illness needs to gain prominence.
3. The efficacy of family treatment will become paramount as the type of health services most appropriate for specific situations are determined.

Chapters 2 and 3 of this textbook pertain to family nursing theory and family research.

Family Nursing Education

Family nursing education has come of age in the U.S. and Canada. Hanson and Heims (1992) reported a research study conducted in the late 1980s in which they looked at the status of family nursing education in all schools of nursing in the United States. Wright and Bell (1989) modeled a Canadian study after the American study. The following list represents those findings and recommendations:

- In general, more family content is being included in undergraduate and graduate nursing curricula, but it could be made more explicit. These clinical courses should be both family-specific and integrated into other coursework.
- An eclectic approach to family assessment is now being taught rather than the use of specific models. Nurses need to learn several models and assessment strategies to be more systematic and thorough in family assessment.
- Clinical practicums in a variety of settings are still focused on individuals rather than families as a whole. Family systems experiences that focus on relationships and interactions must be developed by faculty.
- The methods of supervision for students are primarily through case discussion and process recordings. The use of audiotapes and videotapes for reviewing case material is becoming more common in nursing. There is a need for more direct and live supervision through the use of one-way mirrors.
- There appears to be a deficit of advanced knowledge and skill level in faculty members responsible for advanced family nursing practice courses. More faculty members need to seek graduate work in family nursing, as well as the family social sciences, family therapy, sociology, and psychology, to fill this gap.
- Schools are better at teaching family assessment than family intervention strategies, which explains the fact that family nursing intervention strategies are still in the early stages of development. More emphasis and resources should be focused on nursing intervention strategies with families.
- Faculty members who teach family nursing originate from varied backgrounds and include maternal-child, community, and psychiatric and mental health nursing. There is a growing number of trained and identified professionals with expertise in teaching family nursing. These faculty members need to be teaching the family content, regardless of the territorial traditions of the specialties.
- Schools of nursing across the different regions of the country do not vary significantly in terms of the amount of family-oriented content in their curricula, nor were there differences in what was being taught in family nursing between schools that had undergraduate programs only and those that also had graduate programs.

Education for Family Nursing

Education for family nursing begins during undergraduate nursing education and may continue through postdoctoral training. The question of whether family nursing education prepares the nurse for a generalist or specialist practice is paramount today. The American Nursing Association (ANA, 1995) stated that nurse generalists practice with a comprehensive approach to health care and can meet the diversified health concerns of individuals, families, and communities, whereas nurse specialists are expert in providing care focused on specific clusters of phenomena representing a refinement of interests. In the area of general versus specialist, Gilliss (1993) wrote that a nurse who views the family in context could be a generalist in family nursing and a specialist in another field of practice. Conversely, those nurses who practice family nursing are specialists in family care and generalists in other areas of practice.

Gilliss (1993, p. 36) and others have proposed a schema to conceptualize the levels of preparation for family nursing education (see Figure 1–8). At the baccalaureate level, students should receive preparation for working with the family as context and the family as a component of society. This is consistent with the generalist orientation of undergraduate nursing education. This approach is more commonly addressed in undergraduate nursing courses that deal with children's, women's, or community health issues. However, family content to prepare nurses to work with families in all areas of practice is needed in other coursework as well.

Master's level preparation is required for specialty practice in family nursing, such as working with the family as a client or the family as a system. This preparation consists of courses pertaining to family theory, nursing intervention with families, advanced practice, and clinical supervision. At one school of nursing, many master's students (nurse practitioners and clinical nurse specialists) are required to take this kind of

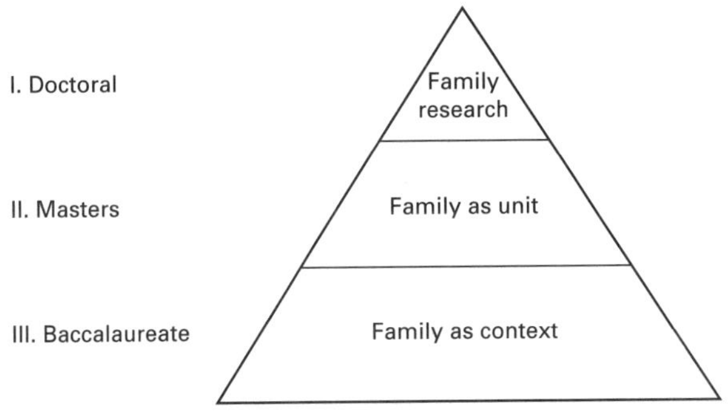

FIGURE 1–8
Levels of preparation for family nursing.
(From Gilliss, C.L. (1993). (eds.), *Readings in Family Nursing.* Philadelphia: JB Lippincott, p. 36.)

coursework. As in much of nursing education, master's preparation has a clinical specialty focus.

Finally, there is doctoral and postdoctoral education in nursing. The focus of doctoral study is usually on family theory development and research and, in some schools, that focus is on family nursing. Again, at the same school of nursing mentioned just previously, one of the two tracks in the doctoral program is focused on the family while the other is on gerontologic nursing and family caregiving. The National Institute of Nursing Research (NINR) is now funding institutional and individual National Research Service Awards (NRSAs) to support graduate and postdoctoral students in family nursing research.

CONCEPTS FOR FAMILY HEALTH CARE

Theorists from other family social sciences have been involved in developing some important ideas about family health care that are pertinent for family nursing. Four of these ideas are presented below: the family health and illness cycle, levels of family care, when to assemble the family in health care, and the therapeutic triangle in health care (Doherty, 1985; Doherty and McCubbin, 1985; Doherty and Campbell, 1988).

The Family Health and Illness Cycle

The family health and illness cycle (Figure 1–9) represents an outline of a series of temporal phases in the family's efforts to reduce the risks of illness, to manage the initial onset of illness, and to adapt to death or illness. There is no unilateral direction in the model, but rather each phase in the cycle represents a different aspect of health and illness. Also, each phase of the cycle represents an arena around which a body of theory, research, and clinical observations have been built. The function of the model is to show how different topics pertaining to family and health research, theory building, and practice are interrelated.

One area of the cycle in which family nurses work is in *family health promotion and risk reduction.* This area emphasizes the environmental, social, psychological, and interpersonal factors surrounding the family that help promote health and reduce health risk. This includes family beliefs and activities that help family members maintain good health through avoiding behaviors that increase their likelihood of becoming ill, such as diet, exercise, or smoking. Nurses can do a lot to promote family health that will in turn reduce risk.

Another part of the cycle that nurses get involved with is *family vulnerability and illness onset.* This includes life events and experiences that render family members' susceptible to new illness or relapses of chronic illness. For example, nurses work with family stress responses related to relapses or exacerbations of chronic disorders (for example, diabetes, multiple sclerosis, or schizophrenia), which have been found to be associated with the number of visits to health care providers, hospitalizations, and accidents. The development of support groups would be one nursing strategy for dealing with family members who have chronic illness (for example, a cancer support group for women).

The third part of the cycle pertinent to family nurses is the *family illness appraisal,* which includes the meaning that families give to the individual's symptoms of illness and whether the family is amenable to intervention. An example of a strategy that nurses may use to help families cope with a situation before the situation becomes more acute includes leading groups for depressed adolescents before they consider or attempt suicide, thus intervening in suicidal behaviors.

The *family acute response* refers to the immediate aftermath of illness and is an important area of intervention. The acute response occurs during the crisis period after an extraordinary event, such as a heart attack or a diagnosis of cancer. Families go through disorganization for a while, and family nurses can intervene by helping them cope with the crisis.

Next, there is the *family adaptation to illness,* which refers to the long-term effects of illness on the family and

Family Health and Illness Cycle

Phase 1. Family health promotion and risk reduction
Phase 2. Family vulnerability and disease onset/relapse
Phase 3. Family illness appraisal
Phase 4. Family acute response
Phase 5. Adaption to illness and recovery

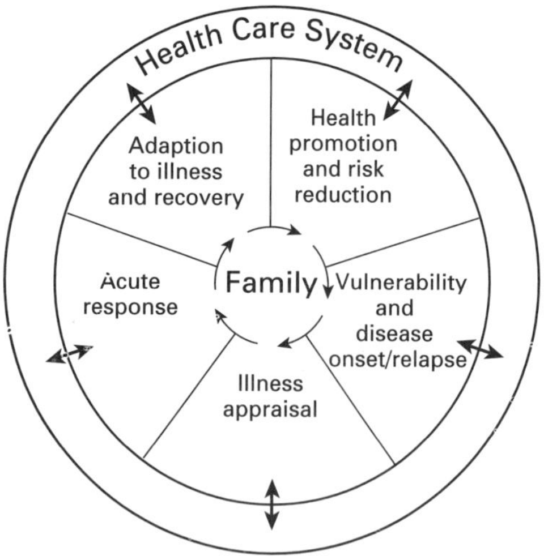

FIGURE 1–9
Family health and illness cycle. (From "Families and Health Care: An Emerging Arena of Theory, Research, and Clinical Intervention," by W. J. Doherty and H. I. McCubbin, 1985, *Family Relations*, 349, pp. 5–11, with permission.)

the role of families in facilitating recovery of individual members. Families must adapt to the demands of the chronic condition; thus, a whole body of information has evolved around family coping and family compliance with medical regimens. How do families promote the recovery of ill members while preserving their energy to nurture other family members and perform other family functions? An example of an appropriate intervention would be to help families find respite care for family caregivers so that caregivers do not "burn out."

Finally, the *family and health care system* refers to the family's decision regarding whether to seek outside help for the illness or handle it within the family. This family help-seeking behavior can take place at any phase of the family health and illness cycle, and the resources sought can include everything from Western medical protocols to nontraditional New Age health care providers.

Levels of Family Care

The next concept derived from family social scientists and useful for family nursing are levels of family care as described by Doherty (1985). They proposed a continuum of health provider involvement when caring for families.

Level 1: Minimal emphasis on the family involves contacting families only when necessary for practical or legal reasons. Nurses require little knowledge or skill to handle this level of care. An example might be a hospital intensive care nurse contacting the family to get a code or no code signed.

Level 2: Ongoing medical information and advice is given by generalist family nurses to families through regular contact. The nurse may be answering questions or advising families on care management. An example might be a clinic nurse working with a family on diabetic foot care of an elderly patient.

Level 3: Providing support and addressing feelings is given to families based on knowledge about normal family development and how families react to stress. The family nurse encourages family members to discuss their reactions and supports them in their coping efforts. Care is more individualized to that particular family. For example, a community health nurse may make a home visit to a newly discharged paraplegic patient who is going home for the first time.

Level 4: A systematic way of assessing families and planning interventions involves a good understanding of family systems and awareness of the nurse's own family systems and the larger systems in which families and health care providers operate. More knowledge and skill are required for this level of activity and it usually involves graduate training in a specialty that incorporates family into the paradigm of care. An example would be a clinical nurse specialist who is coordinating care for a trauma patient with multiple injuries in a tertiary setting.

Level 5: Finally, this level of care requires a high level of knowledge and skill with family systems and patterns of dysfunctional interaction. The nurse prepared to work at this level is a specialist in psychiatric mental health nursing, family therapy,or both. The generalist nurse either refers a family to or consults with a psychiatric mental health liaison nurse who is a clinical nurse specialist or nurse practitioner in this area. An example of this level of care: The specialist nurse is consulted concerning a difficult and complex family structure in which some members of the family want resuscitation of a dying family member and other members do not. This situation would require structuring a family conference, assessing the function of the family, and mediating a decision.

When to Assemble the Family in Health Care

The next concept that is derived from family social science and is useful for family nursing is Doherty's (1985) guidelines to assist health providers in knowing when to involve whole families while providing care. Figure 1–10 shows a two-sided continuum. One upper half of the continuum ranges from the individual patient being seen alone to whole family conferences being essential. The bottom half of the continuum speaks to the kind of health care problem being addressed and ranges from minor acute problems (minor suturing) to a serious acute illness (heart attack). The benefit of this idea is that it assists nurses in making decisions about the level or degree of family involvement for any given situation and reassures nurses that "family nursing" can take place even when the whole family is not assembled.

The Therapeutic Triangle in Health Care

The third concept of importance to nurses in providing family care is the notion of the therapeutic triangle (Figure 1–11). It is a concept derived from family systems theory, but it applies to all approaches to health care.

In the provision of health care, there are three main actors in the therapeutic triangle: the identified patient, the health care professional, and the family of the identified patient. Relationships exist primarily between the dyads in the triangle with the third party in the triangle in the background. Triangulated relationships are those in which a third party becomes involved to stabilize tensions that exist in the dyadic relationship. The third party distracts from the anxiety level that is based in the dyad. As the given dyad changes, so does the third party; for example, a patient-family dyad with the health care professional as the third party, or a health care professional-identified patient dyad with the family as third party.

Situations occur in which there is difficulty in a nurse-patient relationship and the patient engages their family to communicate with the nurse instead of directly confronting the nurse, or in which the health care provider provides a listening ear to a disgruntled patient complaining about his or her family's caregiving ability. Often health care providers find themselves positioned between family members. A more thorough discussion of this concept can be found in Broderick (1983).

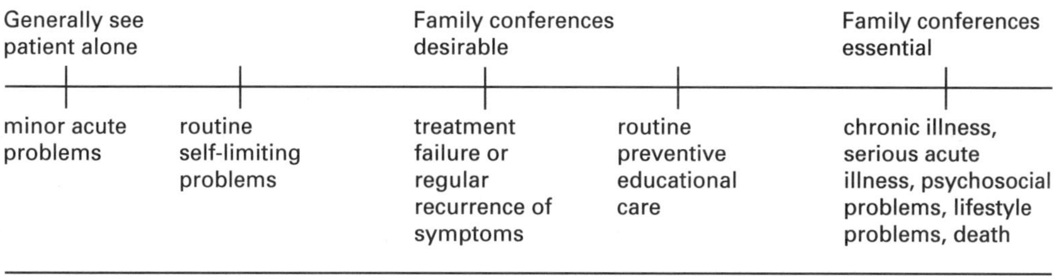

FIGURE 1–10
When to assemble the family in health care. (From Doherty, W. (1985). Family Intervention in Health Care. *Family Relations, 34*, 129–137.)

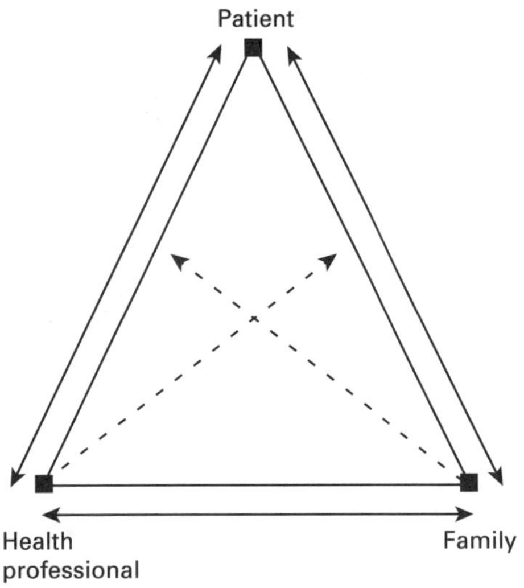

FIGURE 1–11
The therapeutic triangle in health care. (From Broderick, C.B. (1983) *The Therapeutic Triangle.* Beverly Hills: Sage Publications.)

FAMILIES

History of Families

A brief macroanalytical history of families is important for understanding family nursing. The past helps to make the present realities of family life more understandable, because the influence of the past is evident in the present. This historical approach provides a means of conceptualizing family over time and within all of society. Finally, history helps to dispel preferences for family forms that are only personally familiar and broaden nurses' view of the world of families.

Prehistoric Family Life

Archaeologists and anthropologists have found evidence of prehistoric family life, that is, existing before the time of written historical sources. These family forms varied from present day forms, but the functions of the family have remained somewhat constant over time. Families were then and are now a part of the larger community and constitute the basic unit of society.

Family structure, process, and function were a response to everyday needs. As communities grew, families and communities became more institutionalized and homogeneous as civilization progressed. Family culture was that aspect of life derived from membership in a particular group and shared by others. Family culture was composed of values and attitudes that allowed early families to behave in a predictable fashion.

The earliest human matings tended toward permanence and monogamy. Man and woman dyads are the oldest and most tenacious unit in history, which is perhaps why the "nuclear" family dominates modern experience. Biologically, human children need care and protection longer than other animals' offspring. This necessity led humans to marriage and permanent relationships—it did not dictate family structure, but it was essential for the activity of parenting.

Economic pairing was not always the same as reproductive pairing, but it was a by-product of reproductive pairing. A variety of skills were needed for living and no single person possessed all skills, so male and female role differentiation began to be more clearly defined. Early in history, children were part of the economic unit. In most societies, reproductive pairing merged also with the nurturing pair and the economic unit, as well as into respective gender role differentiation, and ultimately into socialization (education).

As small groups of conjugal families formed communities, the complexity of the social order increased. This, in turn, changed the definition of the family.

European History

Many Americans are of European ancestry and come out of the family structure that was present there. Social organizations called families emphasized consanguineous (genetic) bonds. The tendency toward authority was concentrated in few individuals at the top of the hierarchical structure (kings, lords, fathers). The heads of families were males.

Property of family transferred through the male line. Females left home to join their husbands' families. Mothers did not establish strong bonds with their daughters because the daughters eventually left their home of origin to join their husband's family of origin.

Women and children were property to be transferred. Marriage was a contract between families, not individuals. Extended patriarchal family characteristics prevailed until the advent of industrialism.

Industrialization

There was great stability within family systems until the Industrial Revolution. The revolution first appeared in

England aaround 1750 and spread to Western Europe and North America. Some believe that the nuclear family idea started with the Industrial Revolution. Extended families had always been the norm until families left farms, moving into the cities, where men left home to work in the factories. This left women at home maintaining the home and caring for the children. Extended families were left behind. There is some evidence that English families were nuclear from the 1600s, because family size has stayed constant at 4.75 people per family ever since.

Out of the religious Reformation came a strong movement for individuation, in which the Protestant ethic promoted the idea that the family unit was no longer paramount, but rather the individual within the family. This paradigm shift had a lot to do with the message of personal salvation of the Reformation and Protestantism.

When factories of the Industrial Revolution started to be built, people began moving about. The state had begun to provide services that families previously had performed for their members. Informal contractual arrangements between public and state power and nuclear families took place, in which the state gave fathers the power and authority over their families in exchange for males giving the state their loyalty and service. This may be one of the ways in which families became controlled by patriarchy.

Women were not expected to love husbands but to obey them. Some feminists believe that the introduction of love into human consciousness was done as a purposeful and powerful force to limit female activity and that it is hard to separate love and submission. This notion is very controversial.

Society today is still living with bequests of patriarchal family life. Women are still struggling to get out from under the rules and expectations of the state and of men. The women's movement and the National Organization for Women (NOW) are two of the forces that have improved the level of equality of women in modern society. A lot more work needs to be done on the issues of equality for all Americans, including gender differences.

In recent years, men have also begun identifying the bondage they experience. They cannot meet all of the needs of families and feel inadequate for failing to do so. This is especially true of men who cannot access the resources of money, occupation, and occupational status through education. There is a men's movement afoot that is promoting male causes, although this movement is not as dynamic as it may be in the future. One of the organizations supporting this work is the National Congress for Men.

American Families

American society and families were molded from the beginning by economic logic rather than consanguineous logic. America does not have the history of Europe's preindustrial age. English patriarchy was not transplanted in its pure form to America.

Women as well as men had to labor in the New World. This gave women new power. Also, the United States had an ethic of achieved status rather than inherited status through familial lines. Female suffrage was easier to obtain on the frontier, as is evidenced by Wyoming being one of the first states to give women the vote.

Children were also experiencing a changing status in American families. Originally, they were part of the economic unit and worked on farms. Then with the great immigration of the early 1900s, the expectation shifted to parents creating a better world for their children than they themselves had. To do this, children had to become more educated to deal with the developing society. Each generation of children obtained more education and income than their parents; they left the family farms and moved to distant cities. As a result of this change, parents lost assurance that their children would take care of them during their old age. This phenomenon is occurring in developing countries today. For example, the city of Seoul, Korea, has grown from 2 to 14 million people in one decade, largely due to young people coming into the cities for work and education.

In addition, the functions of families were changing greatly in earlier American society. The traditional roles that families played were being displaced by the growing numbers and kinds of social institutions. Families have been increasingly surrendering to public agencies many of the socialization functions they previously had performed.

Historically, adolescents worked on the family farms. With the burgeoning of cities in the industrialized world, adolescents lost their productive function on the farm. Teenagers could not be kept from jobs in the cities. The public school system was largely created to help keep adolescents off streets. The concept of the generation gap occurred when the family economic and social functions no longer merged.

Families Today

Today, families cannot be separated from the larger system of which they are a part, nor can they be separated from their historical past. Some people argue that families are in terrible shape, like a rudderless ship in the dark. Other people hail the changes that continue to occur in families and approve the diversity and options that address modern needs. Idealizing past family arrangements and decrying change has become commonplace in the media. Just as some families of both the past and present engaged in behaviors that are destructive to individuals and other social institutions, there are families of the past and present that provide healthy environments. Certainly, the sphere of activity for families is diminishing the strength of the family and lessening their ability to both influence and react to the direction of social change.

If nurses believe that the family as an institution is essential to individuals and society, they can become anxious that the family's traditional tasks are co-opted by other institutions. Many of these institutions (churches, schools, social agencies) actually exert further strain on families even as they attempt to strengthen families. For example, employers (military or business) move families around for the sake of optimizing production. This results in frequent relocations and loss of social support and security, creating a circumstance in which people in families can turn only to each other instead of feeling a part of the larger family or community. These circumstances promote the intensity of familial interaction that results in unrealistic expectations of each other. Isolation is one of the contributing factors to the high incidence of abuse among military families.

The author believes that the structure, function, and processes of families have changed, but the family unit will continue to survive. It is, in fact, the most tenacious unit in society, and the last stronghold over which families have some control. More discussion about the future of families occurs in the last chapter.

Functions of Families

Traditional Families

Down through history, there have been a number of traditional functions that are performed by families. What are the functions that families previously performed for their members? Six functions are summarized in the following section, but not necessarily in their order of importance.

First, families existed to *achieve economic survival.* Fathers were breadwinners, going out into the world to "bring home the bacon," either by self-employment or working for others. Mothers were helpmates, homemakers, and nurturers of children. Families had many children for economic reasons—more children meant more wealth, an opportunity to work more land, and care for their parents into old age. Children of earlier centuries did not experience what we now know as the teen years. Instead, they worked in the family business as mini-adults and stayed home until they married. The family was an economic unit to which all members contributed and from which everyone benefited.

Second, families existed *to reproduce the species.* In earlier times, parents traditionally married before having sex and children. If women became pregnant outside of marriage, they were stigmatized and sent away to homes for unwed mothers. Not many people elected to stay childless and instead had children of their own or adopted children.

Third, *providing protection* from hostile forces was an important family function. Family members needed each other to protect those who could not protect themselves, such as the very young, the very old, and disabled individuals. Indeed, family groups immigrated together to avoid facing hostile cultures alone and formed ethnic blankets (ghettos) in which an "us against them" world prevailed.

Fourth, *passing along the religious faith (culture)* was an important function for families. Families were the primary medium for passing on religious stories, doctrines, traditions, and values. Only candidates for ordination or rich children received formalized religious training. Significant family events were ritualized, such as births, baptisms, marriages, and death. Faith was an integral part of daily family life.

The fifth function of families was *to educate (socialize) their young.* Boys worked with their fathers to learn trades or take over family farms. Girls worked with their mothers, learning homemaking and parenting. Children were largely home-schooled by their parents; reading was learned from religious books—the *Bible* and *Pilgrim's Progress.* The *Bible* and the gun were important family tools in young America. The *Bible* buttressed faith and staved off ignorance, and the gun was used to kill game animals and protect the family.

The sixth function of families was to *confer status.* In the old country, largely Europe, a person *was* the family name. It was difficult to change status in society. If a person's father was a respected blacksmith, the son was expected to become the same. If the father was the town drunk, however, the son had little chance to become something else. An untarnished family name was especially important in a nonmobile society. Many people immigrated to America to seek new opportunities (as well as riches) that their family names could not provide in the old country.

If families met all of these six functions, they were considered healthy, or good. A "good family" was one that was self-sufficient, did not ask for help from others, supported their community institutions, was untainted with failure, starved before they went on welfare, and met "good family" criteria as determined by community and church. That is, they looked good from the outside. People paid little attention to what went on inside the family. Society was not concerned about good communication, emotional support, or trusting relationships. There was more concern about meeting visible family standards set by the community, such as married parents, religious affiliation, affluence, home ownership, and community respect.

Contemporary Families

In contemporary times, historical functions of families have changed. Some functions have changed more than others, and new ones have been added to the list.

First, the *economic function* of families has changed dramatically. Family members do not need each other as they did in the past to stay financially afloat. Government aid, such as Medicare, Social Security, aid for dependent children, and welfare, help subsidize families economically. Women do not need to stay married to a man for food, shelter, or respectability, nor do men marry to have someone cook and clean for them. The spinster aunt was replaced by the career woman.

More than 50 percent of women with young children are now working outside of the home, carrying their own weight in the work place. Children are no longer viewed as economic assets but as costly luxuries. Children do not need parents to survive economically, and the nation has an expansive foster home and welfare program. Some social reformers are even promoting a guaranteed income for all people. Thus, families are not the basic ingredient in economic security anymore.

Second, the *reproductive function* of families has diversified, allowing people many options to have children without marriage and the family. For example, one-third of live births in the United States today occur to women who are not married. Women who were infertile in the past have benefited from in vitro technology and infertility drugs. Sexual activity is more common among all age groups with a whole complement of birth control measures available. So the function of reproduction does not necessarily take place within the boundaries of the traditional family any longer.

Third, *protective functions* of families are no longer as important as they used to be. Social, welfare, and law enforcement agencies have largely taken on this activity for the safety and protection of society. Not all families are willing or able to provide these functions for their offspring. For example, if parents are suspected of child abuse, society removes their children from the home, serving as surrogate parents. Another example is the recent mandate for immunization for children, which occurred because not all families protect their children against these diseases.

Fourth, the *religious (cultural) function* of families has also evolved over time. Instead of families assuming the chief responsibility for passing on the religious faith to the next generation, this activity has been relegated to the churches and synagogues. There has been some counter-activity on the part of churches to pass this responsibility back to families, but for the most part, this has been ineffective. As the citizenry has become more secular, fewer religious values and culture has been passed to the younger generation. Thus, the family structure no longer serves this function in the way of yesteryear.

Fifth, the *educational and socialization function* of families has been transferred to the public and private school system. Educators complain that too much has been placed in the hands of teachers and that families are delinquent in their responsibility and accountability. Home schooling has become slightly more popular with some young parents today, but the majority of mothers are working outside of the home, placing their children in day care centers and preschool. Also, any residual teaching that has traditionally taken place in the home is being eroded by television. Hence, the educational function of the family has lost much of its potency.

Sixth, the family is usually no longer needed to *confer status*. If you are a Rockefeller or Kennedy, your family name may be helpful, but for the majority of Americans, your family heritage is not essential for success. Status today is gained through education, occupation, income, and address. The United States as a country is valued for its "rags to riches" possibilities.

Seventh, the *relationship function* of families has become important in contemporary families, although it was not considered so for families in the past. People marry so that they can love and be loved, instead of for basic needs. Couples join in a search for intimacy, not protection. Parents have children to connect to posterity rather than to be taken care of in their old age.

Maslow (1970) said that this generation of people are sufficiently beyond basic sustenance needs to be able to focus on the quality of their relationships. Families are self-defining, using criteria based on relationships rather than genes or law. If our deepest relationship needs are not met in our families, we search elsewhere. If we are lonely or unhappy in our relationships, we seek alternatives through divorce, infidelity, overwork, volunteerism, chemical dependency, teen alienation, depression, and suicide. The focus on relationships has become paramount in contemporary families.

Eighth, the *health function* of families has been highlighted in contemporary times. Researchers in family health have noted the importance of the interactive effects of the health of individual family members and the health of family. The family can keep its members well by passing along attitudes, beliefs, habits, health promotion, and care of the ill. The family is the genesis of physical and mental health for a lifetime.

In summary, the functions that families serve have evolved over time. Some functions have become more important and others less. It is clear that not all historical families were "good" families and not all contemporary families are having problems. Each type of family over the centuries has had its own problems and strengths that made it the basic unit of all human society.

Changing Demographics of American Families

Major changes are taking place in American families today that are exerting dramatic influences on family life and family health (Ahlburg & DeVita, 1992). The U.S. Bureau of the Census (1991a, 1991b, 1992a, 1992b, 1992c, 1992d, 1994a, 1994b, 1995a, 1995b, 1995c) and the National Center for Health Statistics (1994) report that increases in divorce, remarriage, age at first marriage, labor force participation of women, and delays and declines in childbearing are among the more notable trends today. These individual and collective developments, in the span of just one generation, have altered the structure, process, and function of American families. In comparison to 20 years ago, today's families are smaller and more likely to be maintained by a single parent, have multiple wage earners, require child care assistance, and contain stepchildren. Individual and family life trajectories involve many more transitions today as people form, dissolve, and reform families. This section contains a summary of the many changing family forms in America today and some of the implications for family health.

Family Variation

Families in the past were more homogeneous than they are today. Table 1–3 lists the variations in family types. The past norm was a two-parent family living together with their biological children. One- and two-parent families are becoming increasingly heterogeneous. Table 1–4 shows an overall picture of how family demographics have changed from 1970 to 1990 and what we can expect after the year 2000. Married families with children declined from 49 percent in 1970 and will decrease to 34 percent after the year 2000. Married families without children will increase from 37.1 percent to 42.8 percent in the future. All kinds of single-parent families have increased substantially and are discussed in more detail later. Note the increase in births to single mothers, largely unmarried teens (see Table 1–4). Same-sex households stay steady at 2 percent of American families. Many more people are cohabiting or living alone than in the past.

Table 1–5 shows numbers instead of percentages of families in the various categories over the years 1970 to 2000. Again, it is apparent that married-couple families are decreasing, while married couples without children are increasing. Single-parent families are on the increase, with single fathers as head of the household becoming more common. All other family forms are also increasing (for example, foster children, grandparents raising grandchildren, gay families).

Marriages

The total number of marriages in the United States reached an all-time high in 1984 (2.4 million) and has leveled off since. About two-thirds of all marriages are first marriages; one-third are remarriages. Ninety percent of all people marry at some point in their lives, but the percentage of never-married women who eventually marry decreases with age. The median age for first marriage of women (24.1 years) and men (26.3 years) has increased in recent years, approximating the same figures from the turn of the century. One-fourth of women who marry do so by age 20 and three-fourths

TABLE 1–3
Variations of Family Types

Family Type	Composition
Nuclear dyad	Married couple, no children
Nuclear	Husband, wife, children (may or may not be legally married)
Binuclear	Two post-divorce families with children as members of both
Extended	Nuclear family plus blood relatives
Blended	Husband, wife, and children of previous relationships
Single parent	One parent and child(ren)
Commune	Group of men, women, and children
Cohabitation (domestic partners)	Unmarried man and woman sharing a household
Homosexual	Same-gender couple
Single person (adult)	One person in a household

Source: Bomar, P.J. (Ed.). (1996). *Nurses and Family Health Promotion: Concepts, Assessment, and Interventions,* ed. 2. Philadelphia: W. B. Saunders, (p. 37).

by age 28. Thus, marriage for women is becoming a less age-defined event.

Single Life

Postponing marriage is a phenomenon of recent years. The proportion of men and women in their 20s and early 30s who have never married has grown substantially during the past two decades. The number of single persons in these age groups have nearly tripled for both women and men, and never-married status is even higher for black and Hispanic persons. Postponing marriage suggests that higher proportions of people will never marry. Married persons declined from 72 percent to 61 percent between 1970 and 1991, while the proportion of unmarried persons rose from 28 percent to 39 percent.

This vast rise in singleness among adults today is greater than it was earlier in history. Young adults are postponing marriage, and many are becoming single more than once because of divorce. Elderly married persons find themselves single once again as a result of the death of a spouse or the increasing divorce rate among older couples. Although singleness may be viewed as a temporary state, 90 percent of people marry and of those who divorce, about 75 percent remarry. Single people have a set of unique needs for public- and private-sector services. Issues involving child care and economic equity for single parents, education and work opportunities for young adults, and housing and health care for elderly persons are all important factors in the well-being of the American people.

The rise in singleness among young adults is also associated with various demographic and economic factors, such as educational level, income level, and housing costs. Many more young adults are now living with their parents than previously. Three out of 10 unmarried adults aged 25 to 29 live in the home of their parents (U. S. Bureau of the Census, 1992a). Postponement of first marriage is the major factor in the increase in the proportion of young adults living at home. This is creating a new kind of multigenerational family than that of recent years.

Divorces

The total number of divorces in the United States has been increasing for years. As of 1995 (U.S. Census Bureau, 1995b) there were more than 1.1 million divorces per year. Black and Hispanic Americans have higher divorce rates than white Americans. These figures include not only young adults, who experience divorce

TABLE 1–4
Family Demographics

Family Type	1970	1990	2000 (Projected)
Married with children (%)	49%	36.9%	43%
Married without children (%)	37.1%	41.7%	42.8%
Single-parent families (total) (%)	5.77%	12.00%	12.4%
Female (88% of total)	5.7%	10.20%	9.7%
Male (12% of total)	.07%	1.80%	2.7%
Same-sex households	2.00%	2.00%	—
Single persons (%)	20.00%	30%	—
Births to single mothers (% of all births)	11.00%	27%	—
Unmarried couples (cohabitation)	520,000	3,000,000	—

Source: U.S. Bureau of Census. (1991). Current Population Reports No. 461, (p. 20).

most commonly, but also elderly adults, whose marriages survived for many years before divorce. In recent years, an increasing number of couples over age 60 have been divorcing. Teenaged marriages have the highest risk of divorce. The mean age at divorce is 34 years, and divorce occurs most often in the first 7 years of marriage. About 75 percent of divorced persons remarry after a median interval of about 2 years, and about 75 percent of the second marriages end in divorce. If current divorce levels persist, approximately 50 percent to 60 percent of all recent marriages will end in divorce. About two-thirds of all divorced families involve one or more children, so more than 660,000 children become children of divorce each year. Most of these children are toddlers, preschoolers, or school-aged children.

Remarriages and Stepparenting

An increasing number of children are living in stepfamilies (remarried families) by the time they reach 16 years of age. One-fourth (4.5 million) of American families have at least one stepchild living in the household. Remarried-couple families with stepchildren are

TABLE 1–5
Family Composition in the United States, 1970–2000

Type of Family	1970	1990	1995	2000
All families (in millions)	51.2	64.5	68.0	71.7
Married couples with children (%)	49.6%	36.9%	36.2%	34.5%
Married couples without children (%)	37.1%	36.9%	41.8%	42.8%
Female head of household with children (%)	5.7%	10.2%	10.0%	9.7%
Male head of household with children (%)	0.7%	1.8%	2.2%	2.7%
Other family types	6.9%	9.4%	9.8%	10.3%

Source: Ahlburg, D.A. & DeVita, C.J. (1992). *New Realities of the American Family.* Population Bulletin, 47(2):7.

equally divided between those containing biological children of the couple and children from a previous relationship. Most stepchildren live with their biological mothers and stepfathers rather than vice versa.

Skip-Generation Families

The increase in what has been termed the "skip-generation" family is a phenomenon of the 1990s. This means that children are being raised by their grandparents as a result of both parents working, having chemically dependent parents, or having become "throwaway" kids. The number of grandchildren raised by their grandparents was 2.9 million, or 5 percent of all children under 18 years (U.S. Census Bureau, 1995c). Black children are more likely to live with grandparents than white children.

Single-Parent Families

Single-parent families are considered separately from single personhood. Single-parent families are created in one of five ways: (1) divorce, (2) births out of wedlock, (3) spousal absenteeism, (4) death of a parent, or (5) adoption (Hanson and associates, 1995b). This family structure greatly affects the living arrangements of children. The proportion of single-parent households has doubled from 1970 (12 percent) to 1992 (27 percent).

Today, almost 4 of every 10 children in the United States are either currently living with a single parent or have in the past (Bianchi, 1995). In addition to the 27 percent of children living with a single parent, another 11 percent are living with one biological and one stepparent. Although the increase in divorce fueled the growth in one-parent families in the 1960s and 1970s, delayed marriage and childbearing outside marriage contributed far more to the growth in mother-child families during the 1980s than did marital disruption. Eighty-six percent of single-parent households are headed by women. During the 1980s, however, father-child families increased more than mother-child families. By 1990, almost one in five single-parent families was maintained by a father, although only 3 percent of all children lived in this type of household (Bianchi, 1995). Projections are that one-half of children born today will spend time living apart from one or both biological parents.

Ethnically, single-parenting on the part of unmarried mothers is much higher within the black than white community, and racial differences were greater at the beginning of the 1990s than a generation earlier. Whereas two-thirds of white children currently live with both biological parents, only one-quarter of black children do so (Bianchi, 1995). More black (54 percent) and Hispanic American children (30 percent) than white children (19 percent) live in single-parent households.

Economics and the Single-Parent Family

Single-parent families remain disadvantaged compared with two-parent families in economic status, health status, and housing conditions. Children living with never-married mothers are the most economically disadvantaged group of children in single-parent families (Bianchi, 1995). Single-mother households have lower annual incomes than single-father households ($13,092 and $25,211, respectively). The average income for families with both parents in 1990 was $41,260. Children of poverty were the theme of the 1980s and the theme continues into the 1990s; 33 million American people are poor and, of these, 13 million are children. Of poor children, more than 500,000 are homeless. The gender gap in income level persists; women make two-thirds of what men make. Many single-mother households are poor.

Ten million mothers were living with their children but without the children's fathers. About 58 percent were awarded child support (U. S. Bureau of the Census, 1991a). Of women who are due payments, about half received the full amount. More than 5 million women received child support with the average level of payment approximately being $2,995 yearly, which represented about 11 percent of their family income (U.S. Bureau of the Census, 1991a). In this census, the remaining single-mother families were divided between partial payment and receiving nothing. The poverty rate for all women with children from absent fathers was 32 percent. The majority of absent fathers (55%) had visitation privileges, 7% had joint custody, and 38% had neither visitation nor custody (U.S. Census Bureau, 1991a).

The reader is referred to a special volume recently published on single-parent families that summarizes the latest theory, practice, and research on the various kinds of single parent families (Hanson and colleagues, 1995a, 1995c).

SUMMARY

This chapter provides a broad overview of family health care nursing. First, why is it important to teach nurses about family health care? The focus is on what are families, what is family health care nursing, and where is the profession of nursing in relationship to nursing care of families. Next, concepts for family health care are introduced—what is the family health/illness cycle, what are levels of family care and conceptual models of how nurses assume and work with families in the health care setting. Finally, this chapter ended on a focus pertaining to the history of families, the functions of families and the changing demographics of families. It becomes clear from this chapter that family health care nursing is evolving as the discipline moves forward and as families in society change and grow.

Study Questions

1. Define family.
2. Define family health.
3. List five traits that are common in healthy families.
4. Define family health care nursing.
5. Which of the following statements are true about family nursing practice?
    a. Family care is concerned with the experience of the family over time.
    b. Family nursing is directed at families whose members are both healthy and ill.
    c. The family nurse is responsible along with the family itself for defining who belongs to the family.
    d. If family nursing practice is successful, the family members will simultaneously achieve maximum health.
6. Describe the difference between family as a client and family as a system.
7. Name and describe three of the many roles that nurses can assume with families.
8. The primary mode of supervising students studying family nursing is through
    a. Audiotapes of interactions between students and families.
    b. Videotapes of interactions between students and families.
    c. Process recordings developed by the student.
    d. Direct supervision of student and family interactions.
9. Which of the following nursing specialties have historically focused on the quality of family health?
    a. Maternity nursing
    b. Pediatric nursing
    c. Public health nursing
    d. All of the above
10. True or False: Family health care nursing is a specialty that originated near the end of the 20th century.
11. Discuss three traditional functions performed by families over history that still exist today. What are two functions that have become more meaningful in modern times.

References

Ahlburg, D.A., and DeVita, C. J. (1992, August). *New Realities of the American Family*. Population Bulletin, 47(2):1–44. Washington, DC: Population Reference Bureau, Inc. (Write for permission to reproduce: Population Reference Bureau, Inc., Permissions, 1875 Connecticut Ave., NW, Suite 520, Washington DC 20009-5728).

American Medical Association. (1997). *International Classification of Diseases:* Clinical Modifications (ICD-9-CM), Volumes 1 and 2, ed 9. Dover, DE.:American Medical Association.

American Psychiatric Association. (1994). *Diagnostic and Statistical Manual of Mental Disorders* (DSM-IV), ed 4. Washington, DC: American Psychiatric Association.

American Nurses Association. (1995). *Nursing's Social Policy Statement*. Washington, DC: American Nurses Association.

American Nurses Association. (1996). *Statement on the Scope and Standards of Pediatric Clinical Nursing Practice*. Washington, DC: American Nurses Association.

Anderson, K. H., and Tomlinson, P. S. (1992). The family health system as an emerging paradigmatic view for nursing. *Image: Journal of Nursing Scholarship, 24*:57–63.

Bell, J. M., Watson, W. L., and Wright, L. M. (Eds.). (1990). *The Cutting Edge of Family Nursing*. Calgary, Alberta: University of Calgary.

Berkey, K. M., and Hanson, S. M. H. (1991). *Pocket Guide*

to Family Assessment and Intervention. St. Louis: Mosby Year Book.

Bianchi, S. M. (1995). The changing demographic and socioeconomic characteristics of single-parent families. *Marriage and Family Review, 22*(1–4).

Bomar, P. J. (Ed.). (1989). *Nurses and Family Health Promotion: Concepts, Assessment, and Interventions.* Baltimore: Williams & Wilkins.

Bomar, P. J. (Ed.). (1996). *Nurses and Family Health Promotion: Concepts, Assessment, and Interventions,* ed 2. Philadelphia: W. B. Saunders.

Broderick, C.B. (1983). *The Therapeutic Triangle.* Beverly Hills, CA: Sage Publications.

Burgess, E. W., and Locke, H. J. (1953). *The Family: From Institution to Companionship.* New York: American Book Company.

Broome, M.E., Knafl, I.K., Pridham, K., & Feetham, S. (Eds).(1998). *Children and Families in Health and Illness.* Thousand Oaks: Sage Publications.

Campbell, T. (1987). *Family's impact on health: A critical review and annotated bibliography* (DHHS Publication No. ADM861461). Washington, DC: U.S. Government Printing Office.

Curran, D. (1983). *Traits of a Healthy Family.* Minneapolis: Winston Press (Harper and Row).

Curran, D. (1985). *Stress and the Healthy Family.* Minneapolis: Winston Press (Harper and Row).

Danielson, C. B., Hamel-Bissell, B., & Winstead-Fry, P. (Eds). (1993). *Families, Health and Illness: Perspectives on Coping and Intervention.* St. Louis: Mosby.

Department of Family Nursing. (1985). *Philosophy, Conceptual Framework, Objectives and Definitions.* Portland: Oregon Health Sciences University School of Nursing. Unpublished manuscript.

Doherty, W. (1985). Family intervention in health care. *Family Relations, 34:*129–137.

Doherty, W., and Campbell, T. (1988). *Families and Health.* Newbury Park, CA: Sage.

Doherty, W. J., and McCubbin, H. I. (1985). Families and health care: An emerging arena of theory, research and clinical intervention. *Family Relations, 34*:5–11.

Feetham, S. L. (1990). Conceptual and Methodological Issues in Research of Families. In J. M. Bell, W. L. Watson, and L. M. Wright (Eds.), *The Cutting Edge of Family Nursing.* Calgary, Alberta: University of Calgary.

Feetham, S. L., Meister, S. B., Bell, J. M., and Gilliss, C. L. (Eds.). (1993). *The Nursing of Families: Theory, Research, Education, Practice.* Newbury Park, CA: Sage.

Ford, D. Y. (1994). An exploration of perceptions of alternative family structures among university students. *Family Relations, 43:* 68–73.

Friedemann, M. L. (1995). *The Framework of Systemic Organization: A Conceptual Approach to Families and Nursing.* Thousand Oaks, CA: Sage.

Friedman, M. M. (1998). *Family Nursing: Research, Theory and Practice,* ed 4. Norwalk, CT: Appleton & Lange.

Gilliss, C. (1989). *Family Research in Nursing.* In C. L. Gilliss, B. L. Highley, B. M. Roberts, and I. M. Martinson. (Eds). *Toward a Science of Family Nursing* (pp. 37–63). Menlo Park, CA: Addison-Wesley.

Gilliss, C. L. (1990). Foreword. In J. M. Bell, W. L. Watson, and L. M. Wright (Eds.). (1990). *The Cutting Edge of Family Nursing* (pp. iii-v). Calgary, Alberta: University of Calgary Faculty of Nursing.

Gilliss, C. L. (1993). Family Nursing Research, Theory and Practice. In G. D. Wegner and R. J. Alexander (Eds.), *Readings in Family Nursing* (pp. 34–42). Philadelphia: J. B. Lippincott.

Gilliss, C. L., and Davis, L. L. (1993). Does Family Intervention Make a Difference? An integrative review and meta-analysis. In *The Nursing of Families: Theory, Research, Education, Practice* (pp. 259–265). Newbury Park: Sage.

Gilliss, C. L., Roberts, B. M., Highley, B. L., and Martinson, I. M. (1989). What is Family Nursing? In C. L. Gilliss, B. L. Highley, B. M. Roberts, and I. M. Martinson (Eds.), *Toward a Science of Family Nursing* (pp. 64–73). Menlo Park, CA: Addison-Wesley.

Gordon, M. (1994). *Nursing Diagnosis: Process and Application,* ed 2. New York: McGraw Hill.

Ham, L. M., and Chamings, P. A. (1983). Family Nursing: Historical Perspectives. In I. Clements and F. B. Roberts (Eds.), *Family Health Care: A Theoretical Approach to Nursing Care,* Volume 1 (pp. 88–109). San Francisco: McGraw-Hill.

Hanson, S. M. H. (1986). Healthy Single Parent Families. *Family Relations, 35:*125–132.

Hanson, S.M.H. (1996). Family Nursing Assessment and Intervention. In S.M.H. Hanson and S.T. Boyd (Eds). *Family Health Care Nursing: Theory, Practice and Research* (pp. 147–200). Philadelphia: F.A. Davis.

Hanson, S.M.H. and Boyd, S.T. (Eds.)(1996a). *Family Health Care Nursing: Theory, Practice, and Research.* Philadelphia: F.A. Davis.

Hanson, S.M.H. and Boyd. S.T. (Eds.) (1996b). Family Health Care Nursing. In S.M.H. Hanson and S.T. Boyd, S.T. (Eds.) (1996). *Family Health Care Nursing:Theory, Practice, and Research.* (pp. 5–40). Philadelphia:F.A. Davis.

Hanson, S. M. H., and Heims, M. L. (1992). Family nursing curricula in U.S. schools of nursing. *Journal of Nursing Education, 31(7),* 305–308.

Hanson, S. M. H., Heims, M. L., Julian, D. J., and Sussman, M.B. (Eds.). (1995a). *Single-parent Families: Diversity, Myths, and Realities.* New York: Haworth.

Hanson, S. M. H., Heims, M. L., Julian D. J., and Sussman, M. B. (1995b) Single Parent Families: Present and Future Perspectives. In S. M. H. Hanson, M. L. Heims, D. J. Julian, and M. B. Sussman (Eds.), *Single Parent Families: Diversity, Myths and Realities.* New York: Haworth.

Hanson, S. M. H., Heims, M. L., Julian, D. J., and Sussman, M. B. (Eds.). (1995c). Single Parent Families: Diversity, myths and realities. *Marriage and Family Review, 22*(1–4).

Hanson, S. M. H., Heims, M. L., Julian D. J., and Sussman, M. B. (Eds.). (1995d). Single Parent Families: Present and Future Perspectives. *Marriage and Family Review, 22*(1–4).

Hanson, S. M. H. and Mischke, K., (1996). Family Health Assessment and Intervention. In P. J. Bomar (Ed.), *Nurses and Family Health Promotion: Concepts, Assessment and Interventions,* ed 2, (pp. 165–202). Philadelphia: W. B. Saunders.

Kirschling, J. M., Gilliss, C. L., Krentz, L., Camburn, C. D., Clough, R. S., Duncan, et al. (1994). "Success" in Family Nursing: Experts describe phenomena. *Nursing and Health Care, 15:*186–189.

Loveland-Cherry, C. J. (1989). Family Health Promotion and Health Protection. In P. J. Bomar (Ed.), *Nurses and Family Health Promotion: Concepts, Assessment and Interventions* (pp. 13–25). Baltimore: Williams and Wilkins.

Martin, K.S., and Scheet, N.J. (1992). *The Omaha System: Applications for Community Health Nursing.* Philadelphia: W.B. Saunders Company.

Maslow, A. (1970). *Motivation and Personality.* NY: Harper & Row.

McCubbin, M. A., and McCubbin, H. I. (1993). Families Coping with Illness: The Resiliency Model of Family Stress, Adjustment, and Adaptation. In C. B. Danielson, B. Hamel-Bissell, and P. Winstead-Fry. *Families, Health and Illness: Perspectives on Coping and Intervention,* (pp. 21–65). St. Louis: Mosby.

McEwan, P. J. M. (1974). The social approach to family health studies. *Social Science and Medicine, 8:*487–493.

Mischke-Berkey, K., Warner, P., and Hanson, S. M. H. (1989). Family Health Assessment and Intervention. In P. J. Bomar (Ed.), *Nurses and Family Health Promotion: Concepts, Assessment And Interventions* (pp. 115–154). Baltimore, MD: Williams & Wilkins.

Moriarty, H. J. (1990). Key issues in the family research process: Strategies for nurse researchers. *Advances in Nursing Science, 12*(3):1–14.

Murphy, S. (1986). Family Study and Nursing Research. *Image: Journal of Nursing Scholarship, 18:*170–174.

NANDA: *Nursing diagnosis: Definitions and Classification 1999–2000.* (1999). Philadelphia: North American Nursing Diagnosis Association.

National Center for Health Statistics. (1994). *Births, Marriages, Divorces and Deaths for 1993.* Monthly Vital Statistics Report, 42(12). (DHHS Publication No. 94–1120). Hyattsville, MD: Public Health Service.

Neuman, B. (1989). *The Neuman Systems Model. Application to Nursing Education and Practice,* ed 2. Norwalk, CT: Appleton & Lange.

Nightingale, F. (1979). *Cassandra.* Westbury, NY: The Feminist Press.

Olson, D. H., and Hanson, M. K. (Eds.). (1990). *2001: Preparing Families for the Future.* Minneapolis: National Council on Family Relations.

Orem, D. (1995). *Nursing: Concepts of Practice,* St. Louis: C.V. Mosby.

Otto, H. (1963). Criteria for assessing family strengths. *Family Process, 2:*329–338.

Pender, N. (1996). *Health Promotion in Nursing Practice,* ed. 3. Norwalk, CT: Appleton & Lange.

Pratt, L. (1976). *Family Structure and Effective Health Behavior: The Energized Family.* Boston: Houghton Mifflin.

Roy, C. (1984). *Introduction to Nursing. An Adaptation Model,* ed 2. Englewood Cliffs, NJ: Prentice Hall.

Stanhope, M., and Lancaster, J. (1996). *Community Health Nursing: Process and Practice for Promoting Health,* ed 4. St. Louis: Mosby.

Stinnett, N., Chesser, B., and DeFrain, J. (Eds). (1979). *Building Family Strengths: Blueprints for Action.* Lincoln: University of Nebraska Press

U.S. Bureau of the Census. (1991a). Current population reports, Series P-60, No. 173. Child support and alimony: 1989. Washington, DC: U.S. Government Printing Office.

U.S. Bureau of the Census. (1991b). Current population reports, Series P-20, No. 461. Marital status and living arrangements: March 1991. Washington, DC: U.S. Government Printing Office.

U.S. Bureau of the Census. (1992a). Current population reports, Series P-20, No. 458, Household and family characteristics: 1991. Washington, DC: U.S. Government Printing Office.

U.S. Bureau of the Census. (1992b). Current population reports, Series P-23, No. 180. Marriage, divorce, and remarriage in the 1990s. Washington, DC: U.S. Government Printing Office.

U.S. Bureau of the Census. (1992c). Current population reports, Series P-20, No. 468. Marital status and living arrangements: March 1992. Washington, DC: U.S. Government Printing Office.

U.S. Bureau of the Census. (1992d). Current population reports, Series P-23, No. 181. Households, families and children: A 30-year perspective. Washington, DC: U.S. Government Printing Office.

U.S. Bureau of the Census. (1994a). Current Population Reports, Series P-20, Nos. 477 and 478. Washington DC: U.S. Government Printing Office.

U.S. Bureau of the Census. (1994b). Current Population Reports Series P-20, No. 483. Steven W. Rawlings and A. Saluter. Household and Family Characteristics: March 1994. Washington, DC: U.S. Government Printing Office. Table A, p. vii.

U.S. Bureau of the Census. (1995a). Current Population Reports. Series P-60, No. 184. Statistical Abstract of the United States, 1995. Washington, DC: U.S. Government Printing Office.

U.S. Bureau of the Census. (1995b). Marital Status and Living Arrangements, March 1995. U.S. Government Printing Office.

U.S. Bureau of the Census. (1995c). Statistical Abstract of the United States. Washington, D.C.: U.S. Government Printing Office.

U.S. Department of Health and Human Services. (1990). Healthy People 2000: National Health Promotion and Disease Prevention Objectives. Washington DC: U.S. DHHS (DHHS Pub No. (PHS) 91–50212).

Vaughan-Cole, B., Johnson, M.A., Malone, J.A., Walker, B.L. (1998).(Eds.) *Family Nursing Practice.* Philadelphia: W.B. Saunders Company.

Wegner, G. B., and Alexander, R. J. (Eds.). (1999). *Readings in Family Nursing,* ed 2. Philadelphia: J. B. Lippincott.

Whall, A. L. (1993). The Family as the Unit of Care in Nursing: A Historical Review. In G. D. Wegner and R. J. Alexander (Eds.), *Readings in Family Nursing* (pp. 3–12). Philadelphia: J. B. Lippincott.

Whall, A. L., and Fawcett, J. (Eds.). (1991). *Family Theory Development in Nursing: State of the Science and Art.* Philadelphia: F. A. Davis.

Wright, L. M., and Bell, J. M. (1989). A Survey of Family Nursing Education in Canadian Universities. *Canadian Journal of Nursing Research, 21*(3):59–74.

Wright, L. M., and Leahey, M. (1984). *Nurses and Families: A Guide to Family Assessment and Intervention.* Philadelphia: F. A. Davis.

Wright, L. M., and Leahey, M. (1993). Trends in Nursing of Families. In G. D. Wegner and R. J. Alexander (Eds.), *Readings in Family Nursing* (pp. 23–33). Philadelphia: J. B. Lippincott.

Wright, L.M., and Leahey, M. (1994). *Nurses and Families: A Guide to Family Assessment and Intervention,* ed 2. Philadelphia: F.A. Davis.

Additional Bibliography

Altergott, K. (Ed.). (1993). *One World, Many Families.* Minneapolis, MN: National Council on Family Relations, 3989 Central Avenue NE, Suite 550, Minneapolis, MN 55421, Tel: 612-781-9331.

Boss, P.G., Doherty, W.J., LaRossa, R., Schrumm, W.R., and Steinmetz, S.K. (Eds.). (1993). *Source Book of Family Theories and Methods: A Contextual Approach.* New York: Plenum.

Bozett, F.W., and Hanson, S.M.H. (1991). *Fatherhood and Families in Cultural Context.* New York: Springer.

Candib, L.M. (1995). *Medicine and the Family: A Feminist Perspective.* New York: Basic Books.

Draper, T.W., and Marcos, A.C.: (1990). *Family Variables: Conceptualization, Measurement And Use.* Newbury Park, CA: Sage.

Feetham, S.L., Meister, S.B., Bell, J.M., and Gilliss, C.L. (Eds.). (1993) *The Nursing Of Families: Theory/Research Education/Practice.* Newbury Park, CA: Sage.

Gilliss, C.L., Highley, B.L., Roberts, B.M., and Martinson, I.M. (Eds.). (1989). *Toward A Science Of Family Nursing.* Menlo Park, CA: Addison-Wesley.

Hinshaw, A.S., Feetham, S.L., and Shaver, J.L.F. (1999) *Handbook of Clinical Nursing Research.* Thousand Oaks, CA: Sage Publications.

Kissman, K., and Allen, J. A. (1993). *Single-Parent Families.* Newbury Park, CA: Sage.

Leahey, M., and Wright, L.M. (Eds.). (1987). *Families And Life Threatening Illness.* Springhouse, PA: Springhouse.

Leahey, M., and Wright, L.M. (Eds.). (1987). *Families and Psychosocial Problems.* Springhouse, PA: Springhouse.

Leavitt, M. B. (1982). *Families At Risk: Prevention In Nursing Practice.* Boston: Little, Brown.

Levinson, D. (Ed.). (1996) *Encyclopedia Of Marriage And The Family, Volumes 1 and 2.* New York: Macmillan.

Pearson, A., and Vaughan, B. (1986). *Nursing Models For Practice.* Rockville, MD: Aspen.

Pender, N., Barkauskas, V., Hayman, L., Rice, V., and Anderson, E. (1992). Health promotion and disease prevention: toward excellence in nursing practice and education. *Nursing Outlook, 40:*106–109.

Price, S., and Elliott, B. (Eds.). (1993). *Vision 2010: Families And Health Care.* Minneapolis, MN: National Council on Family Relations.

Ross, B., and Cobb, K.L. (1990). *Family Nursing: A Nursing Process Approach.* Redwood City, CA: Addison-Wesley.

Sawa, R.J. (Ed.). (1992). *Family Health Care.* Newbury Park, CA: Sage. More medical than nursing content, but this book helps to see what the doctors are thinking about family health care.

Stanhope, M., and Lancaster, J. (in press) *Community Health Nursing: Promoting Health of Aggregate Families and Individuals.* St. Louis: C.V. Mosby.

Sussman, M. B., and Steinmetz, S. K. (1987). *Handbook of Marriage and the Family.* New York: Plenum Press.

Whall, A.L. (1986) *Family Therapy Theory For Nursing: Four Approaches.* Norwalk, CT; Appleton-Century-Crofts.

Wright, L.M., and Leahey, M. (Eds.). (1987). *Families and Chronic Illness.* Springhouse, PA: Springhouse.

Wright, L.M., Watson, W.L. and Bell, J.M. (1997). *Beliefs: The Heart of Healing in Families and Illness.* New York: Basic Books.

Focus On

THEORETICAL FOUNDATIONS FOR FAMILY NURSING

This chapter on family nursing theory answers questions related to the theoretical foundations of family nursing and how these foundations drive current nursing practice with families. Theories assist nurses in understanding the structure, function, and process of how families are created, maintained, and changed and how families conduct their business. The chapter challenges you to think soundly and systematically about families in relation to your practice. This chapter provides you with the theoretical and conceptual bases for understanding the rest of the chapters in this book.

The first part of the chapter explains important theoretical and conceptual frameworks for the practice of nursing with families. Definitions of theories, concepts, propositions, and theoretical and conceptual models are provided for clarification of how they build on one another. The importance and function of theory are summarized.

In the second part of the chapter, family nursing conceptual frameworks are presented as an evolving synthesis of scholarship from three major traditions and disciplines: family social science, family therapy, and nursing. Six theories from family social science are summarized: structural and functional theory, systems theory, developmental theory, interactional theory, stress theory, and change theory. Three theories from family therapy are outlined: structural, systems, and interactional theories. Selected nursing models and theories are briefly described as they relate specifically to family nursing: they are organized by their originators, King, Roy, Neuman, Orem, Rogers, and Friedemann. Finally, there is a brief discussion of integrated approaches to the nursing of families. Since no single theory from any discipline is the perfect answer for nursing care of families, some family nursing theorists have developed integrated models, which draw on assumptions from family social science, family therapy, and nursing concepts. Note that a detailed discussion of three of the more fully developed integrated models is contained in Chapter 8.

Chapter 2

THEORETICAL FOUNDATIONS FOR FAMILY NURSING

Shirley May Harmon Hanson, RN, PhD • Joanna Rowe Kaakinen, RN, PhD

OUTLINE

OBJECTIVES

On completion of this chapter, the reader will be able to:

- Explain the advantages inherent in deriving family nursing practice from theoretical frameworks or models.
- Discuss the three sources of family nursing theory and their contribution to the specialty.
- Explain how family nursing theory directs nursing practice of families.
- Describe the basic assumptions of each family social science theory, family therapy theory, and nursing model presented in this chapter
- Summarize the importance of an integrated approach to the nursing of families.
- Discuss the current state of the art for theory development in family nursing.

In all of nursing practice, the nurse-client relationship plays a central role. In many areas of practice, the client is an individual, and nurses expect to develop a relationship with the individual. In family nursing, however, the client in the nurse-client relationship is not an individual but a family. One individual in the family may have a problem or need medical care, but the nurse interacts with the whole family and works with their human responses to actual or potential health problems.

In family nursing, the nurse-client relationship requires nurses to move outside their own worldview and experience and see the situation from the perspective of the client family. Understanding the family's worldview and frame of reference is critical to determining the family's present status, assessing their needs, developing a plan of action, and evaluating the outcomes of interventions. Theoretical views of how families are created, maintained, or changed and of how they function will help nurses understand families' worldview. And the more theoretical approaches with which nurses are familiar, the larger the repertoire they have for supporting families in their choice of actions to resolve health problems or maintain health. Theoretical and conceptual frameworks are especially useful in helping family nurses think interactionally and systemically and shift from the individual-as-client approach to the family-as-client approach.

This chapter discusses the theoretical and conceptual foundations for the nursing care of families. The chapter begins with a definition of theory and then discusses the theoretical foundations for the practice of family nursing. Finally, integrated theoretical approaches to family nursing are presented.

WHAT IS THEORY?

A theory is a set of statements about how some part of the world works (Vogt, 1993, Powers & Knapp, 1990). Theories consist of concepts and relationships among concepts. Concepts, which are the building blocks of theory, are words that are mental images or abstract representations of phenomena. Concepts, or the major ideas expressed by a theory, may exist on a continuum from empirical (concrete) to abstract (Powers & Knapp, 1990). For example, family and health are examples of highly abstract concepts; family breakfast is far less abstract. The more abstract the concept, the greater the range of its definitions. For example, there are many ways in which to define and thus measure the concept of "family," and there are even more definitions and ways to assess the concept of "health."

Propositions are statements about the relationship between two or more concepts (Powers & Knapp, 1990). A proposition might be a statement such as this: The family unit interacts with the health of the individual members of the family. The word "interact" links the two concepts of family and health. A hypothesis is a way of stating an expected relationship between concepts. For example, using the concepts of family and health, one could hypothesize that there is an interactive relationship between family functioning and the health of family members; that is, the family's ability to cope with stress affects the health of individual family members, and in turn, the health of these individual members has an impact on family coping. This hypothesis may be tested by a study that measures family coping mechanisms and family members' health over time and uses statistical procedures to look at the relationships between the two.

All theories are subject to rules of organization; that is, they are composed of concepts, propositions, relationships between propositions, and connections among propositions and the world of empirical observation (Klein & White, 1996). Thus, theories are designed to make sense of the world: to show how one thing is related to another and how together they make a pattern that can predict the consequences of certain clusters of characteristics or events. All theories serve the function of describing, explaining, or make predictions about phenomena (LoBiono-Wood & Haber, 1998). Nursing theories ideally represent logical and intelligible patterns that make sense of the observations a nurse makes in practice and enable the nurse to predict what is likely to happen to clients (Fawcett & Downs, 1992). According to Klein and White (1996), in family nursing the major function of theory is to provide knowledge and understanding that will improve services to families.

Specifically, theories help us to accumulate and organize research findings into coherent patterns and to develop and test hypotheses or predictions of what the world will look like. Theories also make it possible to articulate ideas more clearly and specifically than is possible in everyday language, and they demonstrate how ideas are connected to each other and to other theories. That is, theories are systematic sets of ideas. Finally and most importantly, theories explain what is happening; they provide answers to "how" and "why" questions, help us to interpret and make sense of phenomena, and predict or point to what could happen in the future.

In nursing, the relationship of theory to practice constitutes a dynamic feedback loop rather than a static linear progression. That is, theory grows out of observations made in practice and is tested by research. Tested theory informs practice, and practice in turn facilitates the further refinement and development of theory. Thus, theory, practice, and research related to family nursing are mutually dependent on each other.

As noted above, theories attempt to explain and organize phenomena and are used to describe or predict specific and concrete phenomena (Fawcett, 1995). Theories may be more or less abstract and general, and they vary in the number of phenomena to which they apply. Depending on the level of their abstraction, theories in nursing are generally classified as grand theory, middle-range theory, or low-level (or single-domain) theory.

A conceptual model is a set of general propositions that integrates concepts into a meaningful configuration or pattern (Fawcett, 1995). Conceptual models in nursing are based on the observations and insights of nursing scholars or deductions that combine ideas from several fields of inquiry. Conceptual models provide a frame of reference and a coherent way of thinking about nursing phenomena. A conceptual model is more abstract and more comprehensive than a theory. Like a conceptual model, a conceptual framework is a way of integrating concepts into a meaningful pattern, but conceptual frameworks are often less definite than models. They provide useful conceptual approaches or ways in which to look at a problem or situation, rather than a definite set of propositions.

In this chapter, the terms "conceptual model or framework," "theoretical framework," and "theory" are used interchangeably. In part, that is because there is no single firm theoretical basis for family nursing; rather, nurses' approaches are often eclectic. The interchangeable use of these various terms also reflects the fact that there is considerable overlap of ideas in the various theories, theoretical perspectives, conceptual models, conceptual approaches, and "streams of influence" that are important for family nursing.

As might be expected, there has been a substantial amount of cross-fertilization among disciplines, such as social science and nursing, and concepts originating in one theory or discipline have been translated into similar concepts for use in another discipline. Thus, many of the concepts in nursing theories were adapted from theories in the traditional fields of sociology, anthropology, and psychology and in the more recent fields of family social science and family therapy. For example, concepts such as interaction, stressors, environment, and self-esteem were borrowed from the traditional behavioral and social sciences but have now been integrated into nursing and our notions of health care.

Family social science has also taken concepts from the general social sciences and applied them to families; examples include developmental theory, symbolic interactionism, structural-functional theory, social exchange, and general systems theories. Family therapy theorists have adapted concepts and propositions from the family social sciences and applied them to the new field of family therapy. For example, general systems theory, which is an idea originally developed in the field of engineering, is one of the foundations for family therapy. At present, no single theory or conceptual framework adequately describes the complex relationships of family structure, function, and process. No single theoretical perspective gives nurses a sufficiently broad base of knowledge and understanding to guide assessment and interventions with families. Thus, there is no single theoretical basis for providing nursing care to families; rather, nurses must draw upon multiple theories and frameworks to guide their work with families and take an integrated approach to practice, research, and education in family nursing. Box 2–1 lists the criteria for evaluating family theories that are useful for family nursing.

THEORETICAL AND CONCEPTUAL FOUNDATIONS FOR THE NURSING OF FAMILIES

The conceptual or theoretical frameworks and approaches that provide the foundations for family nursing have evolved from three major traditions and disciplines: family social science, family therapy, and nursing (Figure 2–1, Conceptual Sources of Emerging Family Nursing Theories) (Hanson & Boyd, 1996; Hanson & Kaakinen, 1996; Hanson, Kaakinen, & Friedman, 1998).

Of these three types of theory, the family social science theories are the most well-developed and informative about family phenomena, such as family function, the environment-family interchange, interactions and dynamics within the family, changes in the family over time, and the family's reaction to health and illness. However, it is difficult to use family social science the-

Box 2–1

CRITERIA FOR EVALUATING FAMILY THEORIES

Internal consistency: not containing logically contradictory assertions.
Clarity or explicitness: expressed in such a way that they are unambiguous, defined, and explicated where necessary.
Explanatory power: explains well what it is intended to explain.
Coherence: integrated or interconnected key ideas; loose ends are avoided.
Understanding: provides a comprehensible sense of the whole phenomenon being examined.
Empirical fit: means a large portion of the tests of a theory have been confirmatory or, at least, have not been interpreted as not confirmatory.
Testability: means it is possible for a theory to be empirically supported or refuted.
Heuristic value: has generated or can generate considerable research and intellectual curiosity (including a large number of empirical studies, as well as much debate or controversy).
Groundedness: built up from detailed information about events and processes observable in the world.
Contextualization: gives serious consideration to the social and historical contexts affecting or affected by its key ideas.
Interpretive sensitivity: reflects the experiences practiced and felt by the social units to which it is applied.
Predictive power: successfully predicts phenomena that have occurred since the theory was formulated.
Practical utility: can be readily applied to social problems, policies, and programs of action (i.e., it is useful for teaching, therapy, political action, or some combination of these).

Adapted from Klein, D.M., & White, J.M. (1996). *Family Theories: An Introduction.* Thousand Oaks, CA: Sage Publications.

ories as a basis for assessment and intervention in family nursing because of the abstract nature of the theories, although nursing scholars have made some strides in this regard in recent years (Berkey & Hanson, 1991; Wright & Leahey, 2000; Friedman, 1998; Friedemann, 1995; Hanson & Boyd, 1996; Danielson, Hamel-Bissell, & Winstead-Fry, 1993; Vaughn-Cole, Johnson, Malone, & Walker, 1998).

Family therapy theories are newer and less well-developed than family social science theories, but they are more relevant to family nursing because they emanate from professional practice rather than from an academic discipline, such as family social science. Thus today, family nursing theory, practice, research, and education draw heavily on family therapy theories. Whall (1986), for example, has urged family nurse therapists to reformulate existing family therapy theories to fit the nursing perspective.

Finally, of the three types of theories, *nursing conceptual frameworks* are the least developed in family nursing. During the 1960s and 1970s, nurses placed great emphasis on the development of nursing models. However, these models originated from an individualized medical-model paradigm and few have evolved enough to be useful for family nursing (Berkey & Hanson, 1991). Further, the nursing models, in large part, represent a deductive approach to the development of nursing science (i.e., they move from the general to the specific). Although they embody an important part of our nursing heritage, in the 1990s these nursing frameworks and their deductive approach were being viewed more and more critically. More inductive approaches to nursing theory development (i.e., approaches that move from the specific to the general) are now being advocated. That is, there is more focus today on beginning with empirical observations, whether quantitative or qualitative, and generalizing from those observations to develop abstract propositions and theory.

In the next section of this chapter, the three types of theories that are significant to evolving and integrative family nursing frameworks are briefly summarized (Box 2–2; Table 2–1; Figure 2–1.) First, theoretical perspectives from the family social sciences are presented, because they were derived from the most developed disciplines and serve as a foundation for both family therapy and integrated family nursing models. Second, theories from family therapy are summarized, and their links to the family social science theories are noted. Finally, selected conceptual frameworks from nursing are outlined, with a brief discussion of their links to family social science and family therapy theory. Because family therapy and family nursing are both practice disciplines focused on families and both developed theoretical formulations at about the same time, there are some commonalities between the two fields. The chapter concludes with a brief discussion of integrated models for nursing care of families; these are elaborated in Chapter 8.

Family Social Science Theories

Family social science theories were developed from various social science disciplines, primarily sociology. These theories proliferated during the first half of the 20th century, and by the early 1950s, scholars were beginning to organize the accumulated conceptual knowledge on the family. Although there is still little agreement on what theories constitute the major foundations for family nursing, since the 1960s it has been generally recognized that three conceptual approaches are predominant in the field of marriage and the family. These approaches are (1) structural-functional, (2) interactional, and (3) developmental (Broderick, 1971; Nye & Berardo, 1981). Presently the frameworks of conflict theory, exchange theory, psychoanalysis, social psychology, developmental theory, economics, and law serve as foundations for the study of family.

Family social science theories were originally developed with little thought to their possible use by clinicians. Recently, however, three major books have explored the development of family social science with emphasis on its usefulness for practice. In *Sourcebook of Family Theories and Methods: A Contextual Approach,* Boss, Doherty, Schumm, and Steinmetz (1993) trace the development of family theory from its origins in religion and philosophy through the construction of theory and methodology in the mid-20th century to emerging models; their book emphasizes the interaction between theories and methods. Klein and White (1996), in *Family Theories: An Introduction,* review the major theoretical frameworks from the social sciences used for understanding families: exchange, symbolic interaction, family development, conflict, systems, and ecological. Winton (1995), in *Frameworks for Studying Families,* summarizes the various frameworks used by scholars and researchers in analyzing families. Books such as these have served to make the knowledge base of the family social sciences more accessible for practice disciplines, such as family nursing.

The next section summarizes the major theories from the family social sciences that have been useful to the understanding of families and the practice of family nursing. These include structural-functional theory, systems theory, interactional theory, stress theory, developmental theory, and change theory. Other frameworks that support family nursing include chaos theory, social exchange theory, conflict theory, ecological theory, anthropological and multicultural theories, and phenomenology theory (Nye & Berardo, 1981; Klein & White, 1996; Friedman, 1998; Vaughn-Cole, Johnson, Malone, & Walker, 1998). Unfortunately, we cannot deal with those here in detail.

Structural-Functional Theory

In structural-functional theory, the family is considered a small group that has features common to all small groups. The family is viewed as a social system. Further, this theory assumes that social systems, such as families, carry out functions that serve individuals and functions that serve society. The individuals in the family act in accordance with a set of internalized norms and values, which are learned primarily through socialization.

Family analysis involves examining the arrangement of members within the family, relationships between the members, and relationships of the members to the whole (Artinian, 1994; Hanson, Kaakinen, & Friedman, 1998; Friedman, 1998). The family also is examined in terms of its relationships with other major social institutions, such as medicine, religion, education, government, and the economy. The primary aim is to consider the family in the overall structure of society and see how family patterns fit with other institutions. From this perspective, the basic functions of families are considered to be economic, reproductive, protective, cultural, social, status-conferring, relationship-developing, and health-maintaining (Hanson & Boyd, 1996; Hanson & Kaakinen, 2000). A central

Box 2-2

THEORETICAL FOUNDATIONS USED IN FAMILY NURSING PRACTICE

Family Social Science Theories

Structural-Functional Theory
Systems Theory
Family Developmental Theory
Family Interactional Theory
Family Stress Theory
Change Theory
Others
- Chaos Theory
- Social Exchange Theory
- Conflict Theory
- Ecological Theory
- Anthropological/Multicultural Theory
- Phenomenological Theory

Family Therapy Theories

Structural Family Therapy Theory
Family Systems Therapy Theory
Interactional Family Therapy Theory
Others
- Psychodynamic Therapy Theory
- Experiential Therapy Theory
- Humanistic Therapy Theory
- Strategic Therapy Theory
- Behavioral/Cognitive Therapy Theory
- Narrative Therapy Theory
- Solution-Oriented Therapy Theory

Nursing Models and Theories

Systems Theory
- King
- Roy
- Neuman
- Orem
- Rogers
- Friedemann

Others
- Leininger
    - Watson
    - Peplau
    - Barnard
    - Newman

Integrated
- Hanson & Mischke
- Friedman
- Wright & Leahey
- McCubbin & McCubbin

TABLE 2–1
Differences among family social science theories, family therapy theories, and nursing models and theories

Criteria	Family Social Science Theories	Family Therapy Theories	Nursing Theories
Purpose of theory	Descriptive and explanatory (academic models); to explain family functioning and dynamics	Descriptive and prescriptive (practice models); to explain family dysfunction and guide therapeutic actions	Descriptive and prescriptive (practice models): to guide nursing assessment and intervention efforts
Discipline focus	Interdisciplinary (although primarily sociological)	Marriage and family therapy; family mental health; new approaches focus on family strengths	Nursing focus
Target population	Primarily "normal" families (normality-oriented)	Primarily "troubled" families (pathology-oriented)	Primarily families with health and illness problems

Adapted from Jones, S.L., and Dimond, S.L. (1982). Family Theory and Family Therapy Models: Comparative Review with Implications for Nursing Practice. *Journal of Psychiatric Nursing and Mental Health Services, 20*(10): 12–19.

issue is how well the family structure allows the family to perform its functions. Family theorists who use this approach want to understand the social or family system and its relationship to the overall social system (Nye & Berardo, 1981).

This approach characterizes the family as open to outside influences while maintaining its boundaries. The family, however, is seen as a passively adapting institution rather than an agent of change. This approach tends to take a static view of the societal structure and to neglect change as a structural dynamic.

Nevertheless, this is a useful perspective for assessing families and health. The illness of a family member inevitably brings alterations in the family structure and function. For example, if a single mother is ill, she cannot carry out her various roles, so grandparents or siblings may have to assume child care responsibilities. Clearly, the illness of the single mother changes the power structure and communication patterns of the family. Assessment includes determining whether the changes caused by the mother's illness will affect the family's ability to carry out its functions. The terminal or chronic illness of a family member also affects family structure and functioning. Using the structural-functional perspective, assessment questions during the chronic illness of a family member might include these: What family roles were altered by the onset of the chronic illness? How did the illness alter the family structure? Intervention becomes necessary when changes in family structure alter the family's ability to function. Interventions might include assisting families to use existing support structures and assisting families to modify their organization so that role responsibilities can be redistributed.

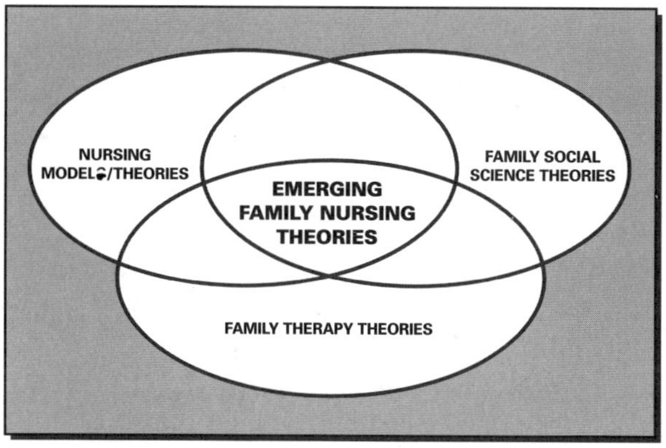

FIGURE 2–1
Conceptual sources of emerging family nursing theories

The major strength of the structural-functional approach to family nursing practice is that it is comprehensive and views families within the context of the broader community. The major weakness of this approach is that it is static and tends to view families at one moment in time rather than as a social system that changes over time.

Systems Theory

Systems theory has over the years been the most influential of all the family frameworks. This approach to understanding families was derived from physics and biology by von Bertalanffy (1950, 1968 as cited in Mercer, 1989). A system is composed of a set of interacting elements; each system is identifiable as distinct from the environment in which it exists. An open system exchanges energy and matter with the environment, while a closed system is isolated from its environment. Systems depend on both positive and negative feedback to maintain a steady state (homeostasis). The systems perspective assumes that family systems are greater than and different from the sum of their parts. The family system is an organized whole, and individuals in the family are interdependent and interactive. There are boundaries, however, in the system, which can be open, closed, or random. Further, there are hierarchies within the family system and logical relationships between subsystems, e.g., mother-child, family-community. Every family system has features designed to maintain stability or homeostasis, although these features may be adaptive or maladaptive. At the same time, the family is considered to change constantly in response to stresses and strains from the external environment, and change in one part of the family system affects the entire system. Causes and effects are modified by feedback loops. The patterns of family systems are circular rather than linear, and the family system increases in complexity over time, evolving to ensure greater adaptability, tolerance to change, and growth by differentiation. Since patterns are circular, interventions to bring change must be directed toward the cycle of change, not toward isolated events.

The family system perspective encourages nurses to see individual clients as participating members of a family system. For example, nurses who are using this perspective assess the effects of illness or injury upon the entire family and the effects of family functioning on the individual with the illness or injury (Wright & Leahey, 2000). Emphasis is on the whole rather than on individuals. Assessment questions that might be asked from this perspective include: Who is in the family system? How has a family member's critical illness affected the family and its members? Interventions by family nurses must address both subsystem and whole family processes and functioning.

The strengths of the general systems framework include the facts that this theory covers a large array of phenomena and views the family within the context of its suprasystems (the larger community in which it is embedded) and its subsystems. Further, this is an interactional and holistic theory that looks at processes in the family, rather than at the content and relationships between parts. The family is viewed as a whole, not as merely a sum of its parts. Unfortunately, the strengths of the theory are also its limitations; that is, because this theoretical orientation is broad and general, it is difficult to apply to practice. Specific concepts and practice guidelines have to be developed outside the theory. Further, this approach may not be as helpful as theories oriented toward individuals in dealing with the concerns of individual family members.

Interactional Theory

The family interactional approach is derived from a major theory in social psychology and sociology called *symbolic interaction.* Hill and Hansen (1960), Turner (1970), Rose (1962), and others have adapted the concepts and propositions of this theoretical perspective to the family. The interactional approach sees the family as a unit made up of interacting personalities and examines internal family dynamics, including communication processes, roles, decision making and problem solving, and socialization patterns (Rose, 1962).

The interactional approach places major emphasis on family roles. That is, each member of the family is considered to occupy formal and informal positions. Family members expect to perform their roles in certain ways, depending on their perceptions of role demands by the family as a whole and by other individuals in the family. Family members judge their own behavior by obtaining feedback from others in the family. The responses of these other family members serve to challenge or reinforce the way that individual family members carry out their roles (Nye, 1976). That is why the theory is called "interactional."

In this approach to the family, the process of role taking is viewed as critical (Turner, 1970). The social interaction between two or more family members leads to role taking (Turner, 1970). Through the process, family members develop informal roles that may or may not be appropriate to the family in the long-run.

This approach to understanding families is particularly useful in family nursing because its focus is on internal processes of social interaction within families, rather than on the outcomes of these interactions. The major problem with interactionism is that the family is seen as existing in a vacuum, with no consideration of the environment or the family's history, culture, or socioeconomic status. In the interactionalist approach, families are considered to be comparatively closed units, and the external world is thought to have little effect on what occurs within the family. However, that view ignores the influence of the external world on the family and interactions within the family.

Working from an interactional perspective, the family health care nurse assesses interaction and communication between family members, family role and power distribution, family coping, and family socialization patterns as well as relationships between marital partners, siblings, and parents and children. The nurse intervenes on the basis of the family's needs for health promotion, health maintenance, or health restoration in relation to these six areas.

Stress Theory

Family stress theory is derived from the work of Rueben Hill (1949), who conducted research on the effects on families of war-induced separations and reunions, during World War II. Hill found that the experiences of families facing separations during war sometimes resembled a roller coaster. The stress of separation often led to crisis, and crisis led to a decline in family functioning or even family disorganization, but this was followed by an upward recovery curve and a new level of family organization. Based on his research, Hill (1965) developed the "ABCX" model of family stress. In this model, "A" is the event or stressor that, with its associated hardships, leads to changes in the family system. "B" refers to the strengths or resources of the family that enable it to deal with stressors. These resources include religious faith, financial resources, social support, physical health, family flexibility, and family coping mechanisms. "C" refers to the way families appraise the seriousness of stressor events or the subjective meaning that the family attaches to such events. The family's definition of an event determines how they will deal with it and how stressful it will be for them. This last point is critical for family nursing. Sometimes nurses cannot understand why families react in certain ways to events; nurses see the reality of the events and the family's reaction seems disproportionate. However, the family is reacting to their appraisal or definition, rather than to the reality of the event. "A," "B," and "C" all influence the family's ability to prevent crisis as a result of stressor events. Changes created by stressors may lead to a crisis, which is "X," or the amount of disruption of the family system caused by the stressful event. Families are more susceptible to crisis if they lack family resources and also if they tend to appraise or define stressors or hardships as crisis-producing.

According to the family stress model (Artinian, 1994), unexpected or unplanned events are usually perceived as stressful and they have the potential to be disruptive of families. However, stressful events within families, such as serious illness, are more disruptive than stressors that occur outside the family, such as floods, economic depression, or war. Further, ambiguous events, that is, events whose meaning for the family is unclear, are more stressful than events that can be easily interpreted. Finally, if a family has not had previous experience with stressor events, the family is more likely to see events as stressful.

Hill's ABCX model has been expanded by McCubbin and Patterson (1983) to include the notion of coping as a major predictor of family adaptation. The latest family stress theory, the resiliency model (McCubbin & McCubbin, 1993) builds on the former two models.

Working from the perspective of family stress, the nurse assesses the stressors, the family's definition of the stressor event, family resources, family coping, and the extent to which the stress has disrupted family functioning. Questions family nurses could ask include these: Did the family have time to prepare for the event, or was it unexpected? (For example, did a family member die suddenly or was the death expected after a long illness?) Has the family experienced similar stressor events? From this perspective, the nurse might intervene to help families enhance their resources and support systems or make more effective use of them.

Family stress theory is widely used in family nursing because it is logical and it fits what nurses see and do in clinical settings. This approach is especially useful in helping nurses recognize that the family's perception of stressors is often more important than objective reality. Thus it is important for family nurses to help families modify their perceptions of stressor events. Stress theory also emphasizes the importance of building on family resources and strengths to enhance coping with stressors.

Developmental Theory

Developmental theory lies at the core of nursing. Developmental stages have been elaborated by Erikson, Piaget, and others, and every nursing student learns these stages for individuals. According to developmental theory, human beings have specific tasks at specific periods of their lives, and successful achievement of the tasks of one stage of life leads to happiness and success with later tasks, while failure to achieve tasks leads to unhappiness, disapproval, and difficulty in achieving later tasks.

Evelyn Duvall (1977), in her classic work, *Marriage and Family Development,* now in its sixth edition (Duvall & Miller, 1985), applies the principles of individual development to the family as a unit. Duvall identifies overall family tasks that need to be accomplished for each stage of family development, beginning with a couple's marriage and ending with death. Development implies movement to a higher level of functioning or unidirectional progression. Disequilibrium occurs during the transitional periods from one stage to the other. The family has a predictable natural history; the first stage involves the simple husband-wife pair and the group becomes more complex over time with the addition of new positions or members. When the younger generation leaves home to take jobs or marry, the group becomes less complex again. Finally the group comes full circle to the original husband-wife pair. At each family life-cycle stage, there are family developmental needs and tasks that must be performed (Duvall & Miller, 1985). However, developmental tasks are general goals, rather than specific jobs that are completed at once. Achievement of family developmental tasks enables individuals in the family to achieve their own tasks.

According to this theoretical approach, every family is unique in its composition and in the complexity of its expectations of members at different ages and in different roles. Families, like individuals, are influenced by their history and traditions and by the social context they live in. Furthermore, families change and develop in different ways because their internal and external demands and stimulations differ. Families may also arrive at similar developmental levels through different processes. However, despite their differences, families have enough in common to make it possible to chart family development over the life span in a way that applies to all families.

Developmental theory, by including the movement of families over time, goes beyond the large-scale view of the family taken in the structural-functional approach and the small-scale analysis used in the interactional framework. It attempts to integrate small- and large-scale analyses while viewing the family as an open system in relation to other configurations and systems in society (Jones & Dimond, 1982, p. 13). Developmental theory explains what changes occur (and how they occur), more or less uniformly, to all human organisms or groups over time.

The developmental approach is extremely useful in practice. A major strength is that it provides a framework for predicting what a family will experience at any period in the family life cycle. It enables family nurses to assess a family's stage of development, the extent to which the family has achieved the tasks associated with that stage of family development, and problems that exist. The nurse can then more easily anticipate clinical problems and identify family strengths and available resources for achieving developmental milestones and handling problems. Thus this conceptualization provides a neat framework, both for assessing families and intervening when necessary. A major weakness of the developmental framework is that it originated when the traditional nuclear family was considered the norm. Today, families vary widely in their makeup and in their roles. The traditional view that a family moves in a linear fashion from marriage through children through the children's adulthood to old age and death is no longer applicable. Families may not involve a marriage, a couple may go through divorce or adopt children, or they may become families with two sets of stepchildren through multiple divorces. Also, families may be made up of single parents and their children or same-sex parents. There are many types of families and many trajectories of families that do not fit within the traditional developmental framework.

Nevertheless, with good common sense and tolerance for diversity, the framework remains useful. In conducting an assessment of families using the developmental model, there are several questions that can be asked: Where does this family lie on the continuum of family life-cycle stages? What are the developmental tasks that are and are not being accomplished? Depending on the assessment, nursing intervention strategies using this perspective might include helping families to understand individual and family growth and developmental stages and helping families recognize the transitions that must occur in moving from one developmental stage to the next (e.g., in moving from the tasks of the school-aged family to the tasks of adolescent family). Interventions might also include helping the family understand the normalcy of disequilibrium in these transitional periods.

Family nurses must also recognize that in every family, both individual and family developmental tasks must be accomplished for every stage of the individual and family life cycle. Therefore, it is important for the nurse to keep in mind the needs and requirements of both the family as a whole and the individuals making up the family.

Change Theory

According to Maturana (1978; Maturana & Varela, 1992), change in the family's structure occurs as compensation for perturbations and, paradoxically, has the purpose of maintaining stability. Watzlawick, Weakland, and Fisch (1974) consider that family changes are either first- or second-order changes. In first-order change, the system itself remains unchanged, although one or several of its parts undergo some type of change. For example, when parents learn a new behavioral strategy to discipline a child, the family remains the same, but with the new approach, the child, a part of the family, changes. Second-order change occurs in the system itself. In second-order change, there are actual changes in the rules governing the system, and therefore, the system is transformed structurally or in its communications. Second-order change may be said to occur when parents begin to treat their teenager as a growing adult instead of as a young child. Because the teenager is no longer viewed as a child, the whole family system is now different.

Families do not change smoothly or in a linear fashion; rather, changes occur in leaps, making a kind of transformation in which patterns appear that did not exist before. Bateson (1979) has said that we are unaware of most changes and become accustomed to a new way of being before our senses advise us. Wright and Watson (1988) have noted that "the most profound and sustaining change [within a family] will be that which occurs within the family's belief system (cognition)" (p. 425).

Wright and Leahey (2000) point out that change is dependent on the perception of the problem. Therefore, family nurses must recognize that there are as many truths or realities as there are members of a given family. The nurse must accept all these perceptions and offer the family another, more comprehensive view of their problems. Change is dependent on context. Efforts to promote change in family systems must take into account the family's context and the connections between the family and the larger community.

A family health care nurse working from the perspective of change theory must realize that helping families change depends on the family goals. These goals must be mutually developed between nurses and families with a realistic time frame for accomplishing them. Without family input, nurses are likely to set unrealistic goals for families. Often the primary goals in family nursing are to change or alter the family's view of the problem and assist the family to find new behavioral, cognitive, and affective responses to the problem. However, understanding alone does not lead to change. While understanding problems is often the first step, change occurs not simply through understanding, but through alterations in beliefs and behaviors. Thus, it is often fruitless to search for answers to "why" with families. Instead, it is more fruitful to focus on "what" is being done here and now to perpetuate the problem and "what" can be done to effect a change.

This approach provides the family with alternative avenues for action. It is the nurse's responsibility to facilitate change in families. However, the nurse cannot make families change; he or she can only create a context that makes change more possible. The nurse must understand, of course, that change does not occur equally in all family members. Some family members change more dramatically and quickly than others, in part because change is the result of many different factors and because it is often difficult to tell what exactly leads to change in one person or in a whole family.

In summary, these various social science theories provide somewhat overlapping conceptual approaches to family nursing. The structural-functional approach views the family as a social system and emphasizes the purposes or functions of the family, its internal organization and its relationship to the larger society. The systems approach also views the family as an open social system within the larger community (or suprasystem) but is more oriented toward family processes. The interactional approach deals primarily with the internal dynamics of the family. The developmental approach sees families as progressing through the life cycle and considers that all families have a predictable history associated with changing ages and member composition. Finally, change theory focuses on family transitions. All of these approaches are useful in that they provide nurses with a framework for understanding families; however, they tend to be abstract, and this limits their applicability to family nursing practice.

Family Therapy Theories

Although family therapy is a relatively new field, over the past 40 years theory development in family therapy has made great strides. Unlike family social science theories, family therapy models are practice-oriented. However, they have been developed to work with troubled families and, therefore, most focus primarily on family pathology (Box 2–2; Table 2–1). Nevertheless, these conceptual models describe family dynamics and patterns that are found to some extent in all families. Because these models are concerned with what can be done to facilitate change in "dysfunctional" families (Whall, 1983), they are both descriptive and prescriptive; that is, they not only describe and explain observations made in practice; they also suggest treatment or intervention strategies.

Family therapy models have all been influenced by theories in psychology and sociology. Just as there is no single approach to family nursing, there is no single approach to family therapy that can be put forth as the "right" or "wrong" approach; different models offer alternative explanations of family phenomena and suggest specific approaches to family assessment, diagnosis, and treatment.

We describe here three prominent family therapy models (Goldenberg & Goldenberg, 1996) based on social science theories: (1) structural family therapy, (2) family systems therapy, and (3) family interactional and communications therapy. Other frameworks and approaches to family therapy that contribute to family nursing theory include the psychodynamic approach (Ackerman, 1966), experiential or humanistic approach (Whitaker & Keith, 1981), strategic approach (Madanes, 1991), behavioral or cognitive approach (Falloon, 1991), the narrative approach (White & Epston, 1990), and solution-oriented therapy (Selekman, 1997). Unfortunately, we do not have space enough to describe these theories here.

The three conceptual models we will discuss all view the family as made up of interdependent subsystems and see the family as greater than the sum of its parts. The models stress the need to view the family as a whole and note that a change in one part affects all other parts of the whole.

Structural Family Therapy Theory

Structural family therapy was developed by Minuchin and his associates (Minuchin, 1974; Minuchin & Fishman, 1981; Minuchin, Rosman, & Baker, 1978). This systems-oriented approach uses spatial and organizational metaphors to describe problems and develop solutions (Goldenberg & Goldenberg, 1996). From this perspective, the family is viewed as an open sociocultural system that is continually faced with demands for change, both from within and from outside the family. Within the context of the family, individuals must learn to adapt to these demands and the resulting stresses. The family's underlying organizational structure (i.e., its enduring transactional patterns and flexibility in responding to demands for change) helps determine how well the family functions.

In structural family therapy, transactional patterns, or the ways in which family members generally interact, are viewed as laws that govern the conduct of family members. Transactional patterns help the family to be stable (or homeostatic). The family structure is a covert (i.e., unspoken) set of functional demands that organize family interactions. The availability of alternative transactional patterns, as well as the ability to mobilize these alternative transactional patterns to meet external and internal demands for change, determines the adaptability of the family. Dysfunctional transactional patterns lead to poor adaptation and in turn to family dysfunction.

The family system differentiates and carries out its affective and socialization functions through subsystems. These subsystems may be individual members of the family or relation or interpersonal subsystems, such as the marital subsystem or the parent/child and sibling subsystems in the two-parent nuclear family. Family subsystems are differentiated by boundaries. The clarity of these boundaries is an indicator of how well the family functions. The two pathological extremes in boundaries are the disengaged family and the enmeshed family. In the disengaged family, boundaries are so rigid that there is little cohesiveness between family members; in the enmeshed family, the boundaries are so diffuse or porous that subsystems do not function autonomously or independently. As Minuchin (1974) explained, in the enmeshed family, when one person sneezes, everyone runs for the Kleenex.

The goal of structural family therapy is to facilitate restructuring of the family. This approach is present-centered, action-oriented, and problem-focused. Clarifying boundaries and power hierarchies (i.e., who is in charge) helps the family to understand their structure and then to restructure to make the family more functional.

The family nurse who is working from this perspective assesses families by asking questions, observing family transactions, and asking family members to interact with each other about a particular situation. It is important to evaluate the whole family system, its subsystems, boundaries, and coalitions as well as family transactional patterns and covert rules. It is also important to show respect for the current family structure. Nurses who intervene to help the family restructure should encourage and reinforce family successes through praise and support (Minuchin & Fishman, 1981).

This approach is a clear, well-integrated, and well-tested approach. However, the approach calls for a very directive, active, and even confrontational role on the part of the family therapist or family nurse. Some practitioners or families may feel uncomfortable with this approach.

Family Systems Therapy Theory

Family systems therapy was first developed by Murray Bowen (1978); Bowen was a pioneer in the field of family therapy and is still recognized as the leading theorist in the field. Since his death in 1990, his work has been continued by David Freeman (1992).

Murray Bowen's particular version of family systems theory begins with the assumption that anxiety is an inevitable, omnipresent part of life (Gladding, 1995; Goldenberg & Goldenberg, 1996). Chronic anxiety is the basic cause of dysfunction in individuals and in families. The only antidote for chronic anxiety is "resolution through differentiation" (Goldenberg & Goldenberg, 1996, p. 169). Box 2–3 lists the eight interlocking concepts of Bowen's family systems theory.

In Bowen's view, the key to healthy function is differentiation of self, or the ability of persons to distinguish themselves from their family of origin, emotionally and intellectually. According to Bowen, there are two counterbalancing life forces, togetherness and individuality, which exist at two ends of a continuum. On one end of this continuum is autonomy, which is an ability to see oneself separately from others, think through a situation without confusing self with others, and separate feelings from rational thought. At the other end of the continuum is undifferentiated ego-mass, which implies emotional dependence on the family of origin, even if one is living away from the family. People can be ranked on a scale of differentiation of self. The more differentiated the individual, the more that individual is able to use logical reasoning and adapt to stress and change in the surroundings. Thus, a well-differentiated person is less apt to experience emotional difficulties.

In Bowen's family systems theory, the nuclear family is viewed as a *family emotional system*. In this system, the coping strategies and patterns that are used tend to be passed on from generation to generation, a phenomenon that Bowen calls the *multigenerational transmission process*. Thus, families who are dysfunctional have usually carried the problematic behaviors over several generations. Further, families tend to perpetuate their level of differentiation. That is, people tend to marry partners at their own level of differentiation and couples tend to produce offspring at the same level of differentiation as themselves. Further, parents who are anxious and have poor differentiation of self tend to transfer their anxiety and low level of differentiation to a susceptible child. This phenomenon is called *the family projection process*.

According to Bowen, *triangles* are a way that families use to deal with anxiety. In a triangle, which Bowen says is a basic building block of any emotional system, the tension between two persons is projected onto another object or person in the family. In particularly stressful situations, anxiety may spread from a triangle within the family to triangles that include persons outside the family.

Box 2–3 BOWEN'S FAMILY SYSTEMS THEORY: EIGHT INTERLOCKING CONCEPTS

Differentiation of Self
Nuclear Family Emotional System
Multigenerational Transmission Process
Family Projection Process
Triangles
Sibling Position
Emotional Cutoff
Societal Regression

Sibling position is another important concept in family systems therapy. From this perspective, people are seen as developing fixed personality characteristics based on their birth order in their family of origin (Toman, 1961). The more closely a marriage replicates the couple's sibling positions in the family of origin, the better chance that couple has of having a successful marriage.

Emotional cutoff occurs when children have unresolved attachments to parents. Children who are emotionally fused to their parents and family of origin may live near or far from them. They may try to withdraw from parents and stay emotionally distanced from the family, but they are fused regardless of their physical proximity.

Societal regression occurs on a community level but is like failure to differentiate the self on an individual level. It occurs when so many toxic forces counter the tendency to achieve differentiation that the society regresses under the stress.

Bowen's family systems therapy focuses on promoting differentiation of self from family and promoting differentiation of intellect from emotion (Becvar & Becvar, 1996). Family members are encouraged to examine the processes described above so as to gain insight and understanding into their past and present. They are thus freed to choose how they will behave in the future. Using Bowen's approach, a family nurse or therapist would have individuals or couples look at their family tree. The nurse would serve as coach and teacher, asking questions about people's history while helping the clients to construct a family tree, called a multigenerational genogram. In this approach, families are encouraged to ask questions of their own family members to gain an understanding of the past and the ways they currently interact. The goal is to help family members stop triangulating, develop relationships with individual family members, and end emotional withdrawal.

Because this approach to the family is objective and neutral, it takes the blame out of what people bring to a family therapist. However, this type of therapy emphasizes understanding the past to deal with problems in the present, and therefore it requires a long commitment. Many people are not inclined to stay with such therapy to completion, and today many health plans are not inclined to pay for it.

Interactional Family Therapy

The interactional or communication therapy approach was originally developed at the Mental Research Institute (MRI) in Palo Alto, California, by Don Jackson, John Weakland, Paul Watzlawick, and Virginia Satir (Becvar & Becvar, 1996; Goldenberg & Goldenberg, 1996). This approach sees the family as a system of interactive or interlocking behaviors or communication processing. Emphasis is on the here-and-now rather than the past. The key question is "what is being processed," not "why." This approach is based on the fundamental rules of communication developed by Watzlawick, Beavin, and Jackson in their book, *Pragmatics of Human Communication* (1967). The first rule is that human beings cannot *not* behave; and therefore, they cannot *not* communicate. All behavior is communication at some level. However, to be fully understood, all behavior (communication) must be examined in its context. Further, all systems, such as the family system, are characterized by rules that maintain homeostatic balance and preserve the system.

This approach to the family is based on the dynamics of interchanges between individuals, and that is why it is called "interactional" analysis. The approach assumes that emotional problems result from the way people interact with each other in the context of the family. In the normal or functional family, rules are clear and communication is clear; this kind of family can maintain its basic integrity even during stressful periods and accommodate change when it is needed. A breakdown in family functioning occurs when dysfunctional communication is predominant and the rules of communication are ambiguous. Dysfunctional families are said to be "stuck."

> Individual symptoms reflect family system dysfunction and these symptoms persist only if they are maintained by that family system (Goldenberg & Goldenberg, 1996, p. 211).

The individual symptoms maintain the family's current equilibrium, and the family avoids change even when it is needed.

Satir (1982), a well-known interactional family therapist, says that the natural movement of all individuals is toward positive growth and development and that a symptom indicates an impasse in the growth process. Satir assumes that all individuals possess the resources necessary for growth and development. Each person, she says, is in charge of his or her own growth. Therapy provides a supportive context for such development and the role of the therapist is to facilitate the process. Primary goals of family therapy are to understand the communication rules and processes that the troubled family uses and to teach the family to use more functional communication rules and processes.

Key interventions focus on establishing clear, congruent communication and clarifying and changing family rules (Jackson, 1965; Satir, 1982). This approach is very useful for family nurses because it stresses the interactions among family members. The weakness of the interactional approach is that it looks only at internal family behavior and not how the family is affected by the larger environment.

Nursing Models and Theories

Nursing theories and models have evolved from practice questions, theories borrowed from other disciplines, and an examination of the philosophical perspectives of nursing. In turn, family nursing draws knowledge from family social science theories, family therapy conceptual models, and nursing theories and models. However, principles and concepts from the borrowed theories are not arbitrarily incorporated into family nursing approaches to practice. These theories are interpreted from a family nursing perspective in nursing situations (Chinn, 1995).

The discipline of nursing is concerned with the concepts of person, environment, health, and nursing. The following three propositions are central to nursing theory:

1. Nursing is concerned with the principles and laws that govern the life process, well-being, and optimum function of human beings, sick or well.
2. Nursing is concerned with the patterning of human behavior in interaction with the environment in normal life events and critical life situations.
3. Nursing is concerned with the processes by which positive changes in health status are effected (Whall & Fawcett, 1991, p. 3).

Originally, nursing theorists looked only at individuals, but the notion of client has now been expanded to include individuals, families, and communities (ANA, 1995). It is not appropriate, however, to simply substitute the word "family" for the word "individual" in nursing theories. As Gilliss (1991) has pointed out, to do so is to ignore the complexity of family systems. Whall and Fawcett (1991) restated the three central propositions in nursing theory from the perspective of family nursing.

1. Family is concerned with the principles and laws that govern family process, family well-being, and optimal function of families in various states of illness and wellness.
2. Family is concerned with the patterning of family behavior in interaction with the environment in normal life events and critical life situations.
3. Family is concerned with the processes by which positive changes in family health status may be effected (Donaldson & Crowley, 1978; Gordner, 1980, cited by Whall & Fawcett, 1991, pp. 3 & 4).

According to Whall and Fawcett (1991), the family nurse must consider environmental influences on family health and the effect of actions taken by nurses on behalf of or in conjunction with the family. In addition, the practitioner must work from a comprehensive biopsychosocial or holistic perspective on health and focus on family well-being, rather than on family pathology (Whall & Fawcett, 1991, p. 4).

Whall and Fawcett (1991) note that there is little evidence of formal family theory in nursing. Yet the importance of the family was noted even by Florence Nightingale, the first major nurse theorist. Nightingale saw the family as potentially both positive and negative (Nightingale, 1859). In 1852, for example, she wrote:

> The family? It is too narrow a field for the development of an immortal spirit, be that spirit male or female. The family uses people not for what they are, not for what they are intended to be, but for what it wants them for—for its own uses. This system dooms some minds to incurable infancy, others to silent misery (Nightingale, 1859, p. 37).

At the same time, Nightingale saw the family as a supportive institution for individual family members, throughout the life span. She firmly believed in home health nursing and maintaining ill persons in the home environment.

The family as client is now fully accepted in nursing (Whall & Fawcett, 1991). The family is addressed in the ANA Social Policy Statement (1995) and in specific ANA standards of clinical nursing practice. Family nursing is clearly a component of the nursing discipline, even though "there remains virtually no evidence of formal middle-range family theory that is unique or distinctive to nursing" (Whall & Fawcett, 1991, p. 15).

In her book, *Nursing Theories: The Base for Professional Nursing Practice,* George (1995) summarizes nursing models and theories. Here we will briefly review those models and theories that are most applicable to family nursing practice. They include the work of King, Roy, Neuman, Orem, Rogers, and Friedemann. Other nursing theories that may be considered in the practice of family nursing include the cultural care theory of Madeline Leininger, the philosophy and science of caring developed by Jean Watson, the theory of psychodynamic nursing by Hildegard Peplau, the parent-child interaction model of Kathryn Barnard, and the model of health by Margaret Newman (Marriner-Tomey, 1998; Meleis, 1997).

King

Imogene King (1981, 1987) derived her conceptual framework of nursing, named the *theory of goal attainment,* from systems theory. In her early work, King viewed the family as simply the context for individual development. She defined the family as a small group of individuals bound together for the socialization of the members. The family was the vehicle for transmitting values and norms of behavior across the life span (King, 1983; Whall, 1986; Frey & Sieloff, 1995).

Later, King came to view the family as both an interpersonal and a social system, and her framework focused on the integration of the personal system, interpersonal systems, and social systems (George, 1995). King's framework includes the concepts of interaction, communication, transaction, role, self, growth and development, time, perception, and personal space; thus her framework is not only a systems theory but can also be viewed as an interactional theory. King especially emphasized the importance of the interaction between nurses and clients.

Roy

In 1976, Sister Callista Roy developed her *adaptation model* (Roy, 1976; Roy & Roberts, 1981), in which the individual is viewed as an adaptive system that responds to environmental stimuli in four response modes: physiological, self-concept, role function, and interdependence. Roy's model was derived primarily from von Bertalanffy's (1968) general systems theory and adaptation theory (George, 1995).

As did other nursing theorists of her time, Roy originally saw the family as the context for individual development and adaptation. Then, in 1981, Roy and Roberts expanded this view and described the "family as an adaptive system that, like the individual, has inputs, internal control and feedback processes and output" (Whall & Fawcett, 1991, p. 23).

Roy's *theory of adaptation* holds promise for describing and explaining the phenomena observed in family nursing. Moreover, Roy's theory stresses health promotion and the importance of assisting clients in coping with their environment, which are important elements of family nursing. Thus McCubbin and Figley (1983) have suggested broadening the adaptation model to include ineffective family coping patterns that lead to problems in family functioning.

Neuman

The *Neuman systems model,* developed by Betty Neuman (1982), is based on several family social science theories, including the systems and stress theories of de Chardin (1955), Cornu (1957), Edelson (1970), Emery (1969), Laszlo (1972), Lazarus (1981), Selye (1950), von Bertalanffy (1968), and Caplan (1964, as cited in George, 1995, p. 282).

Neuman defines the family as "a group of two or more persons who create and maintain a common culture; its most central goal is one of continuance" (Neuman, 1983, p. 241). She views the family as a system composed of family member subsystems; the relationships among individual family members or subsystems are the central focus of her model. In Neuman's model, the family system is threatened when it is exposed to stressors that affect its stability and its state of wellness. The family's primary goal is to maintain its stability by preserving the integrity of its structure (Whall & Fawcett, 1991).

Orem

Dorothea Orem's *self-care deficit theory* (1971, 1983a, 1983b) views the family as the basic conditioning unit, in which the individual learns culture, roles, and responsibilities. Orem's specific focus is on the role of family members in helping the individual family member achieve self-care. Thus she sees the family primarily as supportive of the individual, not as a client or recipient of care. Nevertheless, Orem (1985) has suggested that people receive health care not only as individuals but also as members of a multiperson unit, the family.

The *self-care deficit theory* by Orem has been expanded by Gray (1996) to include families. Gray points to several ways in which the theory is applicable to family nursing:

- Self-care of families can be evaluated in a variety of situations. For example, the self-care potential of families can be assessed as it relates to health promotion and health protection. Each individual family member is a self-care agent who makes continual contributions to his or her own health.
- Self-care reflects the personal values and health beliefs of the family. The family's self-care behavior evolves through a combination of social and cognitive experiences that have been learned through interpersonal relationships, communication, and culture, which are unique to each family.
- Self-care can be administered to families by individual self-care agents. Thus family members, either individually or collectively, can initiate and perform self-care, based on their views of health and their ability to perform self-care behaviors.
- The concept of self-care can be used to promote health in families and to recognize and evaluate areas where diminished health may exist (p. 88).

Rogers

Martha Rogers' (1970, 1986, 1990) *theory of unitary human beings* is an abstract theory based on general systems theory and drawing on many fields of study, including anthropology, sociology, astronomy, religion, philosophy, history, and mythology (George, 1995).

Rogers views the human being as a unitary multidimensional energy field that is engaged in a continuous mutual process with the environment. Rogers primarily addressed the individual in her writings, but Fawcett (1991) has expanded her theory, explaining that the family is a constant open system energy field that is ever-changing in its interactions with the environment. Casey (1996) explains the application of Rogers' theory to family nursing as follows:

- The family unit is a whole; it is composed of subsystems that are interdependent and that together form a unity that is different than the sum of the family subsystems.
- The family is an open system in constant interaction with the environment through exchange of matter and energy.
- Families are continuously influenced by information in the environment and, depending on the degree of permeability of their boundaries, they are constantly responding to this input.
- The family system is subject to change along a space-time axis. The family moves through stages of development in a sequential, unidirectional manner.
- The family has the capacity for feeling, knowing, and comprehending and for using these processes to determine patterns, make choices, and recognize its environment (pp. 56–57).

Friedemann

Marie-Louise Friedemann's (1995) *framework of systemic organization* is built on the view of the family-as-client. She sees the family as a social system that has the expressed goal of transmitting culture to its members. Consistent with general systems theory, her framework is based on the following assumptions:

- The family, which is embedded in the civil or social system, transmits culture (i.e., the total of human patterns and values).
- The family and the civil system and environment at large share responsibility for providing physical necessities and safety, teaching social skills to its members, fostering personal growth and development, allowing emotional bonding of family members, and promoting a purpose for life and meaning through spirituality.
- The family satisfies its members' needs for control over their environment and helps them find their place in the network of systems through spirituality.
- All family processes include collectively accepted and coordinated behaviors or strategies that aim at regulating space, time, energy, and matter in pursuing family stability, growth, control, and spirituality.
- Family processes fall into four dimensions: system maintenance, system change, coherence, and individualization. These dimensions are interdependent but also exist independently in that no single dimension is emphasized at the expense of another in healthy families (pp. 16–17).

The elements that are central to Freidemann's theory are family stability, family growth, family control, and family spirituality. The family offers safety to its members as they learn group values, norms, and acceptable behaviors. As its members grow, the family grows and interacts with other systems, such as schools, church, and work. Family growth is facilitated by communication among its members. By selectively opening or closing its boundaries, the family can serve as a buffer between its members and the demands of society. Family control is maintained through the structure of the family. Family spirituality connects family members emotionally and encourages self-growth of the individual members (Friedemann, 1995).

Integrated Approaches to the Nursing of Families

Families are complex small groups in which multiple processes and dynamics occur simultaneously. Families do not function in one way alone. No single theory or conceptual framework from family social science, family therapy, or nursing fully describes the dynamics of family life. Thus nurses who use only one theoretical approach to working with families are, in essence, limiting the possibilities for families.

Integrating theories allows nurses to view the family from a variety of perspectives, which increases the probability that the interventions selected will be implemented by the family, because they "fit" the structure, processes, and style of functioning for that family. By integrating several theories, nurses acquire different ways in which to conceptualize problems, and this enhances their thinking about interventions. Instead of fragmented knowledge and piecemeal interventions, nursing practice is based on an organized, realistic conceptualization of families. Nurses who use an integrated theoretical approach build on the strengths of families in creative ways.

The Family Assessment Intervention Model and Family Systems Stressor Strength Inventory (FS^{3}I)

Several nursing scholars have taken integrated approaches to working with families. They include Berkey and Hanson (1991) and Hanson and Mischke (1996), who merged general systems theory and the Neuman systems model (Neuman, 1982; Neuman, 1983) to develop the family assessment intervention model and family systems stressor strength inventory (FS^{3}I). Both of these are excellent for investigating and identifying family stressors and creating family interventions from a microscopic view of family. Similarly, Friedman (1998) combined general systems theory, developmental theory, and structural-functional theory into an assessment tool that provides a macroscopic view of families.

Calgary Family Model

Another integrated approach to working with families was developed by Wright and Leahey (2000) and Wright, Watson, and Bell (1997). This approach, which is called the Calgary family model, integrates general systems theory, communication theory, change theory, and cybernetics in a unique approach to working with families. The model draws on sociological theories and other theories, such as Maturana and Varela's (1992) theory of the biology of knowing, Bateson's (1979) theory of the mind, and constructivist and narrative approaches (Wright, Watson, and Bell, 1997). All three of these integrated family assessment models are described in detail in Chapter 8.

Resiliency Model of Family Stress, Adjustment, and Adaptation

Other integrated approaches to family nursing include McCubbin and McCubbin's (1993) *resiliency model of family stress, adjustment, and adaptation* for working with families who are experiencing stress (Chapter 6). McCubbin and McCubbin were interested in why families react in dramatically different ways when they are faced with similar stressors. Their model is based on Ruben Hill's work on stress and adaptation (1949, 1965) and on the double ABCX model developed by McCubbin and Patterson (1983). (A detailed description of this model can be found in Danielson, Hamel-Bissell, and Winstead-Fry [1993], and in Vaughn-Cole, Johnson, Malone, and Walker [1998].

The resiliency model provides a way for nurses to facilitate family adjustment and adaptation by looking at family strengths and capacities for responding to stress. Based on the family's response to health stressors, the nurse and family, working together, create interventions that are more likely to result in positive family adjustment.

The resiliency model incorporates the general systems view that what happens to one part of the family affects the family as a whole. Thus the resiliency model has many similarities to Neuman's systems model of nursing. It is also similar to Rogers's energy field theory of unitary human beings in that nurses work with families to repattern disrupted patterns of functioning by building on the natural processes of resiliency and regenerativity.

Combined Models

Vaughn-Cole, Johnson, Malone, and Walker (1998) have taken an integrated approach to families, using the resiliency model, an ecological model, and a family systems model. Although each model conceptualizes family differently, there are common themes. They suggest that family nursing should use a multidimensional definition of family, regardless of family type. They have also found that nurses use a variety of tools and methods to assess the family and individual family members, and many of their interventions are the same, regardless of the conceptual framework used. Similarly, Kaakinen (1998) has found that regardless of the theoretical approach used to assess problems and develop interventions, family is constant and central to the health care issues of the family members. Health care is not autonomous but is always influenced and carried out by the family. Further, families are extremely knowledgeable about the needs of family members and about the effect that the illness of one member has on the whole.

Clearly, family nursing requires the use of integrated approaches to guide practice, research, and education. One theoretical perspective does not give nurses a sufficiently broad base of knowledge on which to assess and intervene with families. Nurses must draw on multiple theories to be effective in tailoring interventions for specific families with unique needs. The number of possibilities for interventions is increased when nurses use multiple ways of conceptualizing families. We must continue developing integrated approaches that are sensitive to family needs and tested over time.

SUMMARY

Family nursing today draws on three types of theory: family social science theories, family therapy theories, and nursing models and theories. Of the three, the family social science theories are the most well developed and informative with respect to the functioning of families, the environment and family interchange, interactions within the family, family changes over time, and the family's reaction to health and illness. However, there are major problems in using the family social science theories as a basis for assessment and intervention in family nursing, because they remain abstract and clinical applications have not been delineated. Fortunately, recent work has made some strides in this direction (Berkey & Hanson, 1991; Wright & Leahey, 2000; Hanson & Boyd, 1996).

Family therapy theories provide reasonably well developed conceptualizations of the family. Since they come from a professional practice background rather than the academic disciplines, they are more easily applied in family nursing practice. Indeed, as the specialty of family nursing becomes more sophisticated, family nurses are increasingly drawing on family therapy ideas. Not all family therapy theories are applicable to nursing, however. Nursing focuses on the entire health-illness continuum and on health promotion, and because family therapy is intended for families with problems, the conceptualizations are not always applicable to healthy families or families with health problems that are physiological. Also, family therapy theories are more applicable to advanced nursing practice and, thus, may be beyond the level of expertise of baccalaureate-qualified practicing nurses. Whall (1986) has urged family nurse therapists to reformulate existing family therapy frameworks to better fit a nursing perspective.

Finally, of all three types of theories, nursing models and theories are the least well developed. Nearly all of the nursing models originally focused on the individual rather than the family, and only a few have evolved to fit a family nursing focus (Berkey & Hanson, 1991). The importance of the nursing models for family nursing lies in the rich understanding they provide of human responses and the relationships between individuals, health, the environment, and nursing. Nursing theories, however, need to be expanded to include the client as family to make them fully relevant to family nursing practice.

The nursing profession has recently come to recognize that family nursing has roots in all three genres of theory: family social science, family therapy, and nursing (Hanson, Kaakinen, & Friedman, 1998). The next generation of family nurses need to further explore how these three traditions can be used together to formulate concepts and propositions for nursing of families. The efforts of some family nursing scholars to develop integrated models for the nursing care of families have been briefly noted in this chapter and are described in more detail in Chapter 8. The art and science of "family nursing" evolved from a rich background and draws on a multitude of disciplines. Just what this broad theoretical or conceptual background means for theory, practice, research, and education in family nursing is an emerging question.

Study Questions

1. Which of the following statements about theories are accurate?
   a. Theories are subject to rules of organization.
   b. Theories are statements about how some part of the world works.
   c.. Theories represent logical and intelligible patterns that make sense of observations.
   d. All of the above.
2. The conceptual and theoretical frameworks that provide the foundation for family nursing have evolved from the following three major traditions and disciplines: ________________________, ______________, and __________________.
3. Discuss why it is important for nurses to integrate conceptual and theoretical frameworks when working with families.
4. Select a research article that investigates a question or describes family function. Review it to determine the conceptual framework or theoretical approach(s) used to support the study and the findings. Was the article approached from any of the three disciplines and traditions discussed in the chapter? Did the researchers use an integrated approach to make sense out of the concept studied? How did the theoretical concepts they studied contribute or limit the findings about families? How will this knowledge assist nurses in caring for families?

References

Ackerman, N. (1966). *The Psychodynamics of Family Life.* New York: Basic Books.

American Nurses Association. (1995). *Nursing: A Social Policy Statement.* Kansas City: MO.

Artinian, N.T. (1994). Selecting Model to Guide Family Assessment. *Dimensions of Critical Care Nursing, 14*(1):4–16.

Bateson, G. (1979). *Mind and Nature.* NY: E.P. Dutton.

Becvar, D.S. & Becvar, R.J. (1996). *Family Therapy: A Systemic Integration.* Boston: Allyn and Bacon.

Berkey, K.M. & Hanson, S.M.H. (1991). *Pocket Guide to Family Assessment and Intervention.* St. Louis: C.V. Mosby.

Boss, P.G., Doherty, W.J., Schumm, W.R., & Steinmetz, S.K. (Eds.) (1993). *Sourcebook of Family Theories and Methods: A Contextual Approach.* NY: Plenum Publishing Corporation.

Bowen, M. (1978). *Family Therapy in Clinical Practice.* NY: Jason Aronson.

Broderick, C.B. (1971). Behind the Five Conceptual Frameworks: A Decade of Development in Family Theory. *Journal of Marriage and the Family, 33:*129–159.

Casey, B. (1996). The Family as a System. In C. Bomar (Ed.), *Nurses and Family Health Promotion: Concepts, Assessment, and Interventions,* ed 2. Philadelphia: Saunders.

Chapan, G. (1964). *Principles of Preventive Psychiatry.* New York: Basic Books. Out of print.

Chinn, P.L. (1995). *Theory and Nursing: A Systematic Approach,* ed 4. St. Louis: CV Mosby.

Cornu, A. (1957). *The Origin of Marxist Thought.* Springfield, IL: Thomas. Out of print.

Danielson, C. B., Hamel-Bissell, B., Winstead-Fry, P. (1993). *Families, Health and Illness: Perspectives on Coping and Intervention.* St. Louis: CV Mosby.

De Chardin, P.R. (1955). *The Phenomenon of Man.* London: Collins. Out of print.

Donaldson, S.K. & Crowley, D.M. (1978). The Discipline of Nursing. *Nursing Outlook, 26:*103–120.

Duvall, E.M. (1977). *Marriage and Family Development,* ed 5. Philadelphia: Lippincott.

Duvall, E.M. & Miller, B. (1985). *Marriage and Family Development,* ed 6. NY: Harper & Row.

Edelson, M. (1970). *Sociotherapy and Psychotherapy.* Chicago: University of Chicago. Out of print.

Emery. F. (1969). *Systems Thinking.* Baltimore: Penguin Books. Out of print.

Falloon, I.R.H. (1991). Behavior Family Therapy. In A.S. Gurman and P.P. Kniskern (Eds.) *Handbook of Family Therapy.* New York: Brunner/Mazel.

Fawcett, J. (1991). Spouses' Experiences During Pregnancy and the Postpartum: A Program of Research and Theory Development. In A. Whall & J. Fawcett (Eds.), *Family Theory Development In Nursing: State Of The Science And Art.* Philadelphia: F.A. Davis.

Fawcett, J. (1995). *Analysis and Evaluation of Conceptual Models of Nursing,* ed 3. Philadelphia: F.A. Davis.

Fawcett, J. and Downs, F.S. (1992). *The Relationship of Theory and Research.* Philadelphia: F.A. Davis.

Freeman, D.S. (1992). *Multigenerational Family Therapy.* NY: The Haworth Press.

Frey, M. & Sieloff, C. (Eds.). (1995). *Advancing King's Systems Framework and Theory of Nursing.* London: Sage.

Friedman, M.M. (1998). *Family Nursing: Research, Theory and Practice,* ed 4. Norwalk, Conn: Appleton & Lange.

Friedemann, M-L. (1995). *The Framework of Systemic Organization: A Conceptual Approach to Families and Nursing.* Thousand Oaks: Sage Publications.

George, J.B. (1995). *Nursing Theories: The Base for Professional Nursing Practice,* ed 4. Norwalk, CT: Appleton & Lange.

Gillis, C. (1991). *Family Nursing Research.* Image, 23(1): 19–22.

Gladding, S.T. (1995). *Family Therapy: History, Theory, and Practice.* Englewood Cliffs, NJ: Prentice Hall.

Goldenberg, I. & Goldenberg, H. (1996), *Family Therapy: An Overview.* Pacific Grove, CA: Brooks/Cole.

Gordner, S. (1980). Nursing Science in Transition. *Nursing Research, 29*:80–83.

Gray, V. (1996). Family Self-Care. In C. Bomar (Ed.), *Nurses and Family Health Promotion: Concepts, Assessment, and Interventions,* ed 2. Philadelphia: Saunders.

Hanson, S.M.H. & Boyd, S.T. (1996. *Family Health Care Nursing: Theory, Practice and Research.* Philadelphia, PA: F.A. Davis.

Hanson, S.M.H. & Kaakinen, J. (2000). Nursing of Families in the Community. In M. Stanhope and J. Lancaster (Eds.), *Community Health Nursing: Promoting Health of Aggregates, Family and Individuals* ed 5. St. Louis: C.V. Mosby.

Hanson, S.M.H., Kaakinen, J., & Friedman, M. M. (1998). Theoretical Approaches to Family Nursing. In M. M. Friedman, *Family Nursing: Research, Theory and Practice,* ed 4, pp. 75–98. Norwalk: Appleton & Lange.

Hanson, S.M.H & Miscke, K. (1996). Family Health Assessment and Intervention. In P. Bomar (Ed.) *Nurses and Family Health Promotion,* ed 2, pp. 165–202. Philadelphia: Saunders.

Hill, R. (1949). *Families Under Stress.* NY: Harper and Brothers.

Hill, R. (1965). *Challenges and Resources for Family Development: Family Mobility in Our Dynamic Society.* Ames, IA: Iowa State University.

Hill, R., & Hansen, D. (1960). The Identification of Conceptual Frameworks Utilized in Family Study. *Marriage and Family Living, 22(4)*:299–311.

Jackson, D. D. (1965). Family Rules: Marital Quid Quo. Archives of *General Psychiatry,* 12:589–594.

Jones, S.L. & Dimond, S.L. (1982). Family Theory and Family Therapy Models: Comparative Review with Implications for Nursing Practice. *Journal of Psychiatric Nursing and Mental Health Services,* 20(10):12–19.

Kaakinen, J. (1998). *Theories Across Family Nursing Approaches: Family Systems, Resiliency Stress Model, And Ecological Approach.* Unpublished manuscript.

King, I. (1981). *Family Therapy: A Comparison of Approaches.* Bowie, MD: Brady.

King, I. (1983). King's Theory of Nursing. In I.W. Clements & J.B. Roberts. (Eds.). *Family Health: A Theoretical Approach to Nursing* (pp. 177–187). New York: John Wiley & Sons.

King, I. (1987, May). *King's Theory.* Paper presented at Nursing Theories Conference, Pittsburgh, PA. (Cassette recording.)

Klein, D.M. & White, J.M. (1996). *Family Theories: An Introduction.* Thousand Oaks, CA: Sage Publications.

Laszlo, E. (1972). *The Systems View of the World: The Natural Philosophy of the New Development in the Science.* New York: Braziller. Out of print.

Lazarus, R.S. (1981). The Stress and Coping Paradigm. In C. Eisdorfer, D. Cohen, A. Kleinman, & P. Maxim (Eds.), *Models for Clinical Psychopathology,* pp. 177–214. New York: SP Medical and Scientific Books.

Leddy, S. & J.M. Pepper. (1993). *Conceptual Bases of Professional Nursing,* ed 3. Philadelphia: Lippincott.

LoBiondo-Wood, G. & Haber, J. (1998). *Nursing Research: Methods, Critical Appraisal, and Utilization,* ed 4. St. Louis: CV Mosby.

Marriner-Tomey, A. (Ed.) (1998). *Nursing Theorists and Their Work,* ed 4 St. Louis: C.V. Mosby.

Maturana, H. (1978). Biology of Language: The Epistemology of Reality. In G. Millar and E. Lenneberg, (Eds). *Psychology and Biology of Language and Thought,* pp 27–63. NY: Academic Press.

Maturana, H.R. & Varela, F.J. (1992). *The Tree of Knowledge: The Biological Roots of Human Understanding.* Boston: Shambhala (Random House).

McCubbin, H. & Figley, D. (Eds.) (1983). *Stress and the Family: vol 1. Coping with Normative Transitions.* New York: John Wiley and Sons.

McCubbin, H.I. & Patterson, M. (1983). The Family Stress Process: The Double ABCX Model of Adjustment And Adaptation. In H.I. McCubbin, M.B. Sussman, and J.M. Patterson (Eds.) *Social Stress and the Family.* (Special issue.) *Marriage and Family Review, 6*:7–27.

McCubbin, M.A. & McCubbin, H.I. (1993). Family Coping with Illness: The Resiliency Model of Family Stress, Adjustment, and Adaptation. In C. Danielson, B. Hamel-Bissell, & P. Winstead-Fry. (Eds.), *Families, Health and Illness.* St. Louis, MO: C.V. Mosby.

Meleis, A.I. (1997). *Theoretical Nursing: Development and Progress,* ed 3. Philadelphia: Lippincott.

Mercer, R. (1989). Theoretical Perspectives on the Family. In C.L. Gillis, B.L. Highley, B.M. Roberts, & I.M. Martinson. *Toward a Science of Family Nursing,* pp 9–36. Menlo Park, CA: Addison-Wesley.

Minuchin, S. (1974). *Families and Family Therapy.* Cambridge, MA: Harvard University Press.

Minuchin, S. & Fishman, H.G. (1981). *Family Therapy Techniques.* Cambridge, MA: Harvard University Press.

Minuchin, S., Rosman, B.L., & Baker, L. (1978). *Psychosomatic Families. Anorexia Nervosa in Context.* Cambridge, MA: Harvard University Press.

Neuman, B. (1982). *The Neuman Systems Model: Application to Nursing Education and Practice.* Norwalk, CT: Appleton-Century-Crofts.

Neuman, B. (1983). Family Intervention Using the Betty Neuman Health Care Systems Model. In I.W. Clements & F.B. Roberts (Eds.). *Family Health: A Theoretical Approach to Nursing Care.* New York: John Wiley.

Nightingale, F. (1859). *Notes on Nursing: What It Is, and What*

It Is Not. London: Harrison. Reprinted 1980. Edinburgh, N.Y.: Churchill Livingtone.

Nightingale, F. (1979). Cassandra. Westbury, NY: *The Feminist Press.*

Nye, F.I. (1976). *Role Structure and Analysis of the Family,* vol 24. Beverly Hills, CA: Sage.

Nye, F.I. & Berardo, F. (Eds.) (1981). *Emerging Conceptual Frameworks in Family Analysis.* NY: Praeger.

Orem, D. (1971). *Nursing: Concepts of Practice.* NY: McGraw-Hill.

Orem, D. (1983a). The Family Coping with a Medical Illness: Analysis and Application of Orem's Theory. In I. Clements & F. Roberts (Eds.), *Family Health: A Theoretical Approach to Nursing Care.* NY: Wiley.

Orem, D. (1983b). The Family Experiencing Emotional Crisis: Analysis and Application of Orem's Self-Care Deficit Theory. In I. Clements & F. Roberts (Eds.), *Family Health: A Theoretical Approach to Nursing Care.* NY: Wiley.

Orem, D. (1985). *Nursing: Concepts of Practice,* ed 3. NY: McGraw-Hill.

Polit-O'Hara, D., & Hungler, B.P. (1997). *Essentials of Nursing Research.* Philadelphia: Lippincott-Raven.

Powers, B. & Knapp, T. (1990). *A Dictionary of Nursing Theory and Research.* Newbury Park, CA: Sage.

Rogers, M. (1970). *Introduction to the Theoretical Basis of Nursing.* Philadelphia: F.A. Davis.

Rogers, M. (1986). Science of Unitary Human Beings. In V. Malinski (Ed.). *Explorations on Martha Rogers' Science of Unitary Human Beings,* pp. 3–8. Norwalk, CT: Appleton-Century-Crofts.

Rogers, M. (1990). Nursing: Science of Unitary, Irreducible, Human Being: Update, *1990.* In E. Barret, *Visions of Rogers' Science-Based Nursing,* pp. 5–11. NY: National League for Nursing.

Rose, A.M. (1962). *Human Behavior and Social Processes.* Boston: Houghton Millflin.

Roy, C. (1976). *Introduction to Nursing: An Adaptation Model.* Englewood Cliffs, NJ: Prentice-Hall.

Roy, C. & Roberts, S. (1981). *Theory Construction in Nursing: An Adaptation Model.* Englewood Cliffs, NJ: Prentice-Hall.

Satir, V. (1982). The Therapist and Family Therapy: Process Model. In A.M. Horne & M.M. Ohlsen (Eds.), *Family Counseling and Therapy,* pp 12–42. Itasca, IL: F.E. Peacock.

Selekman, M.D. (1997). *Solution Focused Therapy with Children.* NY: The Guilford Press.

Selye, H. (1950). *The Physiology and Pathology of Exposure to Stress.* Montreal, Quebec: ACTA. Out of print.

Toman, W. (1961). *Family Constellation: Its Effects on Personality and Science Behavior.* New York: Springer.

Turner, R.H. (1970). *Family Interaction.* New York: John Wiley and Sons.

Vaughan-Cole, B., Johnson, M.A., Malone, J.A., & B.L. Walker. (1998). *Family Nursing Practice.* Philadelphia: Saunders.

Vogt, W. P. (1993). *Dictionary of Statistics and Methodology.* Newbury Park, CA: Sage.

von Bertalanffy, L.V. (1950). The Theory of Open Systems in Physics and Biology. *Science,* 111:23–29.

von Bertalanffy, L.W. (1968) *General Systems Theory: Foundations, Development, and Applications.* New York, NY: George Braziller.

Watzlawick, P., Beavin, J., & Jackson, D. (1967). *Pragmatics of Human Communication.* NY: W.W. Norton.

Watzlawick, P., Weakland, J., & Fisch, R. (1974). *Change: Principles of Problem Formulation and Problem Resolution.* NY: W.W. Norton.

Whall, A.L. (1983). Family System Theory. Relationship to Nursing Conceptual Models. In J. Fitzpatrick & A. Whall (Eds.), *Conceptual Models of Nursing: Analysis and Application,* pp. 69–93. Bowie, MD: R.J. Brady.

Whall, A.L. (1986) *Family Therapy Theory for Nursing.* East Norwalk, CT: Appleton & Lange.

Whall, A. & Fawcett, J. (Eds.). (1991a). *Family Theory Development in Nursing: State of the Science and Art.* Philadelphia: F.A. Davis.

Whitaker, C.A. & Keith, D.V. (1981). Symbolic-Experiential Family Therapy. In A.S. Gurman & D.P. Kriskern (Eds.). *Handbook of Family Therapy.* New York: Brunner/Mazel.

White M. & Epston, D. (1990). *Narrative Means to Therapeutic Ends.* New York: W.W. Norton.

Winton, C.A. (1995). *Frameworks for Studying Families.* Guilford, CT: Dushkin.

Wright, L.M. & Leahey, M. (2000). *Nurses and Families: A Guide to Family Assessment and Intervention,* ed 3. Phil: F.A. Davis.

Wright, L.M. & Watson, W.L. (1988). Systemic Family Therapy and Family Development. In C.J. Falicox (Ed.), *Family Transitions: Continuity and Change over the Life Cycle,* pp 407–430. NY: Guilford Press.

Wright, L.M., Watson, W.L. & Bell, J.M. (1997). *Beliefs: The Heart of Healing in Families and Illness.* New York: Basic Books.

Additional Bibliography

Barth, R.P. (1990). Theories Guiding Home-Based Intensive Family Preservation Services. In L.M. Tracy, & C. Booth, (Eds). *Reaching High Risk Families: Intensive Family Preservations in Human Services*. NY: Aldine deGruyter.

Boyd, S.T. (1996). Theoretical and Research Foundations of Family Nursing. In S.M.H. Hanson and S.T. Boyd, *Family Health Care Nursing: Theory, Practice and Research,* pp. 41–56. Philadelphia, PA: F.A. Davis.

Broderick, C.B. (1993). *Understanding Family Process*. Newbury Park, CA: Sage Publications.

Broome, M.E, Knaftl, K., Pridham, K., & S. Feetham. (1998). *Children and Families in Health and Illness*. Thousand Oaks: Sage.

Carlson, J. and Lewis, J. (1991). *Family Counseling: Strategies and Issues*. Denver: Love.

Clements, I.W. & Buchanan, D.M. (1982). *Family Therapy: A Nursing Perspective*. NY: John Wiley & Sons.

Day, R.D., Gilbert, K.R., Settles, B. & Burr, W.R. (1995). *Research and Theory in Family Science*. Pacific Grove, CA: Brooks Cole.

Gilliss, C.L., Highley, B.L., Roberts, B.M. & Martinson, I.M. (Eds). (1989). *Toward a Science of Family Nursing*. Menlo Park, CA: Addison-Wesley.

Hanson, S.M.H. & Kaakinen, J. (In press). Nursing of Families in the Community. In M. Stanhope and J. Lancasters (Eds.), *Community Health Nursing: Promoting Health of Aggregates, Families, and Individuals,* ed 5. St. Louis: C.V. Mosby.

Hill, R., Katz, A.M., & Simpson, R.L. (1957). An Inventory of Research Marriage and Family Behavior: A Statement of Objectives and Progress. *Marriage and Family Living, 19*:89–92.

Meleis, A.I. (1992). Directions for Nursing Theory Development in the 21st Century. *Nursing Science Quarterly, 5*(3):112–117.

Meleis, A.I. (1996). Theory Development: A Blueprint for the 21st Century. In P. Walker and B. Neuman, (Eds), *Blueprint for the Use of Nursing Models*. NY: NLN Press.

Nicoll, L.H. (Ed.). (1997). *Perspective on Nursing Theory*. Philadelphia: Lippincott.

Nightingale, F. (1949). Sick Nursing and Health Nursing. In I. Hampton, et al. *Nursing of the Sick: 1893*. New York: McGraw-Hill.

Stanhope, M. (1996). Family Theories and Development. In M. Stanhope and J. Lancaster(Eds.), *Community Health Nursing: Process and Practice for Promoting Health*. St. Louis: C.V. Mosby.

Timpson, J. (1996). Nursing Theory: Everything the Artist Spits Is Art. *Journal of Advanced Nursing, 23:* 1030–1036.

Wegner, G.D. & Alexander, R.J. (Eds). (1993). *Readings in Family Nursing*. Philadelphia: Williams & Wilkins.

Wicks, M. (1995). Family Health As Derived from King's Framework. In M. Frey & C. Sieloff (Eds.), *Advancing King's Systems Framework and Theory of Nursing*. London: Sage.

Focus On

RESEARCH IN FAMILIES AND FAMILY NURSING

The previous chapter provided you with theoretical foundations for family nursing practice and research, including what theory is, the functions of theory, and criteria for evaluating family theory. Theories that help frame research and practice in family nursing were summarized and integrated approaches to family nursing were described.

This chapter is about research in family nursing and addresses methods used to identify and validate family theory. Research methods and issues particular to family research are addressed to enhance the reader's ability to evaluate research on families for use in nursing practice. Specifically, this chapter discusses the central issue of family as a "unit of analysis" and describes how resolution of this issue affects the nature of research questions. An overview of family research designs is provided and several methodological issues are addressed; these issues include sampling, modes of data collection, measurement, and data analysis. Qualitative methods in family research are described. Selected ethical challenges in the conduct of family research are presented for consideration, and criteria for evaluating family research are delineated.

This chapter concludes with an overview of the evolution of family nursing research and a discussion of what is needed next. Together with the theoretical foundations provided in the previous chapter, this chapter should provide readers with a foundation for an informed reading and evaluation of research for use in family nursing.

Chapter 3

RESEARCH IN FAMILIES AND FAMILY NURSING

Gail M. Houck • Sheila M. Kodadek

OUTLINE

OBJECTIVES

On completion of this chapter, the reader will be able to:

- Discuss conceptual distinctions among family-related, family, and family nursing types of research.
- Describe how the unit of analysis influences the nature of research, especially family research, and the types of research questions addressed.
- Identify approaches to family research design.
- Summarize sampling issues related to family nursing research.
- Discuss the relationship between strategies for measurement and data collection.
- Analyze ethical challenges inherent in family nursing research.

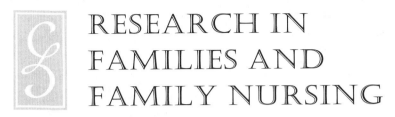

- Discuss challenges presented by addressing the complexity of families in family research.
- Discuss key bodies of literature in family nursing research in light of the historical context for the evolution of this science.

This chapter on research in families and family nursing presents a discussion of conceptual and methodological issues that attend research in this field and provides an overview of the evolution of family research in the nursing discipline. The issues addressed in this chapter provide readers with a foundation for an informed reading and evaluation of research for its use in family nursing. Although the emphasis here is research for application by the discipline of nursing, the research literature synthesized in subsequent chapters is interdisciplinary, and issues that we discuss are relevant considerations in evaluating any family research.

DEFINING FAMILY: THE UNIT OF ANALYSIS

The nursing discipline has a long-standing tradition of concern for the well-being of families and their individual members. Beginning in the early 1970s, nursing's research interest in families and family nursing became a significant focus for the profession (Ganong, 1995), with the goal of strengthening its knowledge base in family practice. As the discipline's interest in and conduct of research on families have grown, so has the need to specify and define what constitutes the family. This is probably the most practical question that faces a family researcher: who to include in the study. However, in family research, it is a complex issue (Copeland & White, 1991).

In the first chapter, Hanson describes four approaches to family nursing: the family as the context for individual development, the family as a client, the family as a system, and the family as a component of society (p. 9–10). To build the science for these approaches, researchers must be certain that who is included in the study and the information collected are consistent with how the findings will be used. In other words, research findings about how a family supports a chronically ill child's psychosocial development (family as context) cannot be used as findings about how the family adapts to a child's chronic illness in terms of family coping and functioning (family as system).

Two sets of distinctions have characterized discussions about research with families. The first set concerns those distinctions between family-related research and family research (Feetham, 1990), and the second set concerns distinctions between individual persons and families in research (Robinson, 1995). These distinctions bear on the issue of the "unit of analysis" in family research. Research that focuses on relationships between family members, using data reported from individuals, often is referred to as family-related research; in contrast, research that focuses on the family unit as a whole is referred to as family research (Feetham, 1990). What is important is whether the researcher obtains information from an individual about the family or from the family as a whole at one time.

Data from an individual family member about the family represent the individual's perspective. The assumption underlying this approach is that the individual's perspective is a valuable source of information about the family (Uphold & Strickland, 1989). In particular, the individual family member is the appropriate unit of analysis when the family is viewed as the context for individual growth, development, well-being, and adaptation. In such cases, the individual's perceptions of the family's influence on his or her development, health, illness, or treatment are the focus of study. From a pragmatic standpoint, this approach to researching families is less expensive and has fewer statistical analysis problems than does collecting data from more than one family member.

Family-level information usually is derived through an interview with the whole family, an observational method, or a method of data analysis, such as combining the responses or test scores of several family members. Family-level data are obtained from multiple family members as informants. Although it is thought that greater insight into families may be obtained through study of the family as the unit of analysis, several problems may be encountered (Uphold & Strickland, 1989). First, a bias may occur if not all members of a given family are willing to participate; however, recruitment, retention, and coordination of whole families can be difficult or even impossible from a practical standpoint. Second, there are scoring problems when data from multiple family members are used. Along this line, it is a problem that most instruments are designed for one person. (However, several approaches to scoring address these problems, which will be discussed later in this chapter.) The important point is that the choice of who should be the source of data collection, or the unit of analysis, should make sense in terms of the purpose of the study, the theoretical orientation and research question, and whether the researcher wants to generalize about the family as a whole or focus on the individual's perceptions about the family.

The second set of distinctions, between research of individuals and research of families, has resulted not only in a call for attention to the family as the unit of analysis but also in a consideration of the whole without consideration of its parts. Robinson (1995) argued against this separation, which takes an either/or approach. Instead, she proposed a schema in which both the individual and the family are considered, with each serving as background for the other. Accordingly, there are four units of analysis or interest in nursing research:

1. Individual family member
2. Individual family subgroup (marital dyad, parents, parent-child, siblings)
3. Family group

and

4. Individual family system (Robinson, 1995)

These distinctions simply clarify differences in research according to area of interest, focus of attention, and kind of data used, but with the explicit consideration of the individual.

Again, the distinctions around the "unit of analysis" have to do with who is included in the studies and to what extent we can generalize the information we learn. Family nurses and other family health professionals have called for defining family in a way that moves beyond the traditional ideas of limiting membership by blood and marriage. Nurse researchers typically have argued for definitions that allow families to define themselves (Bell, 1995; Hanson & Boyd, 1996; Wright & Leahey, 2000).

However we define families, it is clear that they are a special form of small group, with unique dimensions that challenge researchers (Ganong, 1995). Ganong summarized the characteristics that make families difficult to study as follows:

- An ethic of privacy governs nearly every aspect of family life.
- Family systems are value-laden.
- Families, similar to other small groups, have unique attributes, such as organization around gender and generation.
- Families are structurally, ethnically, and culturally diverse.
- Families are "ongoing" and exist multigenerationally over time.
- Families are influenced by the sociocultural context (Ganong, 1995).

All of these characteristics contribute to the complexity of research on families. At the same time, these characteristics speak to the necessity for systematically-derived knowledge about families to guide the practitioner of family nursing. The complexity of families also speaks to the necessity for systematically-derived knowledge about nursing interventions with families. The specifics of caring interventions or intervention programs that affect families in constructive ways require articulation and investigation. In this regard, the unit of analysis is two-fold, including the *outcomes* of family nursing interventions (whether targeted for an individual member, a dyad, or the family system) as well as the *process* of what constitutes the intervention (Bell, 1995b). From a definitional standpoint, it seems crucial to distinguish between treatment provision and caring interventions because, according to Frank's (1995) personal accounts, their respective, consequent family experiences differ considerably. Ultimately, it is in the lives of families that family researchers and family nurses strive to make a difference.

RESEARCH QUESTIONS ABOUT FAMILIES AND FAMILY NURSING

How do research questions vary according to the unit of analysis and how much of the whole family needs to be included to be family research? Fisher and colleagues (1990) concluded a decade ago that family researchers can focus selectively on family subsystems or identifiable parts of the family. They asserted that a family focus is not violated when certain elements within the family are identified and assessed, while other elements are not (e.g., excluded or controlled). Again, this focus is apparent in the four approaches to family nursing described in the first chapter. With these notions in mind, it is useful to consider Robinson's distinctions about family as background; or foreground as a way of categorizing research questions.

Nursing research on the *individual family member*

strives to eliminate the separation between individual and family member. According to this focus, the family is background; and the person as individual, as family member, or as both individual and family member is foreground (Robinson, 1995). The unit of analysis may be individual (e.g., physiological measurements or self-reporting), relational (e.g., data from two or more "related" persons about the individual or family), or transactional (e.g., data from family members in interaction). See Berkey and Hanson (1991) or Robinson (1995) for more detailed discussion of these levels of analysis.

Research questions that characterize the individual family member focus include those pertaining to battered women. In this body of research, family violence is the background and the battered woman, mother, wife, or partner is the foreground. Research questions that pertain to transition to parenthood also reflect this emphasis. For example, family relationships and social support may be the background, and the parenting experience of the mother or father then would be foreground. Alternatively, the focus may be on the parent or family as background and the infant or child as foreground. The points here are that (1) family phenomena serve as the context for the individual, and (2) studies framed by such questions inform us not only about the individual but about the family as well.

When the *individual family subgroup* is the focus of interest, it is possible to focus on persons as individuals and as family members, as well as on their relationship (Robinson, 1995). The focus is on the relationship as a subgroup of the family, from the perspective of persons individually and in interaction. Research questions may concern the marital relationship as perceived by the individual partners (relational data) or as observed by researchers (transactional data), and it may concern individual characteristics (e.g., personality and psychosocial characteristics) that attend the relationship. Research questions about parent-child relationships also reflect this focus, with attention paid both to the assessment of individual characteristics that may contribute to the relationship and to the assessment of the relationship itself. Other examples of this focus are research on individual adjustment or development (child or adult) and marital and parental adjustment to life events (Benson & Deal, 1995).

In research on the *family system or group,* the individual family members and their relationships become background and the family is foreground (Robinson, 1995). In this focus, the family is the unit of analysis and is distinct from individuals and family members.

This emphasis does not represent the "whole" family or a "holistic" perspective because it does not include the parts of the family or the individual's and subgroup's perspectives (Fisher et al, 1990; Robinson, 1995). This focus characterizes much of the family sociological research before the 1970s (Benson & Deal, 1995). Individual and relational levels of data can be used to inform us or to make statements about the family. For measures of the family per se, transactional data would be collected to reflect a characteristic or property of the family without accounting for the contribution of particular family members or relationship patterns between members. Research questions that typify this focus pertain to family functioning during crisis or transition, family adaptation to chronic illness, and family experiences with specific events.

Research on the *individual and family system* involves consideration of the influence of family on individuals and individuals on family (Robinson, 1995). This focus of research, a trend beginning in the 1970s, includes both the individual family member and the family as foreground and of interest. The essential idea is that an integrated focus on the person as individual and family member as well as on the family allows the researcher to question how the individual as a separate, autonomous person contributes to the family system variables and vice versa (Benson & Deal, 1995). Research questions typical of this focus address spousal care givers of persons with Alzheimer's disease or other chronic illnesses and conditions, parental caregivers of children with chronic conditions, and children in families in which the mother has breast cancer. The key is for individual characteristics or other variables to be considered, including those embedded in the family member role, as well as for the family to be conceptualized and assessed as a family system. Again, data from individual, relational, and transactional levels are relevant.

OVERVIEW OF DESIGNS FOR FAMILY RESEARCH

A study is designed to fit the research questions asked about specific phenomena: in this case, families. The research design includes the plan, structure, and procedures for collecting and analyzing the data to answer the research questions. Two issues are central (Miller, 1986): 1) Does the design fit the research question(s)? and 2) Is the design both practical and economical? There are several ways of classifying research designs, none of which is universally accepted. This overview addresses exploratory, descriptive, correlational, longitudinal, and experimental designs.

Exploratory

Exploratory studies are conducted when little is known about a phenomenon of interest. The purpose of exploratory research is to generate ideas, insights, or understandings about family phenomena that are not well understood. Both quantitative and qualitative methods are appropriate for this design. Although such research may be less structured and more flexible in approach, this does not mean that it proceeds without a plan or systematic procedure. A well-executed exploratory study can develop and refine ideas about family phenomena and can build family theory. For example, Oxley and Weekes (1997) used an exploratory design "to explore and describe the meaning African American adolescents give to the experience of being pregnant and strategies they used to manage the pregnancy experience" (p. 168). Among the findings was the importance of identified needs being met by the adolescents' boyfriends and mothers.

Descriptive

Descriptive research is distinguished from exploratory research by its specification of variables about families that it seeks to describe or assess in a population. It is not flexible in the way exploratory research can be and does not rely on subjective insight in the same way (Miller, 1986). A variety of methods are used to describe characteristics of marriages and families, including surveys, structured interviews, and intensive observations in the laboratory, the clinical setting, or in the family home.

Correlational

Correlational family studies assess the relationships among characteristics of families, family relations, and individual family members. The purpose of this research design is to examine specific relationships between two or more variables of interest. Correlational designs typically examine variables that are not under the control of the researcher or cannot be experimentally manipulated. Observations, questionnaires, and interviews are among the methods that can be used to collect data.

Correlational designs are common to family research because they tend to fit the research questions that interest investigators and experimental designs are not usually feasible (Miller, 1986).

Olsen and associates (1999) used a descriptive correlational design to examine how support and communication are related to hardiness in families who have young children with disabilities. They found that perceived family support was a predictor of family hardiness for both parents. Incendiary communication was negatively related to family hardiness for mothers, and income was positively associated with assessments of family hardiness by fathers (p. 275).

Experimental

Experimental designs allow the researcher to control or manipulate causal (independent) variables and to randomly assign families to treatment and control groups. Experiments are designed to allow the inference of a functional or causal relationship between causal factors (independent variables or treatments) and individual or family outcomes (dependent variable). Family intervention research typically involves an experimental design by which one group of families receives or participates in an intervention and another group does not participate or receives a different intervention. In some designs, families who are not selected for the experimental intervention or demonstration program may be placed on a waiting list and, after comparisons can be made on the outcomes, will subsequently receive the effective intervention. Other designs provide the "usual" intervention or program to one group of families and the experimental or demonstration intervention to another group, and the outcomes are compared. The central point in an experimental design is that a comparison can be made between interventions and their respective outcomes, so that cause and effects can be determined.

One example of an experimental design is the use of a randomized clinical trial to evaluate the effectiveness of a nursing support and education support service in improving family functioning after cardiac surgery by Gilliss and colleagues (1990). The service was offered in the hospital and by telephone to 67 pairs of patients and caregivers after cardiac surgery, with family variables included in the study.

Longitudinal

Many family research questions are concerned with continuity, naturally occurring change, and predictability over time; longitudinal designs, in which the same families are studied over time, address such questions (Copeland & White, 1991). Individual development within the family also can be addressed readily through longitudinal design. The defining feature of longitudinal design is that the same families or family members are assessed at two or more points in time. For example, how families adapt to the mother's diagnosis of breast cancer was studied by making a specified number of data collection visits to the same families—involving the same family members—at specified intervals (e.g., Woods, et al, 1989; Lewis, et al, 1993; Lewis, 1993; Lewis, et al, 1996). Research that addresses parent-child interaction and child developmental outcomes at specified ages in infants, toddlers, and preschoolers is another example of longitudinal design (e.g. Barnard, 1979; Barnard et al, 1989; Houck, et al, 1991; Houck, 1999).

Several potential problems require attention with this design. First, if children are involved, appropriate measures for developmental age must be included. As the nature of the measures change according to age, for example, mothers' reports on or observations of preschoolers versus self-reporting by children in middle school, there is concern for how comparable the measures are. Second, the question always must be raised as to whether changes are developmental, evolutionary (or part of a process), or result from some other influence. Finally, attrition is a problem common to longitudinal research studies (Ryan & Hayman, 1996; Motzer, et al, 1997). Many subjects who initially participate will drop out of the study because they move or their circumstances change. Especially problematic for family researchers are changes in family constellations: family members graduate, move away, or refuse to participate, and new members are added through birth or marriage.

METHODS IN FAMILY RESEARCH: ISSUES AND CHALLENGES

Once the study design is identified, the family researcher is faced with the challenge of how to get the information needed to answer the research question. There are significant methodological issues in family research. How these issues are addressed is central to the quality of family research and a central concern for the nurse who is evaluating family research for use in practice. Frequent sampling, data collection, measurement, and analysis issues in family research are now addressed. While all four topics are of concern in both quantitative and qualitative family research, there also are significant differences. Following the discussion of these four topics is an overview of qualitative methods in family research.

Sampling

A primary concern with sampling is whether the families who participate in a study are representative of the populations or groups to whom findings and conclusions can be generalized. Socioeconomic stratification is one way of characterizing a sample. Economic resources, social prestige, power, information, and lifestyle affect many family variables; the variables most frequently used to indicate socioeconomic level are occupation, income, and formal education (Smith & Graham, 1995). Recently, there have been problems with using exclusively male characteristics to assess socioeconomic level and with using women's characteristics separately or along with men's. What is important in the conduct of family research is to identify potentially relevant variables and which individual respondents serve to classify a family's socioeconomic level. In the end, the key issue is whether the sample of participating families (if characterized by these variables) is representative; does it include a reasonable range? Researchers may also be interested in certain groups within a sample and linking certain kinds of interventions accordingly; for example, low education, low income, or "social risk." The ways in which these categories are defined by sampling criteria or demographic data are important.

Another sampling consideration involves restricting the families to those with a specific health condition, diagnosis, or circumstance. For example, researchers may want to investigate family responses to pregnancy in midlife, management strategies for cardiac disease, coping with parental death, or parenting a preschooler. Criteria for including and excluding families from the sample must be clear and ensure that the sample represents the group of interest.

A third sampling issue concerns cross-cultural family research. Family research and theory cannot be assumed to have cross-cultural applicability (Moriarty, et al, 1995). The conduct of cross-cultural research requires collaboration not only across disciplines but among researchers of the ethnic groups under study. Challenges to the investigators include access to the population of interest and cultural competence in the collection and analysis of data. From the standpoint of research evaluation, at issue is whether there is cultural or ethnic representation among the investigators and whether they account for cultural competence in the conduct of the study. Although many researchers have argued for cross-cultural comparisons, such findings often contribute to broad generalizations. Rather, investigators increasingly are urged to explore variation within cultural or ethnic groups rather than to directly compare cultural groups (Kelly, et al, 1992).

Another sampling issue occurs in longitudinal research, which, as mentioned previously, has the problem of attrition. The loss of sample members over time occurs because families move and cannot be located or refuse to continue their participation. With older families or families with ill members, some participants die and others may no longer be able to participate as a result of illness or disability. Thus, there is a potential threat of attrition bias. This bias is assumed to exist when there are significant differences in the sample between the initial and subsequent data collections (Miller & Wright, 1995). It is important that reports of longitudinal research address the issue of attrition, including whether attrition bias was found to exist, any measures were taken to correct the bias, and any cautions were applied in the interpretation of the findings.

Modes of Data Collection

Modes of data collection refer to, in part, which family members participate in the study. One way of classifying the nature of the data is whether it is individual, relational, or transactional (Berkey & Hanson, 1991; Feetham, 1990; Fisher, et al, 1985). Individual data are collected from a single family member and reflect individual perceptions about the phenomenon of interest; there is no reference to the perceptions of other family members. Relational data are collected from individual family members and combined in some way (e.g., using means, sums, and difference scores) to address relationship dimensions or are obtained through the observation of or interview with a dyad. Family level or transactional data typically are obtained from naturalistic observation of family interaction as well as by aggregating data from all individual family members. The primary consideration about the source of data pertains to recognition that responses will differ when the same questions are asked of family members individually and also in the presence of a partner, parent, or the entire family.

Self-reports are useful for obtaining information about subjective events and conditions (Copeland & White, 1991). Also called survey method, data collection by self-report consists of asking people questions directly through questionnaires, face-to-face interviews, or telephone interviews (Miller, 1986).

Questionnaires are surveys that can be mailed to respondents or administered in a group or family setting, and the respondents can mark the answers themselves with complete anonymity. Questionnaire data are cost-effective, but it is difficult or impractical to follow up on missing or incomplete data; in other words, data quality can be a limitation. Face-to-face interviews employ an interviewer to ask the respondent the questions and to record the answers. They can be more flexible, allowing the interviewer to probe for more information, clarify responses, or elicit elaboration; interviews can yield more complete and accurate data. However, these advantages must be considered in light of the costs for training and evaluation of the interviewers. Telephone interviews are inexpensive and have the advantage of being rather quick, yet yielding high-quality data (Miller, 1986).

When self-report methods are used in research, there are several issues to be addressed that pertain to *how the questions are asked*. The investigators usually provide examples of the items on questionnaires or the questions asked in direct or telephone interviews, so the reader can evaluate them. The questions should be clear and unambiguous and should use vocabulary that fits the education and experience of the participants. The questions should focus on a single idea, provide a clear frame of reference so that the responses are relevant, and ask only for information the respondent has, not speculation about how others think or feel. Closed-ended, fixed-response (multiple choice, or true or false) formats are useful in large studies and can be objectively scored, but the responses may not reflect the issues the researcher intended to assess. Open-ended formats, especially useful for interviews, provide the opportunities for clarification and elaboration but are also subject to interviewer bias and require inter-rater reliability to be established (Copeland & White, 1991).

Observational methods are systematic procedures for observing behavior and recording what happens. Direct observation of families and relationship interactions can provide objective information about the behavior of family members. Observational researchers assume that while the presence of an observer or camera may alter family members' behavior in some respects, people cannot change their behavior in any profound way by simply trying to do so (Copeland & White, 1991). To further guard against "impression management," observational coding systems usually are designed to tap behaviors, dynamics, or characteristics that operate below the level of conscious control. The family is asked to engage in a task that is interesting to the members to minimize the artificial nature of the situation and enhance the realism of their behavior.

Of course the task must elicit the behavior or dynamics that represent the construct of interest, for example, planning something together, problem solving, conflict resolution, discussing or interpreting story, or having a meal together.

Coding systems are developed to capture what is going on in the family as it is observed. Coding systems can assess: (a) interpersonal process, or *how* family members interact with each other, regardless of what they say; (b) verbal content, or *what* is said by whom; and (c) affective display, or the nonverbal expression of emotional tone. Within these categories, the researcher can code the interaction at a very specific level or can rate the interaction at a more clinical level.

Specific codes focus on smaller, discrete behaviors that can be counted or timed. The frequency of a few specific behaviors or acts may be counted or the duration of a process may be timed. An observational checklist may require the observer to note whether or not many specific behaviors occur within a task or given time frame. Global ratings, on the other hand, involve entire interactions or larger segments of interaction. A rating or judgment is assigned on a carefully defined scale that assesses a dimension (for example, control or power, communication, reciprocity, enmeshment, or adaptability) of a family or dyadic interaction over the period of observation. Extensive training of observational coders is required to be certain the coding systems are accurately employed. Once accuracy is achieved, intercoder or interrater reliability must be established over a specified number of videotaped or live observations.

Secondary data sources concern a source rather than the collection of data per se. Existing data sources include data sets from completed projects on related topics, family and social archives, large-scale surveys, and public records. *Secondary analysis* involves using previously collected data to answer questions not asked by the original investigator or to ask similar questions in new ways (Copeland & White, 1991). The existing data sets may have been designed for other purposes or may have been collected for both current and future unspecified purposes (e.g., census data or vital statistics). Interviews, written narratives, questionnaires, videotaped observation sequences, and demographic surveys all can be viewed from a new perspective and may even benefit from secondary analysis. Raw data may be available for coding in a new way, which is especially true of interviews, narratives, and observation sequences. In other cases, access to existing data may be available, such as demographic data, scores on questionnaires or tests, and observational codes. These data may be used to address new questions or relationships among different variables or to examine follow-up data or replication. A third source of data is the ongoing records (which can be used by researchers) of society that are collected for legal, medical, or political reasons.

Measurement

Measurement is the process of linking theoretical ideas or concepts to empirical indicators or variables (Miller, 1986). Congruence between concepts and measures is a goal achieved through operational definitions. In other words, the explicit procedures or instructions for linking abstract concepts to measures are operational definitions; they describe the "operations" necessary to produce scores, whereas measurement is the process of obtaining them (Berkey & Hanson, 1991; Miller, 1986). Articulation of the logical linkages between conceptualization, operational definition, and measurement requires both precision and creativity. This has been a challenge to family researchers (see Feetham, 1990) and perhaps stems from the difficulty of finding a way to "measure" systematically (with numbers, observational classifications, or ratings) the dynamic interactions of family life.

To read and evaluate family research, one must be mindful of the levels of measurement. Nominal measurement simply means naming, categorizing, or classifying. If a number is assigned to a category or classification, it is for the purpose of grouping data and does not reflect a numeric value. Gender, ethnicity, and marital status are typical nominal measurements. Observational methods often result in categorizations or classifications, as do several of the family functioning measures that use scores to arrive at classifications.

Ordinal level measurement means that it is possible to rank subjects on the basis of the variable being assessed. Ordinal rankings do not reflect a quantity but rather a general amount or more or less of a characteristic (e.g., controllingness, sensitivity, rigidity). In contrast, interval level measurement does reflect quantity, with equal distance between the points of measurement. Ratio level measurement, in addition to reflecting equal distance between measurement points, includes an absolute zero, which represents that none of the characteristics being assessed is present. The important issue is for the researcher and the practitioner to be clear about the meaning of the measurement used in a given study, especially since many of the measures and observations in family research are also used as clinical assessments (Berkey & Hanson, 1991).

Reliability of measurement is crucial to obtaining meaningful data about families. Reliability essentially refers to the dependability and consistency of a measure. Stability or consistency over time is one aspect of reliability; greater stability is expected for traits or consistent characteristics. Of course, development and growth also affect stability, and the challenge is to tease out what is real change. In general, one hopes for stability in measurement. Internal consistency is another aspect of reliability and reflects how well all parts of the measure are in correspondence or agreement. Finally, as discussed with observational methods, interrater or intercoder reliability is concerned with the dependability of coders (as "instruments") or how consistently two observers agree in their coding of observed family phenomena.

Validity also is central to the meaningfulness of research findings. Validity refers to the appropriateness of the specific use of a given measure. One way of establishing validity is to measure a concept using multiple methods. However, it can be difficult to administer multiple measures for reasons of time, expense, and burden, and the results are not always clear (Polit & Hungler, 1987). The key is for the measure to be related to something conceptually and operationally meaningful.

The issue of validity really raises the question of what to measure. Fisher and colleagues (1990) have advocated strongly for multiple measures; for selecting from several family constructs, dimensions, or domains expected to be related to health; and for sampling each one with multiple indicators to thoroughly describe the domain. Through broader family assessments with multiple indices, more complete descriptions and better predictions of outcomes can be obtained. These authors argued for triangulation or the use of self-report, historical, interview, and observational methods to obtain the unique perspectives of the family, and to integrate cross-method data in analyses to further our understanding of the complexities of the family unit.

Data Analysis

The crux of data analysis in family and family nursing research is embodied in Feetham's (1990) caveat: Selection of a data analysis technique should not be arbitrary but, rather, be linked conceptually to the study and appropriate to the data. Generally speaking, family research is *multivariate* in nature; that is, multiple concepts and, therefore, multiple variables are of interest in our efforts to understand families. Thus, family research typically involves multivariate statistics. As a reader of family and family nursing research, it is important to be mindful that larger samples are needed to support such analyses, unless certain *data reduction techniques* are undertaken. Recognizing the inherent need for multivariate analyses in the face of the challenges in recruiting and retaining target families for research, Fisher and colleagues (1990) explicated several effective strategies for managing large variable sets with relatively small samples.

Multivariate analysis aside, there are three broad approaches to data analysis: descriptive analysis, assessment of relationships, and determination of differences. Descriptive analysis basically describes the sample and the characteristics assessed. For example, families may be described in terms of parental marital status, family income level, education level of the partners or spouses, and number of children. Families may then be described in terms of the number and proportion who experience various types of conflict, presented perhaps as classifications or in terms of a score. The distribution of types or the average scores on a scale may be described in relation to national norms. The goal of such analysis is to describe selected family characteristics in a sample of individuals or families.

If the research questions were concerned with the relationships between family characteristics, the data analysis assesses the relationships between variables. Both correlational and regression analysis may be used. There are several types of correlation (e.g., Pearson's or canonical) and regression (e.g., linear, multiple, or logistic) analyses, but all generally require interval, ratio, or dichotomous (1/0) scores. Measures of association also may be used to assess the relationships among nominal variables and ordinal level data (using nonparametric statistics).

When research questions are concerned with differences between families, data analysis assesses for group differences. The sample—whether individuals, married couples, parents, or families—are grouped on the basis of a classification or nominal characteristic to assess differences between those groups on a measure. The scores are usually at the interval or ratio level of measurement. At the most general level, t-tests determine differences between two groups, and analysis of variance techniques are applied to more than two groups. In both cases, one dependent measure is assessed for differences. When there is more than one dependent or outcome measure, multivariate analyses are used. If measures are applied over time, on repeated occasions, one should expect to see a repeated measures analysis.

These are some broad generalizations about what to expect in the data analysis of family research. However, analysis of such a complex social unit is becoming equally complex, and there are many exceptions to these generalities, many variations within these approaches, and new strategies and techniques for analyzing large data sets. The issue of concern in assessing a study is whether there is a logical consistency between the data analysis and the research questions, the central concepts or domains of concern, the design and measurement, and the conclusions.

QUALITATIVE METHODS AND FAMILY RESEARCH

Qualitative methods are a common approach to family research, and family nursing researchers are recognized both within and outside of the discipline for their knowledge and skill in qualitative research. Qualitative methods often are chosen for exploratory investigations (Miller, 1986) and are most valuable when researchers seek in-depth information about how and why people behave, think, and make meaning as they do (Ambert, et. al, 1995). Qualitative research allows for the discovery or uncovering of perceptions, meanings, understandings, multiple realities, and psychosocial context in families. Although a qualitative approach to family research usually relies on the interview method, content analysis of written materials and participant observation of the family also may be used. Within the qualitative approach, there are distinct methods; each method emphasizes selected aspects of the phenomenon in question, with focus on specific aims and evidence. Sampling plans and data analysis differ markedly from quantitative methods, with effort generally focused on identifying research participants who have experience with the phenomenon under study. Regardless of the specific qualitative method, rigor in qualitative research is assessed in terms of its credibility (faithfulness to the descriptions and interpretations of experience), applicability (fittingness to other contexts), consistency (the ability to audit or to follow the researcher's "decision trail"), and confirmability (Sandelowski, 1986).

Discovering theory about family or individual experiences in families is the aim of the *grounded theory* method in family research. Grounded theory methodology was developed and named in the mid-1960s by Glaser and Strauss (1967). Grounded theory researchers generate or construct theory from data provided by families; thus, the specific theory is connected closely with the data and is said to be "grounded" in data. This approach explicitly acknowledges the family and its members as experts in their own experience and allows nurses to explore areas of nursing experience that have not been adequately addressed by existing theories. Symbolic interaction theory underlies this method, a theory that helps to explain how a group of people—in this case, a family—defines reality through social interaction.

Wilson and Morse (1991) used grounded theory methods to examine the experience of husbands living with a wife who is undergoing chemotherapy. Their analysis of the data resulted in a three-stage model of husbands' perceptions of their experience: Husbands moved from identifying the threat, to engaging in the fight, and finally, to becoming a veteran (p. 227). Recurrence meant the cycle resumed, although with experience.

Hermeneutic phenomenology is an approach to the study of shared family meanings and family concerns (Chesla, 1995). Careful attention to context is essential to this approach; family and cultural history are important to the understandings derived from this research. Hermeneutic study emphasizes the everyday experience of families and focuses on their central concerns in living with life situations (Chesla, 1995).

The perspective of *interpretative phenomenology* embraces both the shared, everyday "lived experiences" of the family and the multiple realities of family members. The individual family member's unique experience of the family and perception of reality is recognized. Thus, the researcher seeks to understand the lived experience of the different family members and their multiple realities (Hartrick & Lindsey, 1995). The focus is not on the facts of a situation but, instead, on the meaning of those facts to the various family members. Hartrick and Lindsey consider the "phenomenological attitude" as central to this method, as a way of coming to question human experience in an effort to uncover deeper meaning.

An example of phenomenological research in family nursing is Chesla's use of hermeneutic phenomenology to guide her study of the caring practices of parents with their adult schizophrenic children (1994). The richness of this method can be seen in her interpretation of the meaning of those practices.

Narrative inquiry is another qualitative method by which the researcher seeks to understand the meanings of experiences from families and their individual members. As families and family members relate about their experiences, they are telling their stories. This form of inquiry analyzes the narratives or created structures of the stories, on the assumption that family members, as narrators telling their stories, select, order, and prioritize events based on their meaning for the individuals involved (Knafl et al., 1995). Narrative inquiry identifies the "plot" or the organizing framework of the story according to the temporal unfolding of the story (Poirier & Ayres, 1997), which reveals the context and meaning of the events and experiences for the narrator (Knafl et al., 1995). The researcher notes inconsistencies, repetitions, and omissions to identify "secrets," or those issues that are to be avoided or that bring discomfort to the narrator (Poirier & Ayres, 1997). Ultimately, the researcher is able to arrive at interpretations of story "types" through careful analysis and comparison of unique story features and similarities across stories. An example of this approach is the application of narrative analysis techniques to parents' stories of the events preceding their child's diagnosis of a serious chronic illness (Knafl et al., 1995). The analysis uncovered five major pathways to diagnosis (direct, delay, detour, quest, and ordeal) and information about what those pathways meant for parents (p. 411).

Leininger (1985), described *ethnography* as the systematic process of observing, detailing, describing, documenting, and analyzing patterns of a culture to understand the patterns of people in their familiar environment (p. 35). Ethnography generally is associated with anthropology but has been used in family research to understand patterns of behavior or lifestyles of families who share experiences. Recent examples of ethnographic research in family nursing include three ethnographic studies on family health of Appalachian families. One study examined the definition and practice of family health, the second examined family health during and after death of a family member, and the third examined family health in an economically disadvantaged population (Denham, 1999a, 1999b, 1999c).

ETHICAL CONSIDERATIONS

A major consideration in the conduct of family research is disclosure of personal information (e.g., marital conflict or satisfaction, sexuality, child-rearing strategies). Further, in family nursing research, we typically ask family members about their responses to another member's illness or health condition or how they experience care giving and other aspects of family life with an ill or disabled member. Often such responses have not been articulated before this research process or perhaps the personal information has not been disclosed to other family members. Therefore, the balance between the risks to the participants by intrusive or threatening data collection procedures and the benefits to family science and society must be sensitively considered (Bussell, 1994).

Informed consent, as with any research, is essential. What is particular to family research, however, is the involvement of young children and adolescents. An important strategy is to include a child *assent* form that describes the purpose of the research and obtains the child's or adolescent's agreement to participate. This consenting procedure is used with children who are able to read.

Another aspect of informed consent pertains to the use of videotaped observations; the faces and voices are recorded and names are usually used in the observation period. Participants must be fully informed about how the videotaped data will be managed and stored, and who will see it. They must be informed when the videotapes will be destroyed and whether they will have access to view the recordings or obtain a copy (i.e., who owns the data?). One valuable strategy is to provide participants with a copy of the recording, if doing so does not violate the integrity of the research procedures.

The research setting presents other considerations. When data collection takes place in the home, several issues emerge. One is the issue of privacy if individual interviews take place or questionnaires are administered. The privacy and confidentiality of the individual member or couple must be maintained and any undue influence by other family members should be avoided. This caution is especially necessary for children, care receivers, and those who are vulnerable to other family members in terms of a power differential. Another consideration in the home setting concerns the visibility of the family's private living space; researchers must be most careful not to draw unwarranted conclusions from the experience.

Working with families does challenge our conceptions of ourselves as researchers who study families and as nurses who intervene with families. As nurses, we are required to report any child or elder maltreatment according to state law and, in some states, we are mandated to report if a child witnesses domestic violence. At a minimum, there is an obligation to be familiar with local statutes regarding not only abuse and violence but suicidality and violent intent as well (Bussell, 1994). However, there are many other situations that we may consider "clinically urgent" and that present a basic ethical dilemma between individual welfare and scientific gains. Many of these difficult conflicts can be avoided by establishing guidelines for when and how to intervene on a subject's behalf before data collection (Bussell, 1994).

Further, if clinical information will be derived from certain measures (e.g., depression level), the consent form can state that subjects will be informed if they have scores that are in a clinical range on a given measure. In this way, participants are aware that they will receive clinically relevant feedback. At the same time, the consent forms typically state, quite clearly, that the investigators' work with the family is for scientific purposes and that they will not be expected to provide treatment.

This blurring of boundaries occurs in a similar way even with self-report data. The process of completing questionnaires about parenting, marital relations, sexuality, conflict, and responses to caring for a family member is likely to trigger consideration of ideas and feelings that may not have been addressed previously. In fact, the process of both participating in interviews and completing questionnaires may facilitate considerable reflection on one's own experiences and family life. Although this reflection may serve as a benefit of the research process, alternatively, it can serve as a risk for unpleasant feelings (e.g., anxiety, anger, or regret) or adverse responses that require professional assistance. It is not uncommon, then, for a research team to be prepared to make referrals for crisis intervention or provide a list of relevant mental health or diagnosis-specific resources.

CRITERIA FOR EVALUATION

There has been a long-standing gap between family nursing research and practice, a circumstance that has limited the extent to which research can enhance practice with individuals and their families. Dialogue between researchers and practitioners of nursing is even more crucial in the era of health-care reform, with much of the care that used to be hospital-based and carried out by professional nurses now carried out by family members in the home. With limited resources, the family itself as a "resource" becomes crucial to the individual patient's well-being and, therefore, their function must be optimized. Further, the "high users" of health-care resources are complex, multiproblem cases that require professional nursing intervention with both individuals and their families, e.g., catastrophic care, chronic illness care, cancer care, and end-of-life care and those issues that may influence care and require attention themselves, such as domestic violence, mental health problems (especially depression), and nonadherence issues. Toward this end, family and family nurse researchers must attend to the context of practice, present findings in clinical journals, and discuss how to apply findings. However, until researchers become adept at doing so, it rests with the practitioners of nursing to evaluate family and family nursing research and to integrate relevant research into their practice. The following evaluation criteria should assist in this effort. They are drawn from those identified by Feetham and colleagues (1990) and summarize much of the discussion thus far in this chapter.

The first issue to be evaluated in family and family nursing research is whether an *explicit family conceptual or theoretical framework* is used. The basic assumptions the investigator holds about individuals and families in the conduct of the research must be clear. Family itself is likely to be the "lens" with which the problem under research is viewed, although the family as a whole may be considered or the family may be the context or environment for an individual's health and illness.

Thus, another criterion for evaluation is a *concept of the family* and this conceptualization must be consistent with the theoretical framework. Recall that the family may be viewed as a system interacting with its environment (health-care system, community), as an environment for the individual members, as a mediator or moderator for individual members, or as the cause of health or illness (Feetham and associates, 1990). The researcher should be explicit about this and, if not, the conceptualization should be made clear to the reader.

It follows, then, that there must be a *definition of the family*. This involves a clear statement about who was included in the data collection process. In other words, the definition of the family should be linked to the participants in the study. Here we are not only talking about a theoretical definition but how the definition of family is operationalized. Look for congruence between the theoretical framework, the concept of the family, the definition of family, and the persons who participate in the study.

There must be a *logical consistency* in the methods of family research. As this chapter has described, the research design, the modes of data collection, the measures, and the data analysis must be consistent with the foregoing criteria; all relate back to the unit of analysis. Throughout the methods section, actual or potential *ethical considerations* should be addressed. Finally, the findings must add to the *knowledge base* about families and should have *relevance* to nursing practice.

These criteria should serve as a guide to reading family and family nursing research and to the interpretation of the findings for practice. Research about families and individuals and their families has the potential to affect nursing practice in an important way. In this era of health care reform, families increasingly take on what once was professional nursing care. To optimize patient and family outcomes, this link between research and practice is crucial.

FAMILY NURSING RESEARCH: PAST AND FUTURE

Nursing's interest in families is not new. Throughout its history, the profession of nursing has been concerned with family influences in the health and well-being of individual members. Perhaps the most enduring example of this is the focus on families that has characterized community health nursing practice for generations. However, in the 1970s, nurses became significantly more appreciative of the influence families exert on the health-related beliefs, attitudes, and behaviors of their individual patients. They systematically began to ask questions about relationships between families, health, and illness.

Consequently, nurse researchers interested in family issues began moving away from individually focused studies, choosing instead to focus on families. As stated earlier in this chapter, discussions about what constituted family research were frequent and lively and continue today.

Classic review articles provide a glimpse of the remarkable upsurge in family nursing research that occurred during the 1970s and early 1980s, and can give the reader an appreciation of the creativity and clinical grounding of the researchers involved. In 1983, Gilliss' paper, "The Family as a Unit of Analysis: Strategies for the Nurse Researcher," was published in *Advances in Nursing Science* (Gilliss, 1983). In this paper, Gillis examined the nature of the family as a research phenomenon, reviewed and critiqued approaches that had been used to study the family, and identified strategies appropriate to the nature of nursing research (pp. 50–51). Gilliss concluded that family research remained flawed, despite creative strategies, and suggested attention to "the logical consistencies among what is measured, about whom, from whom, and for what purpose" (p. 58). In addition, she advocated that theoretical frameworks that are used should be congruent with study variables and data collection procedures, and that data analysis must be theoretically consistent with family research.

In 1984, Feetham's paper "Family Research: Issues and Directions for Nursing" was published in the *Annual Review of Nursing Research.* In this landmark paper, Feetham reviewed research in nursing to date, using the categories of family characteristics, family as environment of the individual, external environment and the family, nursing interventions with families, and family-related research. She suggested that a single definition of family by nurses is not essential, but what is essential is that each investigator define family within the context of the research. She recommended that researchers focus on "how families help each other, how they cope, and how they grow" (Feetham, 1984, p. 20). She also suggested that nursing research that examines concepts common to healthy families or to families who grow and develop in spite of illness within the family help identify predictors of family health (Feetham, 1984, p. 20).

Five years later, Gilliss (1991) wrote that there had been a marked upsurge in activity in family nursing research since Feetham's review (p. 44). However, she identified significant gaps in the literature. She found that there were populations missing or underrepresented in nursing research; specifically, nontraditional families, families from nondominant cultures, family dyads other than parent-child, and siblings were seldom included in family nursing research. In addition, there was little research on interactions between families and communities. Finally, the lack of experimental studies was noteworthy.

In a later paper, Gilliss (1991) advocated setting priorities in family nursing research. She recommended a focus on studies that demonstrated relationships between the practice of family nursing and its outcomes, and she urged further development of methods of data collection to capture family-level data.

In a review of family nursing research from 1984 to 1990, Hayes (1993) also identified a dearth of research with nontraditional families and families from nondominant cultures. In addition, she concluded that families of the elderly and healthy, well-functioning families also were underrepresented in family nursing research.

Whall and Loveland-Cherry (1993) reviewed family unit-focused research published from 1984 to 1991. Like Gilliss, they found there had been a dramatic increase in family-unit studies in nursing since Feetham's 1984 review. In addition they found commonalities beginning to emerge, including a focus on assisting families coping with illness events and a health (rather than illness) perspective. However, family as the unit of analysis still was not defined consistently or even often. Replications of studies that help build trustworthy science were rare. The majority of studies continued to be descriptive or exploratory in nature. Intervention studies were most often focused on illness and hospital care. Whall and Loveland-Cherry joined the authors of earlier reviews in recommending explicit definition of the theoretical frameworks underlying studies.

Ganong (1995, 1996) and Hayes (1995) used the *Journal of Family Nursing* for a lively exchange about trends and issues in family nursing research. Ganong is a not a nurse and brought to the discussion his view from family social science; Hayes came from a family nursing perspective. While they disagreed on some points, including the level of sophistication of family nursing research to date, they did agree that there are "huge gaps in our understanding of families in health care" (p. 93), whatever the discipline, and that family nursing has made unique and valuable contributions to addressing those gaps.

Much work has been done in family nursing research. The following chapters introduce the reader to rich areas of family and family nursing research, which are discussed and applied to specific areas of nursing practice. Family nursing researchers have given the discipline and family science knowledge about interactions among families and health and illness across the life span, including family health promotion, family management of acute illness, and family care giving. Research on aging families and healthy families is increasing steadily. Family nursing can be justifiably proud of this heritage.

However, there is much work to be done. Some of the gaps in family nursing research have narrowed during the last 30 years, while others have widened. The following are areas for future work in family nursing research:

- Family intervention studies, using the wealth of exploratory, descriptive, and correlational studies in the literature
- Studies of families representing diversity in structure, ethnicity, and living situation
- Studies that focus on relationships between families and other social systems
- Increased and consistent attention to the unit of analysis in family studies
- Attention to theory development and theoretical consistency within and across studies
- Attention to biosocial research opportunities in family nursing, including the implications for families of the ever-increasing information on genetics (Feetham, 1999)

SUMMARY

In 1992, Knafl wrote that family research was a field "for those with a pioneering spirit, a tenacious mind set, and high tolerance for ambiguity!" (p. 100). It is also, as she noted more recently, a field for nurses "who can meld their methodological and theoretical sophistication with their clinical grounding" (p. 245). The past 30 years have been exciting ones for family nurses and family nursing research. And the next 30 years promise to be every bit as challenging.

Study Questions

1. How does the unit of analysis in family nursing research influence the nature of the research? How does it influence the type of research questions addressed? How does it influence the data received? Give an example of each.
2. Why is it important for family nurse researchers to define "family" explicitly in a study?
3. Choose one of the research designs used in family research and give an example of a family research question that would be appropriate for that design.
4. Briefly discuss two challenges associated with sampling in family research.
5. How questions are asked can make a significant difference in the quality of data when self-report methods are used in family research. Describe three strategies to improve the quality of the data collected.
6. Distinguish between reliability and validity of measurement in family research.
7. Why is quantitative family research *multivariate* in nature?
8. Give two reasons why a family nurse researcher might choose qualitative methods to answer a research question.
9. Briefly discuss three ethical considerations in family nursing research.
10. List six issues that should be evaluated in family and family nursing research.
11. The authors list seven areas for future work in family nursing research. Which area do you believe should be addressed first if the goal is improvement of family nursing practice? Why?

References

Ambert, A., et al. (1995). Understanding and evaluating qualitative research. *Journal of Marriage and the Family,* 57:879–893.

Barnard, K. E. (1979). Teaching scale/feeding scale. In, *Instructor's Learning Manual, NCAST.* Seattle, WA: University of Washington.

Barnard, K. E., et al. (1989). Measurement and meaning of parent-child interaction. In F. J. Morrison, et al, (Eds.), *Applied Developmental Psychology,* pp. 39–80. San Diego: Academic Press.

Bell, J. M. (1995a). What is "family"? Perturbations and possibilities. *Journal of Family Nursing,* 1:131–133.

Bell, J. M. (1995b). Wanted: Family nursing interventions. *Journal of Family Nursing,* 1:355–358.

Benson, M. J., & Deal, J. E. (1995). Bridging the individual and the family. *Journal of Marriage and the Family,* 57:561–566.

Berkey, K. M., & Hanson, S. M. H. (1991). Family nursing assessment/measurement instrumentation. In *Pocket Guide to Family Assessment and Intervention,* pp. 226–277. St. Louis, MO: Mosby Year Book.

Bussell, D. A. (1994). Ethical issues in observational family research. *Family Process,* 33:361–376.

Chesla, C. A. (1994). Parents' caring practices with schizophrenic offspring. In P. Benner (Ed.), *Interpretive Phenomenology: Embodiment, Caring, and Ethics in Health And Illness,* pp. 167–184. Thousand Oaks, CA: Sage.

Chesla, C. A. (1995). Hermeneutic phenomenology: An approach to understanding families. *Journal of Family Nursing,* 1:63–78.

Copeland, A. P., & White, K. M. (1991). Applied Social Research Methods Series, vol 27. *Studying Families.* Newbury Park, CA: Sage.

Denham, S. A. (1999a). Part 1: The definition and practice of family health. *Journal of Family Nursing,* 5:133–159.

Denham, S. A. (1999b). Part 2: Family health during and after death of a family member. *Journal of Family Nursing,* 5:160–183.

Denham, S. A. (1999c). Part 3: Family health in an economically disadvantaged population. *Journal of Family Nursing,* 5:184–213.

Feetham, S. L. (1984). Family research: Issues and directions for nursing. In H. H. Werley & J. J. Fitzpatrick (Eds.), *Annual Review of Nursing Research,* pp. 3–26. New York: Springer.

Feetham, S. L. (1990). Conceptual and methodological issues in research of families. In J. M. Bell, et al. (Eds.), *The Cutting Edge of Family Nursing,* pp. 35–49. Calgary, AB: Family Nursing Unit Publications.

Feetham, S. L. (1999). The future in family nursing is genetics and it is now. *Journal of Family Nursing,* 5:3–9.

Fisher, L., et al. (1985). Alternative strategies for creating "relational" family data. *Family Process,* 24:213–224.

Fisher, L., et al. (1990). Advancing a family perspective in health research: Models & methods. *Family Process,* 29:177–189.

Frank, A. W. (1995). Further reflections on illness (Review essay). *Journal of Family Nursing,* 1:420–426.

Ganong, L. H. (1996). Intimate outsider or unwelcome intruder? Response to Virginia Hayes's critique of "Current trends and issues in family nursing research." *Journal of Family Nursing,* 2:92–97.

Ganong, L. H. (1995). Current trends and issues in family nursing research. *Journal of Family Nursing,* 1:171–206.

Gilliss, C. L. (1983). The nurse as a unit of analysis: Strategies for the nurse researcher. *Advances in Nursing Science,* 5:50–59.

Gilliss, C. L. (1989). Family research in nursing. In Gilliss, C. L., et al. (Eds.) *Toward a Science of Family Nursing,* pp. 37–63. Menlo Park, CA: Addison-Wesley.

Gilliss, C. L., et al. (1990). Improving family functioning after cardiac surgery: A randomized trial. *Heart and Lung,* 19:648–654.

Gilliss, C. L., (1991). Family nursing research theory and Practice. *Image: Journal of Nursing Scholarship,* 23, 12–22.

Glaser, B., & Strauss, A. (1967). *The Discovery of Grounded Theory.* Chicago: Aldine.

Hanson, J. M. H., & Boyd, G. T. (1996). *Family health care nursing: theory, practice and research.* Philadelphia: FA Davis.

Hartrick, G. A., & Lindsey, A. E. (1995). Part 2: The lived experience of family: A contextual approach to family nursing practice. *Journal of Family Nursing,* 1:148–170.

Hayes, V. E. (1993). Nursing science in family care, 1984–1990. In S. L. Feetham, et al. (Eds.) *The Nursing of Families: Theory, Research, Education, Practice,* pp. 18–29. Newbury Park, CA: Sage.

Hayes, V. E. (1995). Response to L. H. Ganong: "Current trends and issues in family nursing research." *Journal of Family Nursing,* 1: 207–212.

Houck, G. M. (1999). The measurement of child characteristics from infancy to toddlerhood: Temperament, developmental competence, social competence, and self-concept. Issues in *Comprehensive Pediatric Nursing,* 22:101–127.

Houck, G. M., et al. (1991). Maternal depression and locus of control orientation as predictors of dyadic play behavior. *Infant Mental Health Journal,* 12:347–360.

Kelly, M. L., et al. (1992). Determinants of disciplinary practices in low-income black mothers. *Child Development,* 63:573–582.

Knafl, K. A. (1992). Family outcomes: Family-practitioner interface. In U.S. Department of Health and Human Services (Ed.), *Patient Outcomes Research: Examining the Effectiveness of Nursing Practice* (NIH Publication No. 93–3411, pp. 97–102). Proceedings of a conference sponsored by the National Center for Nursing Research, September 1991. Rockville, MD: U.S. Department of Health and Human Services.

Knafl, K. A. (1998). Meeting the challenges of chronic illness for children and families: Research implications and future directions. In M. E. Broome, et al. (Eds.) *Children and Families in Health and Illness,* pp. 236–245. Thousand Oaks, CA: Sage.

Knafl, K. A., et al. (1995). Learning from stories: Parents' accounts of the pathway to diagnosis. *Pediatric Nursing,* 21:411–415.

Leininger, M. M. (1985). Ethnography and ethnonursing: Models and modes of qualitative data analysis. In M. M. Leininger (Ed.) *Qualitative Research Methods in Nursing,* pp. 33–71. Orlando, FL: Grune & Stratton.

Lewis, F. M. (1993). Psychosocial transitions and the family's work in adjusting to cancer. Seminars in *Oncology Nursing,* 9:127–129.

Lewis, F. M., et al. (1993). The family's functioning with newly diagnosed breast cancer in the mother: The development of an explanatory model. *Journal of Behavioral Medicine,* 16:351–370.

Lewis, F. M., et al. (1996). The functioning of single women with breast cancer and their school-aged children. *Cancer Practice: a Multidisciplinary Journal of Cancer Care,* 4:15–24.

Miller, B. C. (1986). Family studies text series, vol 4. *Family Research Methods.* Beverly Hills, CA: Sage.

Miller, R. B., & Wright, D. W. (1995). Detecting and correcting attrition bias in longitudinal family research. *Journal of Marriage and the Family,* 57:921–929.

Moriarty, H. J., et al. (1995). Key issues in cross-cultural family research. *Journal of Family Nursing,* 1:359–381.

Motzer, S. A., et al. (1997). Recruitment and retention of families in clinical trials with longitudianl designs. *Western Journal of Nursing Research,* 19:314–333.

Olsen, S. F., et al. (1999). Support, communication, and hardiness in families with children with disabilities. *Journal of Family Nursing,* 5:275–291.

Oxley, G. M., & Weekes, D. P. (1997). Experiences of pregnant African American adolescents: Meanings, perception, appraisal, and coping. *Journal of Family Nursing,* 3:167–188.

Poirier, S., & Ayres, L. (1997). Endings, secrets, and silences: Overreading in narrative inquiry. *Research in Nursing & Health,* 20:551–557.

Polit, D. F., & Hungler, B. P. (1987). *Nursing Research: Principles and Methods,* ed 3. Philadelphia: Lippincott.

Robinson, C. A. (1995). Unifying distinctions for nursing research with persons and families. *Journal of Family Nursing,* 1:8–29.

Ryan, E. A., & Hayman, L. L. (1996). The role of the family coordinator in longitudinal research: Strategies to recruit and retain families. *Journal of Family Nursing,* 2:325–335.

Sandelowski, M. (1986). The problem of rigor in qualitative research. *Advances in Nursing Science,* 8(3):27–37.

Smith, T. E., & Graham, P. B. (1995). Socioeconomic stratification in family resarch. *Journal of Marriage and the Family,* 57:930–940.

Uphold C. R., & Strickland, O. L. (1989). Issues related to

the unit of analysis in family nursing research. *Western Journal of Nursing Research,* 11:405–417.

Whall, A. L., & Loveland-Cherry, C. J. (1993). Family unit-focused research: 1984–1991. In H. H. Werley & J. J. Fitzpatrick (Eds.), *Annual Review of Research in Nursing,* pp. 227–247. New York: Springer.

Wilson, S., & Morse, J. M. (1991). Living with a wife undergoing chemotherapy. *Image: Journal of Nursing Scholarship,* 23:78–84.

Woods, N. F., et al. (1989). Living with cancer: Family experiences. *Cancer Nursing,* 12:28–33.

Wright, L. M., & Leahey, M. (2000). *Nurses and Families: A Guide to Family Assessment and Intervention,* ed 3. Philadelphia: F. A. Davis.

Focus On

FAMILY STRUCTURE, FUNCTION, AND PROCESS

This chapter provides a foundation for the study of family health care. The family is conceptualized as a social institution, a social system, and a social group (Eshleman, 1997). In our society, these three aspects of the family are constantly evolving. Multiple types of families coexist. Each has its unique strengths and weaknesses. Each affects the health of its members and, in turn, is affected by their health. The nurse needs to understand this relationship to provide effective family health care.

To promote the understanding of the family as a social institution, family structure is analyzed. Family structure refers to the individuals who make up the family, the connections between them, and the connections between the family and other social systems. This chapter includes a cogent discussion of family composition, types of families, family size, and the family's social network.

An analysis of family function promotes the understanding of the family as an institution and as a social system. This chapter explores the purpose or function the family serves in relation to individual family members, to the family as a whole, to other social systems, and to society. The relationship between structure and function is explored. The impact of the family system on health status is emphasized.

Finally, this chapter analyzes the family as a social group. Interactional processes that make families unique are analyzed. The roles of family members are examined. Sources of role strain are identified; means to alleviate role strain are considered. Communication, power, and marital satisfaction are the topics that complete the discussion of family process.

Chapter 4

FAMILY STRUCTURE, FUNCTION, AND PROCESS

Naomi R. Ballard

OUTLINE

Family Structure
Overview
Composition
Types
Size
Marital Dissolution
Social Network
Nursing Implications

Function
Overview
Family as a Social System
Function in Society
Nursing Implications

Family Process
Overview
Roles
Communication
Power
Decision Making
Marital Satisfaction
Coping Strategies
Nursing Implications

OBJECTIVES

On completion of this chapter, the reader will be able to:

- Identify the major limitation underlying the analysis of family structure, function, and process.
- Describe four types of family structure present in the American society in the late 20th century.
- Analyze the relationship between family structure and health status.
- Identify four functional prerequisites of the family system.
- Identify two functions of the American family in the late 20th century.
- Analyze the relationship between family function and health status.

- Describe eight familial roles.
- Identify five sources of role strains and five mechanisms to alleviate the strains.
- Differentiate between effective and ineffective familial communication.
- Analyze the relationship between familial power and decision making.
- Analyze the nursing implications of alterations in family structure, function, and process.

Does the family have a future? This question has preoccupied lay people, social scientists, and health professionals for at least four decades (Bane, 1976: Otto, 1970; Spanier, 1989). The demographic and social changes that the family is undergoing are viewed, by many, as indicators of the family's instability, if not its impending demise. These arguments are based on myths about what a traditional family is supposed to be but, in reality, never was. Coontz's (1988, 1992, 1997) historical analyses of the American family document an ongoing evolution in family structure, function, and processes. Change is the norm, not the exception. This is true both for the family as an institution in society and for individual family units, which undergo dynamic changes throughout their life cycle. Change enables the family to continue to play a viable role in society.

The family is, or should be, the primary unit of health care. The structure, function, and process of the individual family unit influence and are influenced by the health status of the individuals in the family and the health of the family unit. For example, the breadth of a family's social network is a determinant of when and how a child gets chicken pox, and a child with a contagious disease limits the parents' ability to meet their social responsibilities. Family health care requires a multidisciplinary knowledge base. This foundation enables nurses to assess the family's health status, ascertain the effect of the family on individuals' health status, predict the impact of alterations in health status on the family system, and work with the family in the development and implementation of an action plan to improve health.

Nurses also need to understand the role of the family as a social institution. The family is linked to almost every other institution within society; consequently, understanding family change requires knowledge of the historical, social, cultural, economic, political, and psychological context in which change occurs (see Chapter 1). This facilitates understanding the effect of change on the health of the individual, the family, and society.

Any analysis of family structure, function, and process is limited by the knowledge on which it is based. Despite the predominance of nontraditional families in American society, little is known about them. The traditional nuclear family remains the standard by which an individual family is evaluated (Ganong, et al, 1990; Spanier, 1989). Indeed, most of our knowledge about the American family is based on research of nuclear families. In the future, researchers need to focus more on nontraditional families; for example, families of lesbians and gays (Allen & Demo, 1995). This would provide a more comprehensive knowledge base.

This chapter analyzes changes in family structure, function, and process that have implications for the delivery of family health care. The discussion of family structure focuses on the decline of the nuclear family and the emergence of other family types in the American society in the late 20th century. The function of the family in relation to the American society and to the maintenance of the family system is analyzed. In the discussion of family processes, changes in the delineation and enactment of familial roles are examined and the effects of communication, power, and decision making on the enactment of familial roles are explored.

FAMILY STRUCTURE

Overview

The most clear-cut change in the American family during the past few decades has been in its structure. Family structure is the ordered set of relationships among the parts of the family and between the family and other social systems. In determining the family structure, the nurse needs to identify the individuals that make up the family, the relationships between them, and the relationships between the family and other social systems. A family's patterns of organization tend to be relatively stable over time. However, they are modified gradually throughout the family life cycle and radically by divorce or death. In a rapidly changing society, several types of family structure may coexist.

Norms that control family relationships are not clearly prescribed by the culture. They evolve in the process of family interaction. Each family type has its strengths and weaknesses, which directly or indirectly affect the health of the individuals in the family and the family unit.

Composition

When do a set of individuals become a family? Traditionally, the family was organized around the biological function of reproduction; therefore, the family was composed of a father, a mother, and their biological children. Throughout American history, this has been the most common type of family (Bane, 1976; Coontz, 1988, 1992, 1997; Degler, 1980). However, during the past two decades, the reproductive function has become increasingly separated from the family (Robertson, 1991) and defining a family has become more difficult. The criteria most often used to define a family are structure and function (Winch, 1977). When the family is defined according to its structure, the positions that the individuals in the family assume and the relationship between them are emphasized. The U.S. Bureau of the Census uses this criterion in its definition of a household, a concept that overlaps with that of family. When a functional criterion is used to define family, the individuals making up the family must engage in activities that are considered familial; for example, child-rearing. A third option, which ignores both the structural and functional criteria, is that the family is whatever the set of individuals says it is. In reality, the definition of a family may be less important to the individuals who compose a family than it is to the scholars who study families. Basically, individuals organize themselves into families in relation to cultural prescriptions and basic human needs. As cultural prescriptions change, families change.

Types

The traditional family composed of a husband and wife, married for the first time, and their biological children is no longer the predominant type of family in the American society. The U.S. Bureau of the Census (1998) currently uses five variables to describe the various types of households and families: marital status, gender of sexual partners, presence of children, parentage of children, and age of children. For example, a remarried or blended family contains a male and female, at least one of whom has been married before. They may or may not have children living in the household. If they do, the children may be his, hers, or theirs. The children may be under or over age 18. Another type of family may be composed of two unmarried men or women who have no children.

Married Couples

Households headed by married couples are undergoing marked change in their structure. The number of households without children is rising as a result of the increased length of the postparental stage of the family life cycle. Furthermore, in approximately one-third of the households headed by married couples, one or both of the spouses has been married previously (Spanier & Furstenberg, 1987). Remarried or blended families and stepfamilies differ from traditional families both in their interaction with children and in their larger social network.

Single-Parent Families

The single-parent family is one in which the head of the household has never been or is not currently married. Single-parent families make up 27 percent of all families with children under 18 years of age (U.S. Bureau of the Census, 1998). This is because of the high divorce rate, the increase in births to adolescents, and the limited availability of marital partners in portions of the population. Single parenthood is particularly common among African-Americans (Jayakody, et al, 1993). Fifty-seven percent of black children under age 18 reside in households headed by their mothers. This is related, in part, to the lack of black men in the marriage market. The high mortality rate, high level of incarceration, and limited opportunities in the labor market for black men reduce the marital options for black women (Fossett & Kiecolt, 1993). Thirty percent of Hispanic children and 21 percent of white children reside in households headed by their mothers (U.S. Bureau of the Census, 1998). Five percent of African-American children, 7 percent of Hispanic children, and 6 percent of white children live in single-parent families headed by their father. Few differences have been found between children raised in single-parent families headed by mothers and those headed by fathers (Downey et al, 1998). However, the single-parent structure alters the relationship between men and women

(Guttentag and Secord, 1983) and between parents and children (Aquilino, 1994; Cooksey & Fondell, 1996; Dawson, 1991; Demo, et al, 1987; Hanson, et al, 1996; MacDonald & DeMaris, 1995; Thomson, et al, 1992). In addition, single-parent families have high rates of poverty; this has ominous implications both for the children and for the future of the American society.

Cohabiting Couples

An alternative for sexual partners who do not wish to marry or who, because of legal proscription, cannot marry is cohabitation. Since 1970, the number of unmarried heterosexual couples who live together has increased markedly (Cherlin, 1992). By 1986, 6 percent of all unmarried adults in the United States were cohabiting (Glick, 1988). Cohabitation has not resulted in a decrease in the marriage rate: 9 out of 10 Americans eventually marry. However, cohabitation has altered the timing of marriage. Many young adults are postponing marriage until their middle or late twenties or even their thirties. In 1998, the median age for marriage for men was 26.7 years and 25 years for women (U.S. Bureau of the Census, 1998). Cohabitation seems to be a part of the courtship process, not an alternative to marriage. Ross (1995) maintains that cohabitation is just one piece of the continuum that constitutes marital status: no partner, partner outside the household, living with partner in the household, and living with married partner in the household. Cohabitation before marriage is associated with a higher divorce rate; moreover, divorced people are more likely to cohabit (Brown & Booth, 1996). In 1990, 11 percent of the population between ages 40 and 59 were cohabiting (Chevan, 1996); the majority were divorced.

Little is known about the cohabitation patterns of homosexual couples. Since 1950, data on unmarried and unrelated adults of the same sex, aged 25 or older, who share a household have been included in the census. The data are limited, however, because these householders may or may not be sexual partners. Nevertheless, the number of cohabiting homosexual couples is assumed to be half as numerous as unmarried heterosexual couples (Glick, 1988). Currently, marriage is not a legal alternative for homosexual couples.

Size

The size of households has decreased during the past few decades. This is related to the decline in fertility and mortality rates (Santi, 1987; Teachman, 1987). The decline in birth rate has reduced the proportion of large families, and the reduced mortality rate has increased the proportion of postparental families. In addition, more individuals are choosing to live alone. In 1998, approximately 28 million households were composed of one person (U.S. Bureau of the Census, 1998). The only trend that seems to offset this decline in household size is the tendency for adult children to return temporarily to their parents' home. Currently, 59 percent of men and 48 percent of women between 18 to 24 years of age live at home (U.S. Bureau of the Census, 1998). Although this percentage includes college students living in dormitories, it shows a marked increase since 1960.

Marital Dissolution

The change that has had the most impact on family structure is the high rate of divorce. The divorce rate rose from the middle of the 19th century until the 1980s (Cherlin, 1992). By 1974, more marriages ended in divorce than in death. In the 1980s, the divorce rate began to decline slightly but remained higher than in the 1960s. From 1960 to 1980, the rise in the divorce rate was greater than would have been predicted by the trend line. What accounted for this? Divorces tend to increase after wars and decrease in times of economic difficulty. Therefore, the Vietnam War, the burgeoning economy, and a cultural emphasis on individualism probably contributed to the high divorce rate from 1960 to 1980. In addition, the options available for women outside of marriage improved. Certainly, people were not disenchanted with marriage, because the majority remarried. However, their expectations for marriage may have exceeded reality.

At the current divorce rate, about half of all marriages end in separation or divorce. This means that two-fifths of all children will experience disruption in their parents' marriage by age 16. The majority of them will live in a single-parent household headed by their mother for at least 5 years before their mother remarries or they reach age 18. The social and economic consequences of the divorce rate for women and children has been well documented (Weitzman, 1985). The long-term impact of high rates of marital dissolution on the adult children and on society is just beginning to become apparent (Amato & Booth, 1996; Aquilino, 1994; Cherlin, 1999; Spitze, et al, 1994).

Social Network

People outside of the home who engage in activities of an affective or material nature with the members of the household constitute the family's social network. The presence of a strong social network improves the health status and life satisfaction of the family members. For an individual, the best single predictor of the size and richness of the social network is education. That is, better-educated individuals are more likely to have a substantial social network. In turn, this will benefit the family. Familial social networks are altered with changes in marital status, the family's developmental level, and the family's geographical location; for example, an individual's social network declines markedly after divorce or separation. Even remarried or reblended families have a smaller social network than traditional families. The reason for this is unclear. Indeed, because of contact with ex-spouses and their families, remarried or blended families might be expected to have a larger social network.

As social systems, families operate on a continuum from a closed to an open system in their interaction with the outside world (Kantor & Lehr, 1975). A closed family system, functioning in isolation from other social systems and social institutions, is impossible to sustain. However, a few types of families, for example, cult members and survivalists, strive to achieve isolation from the larger society. More commonly, families who operate as a more closed system maintain only essential contact with the outside world. Their primary interaction with the outside world is through their work. They send their children to school, but they do not become involved in school activities. Their drapes remained pulled; their doors closed. They have no visitors and may have only a nodding acquaintance with their neighbors. They may not even have a radio or television. Under ordinary circumstances, the closed family may be able to maintain homeostasis, but it may be poorly equipped to deal with change in a heterogeneous society or with the stress of an illness. At the opposite extreme, an open family system encourages interchange with the outside world. They are involved in multiple activities, both inside and outside the family. Visitors are encouraged, drapes are open, lights on, and doors may be unlocked. Indeed, the open family system's boundaries may become blurred, leaving them vulnerable to breakdown of the family structure. Most families lie somewhere between these extremes. They have clearly defined boundaries, but enough flexibility to be able to capitalize on their contact with the outside world.

The family's social network provides both instrumental and expressive support. This is particularly true of the extended family, which, contrary to popular myth, remains the major source of social support for American families. Intergenerational interaction is the norm, not the exception (Stull & Borgatta, 1987). This source of support is especially important for frail elderly persons and for single parents.

Most elderly people who need either material or affective support are able to depend on family members to provide it. The majority of elderly persons live within a short distance of at least one child. Even those who live 3000 miles from their children usually maintain contact. However, the availability of this support diminishes with increasing age of the recipient. As many as one-third of white urban elderly persons in their eighties and nineties have no family members who can respond when needed (Johnson & Troll, 1996).

Families seem to go out of their way to help single parents (Spitze et al, 1994). This is particularly true for black mothers; an extensive system of kin networks has been documented in black communities. However, the prevalence of aid to black single parents may be overstated. Despite the presence of the extensive network, only one-quarter of never-married mothers receive financial assistance and less than one-fifth receive child care help (Jayakody, et al, 1993). In contrast to single-parent families, married-parent families have the advantage of being able to seek support from both families of origin. To determine the viability of a family's social network, evaluation of data on the type of support provided, the proximity of the network, the interaction within the network, and the affinity of the kin is necessary.

Nursing Implications

Every family experiences strain in dealing with both daily hassles and crises. Households headed by married couples usually have more resources to draw on in dealing with day-to-day strains. Single-parent families, especially those headed by women, are particularly vulnerable to strain because they have fewer resources in terms of time, energy, and money with which to cope. Cohabiting families, both heterosexual and homosexual, have to cope with the additional stressors of social censure and legal restraints. These limit the coping strategies that they can invoke.

Nurses, as citizens and as health professionals, need to play an active role in enacting social policies to reduce strain on families. For example, more available child care would reduce the burden of many families. In addition, families are being asked to assume more responsibilities for health care. They are expected to care for acutely and chronically ill family members, who were once cared for by health professionals. This portends disaster for families already strained to the limit. Until social policies are enacted that reduce the burden of families, nurses, through counseling and education, need to help families develop more adaptive interaction patterns and more effective coping strategies (Bomar, 1996; Leahey & Wright, 1987a, 1987b; Wright & Leahey, 2000, 1987; Vaughn-Cole, et al, 1998).

FUNCTION

Overview

Family function is the purpose that the family serves in relation to the individual, other social systems, and society. However, family function is very difficult to describe. One quickly gets caught in circular reasoning: Family function is a consequence of family structure, but the structure exists to fulfill one or more functions. In everyday life, the function of the family is questioned only when a social need, for example, social control, is not being met. Social control provides an excellent example of the difficulty involved in describing family function. Recently, the family's function as an instrument of social control has been questioned. Several social trends, including the increase in violence in our society, the increase in substance abuse, and the increase in teenage pregnancies, have been attributed to the family's ineffectiveness in transmitting values. Unfortunately, this is a simplistic explanation for complex problems because it ignores the interaction of the family and other social institutions. The complexity of these relationships makes describing the function of the family difficult.

To ascertain the effect of the family on the individual's and the family's health status, the function of the American family must be analyzed at two levels. At the microlevel, the consequences of the function of an individual family unit on the growth and development of its members and on the maintenance of the family system are analyzed. On the macrolevel, the effect of the family as a social institution is examined.

Family as a Social System

Functional Prerequisites

For the family to meet society's needs, the family unit must maintain its integrity as a social system. To survive as a social system, the family as a social system must meet certain functional prerequisites: adaptation, goal attainment, integration, pattern maintenance, and tension management (Parsons, 1951).

Adaptation

Adaptation refers to the necessity for the family to accommodate its external and internal environments. The external environment includes the physical environment, other social systems with which the family interacts, and the predominant culture. The internal environment is composed of the family members as biological organisms and as personalities. To adapt, the family must carry out a range of tasks (Bell & Vogel, 1960). Therefore, the family must obtain the resources, the skills, and the motivation to perform the tasks. For example, one of the basic human needs of the family members is to obtain nourishment. One or more family members has to assume the responsibility for making the money to buy or to grow the food; someone has to purchase and cook food that is compatible with the family members' biological needs and their cultural prescriptions; the family members have to be motivated to eat the food; and someone has to clean up afterwards. Failure to perform these tasks puts the individual family members in physical jeopardy and leads to the breakdown of the family as a social system.

Goal Attainment

The family as a social system needs to define its goals and the means to attain them. This is not always conscious. Sometimes, the goals are inferred from the actions of the family members. At other times, the actions of the family members seem incongruent with identified goals. For example, many parents state that spending quality time with their children is a top priority. However, when caught in the bind between the demands of their job and their family, they may attend to their jobs first. In identifying and attaining goals, the family member who has the most influence in the decision making process may vary from situation to situation. However, over time, the leadership structure of the family is fairly stable. Leadership residing in the parental unit tends to promote goal attainment of the family; however, the commitment and motivation of all family members is required.

Integration

Integration, unlike adaptation and goal attainment, refers strictly to activities within the family system. Integration is the means by which a family acquires the cohesion, solidarity, and identity that enable the family members to maintain close relationships over a period of time. The overt and covert expression of affection promotes family cohesion, as do family rituals and celebrations. Symbols of family solidarity include photograph albums, heirlooms, and favorite jokes. Family ties operate to prevent the disintegration of the family system and to motivate family members to abide by the family's norms.

Pattern Maintenance and Tension Management

Like integration, pattern maintenance and tension management are functional prerequisites that deal primarily with the internal state of the family social system. In their interactions with each other, family members develop expectations about how each other should behave. For a family to survive, the members must agree, to a certain extent, on the values that regulate family activities. They may or may not be conscious; but they must be flexible enough to allow for some deviation. For example, a family who expects everyone to show up for a 6 p.m. dinner must make allowances when a family member is delayed by a traffic jam. Furthermore, the family's value system and behavioral expectations need to be modified as the family develops. For example, the constraints placed on a child's travel outside the home are reduced as the child ages.

In summary, each individual family unit has to meet four functional prerequisites: adaptation, goal attainment, integration, and pattern maintenance and tension management. If the function of the family does not enable it to meet these requirements, the family dissolves and is unable to serve the needs of the society.

Function in Society

Overview

Before industrialization, the family played a much larger role in society. It was the primary source of economic production, education, and health care. Later, other institutions, for example, schools and hospitals, have assumed many of the functions that were once the responsibility of the family. Today, the economic and reproductive functions of the family are undergoing change. The primary functions of the family are the socialization of children and the stabilization of adult personalities (Parsons and Bales, 1955). Through these two functions, the family has a major effect on the health of its members.

Economic Function

During the 20th century, the most obvious change in family function was related to economics. In the early stages of American history, the household was the major source of commodity production (Coontz, 1988). Economic relationships within the household reflected familial relationships. The corporate family worked under the leadership of a household head, usually a man. However, women, who because of death of their husbands or fathers had assumed the position as family corporate head, exerted more power than they had before or have since. With the emergence of capitalism in the early 19th century, the household, with its patriarchal system, served as a source of workers. The household head, who received the wage for the family, contributed family members as workers for the fledgling industries. This left a gap at home; eventually married women returned home to resume their domestic duties. Consequently, young women, unmarried women, and men constituted the labor pool until World War II. With the ascent of capitalism in the late 19th and early 20th centuries, the division between work and home—men's work and women's work—increased. However, during World War II, many women moved back into the labor force. After the war, the majority of women returned home; but some elected to remain in the labor force. With the shift from an industrial to a service economy, the number of women in the labor force has increased. This reflects not only the need for their services, but the inability of many men to earn a family wage in the evolving economy. Young men, in particular, are experiencing a worsening of their economic position and older men are leaving the labor force in record numbers. In 56 percent of married couples, both the husband and wife are in the labor force. Sixty-eight percent of women who have children under 18 years of age in the home work outside the home (U.S. Bureau of the Census, 1998). Families are no longer a source of commodity production. Instead, their economic role is that of consumer of goods and services. This plays an important function in keeping the economy viable.

Reproduction

In the past, the primary function of the family in society was the regulation of reproduction. Families today, however, have less control over reproduction (Robertson, 1991) and seem unable or unwilling to control reproduction even among their family members. In the United States, more than a million adolescents become pregnant each year; approximately half of these pregnancies result in live births (Kalmuss, et al, 1992). This essentially means that children are having children. Because only about 5 percent of pregnant teenagers choose adoption, teen-aged mothers and their babies are either integrated into their families of origin or left to fend for themselves. Adolescent childbearing may increase as religious and legal threats to abortion increase. For centuries, the state, religion, and the family have fought for the right to control reproduction. Almost three decades ago, in the *Roe v. Wade* decision, the U.S. Supreme Court ruled that, during the first trimester of pregnancy, the decision to have an abortion should be left solely to the woman and her physician (Leslie & Korman, 1985). However, the *Roe v. Wade* decision has been consistently challenged. Many argue that it negates the rights of the unborn child and the father. The ethical dilemmas mirrored in the abortion controversy are compounded by technological advances in reproduction. Artificial insemination by husband or donor, in vitro fertilization, and artificial embryonation, in which a woman other than the wife donates an egg for fertilization, further remove the family from control of the reproductive process. In some cases, fertilization has moved out of the bedroom into the laboratory—out of the body and into the petri dish. Gestation may take place within the biological mother, even if she is 60 years of age, or in a surrogate. Religious, legal, and technological challenges to the family's control over reproduction will increase in the years ahead.

Socialization of Children

An important function of the family in the American society is the socialization of children. Through this process, children acquire the social and psychological skills to take their place in the adult world. On the parents' part, this seems to involve a combination of social support and social control. In the American society, traditional families composed of a man, a woman, and their biological children seem to be more effective than nontraditional families in the socialization of children. In 1998, nuclear families with children under 18 years of age constituted 36 percent of all family households (U.S. Bureau of the Census, 1998). These children seem to have fewer health and behavioral problems than children reared in nontraditional families (Aquilino, 1994; Dawson, 1991). Moreover, the hierarchy of the nuclear family, with its formal authority structure, seems to be more effective in preparing children for their adult roles (Nock, 1988). The attitudes and values learned in dealing with authority figures in the family are internalized. Consequently, the child reared in a traditional family is more likely to be effective at school or work, because achievement requires functioning in a hierarchical environment.

According to Nock (1988), children in nontraditional families are less likely to internalize the attitudes and values needed for success. The generational boundaries in single-parent families are not as clearly defined. Single parents tend to be more lax disciplinarians. Indeed, a working single parent of school-aged children is probably too tired to do otherwise. In most cases, support from noncustodial spouses is minimal. Children from single-parent homes have less success in school, lower earnings, and lower occupational prestige than children from intact, two-parent families (Nock, 1988). They also have a higher rate of divorce and out-of-wedlock births. Of course, the effects of the nontraditional structure on the socialization process needs to be considered in the context of economic deprivation and psychological stress. The presence of a second adult in the home, for example, a grandmother, helps offset the deleterious effects of being reared by a single parent (Thomson, et al, 1992).

Remarried or blended families also seem to experience more problems with child-rearing. The role of a stepparent is not clearly defined and, frequently, has many negative connotations. Stepparents show less warmth and communicate less well with stepchildren (Thomson, et al, 1992). They participate in fewer child-related activities. This does not seem to change over time. The lack of engagement of stepparents may contribute to the development of more behavioral problems in children from remarried or blended families. However, it does not seem to affect the achievement levels of the offspring. Most likely, remarried or blended families have a hierarchical structure that is similar to traditional families.

Stabilization of Adult Personalities

Another function of the American family is the stabilization of adult personalities. Married men and women have better physical and mental health than never-married, separated, divorced, or widowed persons (Barnett, et al, 1992; Gove, 1973; Hahn, 1993; Verbrugge, 1979). Older persons who have never married have a higher rate of mental disorders than married individuals of similar age. Widows are five times more likely to be institutionalized in long-term care facilities; separated or divorced persons are ten times more likely (Stull & Borgatta, 1987). Married persons have much lower age-standardized death rates. Unmarried persons have death rates above average from cirrhosis of the liver, pneumonia, motor vehicle accidents, suicide, and homicide. However, the cause of the inverse relationship between marriage and poor health for both men and women is unclear.

Are healthier people more likely to get and stay married? Or, does the psychological stress from the loss of a marriage increase one's susceptibility to illness? Marriage seems to have a buffering effect on the health status of both men and women, but the effect seems stronger for men. The marital role, both as spouse and as father, may be more important to men's physical and mental health (Barnett, et al, 1992) than to women's. In a satisfactory marriage, both men and women receive psychological support from each other, which may improve their immunological response. In addition, married men and women are more likely to engage in health-enhancing activities (Hahn, 1993). This is particularly true of married men, who tend to rely on their wives in many health-enhancing activities; for example, the provision of a balanced diet. Married women have a higher family income, are more likely to own a home, and are more likely to have health insurance than single women. Because socioeconomic status is positively related to health status, it may be a confounding variable in the relationship between marriage and health (Rogers, 1995).

What effect does individual happiness have on the relationship between marriage and health? A decrease in marital satisfaction may offset the buffering effect of marriage on health status. Traditionally, personal happiness has been positively correlated with marriage. However, in the past two decades, the difference in happiness between married and never-married persons has decreased (Lee, et al, 1991). Among never-married persons, both men and women demonstrate an increase in personal happiness. Among married persons, women, particularly young women, report a decrease in personal happiness. This change is most pronounced among employed mothers, who are trying to balance multiple demanding roles. However, married people still tend to be happier than unmarried people. The increased economic, psychological, and social support available to married people serves to stabilize their personalities and, consequently, to enhance their health.

Nursing Implications

Nursing interventions to promote family functioning vary with the degree of strain faced by the family. A family that is unable to meet the functional prerequisites of a social system—adaptation, goal attainment, integration, and pattern maintenance and tension management—is in danger of disintegrating. Family therapy by a nurse in advanced practice or another health professional is necessary (Bolechek & McCloskey, 1992). Most families benefit from health teaching or counseling that promotes family health. Instruction on safety, nutrition, exercise, stress management, sleep hygiene, child-rearing, and sexuality should be included (Bomar, 1996; also see Chapter 9). However, health teaching is unlikely to enhance the family's protective health function, unless it is tailored to the specific learning needs of the family and the cultural context. Nurses may also strengthen the family's social support system through the use of themselves as therapists and through the identification of other support services. This is particularly important during times of family transition; for example, the onset of chronic illness.

FAMILY PROCESS

Overview

Family process is the ongoing interaction between the family members, through which they accomplish their instrumental and expressive tasks. In part, this is what makes families unique. Families with the same structure and function may interact differently. Family process, at least in the short term, seems to have a greater effect on the family's health status than family structure and function and, in turn, to be more affected by alterations in health status. It certainly has the most implications for nursing action. For example, for chronically ill persons, the most important determinant of a successful rehabilitation is the ability to assume one's familial roles. This often requires a great deal of adaptation from all family members, which is accomplished through communication, decision making, and other coping strategies. The familial power structure may or may not enhance this process. The success or failure of the adaptation process has an effect on marital satisfaction.

Roles

Role Delineation

Within the nuclear family, each position within the family, for example, husband or wife, has a number of roles attached to it. Each role is comprised of a set of expectations about what one *should* do. After a review of the family literature, Nye (1976) identified eight roles attached to the position of spouse:

1. Provider
2. Housekeeper
3. Child care giver
4. Socializer
5. Sexual partner
6. Therapist
7. Recreational organizer
8. Kinship member

Traditionally, the provider role has been assigned to the husband and the housekeeper and child care giver roles to the wife. However, with the changes in society and in family structure, the traditional enactment of these roles is not viable for many families. Consequently, in interacting with each other, the members of the family have to negotiate and to decide on their behavioral expectations. For example, a newly married couple has to decide who writes the thank-you notes after the wedding. According to the majority of the etiquette books, this is the bride's responsibility. Today, many couples decide that the bride writes thank-you notes to her kin; and the groom, to his. However, they do not make these decisions in isolation; they are influenced by the culture in which they live. For the nuclear family, many culturally prescribed behavioral expectations exist. When the norms are not met, social sanctions may occur; for example, the bride's grandmother may express her displeasure at what she perceives as a lack of social grace. At other times, legal sanctions are incurred, for example, when the parents leave their children alone while they are on vacation without arranging for their care. Nontraditional families, in which the roles are not traditionally proscribed, may actually have more freedom in the negotiation process. However, too often, they are subjected to social sanctions for even existing.

Role Enactment

PROVIDER ROLE

The actual behavior demonstrated by the family members in their various roles are not necessarily congruent with their expectations. The enactment of the provider role has undergone the most change in the past few decades. The proportion of households in which men were the sole breadwinners declined to 15 percent in 1988 (Wilkie, 1991). This is related to a decrease in the proportion of families with a man living in the house, an increase in number of families with no wage-earners, the growth in multiple-earner families, and the growth in number of families solely supported by someone other than a male householder. In industrialized nations, the participation of women in the labor force has increased dramatically (Kalleberg & Rosenfeld, 1990). Many families need more than one income to meet their basic needs. At the same time, the work conditions have become increasingly stressful for both men and women. Therefore, work obligations outside of the home increasingly impinge on the family members' ability to meet their familial role obligations.

HOUSEKEEPER AND CHILD CARE ROLE

Women, in particular, experience a great deal of role strain in balancing their provider role with other familial roles. That is because women continue to be responsible for most of the housekeeping and child care (Kalleberg & Rosenfeld, 1990; Perry-Jenkins & Folk, 1994; Pittman & Blanchard, 1996; Ward, 1993). Robinson and Milkie (1998, p. 206) state that ". . . many women continue to live as 'drudge' wives working full-time in the labor force and doing more than 60 percent of the housework." Husbands of employed wives spend only a small amount of additional time on housework; however, the proportion of time they spend increases because employed wives spend less time on housework (Kalleberg & Rosenfeld, 1990; McHale & Crouter, 1992). Women with children spend the most time on housework. Although husband's roles in child care are increasing, their focus tends to be on playing with the children, rather than meeting their basic needs. The time women spend fulfilling housekeeper and child care roles may be related, in part, to family income. Women with higher incomes spend less time on housekeeping and child care; they pay others to do it for them. Many women, however, earn less because of their familial responsibilities, and they have more familial responsibilities because they earn less. Thus, they are caught in a vicious circle.

Socialization Role

In relation to socialization of the children, the role expectations tend to be more egalitarian. The involvement of both parents is necessary for the development of healthy children, because the father-child relationship is qualitatively different than the mother-child relationship. However, the wife still assumes the larger share of the responsibility for the socialization of the children. Men seem to take more responsibility for the socialization of boys than of girls (Harris & Morgan, 1991).

After separation or divorce, the majority of children have little or no contact with nonresidence fathers (Seltzer, 1991). Fathers may limit contact with children for whom they do not have custody to protect themselves from loss or to avoid conflict. Fathers who visit and pay child support are more likely to be involved in child-rearing decisions; however, less than half of nonresidence fathers pay child support. When children are born outside of marriage, the fathers are even less likely to be involved.

Sexual Role

The sexual and therapeutic familial roles also require an egalitarian relationship between the adult partners, because, in a satisfactory relationship, each needs to play an active role in meeting the sexual and therapeutic needs of the other. The main predictor of an egalitarian sexual relationship seems to be socioeconomic status; more specifically, education. More highly educated women tend to be more assertive; more highly educated men, more sensitive and emotionally expressive (Francoeur, 1987). They are also more accepting of alternative sexual behaviors and tend to rate their sexual intimacy more positively. Women and men in lower socioeconomic classes are more likely to experience early sexual intercourse and to follow more traditional sexual practices.

Two other variables that alter sexual relationships are becoming more important in the American society. One is the increase in the number of ethnic groups with more traditional sexual values. The other is the decrease in the sex ratio; that is, the ratio of males to females. Guttentag and Secord (1983) argue that the sex ratio is correlated with sexual attitudes, values, and behaviors. The clear surplus of females in American society may contribute to an environment in which adultery is acceptable or normal, marriage is viewed as temporary, sexual liberation is encouraged, and women are encouraged to work outside the home (Francoeur, 1987). The relative impact of these two opposing trends is yet to be determined.

Therapeutic Role

The therapeutic role involves partners helping each other with intrafamilial and extrafamilial problems. This includes a willingness to share one's own concerns, the willingness to listen to others, active involvement in problem solving, and emotional support. It embodies what small-group theorists call the expressive role. However, families cannot depend on one member of the group to assume the expressive and another, the instrumental role. To survive as a unit, all members have to assume both roles at one time or another. One study of family roles found that over 60 percent of husbands and wives believed that they have a duty to enact the therapeutic role (Nye, 1976). Over three-fifths disapproved of a husband or wife who refused to help a spouse with a problem. Sixty-three percent of the men and 80 percent of the women in the study enacted the therapeutic role. The husbands and wives included in the study also thought that a family member who reacted with criticism to the person confiding the problem, who disclosed the problem to third parties, or who imposed solutions on the confider deserved verbal sanctions.

The therapeutic role includes supporting family members in activities that promote health and prevent disease. Individuals are more likely to engage in health-promoting activities, such as exercise, when accompanied by a significant other. When individuals become sick, they turn to family members for validation of their symptoms. One wife knew that it was time to seek medical help when her husband found her with all the doors and windows open despite freezing temperatures outside and said, "You're screwed up." This verified her own perceptions. Hyperthyroidism was her eventual diagnosis. In addition to supporting each other in seeking health care, family members also play a therapeutic role in helping the sick person to decide on treatment options. They frequently assist in the administration and evaluation of long-term treatments. Family support is a major determinant in rehabilitation. Individuals who are able to retain their familial roles are more likely to succeed in the rehabilitation process.

Recreational Role

Most recreation occurs with other family members (Hawks, 1991). However, the recreational role is not as culturally prescribed as many other familial roles. Families do not assign recreational responsibilities to a particular member. They do not care who does the planning, as long as it gets done. The quantity and types of recreation engaged in vary with the stages of the family life cycle. Families with a higher socioeconomic status are more active in formal, organized, and expensive activities; families with a lower socioeconomic status tend to rely more on inexpensive activities; for example, visiting relatives (Hawks, 1991). Recreation is also affected by the wife's participation in the labor force. When the woman works outside the home, social activities outside the family decrease, but intrafamily activities and commercial recreation are not as greatly affected (Carlson, 1976). The major complaint about recreation is the lack of time available for it (McCown, et al, 1989). Perceived satisfaction with leisure time is positively associated with marital sociability, satisfaction, stability, and intimacy (Hawks, 1991). The family's involvement in leisure time activities promotes integration of the family system. However, the recreation role is often the first to be dropped when the family is under stress.

Kinship Role

Enactment of the kinship role involves maintaining contact with the extended family and friends. According to Marks and McLanahan (1993, p. 482), "Women continue to function as family 'kinkeepers.'" Women maintain a higher level of interaction with the extended family than men; they give and receive more family help; and they tend to rely on parents, children, or siblings for support. Fathers in traditional families are more likely than men in nontraditional families to give instrumental social support to their parents and their children, including child care, transportation, and repairs to home or car. Nontraditional two-parent families tend to operate in a similar manner. Single fathers and single mothers are more likely to receive support from parents. On the other hand, mothers with a cohabiting partner are less likely to receive social support from parents. Cohabiting homosexual couples rely more heavily on networks of friends. Middle-aged and elderly parents receive help from and give help to their children. A high level of exchange occurs between middle-aged and elderly parents and daughters, even when the daughter is not a care giver (Walker & Pratt, 1991). Older adults tend to limit their help to their primary kin (Gallagher, 1994).

Role Competence

The competent performance of familial roles is a determinant of marital success. Blood and Wolfe (1960) hypothesized that the source of power in the marriage was related to the comparative resources that the husband and wife bring to the marriage. Competent enactment of familial roles is one of the primary resources that one brings to marriage (Bahr, 1976). It constitutes a reward to one's partner. The more rewards, for example, money, love, and status, one receives from a spouse, the more likely one is to comply when differences in opinions arise. Furthermore, the more rewards one receives from a spouse, the more likely one is to be satisfied in the marriage. If the exchange is inequitable, one or both spouses may seek other alternatives.

Role Strain

Sources

Lack of competence in role performance may be a result of role strain. Sources of role strain are cultural and interactional. According to Marks (1994), cultures that encourage equally positive commitments to all of one's roles generate less role strain. For example, if a culture values both work and parenting equally, little role strain occurs. However, O'Neill and Greenberger (1994) studied patterns of commitment to work and parenting and the study did not support Mark's hypothesis. Men experienced less role strain if they had low commitment to work and high commitment to parenting. O'Neill and Greenberger found no relationship between women's patterns of commitment to work and parenting and role strain, although women in professional and managerial jobs experienced less role strain. Interactional sources of role strain are related to difficulties in the delineation and enactment of familial roles. Heiss (1981) identified five sources of difficulties in the interaction process:

1. Inability to define the situation
2. Lack of role knowledge
3. Lack of role consensus
4. Role conflict
5. Role overload

All of these problems place a strain on the family system, but solutions to the problems differ greatly.

Inability to Define the Situation

The first source of role strain is the inability to define the situation. With changes in family structure and gender roles, family members increasingly encounter situations in which the guidelines for action are unclear. For example, a couple who has just begun dating has to decide who opens the car door. In the 1950s, the man automatically opened the door.

Single parents, stepparents, nonresident fathers, and cohabiting partners deal daily with situations for which there are no norms. What right does a stepparent have to discipline the new spouse's child? Is a nonresident father expected to teach his child about AIDS? What name or names go on the mailbox of cohabiting partners? Whether or not the issues are substantive, they present daily challenges to the people involved. One method of dealing with the difficulty is withdrawing from the situation, an alternative that many nonresident fathers choose. A second way of handling the problem is to redefine the situation. For instance, a newly blended family might decide to operate in the same way as a traditional family. Finally, family members might resort to trial and error. The cohabiting couple might put only one name on the mailbox. If this presents problems, the option to change their strategy exists. If a solution cannot be found, family members suffer the consequences of role strain.

Lack of Role Knowledge

A second source of role strain is the inability to choose a role, either because the family members do not know a role appropriate to the situation or they know several and have no basis for choosing among them. For example, in the American society, many people are not taught how to be parents. They may not know how to keep their children from running over the neighbor's dog with their bicycles. Anticipatory socialization in the care of chronically ill family members is also inadequate. Whether the individual is learning how to be a parent or a care giver, "on the job" training may be required. Knowledge may be acquired by observation of peers; reflexive role-taking, in which individuals deduce what others expect them to do in the situation; or explicit instruction. In the case of parents and care givers, opportunities to observe peers may be limited and other family members may not have the knowledge to help; therefore, other means of obtaining the information must be explored. These might include classes in child care, self-help groups, and instruction from health professionals. If individuals are unable to figure out their roles in a situation, their problem-solving abilities are limited.

Lack of Role Consensus

The third source of role strain is a lack of role consensus. Family members may be unable to agree on the expectations attached to a role. The role that currently seems to be the source of the most dissensus in families is the housekeeping role. This is a major problem for dual-career couples. Men who have been socialized into the traditional male role do not seem inclined to increase the amount of time that they spend on household activities. If they do participate actively, their performance may not meet the wife's standards, because she has been socialized into the traditional housekeeping role. This lack of agreement is associated with decreased marital satisfaction. Negotiation is required to reach a working consensus. Persuasion, manipulation, and coercion are other options used to reduce role dissensus. However, over the long term, they are less likely to be effective.

Role Conflict

A fourth source of role strain is role conflict. This occurs when the expectations between the familial roles or within a familial role are incompatible. For example, the therapeutic role might involve being a care giver to an elderly parent. The expectations attached to this role may be incompatible with that of provider, housekeeper, and child care provider. Does one go to the child's baseball game or to the doctor with the elderly parent? Most often, individuals have to set priorities. The care giver and provider roles are maintained to the detriment of other familial roles. The first role to be limited is the recreational role. The caregiver withdraws from activities that, in the short term, seem superfluous but that, in the long term, are sources of much needed energy.

Role Overload

A source of role strain that is closely related to role conflict is role overload. In role overload, the individual lacks the resources, time, and energy to meet the demands of the role. As with role conflict, the first option usually considered is withdrawal from one of the roles. An alternative might be to add roles that are energy-producing; for example, the role of bridge-player, artist, or tennis player. Maintaining a balance between energy-enhancing and energy-depleting roles reduces role strain (Marks & MacDermid, 1996). The individual who experiences either role conflict or role overload might also consider delegating some of the responsibilities to others. This requires skill in negotiation.

Communication

The negotiation of familial roles requires effective communication. Communication, in healthy families, occurs among autonomous individuals in an environment that is relatively free of unresolved conflicts. Healthy communication is characterized by clear, but flexible, rules governing verbal and nonverbal communication, clarity in the verbalization of feelings and thoughts, freedom to express a wide variety of feelings, and receptivity to and acknowledgment of the other person's communication. The psychological defense mechanisms of projection, denial, blaming, and scapegoating are infrequent.

Communication difficulties are probably the most common type of problem in families who seek help to improve their interaction. Differences in the cultural or developmental makeup of the family members may lead to various forms of miscommunication (Varenne, 1992). Communication difficulties may also be related to the different communication styles of men and women. Men's and women's preference for and perception of communication styles vary (Hawkins, et al, 1984). Wives prefer a communication style that conveys interest in, respect for, and validation of the internal realities of self and other, but many wives believe that their husbands' communication styles prohibit this openness. Husbands prefer to explore various facets of an issue, but they believe that their wives tend to avoid or gloss over the issues. These findings, however, may reflect differences in familial power, rather than gender. More study is needed to ascertain whether differences between men's and women's communication styles really exist.

Power

Power is one of the most important, albeit controversial, family processes. According to Szinovacz (1987, p. 652), power is defined as:

> . . . the net ability or capability of actors (A) to produce or cause (intended) outcomes or effects, particularly on the behavior of others (O) or on others' outcomes.

The exercise of power is a dynamic and multidimensional process. Its antecedents include the structural context and the characteristics of the individuals or groups involved. Gillespie (1984) argues that the class or caste system operating in the American society always gives the power to the man of the family. She says (p. 208) that ". . . women are structurally deprived of equal opportunities to develop their capacities, resources, and competence in competition with males." Gillespie cites three sources of men's marital power: (1) the socialization process; (2) the marriage contract, which, in many states, legally favors men; and (3) economic resources. Married women have less sense of control over their lives than unmarried women. If income is constant, marriage decreases a woman's sense of control (Ross, 1991).

Blood and Wolfe (1960) studied individual and family characteristics that determined power in the decision making process. Individual characteristics that contributed to their power included economic resources, education, and organizational participation. A characteristic of the family that tends to give power to the husband is suburbanization. This may reflect the economic power of a husband who is able to provide a home in the suburbs; the isolation of the wife from her family of origin; or, simply, the isolation of the suburban family from others, which allows the stronger individual to assume power. Another important family characteristic affecting power is race; African-American families are more egalitarian than white families.

This probably reflects the African-American man's lack of access to sources of power. These conceptualizations of marital power ignore the emotional interdependence between the spouses. Godwin and Scanzoni (1989) maintained that love and caring, commitment to the marriage, and cooperativeness are also antecedents to exercise of control in the decision making process.

Decision Making

Since the norms governing familial interactions have become outmoded, decision making has become increasingly important in identifying and attaining family goals. Family decision making is not an individual effort but a joint effort. Each decision has at least five features (Scanzoni & Szinovacz, 1980, p. 54):

1. *Who* raises the matter?
2. *What* is being said?
3. What are the *supporting actions* to what is being said?
4. What is the *importance* of what is being said to the party saying it?
5. What is the *response* of the other party?

For example, a 2-year-old boy who refused to eat his spinach until after he had dessert involved the mother in the decision-making process. She had to decide whether the real issue was spinach, dessert, or control. If she defined the issue as the child's dislike of spinach, she could choose to omit it, substitute carrots, or coerce him into eating it. Instead, she defined the issue as control. Rather than withholding dessert until he had eaten his spinach, she decided that she did not want to get into a power struggle over this issue. She chose to let the child decide. Subsequently, he ate both his spinach and his dessert. This example emphasizes the importance of looking at the decision-making process. If one looked only at the outcome, one could conclude that the child controlled the situation. By looking at the process, one sees that the mother made the decision to give the child control.

Communication and power are basic to decision making. Members of the family may have defined spheres of power. The father may choose the car; the mother, the house; and the child, the toy. Or, the allocation and the exercise of power may vary from situation to situation. In a healthy family, the balance of power resides in the parent coalition. Their relationship may be complementary in that each person does the opposite or reciprocal of the other; or, it may be symmetrical, that is, based on similarities rather than differences. Symmetrical participation in decision making is more likely to be satisfactory.

Communication style is a strong predictor of decision-making outcomes (Godwin & Scanzoni, 1989). Certain interactional strategies disrupt, while others enhance, problem solving. The expression of negative emotions is a disruptive factor (Forgatch, 1989). Anger is not necessarily destructive; but contempt, belligerence, and defensiveness are (Gottman et al, 1998). The expression of negative emotions tends to lead to conflict as an outcome of decision making. Consensus or, at the least, continuation of negotiations are the preferred outcomes.

Marital Satisfaction

Even with the leveling off of divorce rates in the United States, marital satisfaction has continued to decline (Glenn & Weaver, 1988; Glenn, 1991). This may be related to higher expectations of marriage or to the breakdown in consensual norms. Although the research findings are contradictory, a curvilinear relationship seems to exist between marriage and the life cycle (Suitor, 1991; Vannoy & Philliber, 1992). Marital satisfaction is relatively high among newly married and older couples. The presence of children in the home reduces marital satisfaction, particularly for husbands (Vannoy & Philliber, 1992). Increased marital satisfaction in aging people may actually reflect cohort differences (Glenn, 1998). Older couples may experience less role strain because of their commitment to enactment of the traditional familial roles. Overall, wives with nontraditional role orientations seem to experience more dissatisfaction with marriage; and wives of husbands with nontraditional role orientations experience more marital satisfaction.

The quality of marital interaction is related to the spouses' involvement and responsibilities both within and outside of the household (Ward, 1993). Satisfaction with the division of household labor has become increasingly important in the explanation of marital quality (Suitor, 1991). Indeed, the curvilinear relationship between marital satisfaction and the family life cycle also reflects wives' involvement in child care and housekeeping (Suitor, 1991). That is, newly married and aging wives have less child care and housekeeping responsibilities and are more satisfied with their marriage. Yet Ward (1993) found that the number of hours spent on household tasks were not related to marital satisfaction. Instead, the marital happiness of wives was associated with the perceived fairness of household labor. Employment outside the home of the wife, in and of itself, does not seem to affect marital satisfaction. Husbands of employed wives do not appear to experience less marital satisfaction than others (Vannoy & Philliber, 1992). Instead, the relative occupational attainment of the spouses seems to be significant. Couples are less satisfied when the wife's occupational attainment is higher than the husband's.

Time constraints are an underlying factor in the relationship between marital satisfaction and child care, household labor, and employment (Zuo, 1992). Marital interaction promotes marital happiness and marital happiness promotes marital interaction. This holds true for both men and women throughout the life cycle. When there is less time for interaction, there is less marital happiness.

Coping Strategies

According to Lazarus and Folkman (1984, p. 141), coping consists of:

> . . . constantly changing cognitive and behavioral efforts to manage specific external and/or internal demands that are appraised as taxing or exceeding the resources of the person.

Each family has its own repertoire of coping strategies, which may or may not be adequate in times of stress. Although coping strategies are almost as numerous as individuals, they may be classified in three broad categories (Pearlin & Schooler, 1982): (1) responses that change the stressful event, (2) responses that control the meaning of the stressful event, and (3) responses that control the stress itself. The family's structure, function, and process; the family's resources of time, energy, money, knowledge, and skills; and the family's past experience with crisis influence family coping. Even functional families may experience difficulty coping when stressful events pile up. By definition, ineffective coping does not reduce or control stress (Measley, et al, 1989). The outcomes of coping are difficult to evaluate in the short term; the long-term results of various coping strategies must be analyzed. For example, an individual's grieving may appear adaptive during the first few weeks after a loss. Others may comment that the mourner is "taking it well." Years later, however, another loss may evoke a disproportionate grief response, reflecting the fact that the mourner did not effectively grieve in the earlier situation.

Nursing Implications

Because of the effect of variables operating on the macrolevel on family structure and function, they may not be directly amenable to interventions by the individual nurse. Rather, the individual nurse usually deals with the sequelae of the family's structure and functional level. These sequelae may result in alterations in family processes, which may be modified by interventions on the microlevel. An individual nurse, even a novice, may be able to improve family interaction.

Alterations in family processes are most likely to occur when the family faces a transition brought about by developmental change, an illness, or another crisis. The family's current mode of operation may no longer be effective and family members need to learn new ways of dealing with the change. For example, in coping with the stress of an illness, particularly a chronic illness, the family experiences alterations in role performance and in power. Incompetent role performance results in dependency; dependency, in turn, results in loss of power for the individual. To help the family adapt to the changes, the nurse needs to facilitate communication, enhance decision making, promote coping, and reduce role strain (Bomar, 1996; Leahey & Wright, 1987a, 1987b; Wright & Leahey, 2000, 1987; and Vaughn-Cole, et al, 1998).

SUMMARY

An understanding of family structure, function, and process provides a foundation for nursing practice and enables the nurse to provide nursing care that is tailored to the uniqueness of the individual family. Because information on nontraditional families is still limited, the nurse needs to maintain an open, inquiring mind. Families will provide guidelines for action. The nurse's role is to promote the health of the individual family members and of the family system. Because the interaction between the two is reciprocal, neither can be ignored.

RESEARCH BRIEF

This chapter is a synthesis of a number of research findings over two decades. Many of the research studies contain secondary analyses in that they use data from another source. The most frequently used source of data in these studies is the U.S. Census Bureau, the origin of a substantive portion of demographic data in the United States.

Demography is the study of characteristics of human populations, including size, growth, density, and distribution of the population as well as the vital statistics of its members. Every 10 years, the U.S. Census Bureau attempts to study the entire population of the United States. This undertaking is beset by many methodological problems; particularly sampling errors. Currently, many statisticians advocate taking a representative sample of the population and extrapolating the findings to the total population. This approach would be cheaper and, many think, more accurate. However, this idea proved to be a political bombshell; it was not approved by the U.S. Congress by the 2000 census.

Representative samples are used in the annual March Current Population Survey (CPS) to obtain the demographic characteristics of households and families for the nation. Findings from these studies are very helpful in identifying trends in the establishment, composition, and size of the nation's families. More details on household and family characteristics for states, metropolitan areas, and other geographic locations are available from the decennial census. To date, these resources have been underused by nurses. For a long time, the data have been available in many libraries on CD-ROM or magnetic tape reels or cartridges. Now, they are as close as your computer keyboard; contact http://www.census.gov on the Internet.

Case Study

THE BLANCHARD FAMILY

The Blanchard family consists of John, age 72; Mary, age 68; David, age 45; Judith, age 43; and James, age 35; and five grandchildren. John and Mary will celebrate their 50th wedding anniversary next year. David lives about three miles from his parents; Judith lives 3000 miles away. Since his divorce one year ago, James and his 3-year-old daughter have been living with his parents.

John and Mary are retired school teachers; they have an annual income of $60,000 from pensions and Social Security. They own their home in the suburbs. So far, they have not had to touch their savings. All of the children are college-educated and self-supporting. However, James has had difficulty retaining a job. He has, on occasion, needed financial help from his parents. Currently, he pays his and his daughter's share of the household expenses. However, his mother and father babysit their granddaughter while James works.

John and Mary both remain active in the community. They frequently volunteer at community activities. They square dance once a week at the local center for senior citizens. They play bridge regularly with their best friends, a couple they have known for 45 years. They get regular health care. They are covered by Medicare and a supplemental insurance.

Three days ago, John had a cerebrovascular accident on the right side of his brain secondary to hypertension. He is right-handed. His left arm is completely paralyzed; his left leg is weak. He does not have any difficulty swallowing or communicating. He will be discharged in 2 days. What does the nurse need to consider in preparing John and his family for his discharge?

Discussion Questions

1. What characteristics of the family's structure promote the family members' ability to handle the stress of a chronic illness? What characteristics inhibit their ability?

2. What is the relationship between marital status and health status?
3. What resources does this family have to cope with the stress of a chronic illness?
4. What support networks might be helpful to this family during this time?
5. How will the enactment of familial roles be altered by this illness?
6. How will the power allocation be altered in this family?
7. What types of communication patterns will facilitate the family's decision making during this illness?
8. How does illness alter marital satisfaction?
9. What other information is needed to help this family with the discharge process?
10. What interventions might be useful in helping this family deal with this transition?

Questions Requiring Additional Knowledge

1. What behavioral problems might be anticipated following a right-sided brain injury?
2. What health teaching will the family need to prevent another stroke?

Study Questions

1. Analyses of family structure, function, and process are limited because the majority of family studies focus on
   a. Extended, multigenerational families.
   b. Nontraditional family structures.
   c. Poor, black, single-parent families.
   d. White, middle-class, two-parent families.
2. Which of the following family types is most likely to have the fewest resources to cope with stress?
   a. Blended families
   b. Cohabiting families
   c. Extended families
   d. Single-parent families
3. Married men are healthier than single men because they
   a. Are less readily sanctioned.
   b. Engage in more healthy activities.
   c. Experience fewer stressors.
   d. Tend to be much happier.
4. Which of the following is a functional prerequisite for the family system?
   a. Adaptation
   b. Determination
   c. Recreation
   d. Socialization
5. Which of the following familial roles has undergone the most change in the last two decades?
   a. Housekeeper
   b. Provider
   c. Recreation organizer
   d. Therapist
6. What is the most common source of role strain in young women with children under 6 years of age?
   a. Definition of the situation
   b. Lack of role consensus
   c. Lack of role knowledge
   d. Role overload
7. The woman is most likely to influence the outcome of familial decision making when she is
   a. Educated.
   b. Rich.
   c. Pregnant.
   d. White.
8. In a healthy family, power
   a. Is equally divided among family members.
   b. Is the purview of the husband.
   c. Resides in the parental coalition.
   d. Is an outmoded notion.
9. A healthy family system is characterized by
   a. Absence of disease.
   b. Parent-child coalitions.
   c. Open communication.
   d. Stereotyped interactions.

References

Allen, K. R., & Demo, D. H. (1995). The families of lesbians and gay men: A new frontier in family research. *Journal of Marriage and the Family, 57*:111–127.

Amato, P. R., & Keith, B. (1991). Parental divorce and adult well-being: A meta-analysis. *Journal of Marriage and the Family, 53*:43–58.

Aquilino, W. S. (1994). Impact of childhood family disruption on young adults' relationships with parents. *Journal of Marriage and the Family, 56*: 295–313.

Bahr, S. J. (1976). Role competence, role norms, and marital control. In F. I. Nye (Ed.) *Role Structure and Analysis of the Family*, pp. 179–189. Beverly Hills: Sage.

Bane, M. J. (1976). *Here to Stay: American Families in the 20th Century*. New York: Basic Books.

Barnett, R. C., et al. (1992). Men's multiple roles and their relationship to men's psychological distress. *Journal of Marriage and the Family, 54*:358–367.

Bell, N. W., & Vogel, E. F. (1960). *A modern introduction to the family*. Glencoe, IL: Free Press.

Blood, R. O., Jr., & Wolfe, D. M. (1960). *Husbands and wives: The dynamics of married living*. New York: The Free Press.

Bolechek, G.M., & McCloskey, J.C. (Eds.) (1992). *Nursing interventions: Essential nursing treatments*, ed 2. Philadelphia: Saunders.

Bomar, P. J. (Ed.). (1996). *Nurses and Family Health Promotion: Concepts, Assessment, and Interventions*, ed 2. Baltimore: Williams & Wilkins.

Brown, S. L., & Booth, A. (1996). Cohabitation versus marriage: A comparison of relationship quality. *Journal of Marriage and the Family, 58*:668–678.

Carlson, J. (1976). The recreational role. In F. I. Nye (Ed.), *Role Structure and Analysis of the Family*, pp. 131–147. Beverly Hills: Sage.

Cherlin, A. J. (1992). *Marriage, Divorce, and Remarriage*, revised and enlarged edition. Cambridge, MA: Harvard University Press.

Cherlin, A. J. (1999). *Public and Private Families: An Introduction*, ed 2. Boston: McGraw Hill.

Chevan, A. (1996). As cheaply as one: Cohabitation in the older population. *Journal of Marriage and the Family, 58*:656–667.

Cooksey, E. C., & Fondell, M. M. (1996). Spending time with his kids: Effects of family structure on fathers' and childrens' lives. *Journal of Marriage and the Family*, 58:693–707.

Coontz, S. (1988). *The Social Origins of Private Life: A History of American Families* 1600–1900. New York: Verso.

Coontz, S. (1992). *The Way We Never Were: American Families and the Nostalgia Trap*. New York: Basic Books.

Coontz, S. (1997). *The Way We Really Are: Coming to Terms with America's Changing Families*. New York: Basic Books.

Dawson, D. A. (1991). Family structure and children's health and well-being: Data from the 1988 National Health Interview Survey on Child Health. *Journal of Marriage and the Family, 53*:573–584.

Degler, C. N. (1980). *At Odds: Women and the Family In America from the Revolution to the Present*. New York: Oxford University Press.

Demo, D. H., et al. (1987). Family relations and the self-esteem of adolescents and their parents. *Journal of Marriage and the Family, 49*:705–715.

Demo, D. H. (1992). Parent-child relations: Assessing recent changes. *Journal of Marriage and the Family, 54*:104–117.

Downey, D. B., et al. (1998). Sex of parent and children's well-being in single-parent households. *Journal of Marriage and the Family, 60*:878–893.

Eshleman, J. R. (1997). *The Family: An Introduction*, ed 8. Boston: Allyn & Bacon.

Forgatch, M. S. (1989). Patterns and outcome in family problem solving: The disrupting effect of negative emotion. *Journal of Marriage and the Family, 51*:115–124.

Fossett, M. A., & Kiecolt, K. J. (1993). Mate availability and family structure among African Americans in U.S. metropolitan area. *Journal of Marriage and the Family, 55*:288–302.

Francoeur, R. T. (1987). Human sexuality. In M. B. Sussman & S. K. Steinmetz (Eds.), *Handbook of Marriage and the Family*, pp. 509–534. New York: Plenum.

Gallagher, S. K. (1994). Doing their share: Comparing patterns of help given by older and younger adults. *Journal of Marriage and the Family, 56*: 567–578.

Ganong, L. H., et al. (1990). A meta-analytic view of family structure stereotypes. *Journal of Marriage and the Family, 52*:287–290.

Gillespie, D. (1984). Who has the power? The marital struggle. In B. N. Adams & J. L. Campbell, (Eds.), *Framing the Family: Contemporary Portraits*, pp. 206–228. Prospect Heights, IL: Waveland Press.

Glenn, N. D., & Weaver, C. N. (1988). The changing relationship of marital status to reported happiness. *Journal of Marriage and the Family, 50*:317–324.

Glenn, N. D. (1991). The recent trend in marital success in the United States. *Journal of Marriage and the Family, 53*:261–270.

Glenn, N. D. (1998). The course of marital success and failure in five American 10-year cohorts. *Journal of Marriage and the Family, 60*:569–576.

Glick, P. C. (1988). Fifty years of family demography: A record of social change. *Journal of Marriage and the Family, 50*:861–873.

Godwin, D.D., & Scanzoni, J. (1989). Couple consensus during marital decision-making. A context, process, outcome model. *Journal of Marriage and the Family, 51*, 943–956.

Gottman, J. M., et al. (1998). Predicting marital happiness and stability from newlywed interactions. *Journal of Marriage and the Family, 60*:5–22.

Gove, W. R. (1973). Sex, marital status, and mortality. *American Journal of Sociology*, 79:45–67.

Guttentag, M., & Secord, P. G. (1983). *Too Many Women? The Sex Role Question.* Beverly Hills: Sage.

Hahn, Beth A. (1993). Marital status and women's health: The effect of economic marital acquisitions. *Journal of Marriage and the Family, 55*:495–504.

Hanson, T. L., et al. (1996). Double jeopardy: Parental conflict and stepfamily outcomes for children. *Journal of Marriage and the Family, 58*:141–154.

Harris, K. M., & Morgan, S. P. (1991). Fathers, sons, and daughters: Differential paternal involvement in parenting. *Journal of Marriage and the Family, 53*:531–544.

Hawkins, J. L., et al. (1984). Spouse differences in communication style: Preference, perception, behavior. In B. N. Adams & J. L. Campbell (Eds.) *Framing the Family: Contemporary Portraits*, pp. 229–240. Prospect Heights, IL: Waveland Press.

Hawks, S. R. (1991). Recreation in the family. In S. J. Bahr, (Ed.), *Family Research: A Sixty-Year Review*, 1930–1990, vol. 1, pp. 387–433. New York: Lexington Books.

Jayakody, R., et al. (1993). Family support to single and married African American mothers: The provision of financial, emotional, and child care assistance. *Journal of Marriage and the Family, 55*:261–276.

Johnson, C., & Troll, L. (1996). Family structure and the timing of transitions from 70 to 103 years of age. *Journal of Marriage and the Family, 58*:178–187.

Kalleberg, A. L., & Rosenfeld, R. A. (1990). Work in the family and in the labor-market: A cross-national, reciprocal analysis. *Journal of Marriage and the Family, 52*:331–346.

Kalmuss, D., et al. (1992). Short-term consequences of parenting versus adoption among young unmarried women. *Journal of Marriage and the Family, 54*:80–90.

Kantor, D., & Lehr, W. (1975). *Inside the Family: Toward a Theory of Family Process.* San Francisco: Jossey-Bass.

Lazarus, R.S., & Folkman, S. (1984). *Stress, appraisal, and coping.* New York: Springer.

Leahey, M., & Wright, L. M. (Eds.) (1987a). *Families and Life-Threatening Illness.* Springhouse, PA: Springhouse.

Leahey, M., & Wright, L. M. (Eds.) (1987b). *Families and Psychosocial Problems.* Springhouse, PA: Springhouse.

Lee, G. R., et al. (1991). Marital status and personal happiness. *Journal of Marriage and the Family, 53*:839–844.

Leslie, G. R., & Korman, S. K. (1985). *The Family in Social Context*, ed 6. New York: Oxford University Press.

MacDonald, W. L., & DeMaris, A. (1995). Remarriage, stepchildren, and marital conflict: Challenges to the incomplete institutionalization hypothesis. *Journal of Marriage and the Family, 57*:387–398.

Marks, S. R. (1994). What is the pattern of commitments? *Journal of Marriage and the Family, 56*:112–114.

Marks, S. R., & MacDermid, S. M. (1996). Multiple roles and the self: A theory of role balance. *Journal of Marriage and the Family, 58*:417–432.

McHale, S. M., & Crouter, A. C. (1992). You can't always get what you want: Incongruence between sex-role attitudes and family work roles and its implications for marriage. *Journal of Marriage and the Family, 54*:537–547.

Nock, S. L. (1988). The family and hierarchy. *Journal of Marriage and the Family, 50*:957–966.

Nye, F. I. (1976). *Role Structure and Analysis of the Family.* Beverly Hills: Sage.

O'Neill, R., & Greenberger, E. (1994). Patterns of commitment to work and parenting: Implications for role strain. *Journal of Marriage and the Family, 56*:101–108.

Otto, H. A. (Ed.). (1970). *The Family in Search of a Future: Alternate Models for Moderns.* New York: Appleton-Century-Crofts.

Parsons, T. (1951). *The Social System.* New York: Free Press.

Parsons, T., & Bales, R. F. (Eds.) (1955). *Family, Socialization, and the Interaction Process.* Glencoe, IL: Free Press.

Pearlin, L.I., & Schooler, C. (1982). The structure of coping. In H. J. McCubbin, A. E. Cauble, & J. M. Patterson (Eds.), *Family stress coping and social support.* Springfield, IL: Charles C. Thomas.

Perry-Jenkins, M., & Folk, K. (1994). Class, couples, and conflict: Effects of the division of labor on assessments of marriage in dual-earner families. *Journal of Marriage and the Family, 56*:165–180.

Peterson, R. R., & Gerson, K. (1992). Determinants of responsibility for child care arrangements among dual-earner couples. *Journal of Marriage and the Family, 54*:527–536.

Pittman, J. F., & Blanchard, D. (1996). The effects of work history and timing of marriage on the division of household labor: A life-course perspective. *Journal of Marriage and the Family, 58*:78–90.

Robertson, A. F. (1991). *Beyond the Family: The Social Organization of Human Reproduction.* Berkeley: University of California Press.

Robinson, J. P., & Milkie, M. A. (1998). Back to the basics: Trends in and role determinants of women's attitudes toward housework. *Journal of Marriage and the Family, 60*:205–218.

Rogers, R. G. (1995). Marriage, sex, and mortality. *Journal of Marriage and the Family, 57*:515–526.

Ross, C. E. (1991). Marriage and the sense of control. *Journal of Marriage and the Family, 53*:831–838.

Ross, C. E. (1995). Reconceptualizing marital status as a continuum of social attachment. *Journal of Marriage and the Family, 57*:129–140.

Santi, L. L. (1987). Change in the structure and size of American households: 1970 to 1985. *Journal of Marriage and the Family, 49*:833–837.

Scanzoni, J., & Szinovacz, M. (1980). *Family Decision-Making: A Developmental Sex Role Model.* Beverly Hills, CA: Sage.

Seltzer, J. (1991). Relationships between fathers and children who live apart: The father's role after separation. *Journal of Marriage and the Family, 53*:79–101.

Spanier, G. B. (1989). Bequeathing family continuity. *Journal of Marriage and the Family, 51*:3–13.

Spitze, G., et al. (1994). Adult children's divorce and intergenerational relations. *Journal of Marriage and the Family, 56*:279–293.

Stull, D. E., & Borgatta, E. F. (1987). Family structure and proximity of family members. In T. H. Brubaker (Ed.). *Aging, Health, and Family: Long-Term Care*, pp. 247–261. Newbury Park, CA: Sage.

Suitor, J. J. (1991). Marital quality and satisfaction with the division of household labor across the family life cycle. *Journal of Marriage and the Family, 53*:221–230.

Szinovacz, M. E. (1987). Family power. In M. B. Sussman & S. K. Steinmetz (Eds.), *Handbook of Marriage and the Family*, pp. 651–693. New York: Plenum.

Teachman, J. D., et al. (1987). Demography of the family. In M. B. Sussman & S. K. Steinmetz (Eds.), *Handbook of Marriage and the Family*, pp. 3–36. New York: Plenum.

Thomas, E. J. (1977). *Marital Communication and Decision Making: Analysis, Assessment, and Change*. New York: The Free Press.

Thomson, E., et al. (1992). Family structure, gender, and parental socialization. *Journal of Marriage and the Family, 54*:368–378.

U.S. Bureau of the Census. (1998). Households and Families. Current Population Survey. URL: http://www.census.gov/population/socdemo/hh-fam.

Vannoy, D., & Philliber, W. W. (1992). Wife's employment and quality of marriage. *Journal of Marriage and the Family, 54*:387-398.

Varenne, H. (1992). *Ambiguous Harmony: Family Talk in America*. Norwood, NJ: Ablex.

Vaughn-Cole, B., et al. (Eds.), (1998). *Family Nursing Practice*. Philadelphia: Saunders.

Verbrugge, L. M. (1979). Marital status and health. *Journal of Marriage and the Family, 41*:267–285.

Verbrugge, L. M. (1983). Multiple roles and physical health of women and men. *Journal of Health and Social Behavior, 24*:16–30.

Walker, A. J. & Pratt, C. C. (1991). Daughters' help to mothers: Intergenerational aid versus caregiving. *Journal of Marriage and the Family, 53*:3–12.

Ward, R. A. (1993). Marital happiness and household equity in later life. *Journal of Marriage and the Family, 55*:427–438.

Weitzman, L. J. (1985). *The Divorce Revolution: The Unexpected Social and Economic Consequences for Women and Children in America*. New York: The Free Press.

Wilkie, J. R. (1991). The decline in men's labor force participation and income and the changing structure of family economic support. *Journal of Marriage and the Family, 53*:11–122.

Winch, R. F. (1977). *Familial Organization: A Quest for Determinants*. New York: The Free Press.

Wright, L. M., & Leahey, M. (2000). *Nurses and Families: a Guide to Family Assessment and Intervention*, ed 3. Philadelphia: F.A. Davis.

Wright, L. M., & Leahey, M. (Eds.). (1987). *Families and Chronic Illness*. Springhouse, PA: Springhouse.

Zuo, J. (1992). The reciprocal relationship between marital interaction and marital happiness: A three-wave study. *Journal of Marriage and the Family, 54*:870–878.

Additional Bibliography

Amato, P. R. & Booth, A. (1996). A prospective study of divorce and parent-child relationships. *Journal of Marriage and the Family, 58*, 356–365.

Bird, Gloria W. & Sporakowski, M. J. (Eds.). (1997). *Taking sides: Clashing views on controversial issues in family and personal relationships* (3rd ed.). Guilford, CN: Duskin Publishing.

Cochran, M., Larner, M., Riley, D., Gunnarson, L., & Henderson, C.R., Jr. (1990). *Extending families: The social networks of parents and their children*. Cambridge University Press.

Lewis, J. M. (1986). *The birth of the family: An empirical inquiry*. New York: Brunner/Mazel.

Lewis, J. M., Beavers, W. R., Gossett, J. T., & Phillips, V. A. (1976). *No single thread. Psychological health in family systems*. New York: Brunner/Mazel.

Montgomery, J., & Fewer, W. (1998). *Family systems and beyond*. New York: Human Sciences.

Matthews, L. S., Wickrama, K. A. S., & Conger, R. D. (1996). Predicting marital instability from spouse and observer reports of marital interaction. *Journal of Marriage and the Family, 58*:641–655.

Skolnick, A. S., & Skolnick, J. H. (Eds.). (1992). *Family in transition: Rethinking marriage, sexuality, child rearing, and family organization* (7th ed. New York: Harper Collins

Spanier, G. B., & Furstenberg, F. F., Jr. (1987). Remarriage and reconstituted families. In M. B. Sussman & S. K. Steinmetz (Eds.), *Handbook of marriage and the family* (pp. 419–434). New York: Plenum Press.

Sprey, J. (Ed.). (1990). *Fashioning family theory: New approaches*. Newbury Park, CA: Sage.

White, L., & Peterson, D. (1995). The retreat from marriage: Its effect on unmarried children's exchange with parents. *Journal of Marriage and the Family, 57*:428–434.

Focus On

SOCIOCULTURAL INFLUENCES ON FAMILY HEALTH

The influence of culture is pervasive: It shapes choices about what we eat, drink, and wear; how we are entertained; how we determine health and illness; and what we study in school as well as a myriad of other aspects of our daily lives. The family's socioeconomic or social class status also plays a primary role in shaping family behavior, particularly family lifestyle. This chapter discusses and explicates some of the complex sociocultural influences on family health. Sociocultural influences refer to both the family's social class background and the family's culture. These influences shape family behaviors, including health behaviors.

In this chapter, we define essential concepts of culture and ethnicity, social class, and family health and discuss the growth in cultural diversity and the disparity between social classes in the United States. We also examine the extent to which health beliefs and practices, family values, patterns of communication, family power, family roles, and family coping styles influence family health. This is followed by an exploration of social class structure in the United States and poverty as a decisive factor in family health. The interaction of culture and social class and its effect on family health are then discussed. Finally, implications for family nursing practice are suggested.

Chapter 5

SOCIOCULTURAL INFLUENCES ON FAMILY HEALTH

Eleanor G. Ferguson-Marshalleck • J. Kim Miller

OUTLINE

OBJECTIVES

On completion of this chapter, the reader will be able to:

- Identify two prime molders of family values, family behaviors, and family structure and function.
- Discuss the growth in cultural diversity and the increasing disparity between social classes in the United States.
- Define culture and discuss its relationship to health beliefs and practices, family health, and family coping behaviors.

- Differentiate between the terms culture, ethnicity, social class, and acculturation.
- Describe the social class structure of the United States.
- Explain cultural (ethnic) differences in family and family members' health status.
- Analyze the differences in family health status and health-related behaviors of families from different social classes.
- Discuss the separate influences of culture and social class and the influence of the interaction of these two variables on family health.
- Discuss the importance of incorporating cultural and socioeconomic assessment in the care of families.
- Describe some nursing intervention strategies that can be used to enhance ethnic and social class sensitivity and competency in the care of culturally and socioeconomically diverse families.

Every student who reads this text comes from a unique sociocultural background, with differences greatly influenced by the social class and the predominant cultural group from which he or she comes. Look around you. What sort of cultural and ethnic variations do you see? What influence do you think those variations have on study habits, food choices, family relationships, or health habits?

Sociocultural influences on family health include both the family's socioeconomic or social class background and the family's culture. A family's cultural legacy plays a central role in influencing the family's value system, function, and behavior. The influence of culture is pervasive; it permeates and circumscribes individual, familial, and social actions (Friedman, 1998). It shapes choices about what we eat, drink, and wear; how we are entertained; how we determine health and illness; and what we study in school as well as a myriad of other aspects of our daily lives.

The family's socioeconomic or social class status also plays a primary role in shaping family behavior, particularly family lifestyle. Families are subjected to very different experiences, both stress-producing and growth-promoting, which exert great influence on family behavior and lifestyle. Family lifestyles vary as a result of these different exposures. Basic to the discussion of sociocultural influences are the essential concepts of culture and ethnicity, socioeconomic status or social class, and family health. Family health is viewed here as an outcome not only of sociocultural influences, but also of the family's developmental stage, its historical experiences, and the family's own idiosyncratic culture.

This chapter discusses and explicates some of the complex sociocultural influences on family health. It focuses on culture and social class, two prime molders of family behavior and values. The chapter begins with basic definitions of the chapter's key concepts, followed by a description of the growth in cultural diversity and the disparity between social classes in the United States.

The discussion continues by examining the influence of culture on family health and moves on to discuss the extent to which health beliefs and practices, family values, patterns of communication, family power, family roles, and family coping styles influence family health.

The influence of social class on family health is then discussed, with demographic data illustrating the widening gap between the affluent and poor in the United States. Selected ethnic groups, social class structure, and poverty as a decisive factor in family health are explored, identifying how the health status of socially disadvantaged and minority populations differs from that of the dominant culture. The interaction of culture and social class and its impact on family health are then covered. These observations raise important questions for nurses and nursing students regarding social justice and the role of the family nurse as client advocate. Finally, implications for family nursing practice are suggested.

KEY CONCEPTS

Culture and Ethnicity

All families are bearers of the culture of the society in which they live (Ablon & Ames, 1989) and of the culture with which they identify. In this sense, many families are multicultural because they are part of both the dominant culture or society and part of their particular subculture. The term *culture* refers to:

> . . . those sets of shared world views and adaptive behaviors derived from simultaneous membership in a variety of contexts, such as ecological setting (rural, urban, suburban), religious background, nationality and ethnicity, social class, gender-related experiences, minority status, occupation, political leanings, migratory patterns, and stage of acculturation; or values derived from belonging to the same generation, partaking of a single historical moment, or particular ideologies (Falicov, 1988, p. 336).

Purnell and Paulanka (1998) also define culture as "the totality of socially transmitted behavioral patterns, arts, beliefs, values, customs, lifeways, and all other products of human work and thought characteristic of a population of people that guide their worldview and decision making" (p. 2). Patterned lifeways, values, ideals, beliefs, and practices are embedded in these definitions. Patterns of learned behaviors, values, and beliefs are transmitted from one generation to the next by the family. *Ethnicity,* a major component of culture, is defined as a group's sense of "peoplehood" based on a combination of race, religion, ancestral history, and nationality. It involves a multilayered sense of shared values and understandings within groups that fulfill a deep psychological need for identity and historical continuity (McGoldrick, 1993).

Socioeconomic Status or Social Class

The terms "socioeconomic status," "social status," and "social class" (which are often used interchangeably in the sociological literature) are used to refer to large groups of persons who have relatively similar incomes, amounts of wealth, life conditions, life chances, and lifestyles (Ropers, 1991). A person's social class status is often determined by the family's social class; and the family's social class, in turn, is determined by the spouses' (traditionally, the husband's or father's) occupational prestige, level of education, income, employment status, or a combination of these.

Socioeconomic status is a major component within the chapter's broad definition of culture. Because this variable is so crucial in understanding families, it is addressed explicitly. Social class has a pervasive effect on family life and each family member's life, especially within complex, heterogeneous societies such as the United States. A family's social class affects the family's lifestyle (where and how the family lives), family members' health status and longevity, their educational and occupational opportunities, and a multitude of other life conditions (Lee & Estes, 1997). Differences in social class are associated with differences in power, privilege, and prestige, which are all resources vital to life conditions (Erickson & Gecas, 1991). For example, Hussey (1997) in a study using data from the National Longitudinal Mortality Study found that injury mortality in young persons was closely linked with family income, education, household structure, and residential location. This study supports the evidence linking socioeconomic differential to inequality in life chances.

Family Health

The term "family health" refers to the health of both individual family members and the family as a whole. Because the health of individual family members affects the health of the whole family system and vice versa, it is difficult to separate the family and its health status from that of its members and their personal health status. Therefore, this chapter focuses on sociocultural influences on both individual family members' health and the family unit's or system's health.

ETHNIC AND CULTURAL DIVERSITY AND DISPARITIES BETWEEN SOCIAL CLASSES

Growth in Ethnic and Cultural Diversity

Since the 1960s and 1970s, there has been a steady growth in racial and ethnic diversity (also referred to as cultural diversity) in the United States. More than one resident in four is nonwhite or of Hispanic origin (U.S. Bureau of the Census, 1992b). The white majority is shrinking and aging, while the African-American, Hispanic American, Asian and Pacific Islander American, and Native American populations are young and growing (U.S. Bureau of the Census, 1992b). If the present rate of births and immigration to the United States continues, by the turn of the 21st century, the Asian-American presence will increase by 22 percent, Hispanic Americans by 21 percent, African-Americans by 12 percent, and Americans of European descent by only 2 percent (Henry, 1990).

Dramatic changes have taken place in the American population over the past decade, as depicted in

Table 5–1 and Table 5–2. Table 5–2 summarizes the changes in the growth patterns of selected racial and ethnic minorities between 1980 and 1990. Although the sizes of the groups vary, the number of racial and ethnic groups profiled attests to the increasingly diverse nature of the population in the United States.

Ethnic minorities such as African-Americans, Asian and Pacific Islander Americans, Hispanic Americans, and Native Americans make up a far larger proportion of the United States population than they did in the past. Representing 12 percent of the American population, African-Americans remain the largest minority group within the United States. This population showed a modest growth from 1980 to 1990, increasing in size from 26.5 million (11.7 percent of the total population) in 1980 to 30 million (12.1 percent) in 1990 (U.S. Bureau of the Census, 1992b). African-Americans are not considered a homogeneous group, as is widely assumed. Although their ancestry is African and many descended from people who were enslaved, there are a number of blacks who immigrated (voluntarily) from Africa, Great Britain, the West Indian islands, and Central and South America, who may not identify themselves as being African-American (Hopp & Herring, 1999; Spector, 1996). The present low rate of immigration, a high rate of infant mortality, and shorter life spans are factors that slow the rate of growth in the number of African-Americans (National Center for Health Statistics, 1992; U.S. Bureau of the Census, 1992a).

The Asian and Pacific Islander population grew proportionally by 108 percent, that is, from 3.5 million (1.5 percent of the total population) to 7.3 million (2.9 percent). The rapid growth of this population is the result primarily of immigration, part of whom are refugees from Southeast Asia. Asian-Americans include people from the diverse countries and cultures of Asia and the Indian subcontinent. This group consists of "at least 23 subgroups such as Asian Indian, Cambodian, Chinese, Filipino, Hmong, Japanese, Korean, Laotian, Thai, Vietnamese, and 'other Asian,' with 32 linguistic groups" (Inouye, 1999, p. 338). Despite these diversities, they share many common cultural characteristics that have been deeply influenced by Buddhism, Confucianism, and Taoism. However, many Asians are also greatly influenced by Christianity. Pacific Islanders include people from the Polynesian, Micronesian, and Melanesian groupings of islands in the North and South Pacific, e.g., Hawaiians, Samoans, Tongans, Tahitians, Guamanians, and Fijians. Native Hawaiians form 57.8 percent of the U.S. Pacific Islander population (Casken, 1999).

TABLE 5–1
Major Racial and Ethnic Divisions of the U.S. Population, 1980 and 1990

Race	Number		Percent of Total	
	1980*	**1990***	**1980**	**1990**
Anglo-American	188.4	199.7	83.2	80.3
African-American	26.5	30.0	11.7	12.1
American Indian, Eskimo, or Aleut	1.4	2.0	0.6	0.8
Asian and Pacific Islander	3.5	7.3	1.5	2.9
Other	6.8	9.8	3.0	3.9
Total U.S. Population	226.5	248.7	100.0	100.0
Hispanic†				
Hispanic origin (of any race)	14.6	22.4	6.4	9.0
Not of Hispanic origin (all other ethnicities)	211.9	226.4	93.6	91.0
Total U.S. Population	226.5	248.7	100.0	100.0

Source: U.S. Bureau of the Census, *1980* Census of Population. General Population Characteristics, 1983 (Tables 38 and 39) and *1990* Census of the Population. General Population Characteristics, 1992b (Table 3)
*Data are reported in millions and rounded off to the closest 100,000.
†It should be noted that persons of Hispanic origin may be of any race; hence, there is a separate category for persons of Hispanic origin.

TABLE 5–2
Change In U.S. Population by Race and Ethnicity for Selected Racial and Ethnic Groups, 1980 to 1990

Racial/Ethnic Group	1980* (Millions)	1990* (Millions)	Increase (%)
African-American	26.5	30.0	13.2
American Indian	1.4	1.9	37.7
Asian			
Chinese	0.8	1.6	104.1
Filipino	0.8	1.4	81.6
Japanese	0.7	0.8	20.9
Asian Indian	0.4	0.8	125.3
Korean	0.4	0.8	125.3
Vietnamese	0.3	0.6	134.8
Pacific Islanders			
Hawaiian	0.17	0.2	26.5
Samoan	0.04	0.06	50.1
Guamanian	0.02	0.05	53.4
Hispanic			
Mexican	8.7	13.5	54.4
Puerto Rican	2.0	2.7	35.4
Cuban	0.8	1.0	30.0
Other Hispanic	3.0	5.1	66.7

Source: U.S. Bureau of the Census, *1980* Census of Population. General Population Characteristics (1983, Tables 38 and 39) and *1990* Census of the Population (1992b, Table 3).
*Data reported in millions. Most data are rounded off to the closest 100,000.

From 1980 to 1990, the Hispanic population grew proportionally by 53 percent, that is, from 14.6 million (6.4 percent of the total population) to 22.4 million (9.0 percent). Hispanic Americans are people or descendants of people from Mexico, Puerto Rico, Cuba, and Central and South America. Friedman (1998) explains that Hispanic-Americans are united by their common language (i.e., Spanish except for Brazilians who speak Portuguese), religion (i.e., strong adherence to Roman Catholicism), and their common values and beliefs. The growth of the Hispanic population in the United States has been the result of both legal and illegal immigration and a high fertility rate (Friedman, 1998b).

The Alaskan Indian, Eskimo, and Aleut Native American populations grew by 38 percent, that is, from 1.4 million to 2 million (0.8 percent). Although the actual number of non-Hispanic whites increased in 1990, they declined as a percentage of the total United States population, from 79.6 percent to 75.6 percent (U.S. Census Bureau, 1992b). United States population growth today is overwhelmingly a function of growth within racial and ethnic minority populations. Some states, such as California, Illinois, and New York, have become centers for immigration.

Growth in the Disparity between Social Classes

Recent increases in income inequality in the United States and the implications for working-class and poor families have been widely addressed in the sociological and public health literature (Braun, 1991; Gilbert & Kahl, 1987; Ropers, 1991; Winnick, 1991). In the 1980s and early 1990s, the rich have continued to become richer and the poor poorer (Braun, 1991; Peterson, 1993; Ropers, 1991; United Press International, 1990; Wolff, 1995), a change characterized by the sociologist Winnick (1991) as a shift toward two societies, separate and unequal. The shift in the distribution of income and wealth and the consequent growing gap between rich and poor began in the early 1970s but accelerated during the Reagan administration because of the reduction of all social programs serving poor people. The escalating national debt, sluggish economic growth, rising unemployment rate, and declining wages exacerbated the problems of America's poor families in the 1980s and early 1990s. The increase in income inequality has adversely affected access to education and employment, particularly for lower-class and working-class families. This widening income gap has meant that the middle class has shrunk while both ends of the income continuum have expanded (i.e., there are increased proportions of rich and poor). Recent economic recovery of the nation has led to some growth in domestic programs, although much of the earlier retrenchment is still very evident. This economic disparity and reduction of social programs has also affected the health and health care of families.

Health Status of Socially Disadvantaged and Culturally Diverse Populations

The health status of individuals in the United States differs dramatically among different cultural groups and social classes. There are several reasons for this: family and personal lifestyle differences; differing access to health care resources, including both services and health insurance; and differing exposure to environmental hazards. Unequal distribution of preventive and basic health care resources results in morbidity and mortality rates that vary significantly between white people and nonwhite people and among socioeconomic classes. Major indicators of health status clearly demonstrate that the health status of minority Americans is substantially poorer than that of white Americans (Lee & Estes, 1997; Nickens, 1991; U.S. Department of Health and Human Services, 1985).

Also, ethnic minorities have poorer mental health and more unmet mental health needs than white persons. Not surprisingly, they also receive less extensive and poorer quality mental health services (Jones & Korchin, 1982; Nickens, 1991). The same situation is true in terms of social class differences: health status is poorer among poor Americans. One glaring indication of this is the difference in infant mortality rates between socioeconomic classes. Babies of poor families, regardless of ethnic or racial background, die at twice the rate of babies of families who are not poor (Boone, 1989; Kramer, 1988; Lee & Estes, 1997).

THE INFLUENCE OF CULTURE

Culture and Family

Culture, which is passed on from generation to generation, affects the health status of families. Moreover, a family's level of *acculturation* to the dominant culture in which they live makes a major difference in how important a family's cultural heritage is in shaping family behavior and health. "Acculturation comprises those gradual changes produced in a culture by the influence of another culture which results in an increased similarity of the two" (Kroeber, 1948, p. 425). In the case of ethnic minority families who immigrate to the United States, the influence is predominantly one way. The American culture exerts a greater influence on the ethnic group to conform to the dominant cultural patterns than vice versa (Friedman, 1998).

Acculturation occurs on a continuum that ranges from adhering to the traditional values of an individual's homeland (including traditional religious practices and cultural artifacts) at one end (the unacculturated end) to adopting the mainstream values of the dominant group at the other end (the acculturated end) (Kumabe, et al, 1985; Locke, 1992; Spector, 1996). This process may be influenced by factors such as time, reason for immigration, and education. According to Berry (1990), voluntary immigrants are likely to experience less difficulty with acculturation than those who are forced to immigrate to a new culture. Spector (1996) also comments that in the United States the usual course of acculturation takes three generations.

Ethnic minority families who have recently immigrated to the United States or those who have remained immersed in the culture of their country of origin are often unacculturated to the dominant culture of the United States. That is to say, they have not integrated the dominant American core values and practices into their lives. The ethnic background of recent immigrants, derived from their country of origin, is therefore much more important in shaping their beliefs and behavior than is the ethnic background of acculturated American families. Hong and Friedman (1998) present two examples of differences in acculturation. They explain that few third and fourth generation Japanese-American families are likely to hold traditional values because they have lived in the U.S. for many generations. On the other hand, Southeast Asian refugees typically have a more difficult time adjusting to the life in a new land than other immigrants since their immigration and their refugee status was so recent.

A family's culture affects its health beliefs and practices. The effects of culture on family health status may also be explored by looking at selected family structural dimensions, such as family values, roles, power, communication patterns, and coping.

Health Beliefs and Practices

Every cultural group possesses a system of beliefs and practices about health and illness (Helman, 1990). These include beliefs about what a symptom is and means, when to seek help and who to seek it from when one is ill, what symbolizes relief or cure, and so forth. Cultures provide explanatory models of health and illness, which include the meaning, cause, process, prognosis, and treatment of illness, as well as maintenance of health (Kleinman, 1980). Purnell and Paulanka (1998) state that "culture is largely unconscious and has powerful influences on health and illness" (p. 2). Western societies typically root their explanations of disease and health in natural phenomena and scientific findings: that is, the causes of disease are considered infection, mechanical injury, tumor growth, or stress.

In non-Western societies, families may have explanatory belief systems in which illness and disease are viewed as resulting from social or supernatural causes or from imbalances (such as hot and cold, or yin and yang) in the body. For instance, traditional Asian health care beliefs and practices, according to Hong and Friedman (1998), emanate from the Chinese culture, which teaches that health is a state of spiritual, psychological, and physical harmony and violation of this harmony, or balance, causes illness and disease. The view of what is an effective therapy generally is congruent with the beliefs about the cause of the health problem (Kleinman, 1980). If the root cause of disease is perceived as spiritual, prayer and other spiritual interventions are used. For example, spiritual interventions are sought by Mexican Americans for certain "folk" and mental illnesses. Similarly, the Hmong people, whose health belief system is primarily based on the supernatural, center much of their treatment on spiritual appeasement (Brainard & Zaharlick, 1989). Also, some Filipino-Americans and African-Americans believe that illness happens because of the "will of God" (Campinha-Bacote, 1998; Miranda, et al, 1998). Some African-Americans believe that faith in God and prayer as a communicating link with God will bring them through their illnesses.

On the other hand, if the root cause of disease is believed to be a problem with social interaction, social interventions are favored. For example, some native Hawaiians believe that there is a relationship between sickness and the breaking of social rules (Casken, 1999). Similarly, some Native Americans who believe that illness is a social phenomenon may execute elaborate, ritualized ceremonies, such as "sings" and sand paintings, for therapy (Adair, et al, 1988).

Most traditional health beliefs and practices promote the health of the family because they are generally oriented to family and society. They reinforce family cohesion. For example, in many cultures, when a family member is seriously ill, family members expect to be present, supportive, and protective. This practice serves to bind the family together in an important task in which all family members take part. Less common is the situation in which cultural beliefs and values adversely affect an individual family member's health. For example, a Hispanic family may delay seeking Western medical treatment because its members have identified a health problem as a folk illness, which they expect to be alleviated by folk remedies. In this case, health care may be delayed. However, most traditional health beliefs and practices, if not effective in terms of cure, are benign enough to have no negative consequences, unless they delay the decision to seek effective professional help (Helman, 1990).

Health beliefs are translated into health care practices, which then affect the health status of the family and its members. What constitutes appropriate care for specific health conditions is bound by cultural and social class expectations. Use of both Western and indigenous health care treatment is found among many Asian and Hispanic families. For example, some Asian-Americans use both Western and traditional medicine. This is especially common when they are dealing with a chronic or serious illness that Western medicine has little hope of curing. In her study of Korean immigrants, Miller found that some Korean immigrants (regardless of their level of acculturation) used traditional Eastern medicine (herbs and acupuncture) for the purpose of health promotion and disease prevention. In addition, these same Korean immigrants sought Western practitioners (physicians) when they needed more accurate diagnosis or fast relief from symptoms such as pain (Miller, 1988).

In seeking Western health care, treatment may be delayed because of the high value placed on self-control, not complaining about pain, and suppression of feelings (Hong & Friedman, 1998). African-American families who tend to be suspicious of health care professionals and who may feel socially and culturally alienated from available health care may delay seeking care. Because of their strong family ties, individual members are more likely to seek health care from the family than from the health care system (Campinha-Bacote, 1998). They will often withstand obvious symptoms of ill health and exhaust all home remedies known to family and friends before feeling forced to turn to the health care system for assistance (Friedman, 1998).

Conflicts between family members about health care beliefs and practices may adversely affect family health. These conflicts are often created by generational differences. The older generation in the family may maintain their traditional views of illness and appropriate interventions, whereas the younger generation may adopt Western health notions and health care practices. The two sets of beliefs and practices may clash, leaving the family divided and less adaptive and able to care for a family member with a major illness.

Values

A family's values guide the development of its norms and rules and serve as general guides to its behavior. *Family values* refer to shared systems of ideas, attitudes, and beliefs about the worth or priority of entities or ideas that bind the members of a family in a common culture (Parad & Caplan, 1965). They are a reflection of the society and the subculture(s) with which the family identifies. Values involve the time dimension, relationships between people, the relationship of human beings to nature, individuals' prevailing orientation in life activities (Kluckholm & Strodtbeck, 1961), and views of independence and interdependence (Lin & Liu, 1993). Some values are more central and influential than others. Given a competing set of demands, central or core values typically determine a family's priorities.

In families that are not acculturated to the society's dominant culture, values are largely based on the family's cultural background, and these are referred to as "traditional" values. But even traditional values are not static; they are shaped and modified to fit social and economic conditions (Mirande, 1991).

Culturally derived values influence family health by setting priorities for making decisions and coping with life's stressors. For example, the value placed on relationships between people in part determines how the family and its members function in crisis. In some cultures, family needs and goals take precedence over individual needs and goals. Asian-Americans and Hispanic Americans, in general, place greater emphasis than Anglo-Americans on the needs of family before the needs of individuals. Filial piety, ancestor worship, and respecting authority are important family core or central values for Asian-American families. Saving face (maintaining family honor) is another important Asian-American family value (Hong & Friedman, 1998; Friedman, 1998). Among Latino families, *familism* is seen as a core value (Suarez & Ramirez, 1999). Members generally pull together, with primary and secondary kin supporting the family member(s) in need. Generally, this practice has positive effects on family functioning and health, although in some families there may be a dark side to familism. De Vore and London (1993) note that "while ethnicity provides individuals with a sense of cohesion and identity drawn from the strength of the group, it also may be the source of strain, discordance, and strife" (p. 323). For instance, extended family obligations, for example, financial or caregiving, may reduce a nuclear family's ability to meet its own needs and goals.

Another family value that may affect family health is orientation to time. When present time is the focus rather than future time, family members may find it hard to change their lifestyles to avoid a potential health problem. For example, when family members appear well and the consequences of an unhealthy lifestyle are likely to become apparent only years later, necessary lifestyle modifications may be difficult to implement. A common example of this situation is the family in which the husband or father has essential hypertension. If the husband or father is from a culture that is primarily present-oriented and he feels "well" and is able to function, he may deny the need to modify his dietary patterns and lifestyle and fail to adhere to his medication regimen (Friedman & Ferguson-Marshalleck, 1996).

A family's relationship to its community also affects family health and functioning. The greater the congruence between a family's values and the wider community's values, the easier it is for its family members and the family to adjust. Moreover, the greater the congruence, the greater the family's success in relating to its community (Friedman, 1998). When family values clash significantly with the values of the community and society in which the family resides, the family's relationship to their community may be strained. In such cases, families may believe they cannot obtain health and welfare services from their communities and so they "ask and receive little." They also may be discouraged from applying for assistance to community agencies that see them as less deserving or in some way "ineligible" for services. With diminished health or welfare services, family and individual health eventually suffers.

Roles, Power, and Communication Patterns

The impact of culture on family roles, power, and communication patterns is considerable, particularly in unacculturated families. Culture dictates the roles family members play within and outside of the family. This is not to say that culture is static; it is not. Culture changes, and family norms, rules and associated roles, power, and communications are modified to meet the demands and challenges that families face. Our culture has changed in response to technological innovation (Murray & Zentner, 1993) and rapid social and demographic changes. These changes have, in turn, affected family roles, power, and communication patterns.

The traditional culturally derived roles of men, women, and children in families have been and continue to be modified to adapt to new realities and challenges. Two trends that have had a great impact on family roles, power, and communication patterns are the increasing numbers of women who work and the increasing numbers of single-parent families (Rossi, 1986; Friedman, 1998). Table 5–3 shows how family roles have changed as a result of technological changes and women's participation in work outside the home. These role, power relationships, and communication changes have occurred in all types of families (Baca-Zinn, 1980; Mirande, 1991; Pleck, 1985; Spitze, 1988; Wilkinson, 1987).

In those families where marital partners are from the same cultural background and agree on family roles, family power distribution, and communication patterns, the common cultural understanding provides meaning, structure, and continuity. For example, McAdoo (1993b), in a study of 40 middle-income African-American families found that African-American spouses shared equally in the major decisions in the family and were satisfied with their marital lives regardless of family decision-making styles. In families where mates are from different cultures, they may have differing expectations about family roles, communication, and power relationships. In these cases, family functioning may be affected negatively.

Culturally based conflicts frequently arise when family members from immigrant families have differing degrees of exposure to the wider American culture. For instance, some middle-aged immigrant Filipino parents on the West Coast do not expect to live with their children in their old age. A younger group of immigrant and native-born Filipinos, on the other hand, believe that children should take care of elderly parents (Miranda et al, 1998). Children may become more quickly acculturated to "the American way" in school. What and how they are taught in school may conflict

TABLE 5–3
Recent Changes in Two-Parent Nuclear Family Roles and Power

Traditional Role or Power Structure	Changes Caused by Technological Innovations	Changes Caused when Women Join the Labor Force
Husband's roles		
Seen as primary breadwinner		Husband and wife share breadwinner role in most families
"Wears pants in the family"		Shift from male (husband and father) domination to greater shared power between husband and wife
Wife's roles		
Supports husband's efforts and decisions		More egalitarian decision making in marriage
In charge of child care and household	Women have ability to plan family; reduction in length of childbearing and child rearing period	Greater spousal sharing of child care roles and, to a lesser extent, household roles
Communication in the family more complementary and hierarchical	Women's time doing household work substantially reduced	Communication more egalitarian and open

Source: Baca-Zinn, 1980; Chilman, 1993; Erickson and Gecas, 1991; McAdoo, 1993b; Pleck, 1985; Spitze, 1988; and Wilkinson, 1987.

with what and how they have been taught at home. As a result, culturally based conflicts often occur between the generations (Larrabee, 1973; Friedman, 1998). The degree of acculturation in terms of language may also cause conflicts. For instance, parents who do not speak English and children who speak only English may have conflicts or misunderstandings because of the language gap. This is evident in most Asian-American immigrants, especially between the first generation of immigrant parents and the children born in the U.S. or children who immigrated when they were very young (Uba, 1994).

Coping

Culture also influences the ways in which families adapt to and cope with internal and external demands and changes. The strategies that families use to cope influence family health and family functioning. *Family coping* is defined as positive problem-appropriate affective, cognitive, and behavioral responses that families and their subsystems use to solve a problem or reduce the stress produced by the problem or event (Friedman, 1992). Family coping strategies develop and change over time in response to the stressors and demands experienced (Menaghan, 1983) and also differ across the family life cycle (Schnittger & Bird, 1993).

Various coping strategies are used to either eliminate the stressor or demand, control the meaning of the stressor or demand, or reduce the stress or tension created by the stressor or demand. Coping strategies may be internal or external (Friedman & Ferguson-Marshalleck, 1996). Internal coping strategies rely on resources contained within the family and external coping strategies depend on supports and resources outside of the family (McCubbin, et al, 1991). Box 5–1 summarizes examples of both types of strategies.

Traditional or unacculturated ethnic families make extensive use of culturally derived family coping strategies. Chinese and Vietnamese immigrant families provide a good example of ethnic differences in family coping patterns. Both Chinese and Vietnamese families commonly use the coping strategy of family group reliance and family cohesiveness. In China, families' social network connections have been essential for survival. Consequently, in the face of family stressors the

Box 5–1

TYPES OF FAMILY COPING STRATEGIES

Internal Family Coping Strategies

Family group reliance, including delegation
The use of humor and stress management tactics
Increased sharing together: maintaining cohesiveness
Controlling the meaning of the stressor/demand: cognitive refraining and passive appraisal
Joint family problem solving
Role flexibility
Normalizing
Limiting leisure time and recreational activities
Accepting stressful events as a fact of life

External Family Coping Strategies

Seeking information and professional help
Maintaining active links with community groups and organizations
Seeking and using social supports (informal and formal social support systems and self-help groups)
Seeking and using spiritual supports
Sharing concerns and experiences with relatives, friends, and neighbors

Source: Adapted from Friedman (1998).

extended family pulls together. Chinese families encourage interdependence and family loyalty, and the receiving and giving of help between the generations (Lin & Liu, 1993).

Immigrant Vietnamese families use similar coping strategies. Gold (1993) quotes one Vietnamese family member's explanation of how his family deals with problems:

> To Vietnamese culture, family is everything. There are aspects [coping strategies] which help us readjust to this society . . . We solve problems because the family institution is a bank. If *I* need money—and my brother and my two sisters are working I tell them I need to buy a house . . . Now I help them. They live with me and have no rent. The family is a hospital. If mom is sick, I, my children, and my brother and sister care for her (p. 304).

Research on ethnic differences in family coping is limited. One study conducted by Friedman (1985), looked at 55 families who had a child with cancer. Half of the families were Anglo and the other half Latino. Anglo families (mostly middle-class) reported that information seeking and the support of neighbors and friends (external) and the support of spouse (internal) were the most helpful coping strategies. On the other hand, Latino families (mostly working-class and lower-class Mexican-American families) reported that extended family support and spiritual support (external) were most helpful. Latinos relied heavily on religion to cope with their child's cancer. Because culture and religion are so closely intertwined in Latin culture and most of the Latino families in this study were recent immigrants and unacculturated, the differences in coping between the two cultural groups was quite pronounced.

The Latino families in Friedman's study depended on primary and secondary kin to assist and support them with the array of demands created by childhood cancer. In those families who had recently immigrated from El Salvador and had no extended family support, family functioning was poorer. Friedman concluded that the absence of the families' natural social support system (the extended family) left a vacuum for these families and reduced their ability to cope. The inaccessibility of culturally appropriate social support and the reluctance of family members to use substitute social supports (e.g., health personnel, neighbors, friends) created personal and interpersonal difficulties in handling the stress of childhood cancer.

THE INFLUENCE OF SOCIAL CLASS

America's Social Class Structure

Like all other industrialized nations, the United States is stratified by class. A stratified society is marked by inequality, by differences among people that rank them as higher or lower on the scale (Gilbert & Kahl, 1987). Although social classes may be distinguished from each other, the lines of demarcation are not clear-cut. Income and wealth are indicators of social class. Available resources (e.g., natural, material, social, political, economic) determine a person's or family's life conditions. The extent to which persons and families have access to and use resources (which are called "life chances" in the literature) reflects their social class. Power, prestige, and privilege are often manifestations of wealth and, hence, a family's social class (Ropers, 1991).

As the United States has been transformed from an agricultural to an industrial society, and then to a postindustrial technological society, the class structure has correspondingly changed. The components of the new class structure, which came about because of shifts in the types of jobs needed to sustain a postindustrial society, are discussed by sociologists Gilbert and Kahl (1987). They describe American society as being a national capitalist class built on corporate wealth with an upper middle class of college-educated professionals and managers. Technicians, semiprofessionals, blue-collar workers, and clerical and sales workers comprise a lower middle class, and people who are unemployed or engaged in menial and unskilled jobs are considered the lower class. At the bottom of the lower class are an increasingly isolated underclass of families and individuals who are employed in unstable menial jobs or are not working.

Poverty

Families with incomes below the poverty line make up an increasing proportion of families in the United States today. More than 11 percent of families in the country live in poverty. While the proportion of the population living below the poverty level declined from a high of 13.7 percent in 1996 to 13.3 percent in 1997, the number of poor people in 1997, 35.6 million, remained statistically unchanged (U.S. Bureau of the Census, 1998). One need only to look at large cities to see how poverty has increasingly affected the rate of homelessness, which, a rare sight in the past, is now glaringly apparent (Berne et al, 1990).

Who are the Poor?

The individuals and families who have suffered most from deterioration or stagnation in the economy and reductions in the level of governmental assistance are children, young families, older adults, and poorly educated and unskilled persons. Other individuals and families who may be affected by the same economic conditions are African-American men, illegal immigrants, families headed by women, and residents of inner cities and economically depressed small towns and rural areas (Chilman, 1991; Wilson, 1987).

One popular misconception about the poor in America is that they are concentrated in inner cities. This is not true. In 1997, only 18.8 percent of poor persons in the United States lived in central cities; 9 percent lived in suburban areas within metropolitan areas (U.S. Bureau of the Census, 1998). The majority (59.2 percent) of poor African-American families and the majority (62.9 percent) of poor Hispanic families do, however, live in central city areas. Because poverty is as much a problem in rural areas as in the inner cities, the problem of poverty and its consequences for health must be addressed in both areas (Winnick, 1991).

There are two groups of poor families: those in temporary poverty and those in persistent poverty. The majority of those who are in temporary poverty escape it by obtaining jobs with wages sufficient for living or by joining extended family units to gain a combined income that will ameliorate the worst effects of poverty. Those in persistent poverty, who are primarily women and children, have a much more difficult time escaping from it (Friedman & Ferguson-Marshalleck, 1996).

Underclass is a term used to describe people in persistent poverty. People in the underclass are described as having attitudes, values, and lifestyles that do not conform to the values of mainstream American society (McAdoo, 1993a). Because of the clash in values and behaviors between underclass families and the mainstream dominant culture, these families have a strained relationship with the wider community. This conflict makes it difficult for underclass families, who are stigmatized by the wider society, to obtain the resources needed to function at even a minimally acceptable level. Poor persons, particularly those in the underclass, are a vulnerable population who are living in poverty conditions with multiple persistent stressors that undermine the physical, psychological, and economic health of the family and its members (Chilman, 1991).

Homelessness is another growing, significant family stressor for poor people. Homelessness is defined as losing one's possessions, living with relatives during hard times, or simply having no home. In the latter instance, families or individuals may or may not have temporary housing in a shelter. In the 1950s through the 1970s, most homeless persons had some shelter: "flophouses," single room-occupancy hotels, or mission shelters. However, many contemporary homeless people are literally sleeping on the streets. Being homeless subjects family members to a myriad of physical and psychosocial stressors. Homeless families are likely to be socially isolated, with no regular or strong ties to family, friends, or other social networks. Their lack of social support magnifies their vulnerability to disabilities and deprivations (Rossi et al, 1987). Single-parent families with children are, tragically, an increasingly visible, vulnerable component of the homeless population. Single women and minorities are also particularly vulnerable homeless groups. Compared with those who have homes, the prevalence of mental illness is greater among homeless women, while the prevalence of alcoholism and other forms of substance abuse is greater among homeless men (Aday, 1993; U.S. Department of Health and Human Services, 1998).

Social Class Effects

Social status is strongly correlated with health. The more affluent an individual or family, the better their life conditions, the greater their access to preventive and therapeutic health care services, and the better their health status. Further, families from the upper and middle classes, regardless of ethnic background, tend to have better self-care behaviors. Because of numerous stressors, poor people find it difficult to be future-oriented and concerned about healthy lifestyles.

The correlation between social class and health holds true for both adults and children. For example, Starfield (1992) found that poor children are more likely to become ill and to have serious illnesses than children from higher-income families. The higher rates of serious health problems and the increased death rates from disease in children of all ages from poor families reflect exposure to environmental hazards, poor nutrition, inadequate preventive care, and poor access to medical care, all of which are a part of social class inequalities in "life conditions" and "life chances." Research findings since the 1930s have consistently demonstrated that lower-class, economically distressed families are more likely to have poorer family health, less family stability, poorer marital adjustment, greater problems in family coping, and troubled family relationships (Voydanoff & Donnelly, 1998).

THE INTERACTION OF CULTURE AND SOCIAL CLASS

The Effects of Culture and Social Class Interaction

While the separate influences of culture (particularly ethnicity) and social class on family health are considerable, the influence of these two variables together may be profound. Certain groups in the United States, largely because of ethnic or racial inequalities and social stratification, have become entrenched in poverty. Institutional racism often locks families into a state in which social class mobility is practically nonexistent. Therefore, these families tend to pass on their "inherited" class disadvantages from one generation to the next.

Gordon (1964) described the pronounced association between ethnic group membership and social class as *ethclass*. This intersection of ethnicity and social class produces identifiable dispositions and behavioral patterns in families and individuals. Social class and ethnicity in interaction define the basic conditions of life and simultaneously account for differences among ethnic groups with different social class positions. For instance, important commonalities are created among families because of their common cultural heritage and by virtue of being black in America. Despite these important commonalities, lifestyles and life chances vary drastically between affluent African-American families and poor African-American families. Ethnic families, especially those of color, are much more likely to be poor than white families of European descent. Among the major ethnic and racial groups in the United States, the percentage of those persons living in poverty in 1997 varied from a low of 11 percent among non-Hispanic whites and 14 percent for Asians and Pacific Islanders to 27.1 percent among Hispanics and 26.5 percent among African-Americans (U.S. Bureau of the Census, 1998).

Being from an ethnic family of color and being poor pose greater hazards to family and individual health than being either from an ethnic family of color that is not poor or from a poor white family. African-American and Hispanic children are nearly four times more likely than Anglo-American children to live in poverty, and indicators of poorer health status are clustered among these poor minority children (U.S. Bureau of the Census, 1997).

However, it must be understood that race and ethnicity have a significant impact on health status primarily because ethnically and racially diverse families are more frequently disadvantaged socioeconomically (Cockerham, 1987). Hence, even though cultural background is linked to differences in individual health status, social class is more important in producing such variation. Spector (1996) agrees when she points out that being poor is the major barrier to obtaining access to the health care system. Lack of health insurance is a major barrier, according to a recent national survey of health care and health insurance coverage. Almost 40 percent of working-age Latinos have no health insurance (de la Torre, 1993). Many Asian-Americans also lack health insurance (Johnson et al., 1995; Louie, 1995; Samani, 1994).

The interaction of culture and social class may also substantially influence health care practices. For example, de la Torre (1993) speculates that ethnic families in the United States who are poor use folk medicine and home remedies more often than they would prefer, simply because they lack access to professional health care. Evidence to support this idea comes from a large survey of Mexican-Americans in Southern California (Keefe, 1981). Among Keefe's sample of Mexican-Americans, it was only the unacculturated, poor Mexican-American families who still used folk medicine to any great extent, and this was primarily in the treatment of folk illnesses. Among the middle-class and more affluent Mexican-American families, the use of folk medicine had practically disappeared. However, contrary to Keefe's sample of Mexican-Americans, Korean immigrants relied on Eastern (herb and acupuncture) medical treatment, regardless of their income and education. Miller (1990) in her study of 102 Korean immigrants reported that respondents with higher income ($40,000 and higher) made more visits to the Eastern doctors' offices for herbal medicines than their poor counterparts. This may have been because most herbs are rather expensive and poorer Korean immigrants could not as easily afford to buy them.

IMPLICATIONS FOR FAMILY NURSING PRACTICE

Social Cultural Assessment and Intervention

The family's sociocultural background is central in shaping family values, beliefs, and behaviors, and in shaping specific health beliefs and practices. Social class and ethnic background (ethclass), both singly and in combination, also affect families' health status. Because of the centrality of sociocultural influences on family life and health, sensitivity to ethnicity, social class, and culture are imperative to nurses who are working with families. In the words of De Vore and London (1993), "practice skills and techniques must be adapted to respond to the needs or dispositions of various ethnic [and class] groups" (p. 324). Further, cultural and socioeconomic assessments must be an integral component of family assessments (Table 5–4 and Table 5–5).

To illustrate the importance of integrating a family's sociocultural aspects to nursing interventions, the Lindero family will be discussed as a case in point (refer to Case Study). The Lindero family provides a case situation that contains some of the components discussed in this chapter. At first, the nurse may consider the family's lack of response to seeking medical intervention for Ernesto as a knowledge deficit related to the infant's state of health. However, it is important in the assessment phase that the nurse considers the social and cultural implications inherent in the family situation that may be contributing to the family's refusal to bring the infant in for medical care.

Using the assessment instruments that appear in this

TABLE 5–4
Cultural Assessment Guidelines

Assessment Criterion	Questions
Ethnic or racial identity	How does the family identify itself in terms of ethnicity and racial background? Are the parents both from the same ethnic background?
Languages spoken	What languages are spoken in the home? By whom? What language is preferred when speaking to outsiders?
Place of birth and immigration history	Where were the parents and children born? If they emigrated from another country, when and why did they immigrate to the United States?
Geographic mobility	Where have the parents lived? When did they move to their present residence?
Family's religion	What is the family's religion? Are both parents from the same religious background? How actively involved is the family in religiously based activities and practices?
Ethnic group affiliation	What are the characteristics of the family's friends and associations? Are they all from the family's ethnic group? Do recreational, political, educational, and other social activities take place within the ethnic group, the wider community, or both? To what extent does the family use services and vendors within the family's ethnic community and within the wider community?
Neighborhood affiliation	What are the characteristics of the family's neighborhood? Is it ethnically heterogeneous or homogeneous?
Dietary habits and dress	What are the family's dietary preferences and prohibitions? Do the family members dress in traditional clothing?
Household appearance	Are the family's home decorations, art, and religious objects culturally derived?
Use of alternative and folk systems	What are the family's health and illness beliefs and practices? What cultural or ethnic healing practices and health promotion activities are used by the family? What types of practitioners are used for health care? Who does the family seek initially for health care services?
Family life transitions	What are the customs and beliefs about family life transitions, such as birth, illness, mourning and death, pregnancy, well-baby care, and elder care?
Acceptance by community	To what extent is the family affected by discrimination?

Source: Friedman (1998), modified with permission.

TABLE 5–5
Socioeconomic Assessment Guidelines

Assessment Criterion	Questions
Family composition and educational level	How many members does this family's constellation have? Who is the head of the household? How many members are under age 18 and over age 65? What are the educational levels of the family members?
Family perceptions of their housing and finances	How do family members feel about the adequacy of their housing arrangements and their finance situation?
Family financial resources	How many members are gainfully employed full-time or part-time? What are their occupations? What is the household annual income? Who are the breadwinners in the family? What are other financial resources (e.g., government, public funds, or assistance)? How does the family pay for health services? How well is the family managing financially?
Family expenses	How much is spent, on average, per month for the following? Rent or mortgage Food Child and elder care Health and dental care Recreational and leisure activities Transportation Utilities Other

Source: Adapted from Friedman (1998).

chapter, the nurse would maintain open communication with the family by using appropriate questions from these instruments. While engaged on the phone with Mrs. Lindero, the nurse would inquire as to how best she could assist the family. Since the Lindero family is Hispanic, the nurse would first consider the health beliefs and practices of the family by asking how they have managed the health problems of family members in the past and whether they have used home remedies or alternative practitioners. The nurse would want to explore approaches that are being used presently by the family to treat the infant. Further, the nurse would need to query about the beliefs that are associated with the infant's physical condition and with not exposing the infant to the elements external to the home.

Because, in traditional Hispanic families, the father is the major decision maker, it becomes necessary to inquire as to the family's decision-making process regarding the medical care and management of family members. Because grandparents are highly regarded, the role of the grandmother is also integral in the decision-making process. The nurse would request to speak with Mr. Lindero to assess his beliefs regarding the health of the infant, his perception of the urgency for medical follow-up, and his reason for not wanting to have the infant seen in an urgent care clinic. Family dynamics, in terms of decision-making process, must be incorporated into family nursing care.

It is important that the nurse not lose sight of the physical state of the infant. The nurse must assess the physical signs and symptoms reported by the family that would indicate the degree of respiratory distress, dehydration, or further complications. If it appears that medical care is warranted, then the nurse could assist the family in balancing cultural belief systems with the need for medical intervention. Once these options are weighed and the family insists that they wish to keep the infant at home, the most appropriate approach may be for the nurse to consider using a home health care nurse. By conducting a cultural assessment to determine patterns and lifeways for the Lindero family along with their perception of the problem and how best to resolve it, the nurse can advocate on behalf of the family in the development of culturally appropriate services.

To effectively assist in the care of families from diverse cultures, ethnic groups, and social classes, family nurses must have a clear understanding of their own ethnic and social class identification and recognize their own potential and real biases (McAdoo, 1993a). Health professionals are repositories of their own ethnic, religious, racial, and social class subcultures. They often believe that they can nullify their biases. However, it is only with continuing self-exploration and awareness of their preconceptions, attitudes, values, and beliefs that health professionals can develop an understanding and sensitivity to different cultures and social classes. One's awareness and sensitivity are never complete. Interpretations continue to arise that have cultural or social class connotations that may interfere with the process of providing services to clients (McAdoo, 1993a).

SUMMARY

The influence of culture is pervasive. It shapes choices about what we eat, drink, and wear; how we are entertained; how we determine health and illness; what

RESEARCH BRIEF

Families represent the fastest-growing subgroup of the homeless population. Most of the research has focused on urban homeless families and not on rural homeless families. The purpose of this study was to describe the characteristics and health of rural homeless families in Ohio. A descriptive cross-sectional design was used to study 76 families who had 125 children under 12 years of age. An interview schedule, the Denver Developmental Screening Test (DDST), the Child Behavior Checklist (CBCL), and SCL-90-R were used to collect data.

The majority of the mothers perceived themselves and their children as having no physical health problems. Twenty-four of the children were behind on their immunizations. Forty-four (52 percent) of the children under 6 years of age had DDST scores that indicated they might have developmental lags and 15 of the children over 4 years of age had CBCL scores that indicated they might have behavioral problems. The reported use of illegal drugs, alcohol, and cigarettes was high for this group of mothers.

Implications for family nursing practice with rural homeless families are as follows:

- Seek out homeless families and their children to assess their health and other needs. Assess families for signs of substance abuse and emotional distress in children, including suicide ideation, suicide plans, or other types self-destructive thoughts or behaviors.
- Use case-management strategies in finding creative solutions to fill service gaps.
- Encourage interdisciplinary collaboration with professionals from multiple service systems to identify, create, and use scarce resources for the homeless.

In summary, nurses have the power to make the choice to provide assistance to homeless families.

Wagner, J.D., Menke, E.M., & Ciccone, J.K. (1995). What is known about the health of rural homeless families? *Public Health Nursing, 12*(6):400–408.

we study in school; and myriad other aspects of our daily lives. The family's socioeconomic or social class status also plays a primary role in shaping family behavior, particularly family lifestyle.

This chapter discusses and describes some of the complex sociocultural influences on family health. The health status of individuals in the United States differs dramatically across cultural groups and social classes. Major indicators show that the health status of minority Americans compared with whites is substantially poorer. The same is true in terms of social class differences: health status is worse among poor Americans. Although the separate influences of ethnicity and of social class on family health is considerable, the influence of the interaction of these two variables may have a much more profound effect. Social class and culture (ethclass), particularly ethnicity, interact to define the basic conditions of life and simultaneously account for differences between ethnic groups with different social class positions.

The major implication for nursing practice is that to provide quality professional nursing care to families, nurses must be not only knowledgeable about the various sociocultural beliefs, values, and practices, but also sensitive and competent in working with families from the various cultural and social classes. To do this, health practitioners need to assess their own cultural and class biases. Finally, health practitioners must identify the socioeconomic and cultural factors that can be modified to facilitate the desired health-related behavioral change.

Case Study

THE LINDERO FAMILY (HISPANIC FAMILY)

The Lindero family consists of Pedro, age 28; Margarita, his 23-year-old wife, three children, and Mrs. Josefina Lindero, Pedro's mother. Margarita delivered an infant boy, Ernesto, six weeks ago who is currently experiencing upper respiratory distress. Margarita calls the nurse at the doctor's office to determine what to do for her baby. The nurse urges Margarita to bring the infant into urgent care. Pedro who has just returned home from work is informed by Margarita of her need to take Ernesto into urgent care. Josefina Lindero tells Pedro and Margarita that it is not necessary to take Ernesto to the hospital. She believes that it will do more harm to take the infant out of the house. Pedro agrees with his mother. Margarita calls the nurse back and informs her that she will not be bringing the baby to urgent care.

Discussion Questions

1. How would the nurse assist this family to resolve the situation?
2. What cultural factors need to be considered?
3. What family structure and functions need to be assessed?
4. What family nursing interventions would be culturally appropriate?

Study Questions

1. The growing significance of cultural diversity in the United States is emphasized by the fact that more than one in four residents are nonwhite or of Hispanic origin. Which ethnic group experienced the highest increase in growth between 1980 and 1990?
   a. Hispanic
   b. Asian/Pacific Islander
   c. Native American
   d. African-American
2. The country of origin of an individual is primarily related to his or her:
   a. Racial classification.
   b. Social class.
   c. Ethnic classification.
   d. Cultural classification.
3. Factors that contribute to differences in health status in various cultural groups and social classes include all of the following except:
   a. Inadequate access to preventive and basic health care resources.
   b. Family and personal lifestyle differences.
   c. Exposure to environmental hazards.

d. Personality differences.
e. Income inequality and rising unemployment.

4. Which of the following types of families are more likely to experience poor health within their family?
   a. Lower-class families
   b. Middle-class families
   c. Upper middle-class families
   d. Economically affluent families
5. Ethnic families that have integrated dominant American core values and practices in their lives are considered to be
   a. Ethnocentric.
   b. Unacculturated.
   c. Culturally competent.
   d. Acculturated.
6. Culturally derived family values influence family health by setting priorities with respect to making family decisions. "Familism" in the Latino culture is an example of which cultural orientation?
   a. Time orientation
   b. Family versus self-interest
   c. Active versus passive orientation
   d. Past versus present
7. Which of the following three philosophical or religious beliefs and value systems are more likely to influence the majority of Asian Americans?
   a. Judeo-Christian beliefs, Muslim, and Confucianism
   b. Taoism, Buddhism, and Confucianism
   c. Buddhism, Hinduism, and Shintoism
   d. Hinduism, Taoism, and Islam
8. Women's participation in the labor force has contributed to all of the following changes in family roles, power relationships, and communication patterns, except:
   a. More open communication.
   b. Greater sharing of child care roles in family.
   c. Less sharing of power in marital relationships.
   d. Sharing of breadwinner role between husband and wife.
9. Ethnic differences in family coping patterns are seen among traditional or unaccculturated families. Which of the following coping strategies would commonly be used by Chinese families? (You may choose one or more answers.)
   a. Family group reliance
   b. Role flexibility
   c. Spiritual support
   d. Maintaining family cohesiveness
10. Families who live below the poverty line are at greater risk of experiencing which of the following?
    a. Homelessness
    b. Poor health status
    c. Lack of access to health services
    d. Higher mortality rates
    e. All of the above

References

Ablon, J., & Ames, G. M. (1989). Culture and family. In C. L. Gilliss, et al. (Eds.) *Toward a Science of Family Nursing*. Menlo Park, CA: Addison-Wesley.

Adair, J., et al. (1988). *The People's Health: Anthropology and Medicine in a Navaho Community*. Albuquerque: University of New Mexico Press.

Aday, L.A. (1993). *At Risk in America*. San Francisco: Jossey-Bass.

Baca-Zinn, M. (1980). Employment and education of Mexican American women: The interplay of modernity and ethnicity in eight families. *Harvard Educational Review, 50*:47–62.

Berne, A.S., et al. (1990). A nursing model for addressing the health needs of homeless families. *Image, 22*: 813.

Berry, J. W. (1990). Psychology of acculturation: Understanding individuals moving between cultures. In R. Breslin (Ed.), *Applied Cross-Cultural Psychology*. Newbury Park, CA: Sage.

Boone, M. S. (1989). *Capital Crime: Black Infant Mortality in America*. Newbury Park, CA: Sage.

Brainard, J., and Zaharlick, A. (1989). Changing health beliefs and behaviors of resettled Laotion refugees: Ethnic variation in adaptation. *Social Science and Medicine, 29*:845–852.

Braun, D. (1991). *The Rich Get Richer*. Chicago: Nelson-Hall.

Campinha-Bacote, J. (1998). African-Americans. In Purnell, L.D. and Paulanka, B. (Eds.) *Transcultural Health Care: A Cultural Competent Approach*. Philadelphia, PA: F.A. Davis.

Casken, J. (1999). Pacific Islander health and disease: an overview. In Huff and Kline (Eds.) *Promoting Health in Multicultural Populations: A Handbook for Practitioners*. Thousand Oaks, CA: Sage.

Chilman, C. (1991). Working poor families: Trends, causes, effects, and suggested policies. *Family Relations, 40*:191–198.

Chilman, C. (1993). Hispanic families in the United States. In H. R. McAdoo (Ed.), *Family Ethnicity: Strength in Diversity*, pp. 141–163. Newbury Park, CA: Sage.

Cockerham, W. L. (1987). *Medical Sociology*, ed 2. Englewood Cliffs, NJ: Prentice-Hall.

de la Torre, A. (1993, March 31). *Access is vital in health care reform*, p. B7. Los Angeles, CA: Los Angeles Times.

De Vore, W, & London, H. (1993). Ethnic sensitivity for practitioners. In H. R. McAdoo (Ed.). *Family Ethnicity: Strength in Diversity* (pp. 317-331). Newbury Park, CA: Sage.

Erickson, R.J., & Gecas, V. (1991). Social class and fatherhood. In E W Bozett and S. M. H. Hanson (Eds.), *Fatherhood and Families in Cultural Context.* New York: Springer.

Falicov, C. J. (1988). Learning to think culturally. In D. C. Breunlin & R. C. Schwartz (Eds.), *Handbook of Family Therapy, Training, and Supervision.* New York: Guilford.

Friedman, M. (1985). *Family stress and coping among Anglo and Latino families with childhood cancer.* Unpublished dissertation. University of Southern California, Los Angeles.

Friedman, M. (1992). *Family Nursing: Theory and Practice*, ed 3. Norwalk, CT: Appleton & Lange.

Friedman, M. (1998). *Family Nursing, Theory, and Practice*, ed 3. Norwalk, CT: Appleton & Lange.

Friedman, M., & Ferguson-Marshalleck, E. (1996). Sociocultural influences on family health. In S. Hanson & S. Boyd (Eds.) *Family Health Care Nursing: Theory, Practice, and Research.* Philadelphia, PA: F. A. Davis.

Gilbert, D., & Kahl, J.A. (1987). *The American Class Structures New Synthesis*, ed 3. Chicago: Dorsey.

Gold, S.J. (1993). Migration and family adjustment: Continuity and change among Vietnamese in the United States. In H. R. McAdoo (Ed.) *Family Ethnicity: Strength in Diversity.* Newbury Park, CA: Sage.

Gordon, M. M. (1964). *Assimilation in American Life.* New York: Oxford University Press.

Helman, C. G. (1990). *Culture, Health, and Illness: An Introduction for Health Professionals.* London: Wright.

Henry, W. (1990, April 9). *Beyond the melting pot*, pp. 28–31. Time.

Hong, G., and Friedman, M. (1998). The Asian-American family. In M. M. Friedman. (Ed.) *Family Nursing: Research, Theory, and Practice*, ed 4. Stamford, CT: Appleton and Lange.

Hopp, J., & Herring, P. (1999). Promoting health among Black American populations: An overview. In Huff and Kline (Eds.) *Promoting Health in Multicultural Populations: A Handbook for Practitioners.* Thousand Oaks, CA: Sage.

Hussey, J. M. (1997). The effects of race, socioeconomic status, and household structure on injury mortality in children and young adults. *Maternal And Child Health Journal*, 1(4):217–227.

Inouye, J. (1999). Asian American health and disease: an overview of the issues. In Huff and Kline, (Eds.) *Promoting Health in Multicultural Populations: A Handbook for Practitioners.* Thousand Oaks, CA: Sage.

Johnson, K.W., et al. (1995). Panel II: Macrosocial and environmental influences on minority health. *Health Psychology, 14*:601–602.

Jones, E. E., & Korchin, S.J. (1982). *Minority mental health.* New York: Praeger.

Kavanagh, K. H., & Kennedy, R H. (1992). *Promoting cultural diversity.* Newbury Park, CA: Sage.

Keefe, S. E. (1981). Folk medicine among Mexican-Americans: Cultural persistence, change and displacement. *Hispanic Journal of Behavioral Science*, 3:41–48.

Kleinman, A.(1980). *Patients and Healers in the Context of Culture. An Exploration of the Borderland between Anthropology, Medicine, and Psychiatry.* Berkeley: University of California Press.

Kluckholm, E., & Strodtbeck, E. (1961). *Variations in Value Orientations.* New York: Row, Peterson.

Kramer, J. M. (1988). Infant mortality and risk factors among American Indians compared to black and white rates: Implications for policy change. In W. A. Van Home & T. V. Tonnesen (Eds.), *Ethnicity and Health*, pp. 89–115. Milwaukee: University of Wisconsin Institute on Race and Ethnicity.

Kroeber, A. L. (1948). *Anthropology.* New York: Harcourt Brace.

Kumabe, K.I., et al. (1985). *Bridging ethnocultural diversity in social work and health.* Honolulu: University of Hawaii School of Social Work.

Larrabee, E. (1973). Comments to Loretta Ford's Research. An Ethnic Perspective. Community Nursing Research: Collaboration and Completion. Denver, CO: Western Institute of Higher Education Commission.

Lee, P. R. & Estes, C. (1997, Eds.). *The Nation's Health*, ed 5. Sudbury, MA: Jones & Bartlett.

Lin, C., & Liu, W. T. (1993). Relationships among Chinese immigrant families. In H. R. McAdoo (Ed.). *Family Ethnicity: Strength in Diversity*, pp. 271–286. Newbury Park, CA: Sage.

Locke, D.C. (1992). *Increasing Multicultural Understanding: A Comprehensive Model.* Newbury Park, CA: Sage.

Louie, K. (1995). Cultural considerations: Asian-Americans and Pacific Islanders. *Imprint, 42*(5):41–46.

McAdoo, H. R., (1993a). Ethnic families and conclusions.

In H. R. McAdoo (Ed.), *Family Ethnicity: Strength in Diversity*, pp. 3–14, 332–334. Newbury Park, CA: Sage.

McAdoo, J. L. (1993b). Decision making and marital satisfaction in African-American families. In H. R McAdoo (Ed.), *Family Ethnicity: Strength in Diversity*, pp. 109–119. Newbury Park, CA: Sage.

McCubbin, H. I., et al. (1991). F-COPES: Family crisis oriented personal evaluation scales. In H. I. McCubbin & A. Thompson (Eds.), *Family Assessment Inventories for Research and Practice*. Madison: University of Wisconsin-Madison.

McGoldrick, M. (1993). Ethnicity, cultural diversity and normality. In E Walsh (Ed.), *Normal Family Processes*, ed 2, pp. 331–360. New York: Guilford.

Menaghan, E. G. (1983). Individual coping efforts and family studies. Conceptual and methodological issues. In H. I. McCubbin, M. B. Sussman, & J. M. Patterson (Eds.), Social stress and the family (special issue). *Marriage and Family Review*, *6* (112),113–135.

Miller, J. K. (1988). Health beliefs and health utilization patterns of Korean Immigrants. Unpublished dissertation. University of Southern California, Los Angeles.

Miller, J. K. (1990, October). Use of traditional health care by Korean Immigrants to the United States. *Sociology and Social Research*, *75*(1):38–48.

Miranda, B.F., et al. (1998). Filipino-Americans. In Purnell and Paulanka (Eds.), *Transcultural Health Care: A Cultural Competent Approach*. Philadelphia, PA: F.A. Davis.

Mirande, A. (1991). Ethnicity and fatherhood. In E. W. Bozett and S. M. H. Hanson (Eds.), *Fatherhood and Families in Cultural Context*, pp. 53–82. New York: Springer.

Murray, R. B., & Zentner, J. R (1993). *Nursing Assessment and Health Promotion: Strategies across the Life Span*, ed 5. Norwalk, CT: Appleton & Lange.

National Center for Health Statistics. (1992) *Health: United States, 1991*. Hyattsville, MD: U.S. Public Health Service.

Nickens, J. W. (1991). The health status of minority populations in the United States. *Western Journal of Medicine*, *155* (July), 27–32.

Parad, H. J., & Caplan, G. (1965). *A framework for studying families in crisis*. In H. J. Parad (Ed.), Crisis intervention: selected readings, pp 55–60. New York: Family Service of America.

Peterson, J. (1993, April 11). Life in the United States, graded on the curve, pp. Al, AI6. *Los Angeles Times*.

Pleck, J. H. (1985). *Working Wives, Working Husbands*. Beverly Hills, CA: Sage.

Purnell, L.D., & Paulanka, B. (1998). *Transcultural Health Care: A Cultural Competent Approach*. Philadelphia, PA: F.A. Davis.

Rix, S. E. (1990). *The American Woman, 1990–1991: A Status Report*. New York: W.W. Norton.

Ropers, R. H. (1991). *Persistent Poverty*. New York: Plenum.

Rossi, A. S. (1986). Sex and gender in the aging society. In A. Pifer & L. Bronte (Eds.), *Our Aging Society*, pp. 111–139. New York: W.W. Norton.

Rossi, R. H., et al. (1987). The urban homeless: Estimating composition and size. *Science*, *235*:1136–341.

Samani, P. (1994). Myth of model minority. *Asian American and Pacific Islander Journal of Health*, *2*(4): 284–289.

Schnittger, M. H., & Bird, G. W. (1993). Coping among dual-career men and women across the family life cycle. *Family Relations*, *39*:199–205.

Spector, R. E. (1996). *Cultural Diversity in Health and Illness*, ed 4. Norwalk, CT: Appleton & Lange.

Spitze, G. (1988).Women's employment and family relations: A review. *Journal of Marriage and the Famity*, *50*:595–618.

Starfield, B. (1992). Child and adolescent health status measures. In Center for the Future of Children. The Future of Children. The David and Lucille Packard Foundation, (2):24–39.

Suarez, L. & Ramirez, A. (1999). Hispanic/Latino health and disease: An overview. In Huff and Kline (Eds.) *Promoting Health in Multicultural Populations: A Handbook for Practitioners*. Thousand Oaks, CA: Sage.

Uba, L. (1994). *Asian American: Personality, Patterns, Identity, and Mental Health*. New York: Guilford.

United Press International (1990, February 6). Tax report says rich gained, poor lost during the 80s, p A4. *Los Angeles Times*.

U.S. Bureau of the Census. (1983). 1980 census of population. General population characteristics. (Part 1, United States Summary PC 80–1-61). Washington, DC: U.S. Government Printing Office.

U.S. Bureau of the Census. (1992a). Statistical Abstracts of the United States. Washington, DC: U.S. Government Printing Office.

U.S. Bureau of the Census. (1992b): 1990 Census of Population. General Population Characteristics. Washington, DC: U.S. Government Printing Office.

U.S. Bureau of the Census. (1997). Age, sex, household relationship, race, and Hispanic origin and selected statuses: ratio of income to poverty level in 1996 (October 3, 1997). Washington, DC: World Wide Web:http://ferret.bls.census.gov/macro/03197/pov/2_001–3.htm.

U.S. Bureau of the Census. (1998). Poverty: 1997 Highlights. Washington, DC. Retrieved June 9, 1999 from the World Wide Web: http://www.census.gov/hhes/poverty/poverty97/pov97hi.html.

U.S. Department of Health and Human Services. (1985). Report of the Secretary's Task Force on Black and Minority Health, vol 1. Executive summary. Washington DC: U.S. Department of Health and Human Services.

U.S. Department of Health and Human Services. (1998, August). Profile of homelessness, Washington, DC. Retrieved June 9, 1999 from the World Wide Web: http://aspe.os.dhhs.gov/progsys/homeless/profile.htm.

Voydanoff, P., & Donnelly, B. W. (1998) *Economic distress, family coping and quality of family life.* In P. Voydanoff & L. C. Le Majka (Eds.), *Families and economic distress* (pp. 97–115). Newbury Park, CA: Sage Publications.

Wagner, J. D., et al. (1995). What is known about the health of rural homeless families? *Public Health Nursing, 12*(6):400–408.

Wilkinson, D. (1987). *Ethnicity*. In M. B. Sussman & S. K. Steinmetz (Eds.), *Handbook of marriage and the family* (pp. 183–210). New York: Plenum Press.

Wilson, W. J. (1987). *The truly disadvantaged.* Chicago: University of Chicago Press.

Winnick, A. J. (1991). *Toward two societies.* New York: Praeger Press.

Wolff, E. N. (1995). How the pie is sliced: America's growing concentration of wealth. *The American Prospect, 22*(Summer):58–64.

Focus On

FACTORS INFLUENCING FAMILY FUNCTION AND THE HEALTH OF FAMILY MEMBERS

This chapter approaches the family from a slightly different perspective than previous chapters. Here you will acquire an intimate view of family system and health relationships. In addition, you will see how factors within the family (e.g., illness, spiritual beliefs, and values) and outside the family (e.g., legal and ethical decisions and public policies) influence family functioning and the health of individual family members.

This chapter also includes further discussion of one of the conceptual frameworks presented in Chapter 2, the resiliency model of family stress, adjustment, and adaptation (McCubbin & McCubbin, 1993; McCubbin, Thompson, & McCubbin, 1996), and a brief overview of Rolland's work (1994) on types and time phases of chronic illness. The main emphasis of the resiliency model is on the resiliency of families or their ability to recover from stressful life situations. The resiliency model helps identify factors, such as family stressors, family type, family resources, family appraisal of the situation, and family problem solving and coping, that may play a role in family recovery. Rolland's typology of illness provides clinically meaningful and useful categories or types of chronic illness that affect individuals across the entire life span. According to Rolland, each type of illness has a distinct pattern of (a) onset, (b) course, (c) outcome, (d) type and degree of incapacitation, and (e) degree of uncertainty. Each time phase of chronic illness (e.g., crisis, chronic, and terminal) has its own psychosocial demands and developmental tasks, which require significantly different strengths, attitudes, and changes from a family. Assessing the type and time phase of the illness, as well as the family factors described in the resiliency model, provides nurses and other health care providers with a foundation for assisting families in their adaptation to illness and their attainment of a higher level of wellness.

Chapter 6

FACTORS INFLUENCING FAMILY FUNCTION AND THE HEALTH OF FAMILY MEMBERS

Marcia Van Riper

OUTLINE

OBJECTIVES

On completion of this chapter, the reader will be able to:

- Examine the influence of family on the physical and psychological health of family members.
- Describe the influence of spirituality and religion on family functioning and the health of family members.
- Discuss ethical and legal factors that influence family functioning and the health of family members.
- Explore the purpose of family policy and how it may affect the family.
- Examine the role of the nurse in advocating for social change that supports the family unit.

This chapter provides an overview of the factors that influence family functioning and the health of individual family members. Both factors within the family (e.g., illness in the family, spiritual beliefs and values) and outside the family (e.g., legal and ethical decisions and public policies) are addressed. In addition, the resiliency model of Family Stress, Adjustment, and Adaptation (McCubbin & McCubbin, 1993; McCubbin, Thompson, & McCubbin, 1996) is presented as an example of a conceptual framework that may help nurses and other health care providers to identify family factors that play a role in family recovery from illness and other stressful situations. Also, Rolland's work (1994) on how illness characteristics and illness time phases influence family recovery from chronic illness is discussed.

FAMILY SYSTEM AND HEALTH RELATIONSHIPS

The physical and psychological health of family members plays an important role in how the family functions on a day-to-day basis. If a family member is in bed with the flu, the chores and tasks which the individual usually performs for the family may need to be put on hold temporarily, or another family member may need to pitch in to keep things running smoothly until the flu has run its course. It also helps if another family member brings hot soup and a favorite magazine for the flu victim to read. Whereas acute illness usually requires only temporary alterations in family life, chronic illness may bring about more lasting changes. For example, when a family learns that Grandpa has been diagnosed with Alzheimer's disease, they have immediate questions: How long can Grandpa live alone? Will we need to have him move in with us? Where will we find the room? How will this affect the children's activities? Will we need to put him in a nursing home? How will we pay for the care? Many families face situations in which one member is dependent on alcohol or drugs, and they must ask themselves how they will manage this type of behavior. Do they ignore the problem and hope it will go away? Do they confront the family member about it and insist that they seek help? There is increasing evidence that, not only does the health of family members affect how the family functions (Covinsky, et al, 1994; Lewis, Hammon, & Woods, 1993; Wright, Watson, & Bell, 1996), but the family can influence the health of its members (Burman & Margolin, 1992; Campbell, 1986; Doherty & Campbell, 1988; Fisher, et al, 1993; Ross, et al, 1990). According to family systems theory, family members are interconnected and dependent on one another. Thus, when there is a change in the health of one member, all family members will be affected and the family unit as a whole will be altered. The functioning of the family also influences the physical health and psychological well-being of the family members. Kern (1995) has suggested that the family can play a role in determining the course of an illness, symptomology, amount of disability, and affective response or distress of the affected family member.

Family Functioning and Physical Health

To date, research concerning the interaction between family functioning and the physical health of family members is rather limited. Existing research has consistently shown a positive relationship between marriage and physical health; poorer health outcomes are noted in never-married, separated, divorced, or widowed persons than in those who are married. Although there may be a selection factor (many persons with major health problems do not get married or stay married), marriage appears to have a supportive and protective influence on physical health beyond any selection bias, and the additional support and higher incomes found in married households have both been associated with better physical health (Ross, et al, 1990). Families with two incomes have more economic resources and thus may have better access to health care. In addition, married persons are less likely to engage in risky lifestyle behaviors, more likely to have nutritious diets, and less likely to smoke, drink excessively, or take risks that increase the rate of accidents (Strong & DeVault, 1993). Although most relationships between marriage and physical health are positive, married persons are also more likely to be overweight and to exercise less (Venters, 1986).

There is growing evidence that the increased morbidity and mortality noted in individuals who are separated, divorced, or widowed may be the result of changes in immune function (Kiecolt-Glaser & Glaser, 1991). In a study by Irwin and colleagues (1987), widows of men who had died of lung cancer during the previous 1 to 6 months had greater impairments in immune function than women whose husbands were being treated for metastatic lung cancer and women whose husbands were in good health. In a study by Kiecolt-Glaser, et al, (1988), separated or divorced men reported significantly more illnesses and had poorer values on two functional indices of immunity, than did sociodemographically matched married men. Providing care for a spouse with dementia, which has been described as a form of living bereavement, also has been associated with changes in immunity and health (Kiecolt-Glaser, et al, 1991). According to findings reported by Kiecolt-Glaser and colleagues, spousal caregivers had poorer immune function and more days of infectious illness than did sociodemographically matched control subjects.

A spouse or stable partner also may help to protect health. When one partner appears ill, the other partner may encourage seeking treatment and then support taking time off work to recover, using medication as prescribed, and resting. For example, a husband's encouragement to seek early treatment for a breast lump may make a big difference in a woman's prognosis if the mass turns out to be malignant; or, a partner's willingness to take on extra caretaking and household responsibilities may give the new mother with a history of postpartum depression the support and encouragement she needs to avoid the downward spiral of postpartum depression (Wood, et al, 1997).

Parenthood is generally viewed as desirable and rewarding; however, most studies show minimal positive effects of children younger than age 18 on parent's physical health (Bird, 1997; Ross, et al, 1990). According to Bird (1997), there is generally a trade-off between the positive experiences of parenting and the burdens and responsibilities that come with it. Children create economic burdens on the family and also decrease the amount of time parents have for each other (Ross, et al, 1990). Thus, the addition of children to a family often creates tensions and leads to a decrease in the quality of the couple's relationship (Belsky, et al, 1985; Belsky, et al, 1983; White, et al, 1986). Parents who have more economic resources, who support each other in work and parenting roles, and who have access to affordable child care and support from extended family members tend to be healthier (Ross, et al, 1990).

Children have health-promoting behaviors that resemble those of their parents (Schor, 1995). Families influence the amount and type of exercise in which children engage by role-modeling, by facilitating access to equipment and facilities, and by providing opportunities to participate in sports and exercise. Children whose parents smoke, use alcohol or other drugs, or overeat are at higher risk for adopting these behaviors. It remains unclear whether children are mimicking their parents' behaviors or responding to similar social and environmental pressures or inducements. Family relationships also can influence children's health risk behavior. For example, adolescents with weak attachments to their families are more likely to smoke (Foshee & Bauman, 1992).

When, where, and how children use health care services is largely controlled by their parents and, logically, resembles the use pattern of their parents (Schor, et al, 1987). For example, parents are generally the ones who decide which symptoms require medical attention or restriction of activities. Left to their own initiative, children tend to seek health care in the same manner in which their parents have sought health care (Schor, 1995).

Family Functioning and Psychological Health

Over a decade ago, Campbell (1986) noted that research on the family and psychological health was further advanced than research on the family and physical health. This continues to be the case today. Existing research suggests that marriage generally protects and improves psychological health, just as it does physical health (Ross and associates, 1990). Unmarried individuals have more depression, anxiety, and other forms of psychological distress than those who are married (Kiecolt-Glaser & Glaser, 1991; Mirowsky & Ross, 1989). One explanation for this is that married people are more likely to have consistent emotional support, and emotional support is associated with lower levels of depression and anxiety (Ross, et al, 1990). Another explanation is that married people have higher household incomes, and economic well-being is related to psychological health (Ross & Huber, 1985).

Marriage has a more positive impact on men's psychological health than on women's (Ross, et al, 1990). Married women have more depression and anxiety than married men (Gove, 1984). Men seem to benefit most from the emotional support they gain from marriage, while women seem to benefit most from the economic support they gain. In a study by Gerstel, Riessman, and Rosenfield (1985), divorced men suffered from a loss of emotional support, whereas divorced women suffered from a loss of economic support.

For years it was assumed that women who were separated or divorced had higher rates of "psychiatric disease" than married women. In addition, it was often suggested that these psychiatric problems were the cause of the separation or divorce. More recently, it has been argued that researchers and clinicians need to consider the life conditions that women who are separated or divorced face, especially if they are parents (Nelson, 1994). In addition to loss of income or change in socioeconomic status, newly separated or divorced women typically have to deal with increased life strains, such as disruptions in their daily routines, a narrowing of their social network, a reduction in social activities, increased parenting responsibilities, a lack of high-quality child care, and ongoing conflicts with their spouse.

Findings from a study by Nelson (1994) indicate that life strains in the initial period following marital separation predict a woman's psychological health 6 years after the separation. That is, separated women who experience greater life strains during the initial period report lower levels of psychological well-being 6 years after their separation.

There is increasing evidence that parents with children living at home experience more psychological distress than people without children and parents whose children have left home (Bird, 1997; McLanahan & Adams, 1987; Ross, et al, 1990; Umberson & Gove, 1989). According to Bird (1997), these differences are caused, in large part, by differences in social and economic resources. As a result of economic pressures, most mothers are no longer staying home to raise their children. According to the U.S. Department of Labor's Bureau of Labor Statistics (1997), the number of dual-worker families (e.g., families in which both the husband and wife worked) grew by 352,000 between 1996 and 1997, while the number of "traditional" families (i.e., couples in which only the husband was employed) declined by 145,000. The labor force participation rate of mothers increased from 70.8 percent in 1996 to 71.9 percent in 1997, as the rate for unmarried mothers (single, widowed, divorced, or separated) increased by 3.2 percentage points to 75 percent. Among mothers with children under a year old, 57.9 percent were working or looking for work in 1997, compared with 54.3 percent the year before.

Finding affordable, high-quality child care can be a critical issue for families, especially single parent families and dual-worker families. Many families have been forced to come up with creative plans for arranging appropriate child care. For example, in some families, parents juggle their work schedules so that one parent can always be with the child or children. In other families, child care is provided by a number of different individuals within the same day (e.g., a neighbor takes care of the child from the time the parents leave for work to when the child gets on the school bus; when school is over, the child goes to an after school program for latch-key children, or a teenager in the neighborhood provides child care). If everything goes as planned, parents may report low levels of stress and high levels of psychological well-being. In contrast, if one person becomes ill or unavailable to provide child care for whatever reason, parents may experience increased stress and may feel burdened. Umberson (1989) noted that parents who feel burdened by their children experience less psychological well-being than parents who feel fewer demands. According to Bird (1997), if parents were relieved of the economic hardships associated with having children and high-quality child care was made available and affordable, levels of psychological distress for parents of children living at home would be similar to levels for people without children.

A number of researchers have noted that having children has both positive and negative effects on psychological well-being. In a study by Umberson and Gove (1989), parents reported more psychological distress than nonparents, but they also indicated that their life had more meaning. Ross and Huber (1985) found that in addition to creating economic hardships for their parents, children may be "a source of gratification," especially for mothers.

In considering the relationship between the family and psychological health, From-Reichman's (1948) description of the schizophrenic mother stimulated a great deal of interest in the role of the family in schizophrenia and other forms of psychological distress. Since then, hundreds of studies on the family and schizophrenia have been carried out (see Goldstein & Strachan, 1987; Karon & Widener, 1994; Parker & Hadzi-Pavlovic, 1990). Researchers have found that poor parental communication (lack of commitment to ideas, unclear communication of ideas, disruptive speech, and closure problems) is common in families with schizophrenia and is present before the symptoms of schizophrenia appear (Doane, et al, 1981; Goldstein, 1985). Researchers have also found that the emotional climate of the family has a consistent and powerful effect on the course of schizophrenia (Butz-laff & Hooley, 1998; Giron & Gomez-Beneyto, 1998;

Vaughn, et al, 1984). Individuals with schizophrenia appear to have difficulty tolerating critical comments by overinvolved family members. When family interventions are successful in reducing overinvolvement and critical comments, individuals with schizophrenia have fewer relapses and their need for hospitalization is decreased (Anderson, et al, 1986; Basolo-Kunzer, 1994; Hogarty, et al, 1991).

While much of the research on the family and psychological health has focused on the family's role in schizophrenia, there has been growing interest in the family's role in depression, alcoholism, and anorexia nervosa. According to Hooley and Teasdale (1989), the single best predictor for relapse in patients with a history of depression is the patient's view of their spouses "criticalness." In a study by Fichter and colleagues (1997), alcoholics were at greater risk for relapse if they reported high numbers of critical comments and decreased warmth by family members. In another study, alcoholic patients with spouses who expressed emotions at a high rate, compared with their counterparts with spouses who expressed emotion at a low rate, were more likely to relapse, had a shorter time of relapse, and drank on a greater percentage of days in the 12 months after starting behavioral marital therapy (O'Farrell, et al, 1998). Despite ongoing interest in the relationship between the family and conditions such as depression, alcoholism, and anorexia nervosa, current understanding of the family's role in the development and course of these conditions is very limited. Much of what has been written about these families has been based on informal reports by family members and clinicians.

According to Tseng and Hsu (1991), researchers and clinicians have typically viewed the family as either the system of pathology, the cradle of pathology, or the catalyst of pathology. When the family is viewed as the system of pathology, the manifested individual psychopathology is considered to be a part of the display of the total family psychopathology. Individual psychopathology therefore receives minimal attention. The primary focus is on identifying dysfunction in family relationships, such as overprotectiveness, rigidity, or lack of conflict solution. When the family is viewed as the cradle of pathology, early family relationships are thought to be the source of vulnerabilities that appear as pathologies later in life. Researchers and clinicians direct much of their attention to early family relationships and their impact on the individual. When the family is viewed as the catalyst of pathology, the unique environment provided by the family is thought to provoke, maintain, or aggravate individual psychopathology. Modification or removal of the individual from the family situation is strongly encouraged as a way to improve the individual's condition.

Much of the research on the family and psychological health of family members has focused on psychological distress or pathology. In addition, the research has looked at only one side of the problem. For example, some clinicians and researchers are still trying to identify the characteristics of the schizophrenic family and the alcoholic family (see Karon & Widener, 1994). This simple one-to-one correspondence between a particular type of family and a particular type of psychological illness can no longer be assumed; rather, researchers must look at multidirectional interactions. More time and effort should be spent identifying factors that influence how individuals and families who are predisposed or vulnerable to life's hardships and traumas emerge resilient, succeed, and even thrive as they recover from adversities.

Application of a Family Stress Model in Illness

Families theories and models, such as the resiliency model of family stress, adjustment, and adaptation depicted in Figure 6–1 (McCubbin and McCubbin, 1993; McCubbin, et al, 1996), can provide insight into factors that influence how families adjust and adapt to a member's illness. According to the Resiliency model, families are more likely to adapt successfully to an illness if:

- They have fewer other family stressors or demands occurring at the same time.
- They have family types or patterns of functioning that are more adaptive (e.g., there is more emotional closeness among family members and they are more flexible and able to change roles, boundaries, and rules when necessary).
- They define the situation positively and view it as something they can master and have control over.
- They have good coping and communication skills.

A short-term acute illness with a predictable course and cure is usually less difficult for families to manage than longer illnesses, because the changes are not permanent and families may be able to manage without drastically altering their usual patterns of functioning. When the

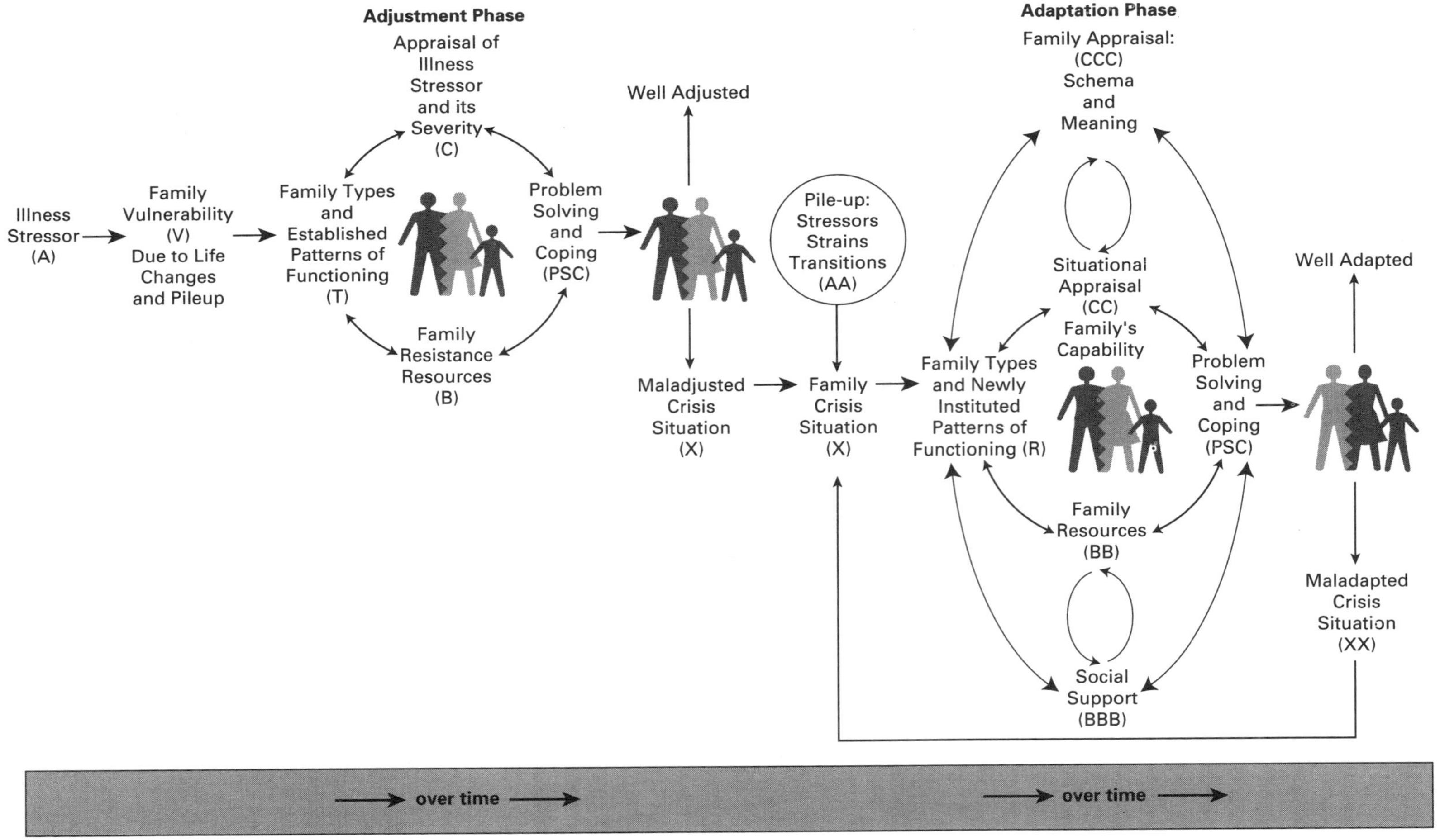

FIGURE 6–1
The Resiliency Model of Family Stress, Adjustment, and Adaptation. (From McCubbin, M. & McCubbin, H. [1993], with permission.)

illness is chronic or in a terminal stage, families usually need to alter their ways of functioning to accommodate the more severe and long-lasting sequelae of the illness. According to the resiliency model (McCubbin & McCubbin, 1993), factors that influence how families respond to a member's illness include family stressors, family types, family resources, family appraisal, and family problem-solving, communication, and coping.

Family Stressors

"A stressor is a demand placed on the family that produces, or has the potential of producing, changes in the family system" (McCubbin & McCubbin, 1993, p. 28). Families are more vulnerable if they experience an accumulation or pile-up of demands at the time that a member becomes ill. Demands on the family unit may include financial problems; work stresses; conflicts among family members, with the extended family, or with former spouses; childbearing or child care strains; transitions of members in and out of the family; other illness or family care strains, such as care of an aging parent; recent losses of close relatives or friends; or legal violations (e.g., family member being arrested, sent to jail, or running away from home). Families rarely have to deal only with one member's illness; they also need to manage other normal expected transitions, as well as work and family demands. Existing strains in the family, such as spousal conflicts or parent-child tensions, may be exacerbated by illness. In addition, the illness itself brings new demands and changes. Negotiation with the health care system and decisions about treatment can go smoothly or become agonizingly difficult. There may be uncertainty about the diagnosis, the treatment options, and the prognosis. Complex conditions may require many types of helpers, who may offer conflicting opinions about what the patient and family should do.

Family Types

McCubbin and McCubbin (1993) have defined family types as "predictable and discernible patterns of family functioning" (p. 29). While there may be many family types, three family types that have been associated with better physical and psychological health for family members and more adaptive functioning of the family as a unit are briefly described.

1. The *regenerative* family is characterized by family hardiness (internal strength and a sense of control) and coherence (view of the situation as manageable and meaningful). These families are more likely to view the illness as a challenge, or something to be managed and mastered, and they are committed to working together to solve problems that arise.
2. The *resilient* family is characterized by greater emotional closeness among family members and by flexibility and the ability to shift roles, rules, and boundaries. These families have strong connections among the members, with feelings of support and affirmation for one another, as well as an ability to take over roles and duties for the ill member, alter family rules of operation, and obtain outside help and information in order to manage the illness.
3. The *rhythmic* family focuses on maintaining and valuing family time and routines that provide stability and predictability in times of illness. These families have established patterns of spending time together at meals, bedtime routines for children, ways of letting members know where they are, and so on. While these routines may be interrupted in times of illness, family time and routines provide a sense of security and consistency in stressful situations.

Family Resources

Family resources are "those attributes and supports that are available for use by the family" (Friedman, et al, 1998, p. 444). McCubbin and McCubbin (1993) have identified three different sources and levels of resources: the individual, the family unit, and the community. Resources from individual family members may include intelligence, personality traits (e.g., optimism), knowledge, skills, physical health, and psychological health (e.g., self-esteem, sense of mastery). Family resources may include cohesion, adaptability, decision-making skills, organization, and conflict-resolution abilities. Resources from the community include personal support (e.g., support from friends and relatives) and institutional support (e.g., support from health care providers and other professionals). To date, social support is the community resource that has received the most attention in the study of family adaptation to illness. McCubbin and McCubbin (1993) have based their definition of social support on Cobb's 1976 definition of social support. Social support includes information exchanged at the interpersonal level that provides:

- Emotional support, leading family members to believe that they are loved and people care for them
- Esteem support, leading family members to believe that they are respected and valued
- Network support, leading family members to believe that they belong to a network of communication in which mutual support and understanding are emphasized
- Appraisal support, allowing family members to assess how well they are doing
- Altruistic support, allowing family members to receive good will from others while giving of themselves

Family Appraisal

The family appraisal of the illness, that is, the way the family sees the illness, is also a critical factor in family adaptation. How do family members define the illness, and what does the illness mean to them? Do they see the illness as having an impact on them? Do they believe they have the resources and capabilities to handle what is happening? Are the family's goals, priorities, and the expectations changed by the illness? Are these changes viewed as temporary or more permanent? Family members will appraise the situation differently depending on their age, gender, role in the family, and experience. Coming to a shared understanding of the situation is difficult and demanding, and it is achieved only through perseverance, patience, negotiation, understanding, and shared commitment (McCubbin & McCubbin, 1993).

Family Problem-Solving, Communication, and Coping

Family problem-solving communication also plays a role in family adaptation to illness. Two types of family communication have been found to predict family adaptation after the diagnosis of a child's congenital heart condition (McCubbin, 1993). Incendiary communication is characterized by bringing up old unresolved issues, failing to calmly talk things through to reach a solution, yelling and screaming at other family members, and walking away from conflicts without much resolution. This type of communication increases the stress. Affirming communication, as the name implies, is more supportive. It is characterized by being careful not to hurt other members emotionally or physically, taking time to hear what others have to say, conveying respect for others' feelings, and ending conflicts on a positive note. Families with more affirming communication and less incendiary communication are better able to adapt to the demands created by a member's illness.

Family coping refers to "family strategies, patterns, and behaviors designed to maintain or strengthen the family as a whole, maintain the emotional stability and well-being of its members, obtain or use family and community resources to manage the situation, and initiate efforts to resolve family hardships created by a stressor" (McCubbin & McCubbin, 1993, p. 30). Families need to balance coping efforts in three areas:

1. Maintaining the functioning of the family unit and optimism about the situation.
2. Managing the tensions of individual members and maintaining their self-esteem, support, and psychological stability.
3. Understanding the health care situation and any treatment regimens for the ill member (McCubbin, 1991).

Nurses and other health care professionals often focus on the third area of family coping by providing education about the disease and its treatment and emphasizing the need to comply with a prescribed regimen. Surprisingly, however, results in a study by Reiss and colleagues (1986) found that patients with end-stage renal disease who were undergoing center-based dialysis and were more compliant with their regimen died sooner. The authors concluded that family members had disengaged from the seriously ill member in an effort to prepare for the anticipated death; the excluded patient then turned to health care professionals for acceptance and was compliant to receive positive feedback from the health care team. Yet, because these patients lacked support from family members, their compliance was not enough to keep them alive. Those patients on dialysis who live longer were not totally noncompliant. They generally followed the regimen but also allowed themselves a day off from diet restrictions and fluid limitations to enjoy a meal out or participate in a family celebration. Thus, these individuals remained more involved with their families and, therefore, they survived longer.

It is important for families who have an ill member to try to balance coping efforts in all three areas to maintain the family as a unit, the health and well-being of all the members, and care and support for the ill member. This may be difficult for families if the health care system emphasizes only the care of the ill member to the detriment of the health of other members and the health of the family unit.

Process of Family Adaptation to Illness

Families make trial-and-error efforts to sort out all the information they receive and decide on strategies to manage the illness situation. All families rely on previously established ways of functioning and coping to manage the initial crisis of a family member's illness. This period is the *family adjustment* phase in the resiliency model. Initially the family may totally reorganize around the member's illness, focusing only on the illness and neglecting other family needs. For short-term acute conditions, where recovery is predictable and complete, this adjustment on the part of the family system can work.

In chronic illnesses and acute illnesses with prolonged recovery times, what seems to work at first may be detrimental to meeting the needs of family members and the family unit as a whole over the long haul. This is called the *family adaptation* phase in the model (Figure 6–1). For example, a mother may take time off from work to spend most of her time at the hospital bedside with an ill child, while the father tries to manage his work and the other children at home. This approach may work at first; but if the child's illness is prolonged, the workplace may not continue to tolerate the mother's absence, problems of reduced income and potential job loss may surface, and the other children may begin to feel neglected. Further, both parents can become exhausted with this arrangement. The family system is then in a state of *crisis*.

This does not mean the family is sick and needs fixing; however, it indicates that change is needed and new patterns of functioning should be tried. Thus, the mother may return to work part-time; the father may spend more time at the hospital; both parents may try to spend time with the siblings left at home; additional help from relatives may be sought to ease the burden on the parents; and if financial resources permit, outside help with household tasks and chores may be obtained. The family thus tries to achieve adaptation. In the resiliency model, this adaptation represents a fit at two levels of functioning: a fit of the individual and the family system (i.e., ensuring the care and well-being of family members and the family unit) and the fit of the family system with the community (including satisfactory relationships in the workplace and hospital).

Influence of Illness Characteristics and Illness Time Phases

The characteristics of the illness itself also influence how the family responds. We have already noted that acute illness usually requires only temporary changes in how the family functions. Chronic illness requires more lasting alterations in how the family operates day to day. Rolland (1994) has proposed that five characteristics of an illness (onset, course, outcome, type and degree of incapacitation, and degree of uncertainty) and three phases of illness (crisis, chronic, and terminal) should be examined to understand the relationship among the chronic illness, the affected family member, and the family unit.

The onset of chronic illness can be acute (e.g., spinal cord injury) or gradual (e.g., AIDS). Although both illnesses may require considerable alterations in family functioning, a gradual onset of illness allows family members more time to mobilize resources and develop ways to cope. Families who experience the sudden onset of a chronic illness in a family member must immediately try to manage their anxiety and tension, alter roles, and try to find ways to manage the situation.

The course of a chronic illness can be progressive, constant, relapsing, or episodic (Rolland, 1994). In progressive illnesses, such as Alzheimer's disease or Huntington's chorea, the affected family member deteriorates over time. The deterioration may occur quite rapidly or very slowly. Caretaking demands increase as the individual's condition worsens, and family caregivers may become exhausted, with deleterious effects on their health. In illnesses with a constant course, such as cerebral palsy or stroke, the family must adapt to the reduced but relatively stable, predictable functioning of the affected family member. Here, too, however, stress on family caregivers is a concern, because the illness brings a permanent change in the individual's functioning. In relapsing or episodic illnesses, such as ulcerative colitis and many forms of cancers, the ill individual and the family as a whole experience relatively stable and normal periods interspersed with flare-ups or exacerbations. This requires a great deal of flexibility so that the family can move into a crisis mode when necessary and then revert back to previous patterns of functioning when all is going well. Because the family needs to be ready to respond to the next relapse, family members are often in a constant state of alertness and tension.

The outcome for the family is affected by whether the illness is inevitably fatal (as in AIDS) or may be fatal (as in many cancers), whether it shortens the expected life span (as in diabetes or emphysema) or has a minimal effect on the life span (as in arthritis or asthma). Rolland (1994) notes that the *initial expectation* of whether the disease is likely to cause death is the most critical factor. The family's perception of whether the illness represents an inevitable loss or a possible loss influences how the family includes or excludes the ill family member in day-to-day family interactions and decision making.

Type and degree of incapacitation also influences how individuals and families respond to chronic illness (Rolland, 1994). The family member can be incapacitated in various ways: cognition (e.g., Alzheimer's disease), sensation (e.g., blindness, deafness), motor functioning (e.g., stroke, spinal cord injury), energy level (e.g., cardiovascular disease, multiple sclerosis), or through social stigma (e.g., mental illness, AIDS). These different kinds of incapacitation require different adaptive strategies by the family. A severe cognitive deficit is usually considered difficult to manage because the family member may be unable to communicate and take part in decision making. The individual's behavior also may be quite unpredictable and disturbing, which can isolate the family from the community. Some conditions, such as a traumatic brain injury, may involve both cognitive and motor impairment.

Rolland (1994) describes degree of uncertainty as a metacharacteristic. That is, degree of uncertainty about a disease overlays and colors the other four characteristics: onset, course, outcome, and incapacitation. The more uncertain or unpredictable the disease is, the more a family has to make decisions with flexible contingencies or back-up plans. This ongoing type of strategic problem solving can exhaust even the most resilient and adaptive families.

Time phases of the illness include the initial crisis, the chronic or long-term care phase, and the terminal or final phase (Rolland, 1994). The initial crisis period includes the time preceding an actual diagnosis and confirmation of the illness and time covered by the expected course of treatment. The family member and the family unit must mourn the loss of health, reorganize to accommodate the changes brought about by the illness, appraise how the illness affects each member and the family unit as a whole, and establish relationships with the health care system and any other outside systems (e.g., special education, insurance providers, vocational rehabilitation) necessary to manage the illness.

The chronic phase can be prolonged and last many years or be quite short, as in a fulminating fatal illness. This is the stage in which permanent alterations are made in family functioning to accommodate the changes brought about by the chronic illness, although most families try to maintain some normality in family life if possible.

The last phase or terminal stage of illness involves coming to grips with the death of a family member, grieving, and letting go. This can be an extremely stressful time, particularly if the family member's death is premature. While the family may feel some relief because the individual is no longer suffering and family caretaking demands have ceased, the irreversible nature of the loss and the permanent change it brings in the family system often require an enormous effort to accept.

SPIRITUALITY, RELIGION, AND FAMILY FUNCTIONING

Although the terms spirituality and religion often are used synonymously in the literature, they are not the same (Dyson, et al, 1997). The word spirituality derives from the Latin word *spiritus,* which refers to breath, air, or wind (O'Neil & Kenny, 1998). The spirit, thus, is "that which gives life to, or animates a person. Figuratively, it connotes whatever is at the center of all aspects of one's life" (Dombeck, 1995, p. 38). The concept of spirituality has a broader meaning than religion and it is considered more inclusive (Fehring, et al, 1997). Spirituality generally encompasses a sense of relation or connectedness within oneself, others, nature, and God, or a higher power that draws one beyond oneself (Emblen, 1992; Miller, 1995; Reed, 1992). It also includes a faith that positively affirms life (Miller, 1995). Religion, on the other hand, has been defined as an organized system of beliefs, practices, and forms of worship (Emblen, 1992). Many individuals, especially older adults, express their spirituality through their religion and religious practices and behaviors (Fehring, et al, 1997).

Three other terms frequently used in discussions about spirituality and religion are spiritual well-being, religiousness, and religiosity. *Spiritual well-being* is defined as a sense of inner peace, compassion for others, reverence for life, gratitude, and appreciation of both unity and diversity (Vaughn, 1986); it includes the conviction that there is a purpose and meaning in life, a relationship with God, and realistic views of adversity and loss (Moberg, 1974). *Religiousness,* originally associated with church attendance and involvement in formal religious activities, has now been defined as adherence to the beliefs and practices of an organized church or religious institution (Shafranske & Maloney, 1990). Religiousness reflects how closely a family believes in and practices the beliefs of particular religious groups, such as Roman Catholicism, Judaism, Islam, or various Protestant Christian denominations. *Religiosity* has been conceptualized as a continuum with intrinsic religious motivation on one end and extrinsic religious motivation on the other end (Allport & Ross, 1967; Hoge, 1972). Intrinsically religious people try to practice religion in their daily lives and they find religion to be the "ultimate" in their motivational systems (Fehring, et al, 1997). On the other hand, people at the other end of the continuum, the extreme, purely extrinsically religious people, find religion and religious practices to be important for sociability, solace, status, or security and as an "instrument" in their motivational system (Fehring, et al, 1997).

Spirituality and religion are important factors in the lives of most individuals and families in the United States. There are nearly 500,000 temples, churches, and mosques in the United States (Weaver, et al, 1998). Over 85 percent of Americans consider religion "very important or fairly important" in their lives and 95 percent profess a belief in God (Gallop, 1993). Individuals described as religiously involved have been shown to have fewer chronic conditions; lower blood pressure; fewer strokes; lower functional disability; less depression, anxiety, suicide, and alcoholism; higher life satisfaction; and greater psychological well-being (Koenig, 1995).

Spirituality and religion can influence every aspect of family life. Transitions in the family life cycle (marriage, birth, and death) are marked by religious ceremonies, observances, and traditions. Many families report new meaning in life and increased depth of spirituality after experiencing a significant illness in a family member. See the "state of the science" article on spirituality and chronic illness (O'Neil & Kenny, 1998). Caregivers of the chronically ill rely on spirituality as a coping mechanism (Herth, 1993; Kaye & Robinson, 1994). Feelings of strength and comfort drawn from religious faith and practices support caregivers and promote psychological well-being (Rabins, et al, 1990). Spirituality and religion also can play a significant role in coping with a family member's death and helping the family to heal after such a loss. According to Thomas and Henry (1984), spiritual hope and peace and belief in the promise of eternal life after the temporary earthly journey can help ease the trauma after the death of a family member.

In a recent study by Fehring and colleagues (1997) concerning elderly people coping with cancer, a consistent positive association was found between intrinsic religiosity, spiritual well-being, hope, and other positive mood states and a consistent negative association was found between extrinsic religiosity, depression, and other negative mood states. That is, elderly people coping with cancer who had high levels of intrinsic religiosity and spiritual well-being had higher levels of hope and other positive mood states and lower levels of depression and other negative mood states than did individuals with low levels of intrinsic religiosity and spiritual well-being.

Research on family strengths has confirmed the importance of religion and spirituality in strong families. DeFrain and Stinnett (1992) note that strong families are not perfect, but they can effectively manage the challenges in their lives. After asking over 3500 family members, over 16 years, about their family strengths, DeFrain and Stinnett (1992) concluded that spiritual well-being was one of six critical qualities of strong families. This spiritual well-being was reflected by family members' sense of optimism, hope, and meaning in their lives. These strong families had a spirituality that went deeper than church attendance and participation in religious activities. Awareness of a higher power gave them a sense of purpose, strength, and support that helped them to be more patient with each other, more forgiving, quicker to get over anger, more positive, and more supportive in their family relationships (Stinnett, 1979). This quality also allowed family members to find goodness and purpose in both the joys and sorrows of daily living and family life.

A shared religious core was found to be one of 15 traits of a healthy family by Curran (1983) in her survey of professionals in education, church, health, family counseling, and voluntary organizations. Two other healthy family traits, a sense of right and wrong and valuing service to others, also were linked to the role of religion and spirituality in the family. Curran stresses that the specific religion a family belongs to is not the important issue. Instead there are three hallmarks that identify a family with a shared religious core. These are (1) a faith in God, which plays a role in family life by giving it purpose, stability, and meaning; (2) a strengthened family support system that encourages nurturing and affirming relationships among family members;

and (3) the feeling of parents that they have a strong responsibility for passing on the faith, which they do in positive and meaningful ways (Curran, 1985).

The aspects of spirituality and religion that contribute to more positive family functioning include religious beliefs related to love, faith, hope, forgiveness, reconciliation, and the worth of human beings; a lifestyle that emphasizes commitment, responsibility, giving, and caring for others; shared beliefs and values; shared religious and church activities; reverence for marriage and family; and affiliation with a support group or network that provides a sense of belonging (Brigman, 1992). Some aspects of spirituality and religion may also be detrimental to families. For example, what constitutes a family may be narrowly defined by religions, with a clear preference for a nuclear family (husband, wife, and children, all living together). Many religions have become more liberal about nontraditional families, sexuality, contraceptive use, divorce, and remarriage. Some religious groups, however, still strongly support only heterosexual unions, consider marriage a lifetime commitment, encourage childbearing, discourage regulation of fertility, and support traditional gender roles. For families whose situation is not congruent with the beliefs and values of their religion, this can be a source of stress rather than support and comfort. Also, a religious emphasis on sin and judgment may produce feelings of guilt and low self-esteem (Brigman, 1992).

The fit between the family's spiritual beliefs and values and the family's situation is critical. Although the inclusion of spiritual beliefs and values in the health care assessment may seem to be an invasion of the family's privacy, it is important for the nurse to be sensitive to how these beliefs and values influence a family's response in illness situations. Even if the family has no formal religious affiliation, nurses need to support the patient's expressions of spirituality or religiosity, help them find meaning and purpose, and in the case of a terminal illness, provide a realistic sense of hope in accordance with their respective belief systems (Fehring, et al, 1997).

ETHICS, THE LAW, AND FAMILY FUNCTIONING

There is no question that ethical and legal factors influence family functioning and the health of family members. What remains unclear is the exact nature of the relationships among ethics, the law, and the family. *Ethics* is "the enterprise of disciplined reflection on the moral intuitions and moral choices that people make" (Veatch, 1997, p.5). It attempts to (a) compare the moral choices that people make for consistency, (b) formulate rules of conduct accounting for these choices, and (c) articulate general principles that might underlie these choices and rules. Ethics confronts questions concerning what is good and bad and what is right and wrong. Ethics is concerned with how people ought to act and how they ought to be in relationships with others.

Law, in contrast, is designed to fulfill its task of social regulation, not to address the full and complex scope of morality (Douglas, 1997). The law is somewhat more constrained than ethics because it must find authority in legal precedent of the past, while at the same time being always aware that it is setting legal precedent for the future. Douglas noted that the United States Constitution, which includes the Bill of Rights, is the "supreme law of the land." Because of this, no state law or court can reduce the guarantees afforded by the Constitution.

According to Douglas (1997), the relationship between ethics and law is similar to a free-spirited dance in which first one partner leads, then the other. Sometimes the partners dance in unison. Other times, the partners dance freely or simultaneously disconnected from one another. Sometimes one partner looks on as the other partner dances alone. Ethics and the law serve to inform one another in a relationship that occasionally is united, but frequently is characterized by tension.

The Patient Self-Determination Act

The Patient Self-Determination Act (PSDA) is an example of a time when a moral principle, the principle of self-determination, or autonomy, was supported by law. According to the PSDA, patients have the right to information about treatment options and the right to express their choices in advance directives, living wills, or durable powers of attorney. The ethical, political, economic, and legal positions represented in the PSDA emerged, in part, from two widely publicized cases concerning the right to refuse treatment: the Quinlan case and the Cruzan case.

The Quinlan case was one of the first highly visible cases to raise the issue of futility in treatment (Douglas, 1997). In addition, the Quinlan case resulted in the development of prognosis committees, which were the precursors of today's hospital ethics committees. The Cruzan case was the first case decided by the United States Supreme Court concerning the right to die and circumstances under which this choice should be honored. In both of these cases, the individuals involved, Karen Quinlan and Nancy Cruzan, had a diagnosis of persistent vegetative state. Quinlan and Cruzan had both lost their decision-making ability, so family members exercised the right to make decisions on their behalf. After a period of careful and deliberate decision making, both families decided to discontinue treatment; the Quinlan family asked for Karen to be removed from the respirator, and the Cruzan family asked that Nancy stop receiving food and fluids via a gastrostomy tube. In both instances, the family's request was denied and the matter had to be settled in court. Undoubtedly, this resulted in a great deal of stress for the families. In addition to dealing with the stressors associated with having a family member in a persistent vegetative state, these families had to deal with the stresses associated with lengthy, widely publicized legal battles. The long-term impact of these stresses on family functioning and the health of family members is not known, but the potential for negative consequences is great.

Ethical Principles

Ethical principles, such as the principle of self-determination, or autonomy, are general action guides specifying moral actions that are prohibited, required, or permitted in certain circumstances (Childress, 1997). Health care providers must consider ethical principles as they make decisions with and about families at all levels; in particular health care settings; at the local community level of providing care; and at the state and national levels, where all types of health care services are organized and funded. Which principles families and health care providers choose to use may have a profound impact on family functioning and the health of family members. The most commonly used ethical principles are described in the following paragraphs.

The *value of life principle* reads that "human beings should revere life and accept death" (Thiroux, 1986, p. 125). This principle holds that life is the most basic possession that humans have. Because life is viewed as so valuable, humans are thought to be morally obligated to preserve and protect it. The value of life principle prompts questions about quality of life. It also stimulates impassioned debates about terminating a pregnancy because the fetus is known to have a genetic disorder, such as Down syndrome or cystic fibrosis.

The *principle of goodness or rightness* demands that humans: (1) promote goodness over badness, (2) cause no harm or badness, and (3) prevent badness or harm (Thiroux, 1986). Beauchamp and Childress (1983) described two ethical principles (e.g., the *principle of beneficence* and the *principle of nonmaleficence*) that are closely related but not exactly synonymous to the principle of goodness or rightness. According to Beauchamp and Childress, the principle of beneficence encourages acts involving the prevention of harm, removal of harmful conditions, and positive benefiting. The principle of nonmaleficence refers to not inflicting harm on others. The principles of beneficence and nonmaleficence encourage behavior that will enhance, or at least not diminish, family functioning and the health of family members. For example, when a community health nurse identifies and reports a possible case of child neglect, the nurse is taking steps to prevent harm. When the nurse works with the family on issues such as proper nutrition, growth and development, age-appropriate discipline, and problem-solving skills, the nurse is taking steps to promote family functioning and the health of individual family members. If the nurse chooses to ignore the signs and symptoms of child neglect, the principle of beneficence has not been upheld and the nurse's action, or lack of action, may negatively affect the child's physical and psychological health.

According to the *priniciple of justice or fairness,* people should treat other humans fairly and justly when distributing goodness and badness among them (Thiroux, 1986). The recent and continuing issue of transforming the current health care system in the United States emerges, in part, from a question concerning whether or not all individuals have a moral right to access health care goods and service (Douglas, 1997). If so, then the question of how goods and services should be distributed fairly among the population becomes a central issue. Noncomparative justice is when equal shares go to all recipients. Comparative justice is when those in greatest need get what they need for survival.

Health care resources are very scarce at the present time, so the principle of justice or fairness has become very important. Health care providers are constantly being confronted with issues such as: Who should receive services first? What type of services should patients and their families receive? Under what circumstances should families be denied services? These are difficult questions and the way in which they are answered will have a powerful impact on family functioning and the health of individual family members. For example, a decision to deny a patient a heart transplant may result in death for the patient and decreased psychological well-being for other family members. A decision to approve a heart transplant may result in improved health for the patient, but over time, it may result in decreased psychological well-being for family members because of the additional stressors associated with chronic conditions.

The *principle of truth telling, or honesty,* is an essential ingredient for trust and meaningful communication between any two individuals (Thiroux, 1986). *Veracity* is the duty to tell the truth. *Fidelity* is the duty to keep promises. *Confidentiality* is the duty to protect privileged information. Despite the merit of veracity, fidelity, and confidentiality, these rights are not absolute. Other societal values, such as a collective need for information or public health and safety of others, may limit individual claims on these rights (Rushton & Infante, 1995). For example, if a 15-year-old girl who is being treated for a sexually transmitted disease asks the nurse not to tell her mother because she "will go ballistic" and the mother calls to inquire about her daughter's treatment, the nurse is faced with an ethical dilemma. If the nurse informs the mother why her daughter is being treated, trust between the 15-year-old girl and the nurse is undermined and the patient-nurse relationship is damaged. In addition, the girl's psychological well-being, as well as her physical well-being may be jeopardized, especially if the mother really does "go ballistic." On the other hand, if the nurse does not tell the mother the truth, the girl's physical well-being may be in danger because of the serious consequences associated with inadequate treatment of her condition. Also, the mother-daughter relationship may be damaged as a result of the element of secrecy.

According to Thiroux (1986), "people, as individuals with differences, must be free to choose their own ways and means of being moral within the framework of the basic principles" (p. 130). This is known as the *principle of individual freedom, or autonomy.* There are two important methods for respecting individual freedom, or autonomy: (a) informed consent and (b) advance directives. Informed consent promotes and respects the autonomy of the patient and the family by expanding their knowledge of available options. Advanced directives are forms of communication in which individuals can give direction on how they would like to be treated when they cannot speak for themselves. Douglas (1997) noted that the principle of autonomy is threatened when others interfere too much (excessive control) or they do not interfere enough (neglect). There is a fine line between autonomy and abandonment, especially in the care of children, persons who are mentally ill, persons with a chronic illness or a developmental disability, and elderly persons. Respect for autonomy also is threatened when the exercise of one person's rights interferes with another person's rights. For example, if a man with an incapacitating illness, such as Huntington's disease, asks to be cared for in the home and health care providers decide that his only living relative, a daughter, should provide the care, her right to individual freedom is threatened. She may be "forced" to quit her job and make other significant life changes to care for her father. Unfortunately, many health care providers believe that the welfare of family members is irrelevant to discussions about "the best thing to do" for a patient with a chronic illness who requires long-term care.

Legal Definition of Family

The question of what constitutes a family has proved to be perplexing to the courts (Liss, 1987). Before the 1960s, legal definitions of family typically reflected prevailing beliefs about the nuclear family (Liss, 1987; Yorker, 1993). With the rapid proliferation of other family forms (e.g., single-parent families, unmarried adults with or without children, blended families, and multigenerational communes), more and more people started to question the existing legal definitions of family. For example, in *Palo Alto Tenants Union v. Morgan* (1970), members of a communal living group challenged a zoning ordinance that defined the family as one person living alone; two or more persons related by blood, marriage, or legal adoption; or a group not exceeding four persons living in a single housekeeping unit. In *Moore v. City of East Cleveland* (1977), a city ordinance was struck down because it made it a crime for a grandmother to live with her grandsons, who were first cousins rather than brothers.

While there have been many attempts to change the way the family is legally defined, definitions that reflect the traditional nuclear family still exist in state and local ordinances. Because of this, nontraditional families may have difficulty finding appropriate housing. In addition, they may be denied food stamps and other welfare benefits (Liss, 1987). This in turn, may have a negative effect on family functioning and the health of individual family members.

It has been suggested that the definition of family used to determine which families qualified for the recently repealed Aid to Families with Dependent Children (AFDC) program was instrumental in breaking up many families (Liss, 1987). While the definition used is not the definition of a nuclear family, it is based on beliefs about the nuclear family. The AFDC program's "man-in-the-house" rule assumed that when no breadwinner (i.e., father) was present, the government should take over the father's role of breadwinner and the mother should be able to stay home with the children (Johnson & Ooms, 1985; Liss, 1987). The man-in-the-house rule became a built in incentive for some poor fathers, even those who are very caring and hardworking, to desert their families. It has been estimated that over 80% of the children who received welfare benefits did so because their father had left the family, not because their father was dead or disabled (Liss, 1987). Children who were deserted by their fathers often found it necessary to take on additional roles in the family. This, in turn, had a negative effect on individual and family functioning. Now that the Personal Responsibility and Work Opportunity Reconciliation Act of 1996 has repealed the 60-year-old AFDC program, the man-in-the-house rule should no longer be a contributing factor to the breakup of families. However, the effect of the new welfare reform bill on the well-being of children and families is yet to be determined (Hofferth, 1999).

Involvement of the Federal Government

The United States Constitution has very little to say about the rights of the family. According to Liss (1987), this omission by our founding fathers may have been intentional, because a basic assumption of the American system is that the rights of the individual outweigh those of the family. In addition, the family has traditionally been viewed as a bastion of privacy, not to be intruded on by the federal government.

Before the 20th century, laws affecting family issues were relatively noninterventionist (Yorker, 1993). The few legal restrictions that existed were based on biblical sanctions (e.g., adultery) and social taboos (e.g., incest). During the late 1800s and the 1900s, state laws that had protectionist and regulatory effects on families were enacted. Many of these laws were paternalistic and based on prevailing notions of morality. Courts at the state and local level used these laws to guide their decisions about family issues, such as marriage, divorce, child support, child custody, and family violence. Ultimately, a confusing patchwork of government actions and services was created (Liss, 1987).

The rights extended to the family vary from state to state. This makes it very difficult when state courts are asked to make decisions about family issues involving individuals living in different states. If there is a question about whether a state law or lower court decision is, in fact, constitutional, the matter goes to the United States Supreme Court (Myers, 1992).

In 1973, the Supreme Court made a landmark decision in *Roe v. Wade* (Liss, 1987). This decision protected the right of women to decide whether to bear a child and thus has had a major impact on family functioning. Over the last 20 years, there have been many unsuccessful attempts to overrule this decision. In 1977 the Supreme Court heard three cases challenging lower courts' decisions that states participating in the Medicaid program could refuse to pay the expenses incidental to nontherapeutic abortions although they were paying the expenses incidental to childbirth. The court ruled that these lower court decisions were not unconstitutional. Three of the Supreme Court justices disagreed with this decision on the grounds that it showed a distressing insensitivity to the plight of impoverished pregnant women. They also noted that it actually forced impoverished women to bear unwanted children, which is likely to have a negative impact on family functioning and the health of individual family members. An unwanted pregnancy is a very stressful experience for the pregnant woman and her family. In addition, unwanted children typically receive less than adequate care and attention, which places them at increased risk for physical and psychological problems.

According to Liss (1987), there are three areas of family-related behavior that have been challenged in the courts, have been reviewed by the highest state courts or the Supreme Court, and have been denied constitutional protection. These include support obligations in marriage, the right to marital privacy in the bedroom, and homosexual relations, including same-sex marriage. Failure of the Supreme Court to intervene in these areas of family life may ultimately lead to poorer individual and family functioning. For example, if one spouse has total control of the family income and refuses to provide other family members with adequate food, shelter, and health care, failure of the court to intervene may further jeopardize the health and well-being of the family members who lack income and power. Ironically, it is only at divorce that the unemployed spouse can claim a proportion of the employed spouse's income.

State and Local Court Decisions Concerning Family Issues

State and local courts are routinely asked to make decisions on family issues such as marriage, divorce, child support, child custody, and family violence (Walker, 1992). The way in which these decisions are made can have profound impact on family functioning and the health of family members. For example, until 1970, when California instituted the first no-fault divorce law, divorce could be obtained only if one party committed a marital offense (e.g., desertion, cruelty, adultery, insanity, or impotence), giving the other party a legal basis or grounds for divorce (Weitzman & Dixon, 1989). The plaintiff's success in obtaining a divorce depended on the ability to prove the defendant's fault in having committed the marital offense. Fault-oriented divorce proceedings were typically very stressful for everyone involved (Strong & DeVault, 1993). In most cases, the proceedings were very time-consuming, and they involved highly charged feelings about custody, property, and children (Liss, 1987; Raschke, 1987; Weitzman & Dixon, 1989). There is growing evidence that the adversarial nature of these proceedings have a negative impact on the psychological health of the children involved (Saayman & Saayman, 1988/1989; Schwartzberg, 1981). At the present time, most states have adopted no-fault divorce laws. While no-fault divorce has been successful in eliminating much of the acrimony and shame that resulted from fault-oriented divorce (Dixon & Weitzman, 1980), there is little research to document whether no-fault divorce reduces the distress and conflict of divorcing couples (Kitson & Morgan, 1991). More research is needed to understand how and under what conditions legal factors affect the adjustment to divorce (Raschke, 1987). For example, more research is needed concerning outcomes for the court-ordered parenting programs for divorcing families. Much of our current understanding of these programs and their impact on family functioning and the health of family members is based on anecdotal reports.

During the past decade, concern over infants born to drug-addicted women has led a number of state and local prosecutors to attempt to impose criminal penalties for maternal substance abuse (Kocsis, 1991; Rhodes, 1992). Initially, the typical strategy was to charge the mother with the crime of "delivering" a controlled substance to the fetus, either before birth, or after birth before the umbilical cord is cut. Most courts ruled that the state statutes related to child endangerment and to delivery of controlled substances did not apply to the unborn child of a pregnant substance abuser, and the criminal charges against the pregnant women were dismissed (Rhodes, 1992). In 1996, the Supreme Court of South Carolina had a different response: the court held that the word "child" as used in the abuse and endangerment statute would include viable fetuses. Because of this landmark decision (Ojeda, 1996), a substance-addicted pregnant woman in South Carolina may be prosecuted for child endangerment if her fetus has reached viability. While most state courts have not adopted this approach, interest in the use of criminal sanctions to deter drug use among pregnant women continues to exist. Many health care providers are concerned that this approach may actually have a negative impact on the health of unborn infants because women who use drugs will fail to seek prenatal care out of fear that they will be subject to criminal charges. Clearly, this is a medical-legal dilemma with ethical implications (Kocsis, 1991).

A juvenile court in Wisconsin took a relatively novel approach toward protecting the fetus of a substance-addicted pregnant woman: they issued a protective custody order (Glaze, 1997). The order directed the fetus be placed in the protective custody of the County Sheriff's Department and taken to the local hospital for inpatient treatment and protection. The court was able to both "punish" the drug abuser and protect the health of the unborn fetus by committing the pregnant substance abuser to the local hospital.

FAMILY POLICY AND FAMILY FUNCTIONING

What is Family Policy?

Policy involves a set of choices or decisions that are made to reach an overall goal through a specific type of action (Zimmerman, 1992). Values and the political process play an important role in setting policies. For example, in the United States, taxes are levied to reach the goal of providing to citizens certain services, such as police and fire protection, road building and maintenance, libraries, schools, and public recreational facilities. Societal values and the negotiation and compromise involved in the political process play a critical role in determining how much tax individuals and businesses have to pay and how the tax dollars are spent.

The term family policy first started appearing in the literature in the United States in the 1960s, but it was not until much later that it was used in public discussion (Kamerman, 1996). Currently, the United States does not have an official stated position on family policy, but family policy is one of the hottest political issues in the United States (Kruger & Nichols, 1997). Hartman (1993) captures the essence of the controversy: "Some have claimed the field of family policy doesn't exist, some say it does, but shouldn't, whereas others argue for a clear and coherent national family policy" (p. 474).

Zimmerman (1992) broadly defines family policy as everything that governments do that affects families, directly or indirectly. Using this definition, any policy that has an impact on families, including those related to housing, health, income maintenance (e.g., Personal Responsibility and Work Opportunity Reconciliation Act, Social Security), education, social services, or employment can be broadly termed a "family policy." Aldous and Dumon (1990) refer to family policy as objectives concerning family well-being and the specific measures taken by governmental bodies to achieve them. This definition, however, limits family policy to those policies designed to positively benefit families (Aldous & Dumon, 1990). Regardless of the specific definition used, it is generally agreed that the overall goal of family policy is to enhance the well-being of individual family members and the family unit (Zimmerman, 1992). This has been defined as individual and family satisfaction with life, meeting the needs of families in the community, reducing the stress of families, providing additional resources to families, and matching resources to the needs of families (Zimmerman, 1988).

Pros and Cons

There has been ongoing debate about whether to establish specific family policies in the United States. Some argue that there is no need, because all policies affect families in some way. Certainly policies related to family planning, abortion, termination of life support, child support, welfare reform, and benefits for the elderly, to name but a few, affect families in some way. Others fear that a family policy will be intrusive and allow government to regulate what many consider to be a very private domain: one's family life. Furthermore, in establishing a family policy, the definition of what constitutes a family becomes quite controversial. If the definition of family is narrow, many individuals in nontraditional family situations will be excluded. For example, many health insurance policies do not recognize domestic partners as family, so these persons are not eligible for coverage under these policies. Cost is always a major concern in the design and execution of any policy, especially if it involves family issues, because of the privacy issue and the many types of family structure that may need to be included. Thus some consider that an overall family policy would be entirely too expensive to implement and maintain, while others maintain that failure to support families in carrying out their societal roles will cost more in the long run.

Supporters of family policy for the United States note that without federal legislation, policies are piecemeal and equitable across the country. Without comprehensive family policies, we leave to chance the care of some of the most vulnerable members of society: children and elderly, mentally ill, and disabled persons. On the other hand, American culture values individualism, or the notion that people need to work hard and be responsible for their own success; that they should rely on family help for assistance and use governmental resources only as a last resort; and that they should be able to live their lives with minimal governmental influence and interference (Zimmerman, 1988). These values have limited the development of an overall family policy.

The Family and Medical Leave Act: A Policy Example

The Family and Medical Leave Act (FMLA) of 1993 is this nation's first venture into a national family policy program (Frank & Zigler, 1996). Over the years there has been growing awareness that family members who need to take time off from work to give birth to a child, adopt a child, or care for an ill family member run the risk of losing their job. When family members return to their place of employment, they may find that they have been demoted to a lower position with less pay. After considerable debate and controversy, the federal FMLA was passed and went into effect in August 1993, during the first months of the Clinton administration. The bill had been vetoed during the previous administration, primarily on the basis of cost. The FMLA provides 12 weeks of leave annually to employees for the birth or adoption of a child; to care for a newborn; to care for a child, parent, or spouse with a serious illness; or to recuperate from a serious illness that does not permit the employee to work. Employees are eligible for this benefit if they have worked at least 1250 hours during the past year (about 25 hours per week). The act applies to companies who have 50 employees or more. Companies do not have to pay workers during this leave but they can allow workers to use their paid vacation and sick leave during this time. For anticipated events (e.g., birth, adoption, scheduled surgery), 30 days' notice to the employer is required. The leave need not be taken all at once but can be used in segments; for example, to accommodate renal dialysis treatments.

When the FMLA was passed in 1993, provisions in the legislation established a commission to examine the impact of FMLA on workers and businesses. In the commission's report, it was noted that overall, the FMLA has had a positive impact on employees. According to the report, the FMLA has succeeded in replacing the piecemeal nature of voluntary employer leave policies and state leave statutes with a more uniform and consistent standard. The FMLA represents a significant step in helping a larger cross-section of individuals meet their medical and family care-giving needs, while still maintaining their jobs and economic security. Also, the FMLA has not been the burden to business that some had feared.

While these findings from the commission concerning the FMLA are very encouraging, there is growing recognition that the FMLA program and its scope are severely limited. For example, more than 25 percent of working Americans should have taken family and medical leave in 1998 but were unable to do so. Forty-four percent of these Americans did not take the leave because they were afraid of losing their jobs or their employers refused to approve the leave. In addition, 43 percent of private-sector employees are not protected by the FMLA because their employer does not meet the current 50-employee threshold.

In January of 1999, Senator Dodd introduced the Family and Medical Leave Fairness Act of 1999. According to Senator Dodd, the purpose of the bill is to extend the FMLA to millions of Americans who remain uncovered. The bill would lower the threshold to include coverage for companies with 25 or more workers. Lowering the threshold would make it possible for 13 million additional workers to have the protection of the FMLA; 71 percent of the private sector workforce would be covered by FMLA. Currently the bill is in the Senate Health, Education, Legal, and Pensions Committee.

The Family and Medical Leave Act is just one example of a national policy that may influence family functioning and the health of individual family members. Another example is the Genetic Information Nondiscrimination in Health Insurance Act that was introduced by Representative Slaughter on January 6, 1999. The purpose of this legislation is to prevent discrimination of individuals and family members on the basis of genetic information or a request for genetic services. Legislation concerning discrimination on the basis of genetic information has also been introduced in the Senate. On March 4, 1999, Senator Snowe introduced the Genetic Information Nondiscrimination in Health Insurance Act. If passed, these two bills could have a positive impact on family functioning and the health of family members by preventing the potentially devastating consequences of discrimination and health insurance denials on the basis of genetic information.

So, what is the future for family policy in the United States? The enactment of family policies is closely tied to the political atmosphere (Zimmerman, 1992). President Carter convened a White House conference on families during his administration in the late 1970s, but fighting between conservatives and liberals on family policy derailed all efforts at establishing family policy goals. During the 1980s, a more conservative political ideology prevailed and the administration supported reducing benefits such as AFDC, reducing funding for family planning and abortions, and decreasing Medicare expenditures through the use of diagnosis-related groups (DRGs). In 1987, the National Commission on Children was created by Congress and President Reagan to evaluate the status of children and families. The Commission unanimously approved a comprehensive and bold blueprint for a national family policy in 1991, and they submitted it to the Congress and President Bush.

During the early part of Clinton's administration, health care reform was a major issue. In 1996, President Clinton signed into law the Personal Responsibility and Work Opportunity Reconciliation Act of 1996. Clinton claimed that this welfare reform bill would provide support and guarantee medical coverage for families moving from welfare to work. Closer analysis suggests an alternative outcome and concern regarding the well-being of children. Currently there is need for descriptive, analytical, and evaluative research to determine the effect of this landmark legislation on family functioning and the health of individual family members, especially children. While Clinton's promises to improve the welfare of families raises hopes and expectations, little progress has been made to date. In addition, minimal progress has been made in the development of a national family policy that is explicit, clear, and coherent. It is clear that many policies have important implications for families, even if they are not family policies per se.

The Role of the Nurse

Nurses can play a key role in informing clients and their families about the FMLA and the new bill if it passes. Many individuals are not aware of their rights in regard to the FMLA. Workers who believe their old job will not be available to them on their return should discuss this with their supervisor or the owner of the company before taking a leave. In 1997, the United States Labor Department established a toll-free phone number to help Americans determine their rights under the FMLA. Complaints about violation of the policy must be filed within 2 years with a private attorney or with the local or regional office of the U.S. Department of Labor's Wage and Hour Division, Employment Standards Administration.

Nurses need to recognize how health care financing and delivery policies influence family functioning. Meister (1989) recommends that nurses analyze how health and social welfare policies are affecting the families they work with. First the economic and social status of each family member should be identified, including the educational level of the family members, the sources and amounts of income, and whether the family can meet their basic needs and unexpected emergencies (e.g., sudden illness, loss of job). The next step is to determine the family's dependence on Medicaid, Social Security, or AFDC; the health services they use; and their social vulnerabilities, such as unemployment, lack of insurance, or lack of a fixed income. Meister (1989) notes that this analysis helps the nurse to identify possible problem areas and risks for families and to determine what policies and programs (or lack of these) are affecting families' well-being. Steps can then be taken to improve an individual family's access to services. This analysis also serves to identify the families' common needs, which may deserve further attention for policy development (Meister, 1989).

SUMMARY

This chapter has addressed some of the factors that influence the health of family members and family functioning. These include both factors within the family (e.g., illness in a family member, spiritual beliefs and values) and factors outside the family (e.g., legal and ethical decisions and public policies). Although illness in a family member may be viewed as something happening within the family, the family also is affected by how that illness is treated in the health care system, what resources are available for financing health care services, and how policies determine who is eligible for these services on the basis of legal and ethical principles. Not only are family members interdependent but so are families and the communities.

What is the role of the nurse in relation to all of the factors discussed in this chapter? The nurse has a role not only in managing health and illness situations in the individual families but also in advocating for social change that supports family integrity. As nurses work with individuals and families, they will recognize how the health of the individual family members influences the family unit and how the family unit influences the health of the individual members and incorporate these into their plan of care. For example, how is a mother's depression affecting the care of the children? How does the father respond to the mother's depression? Does the father help out or completely take over the mother's role? Does the father stay aloof and criticize the way the children are being raised? How is family function affected by the mother's depression? Is the family willing to use community resources that might be of help?

The legal, ethical, and public policy influences on individual families also must be addressed at a larger societal level. Changing policies at this level is a challenging task; however, evidence from the nurse's experience with families can be a powerful tool for informing and influencing policy makers and the legal system. Nurses need to become more politically active, provide testimony about necessary changes in health care delivery, and advocate for families who may be too vulnerable to speak for themselves, and to promote positive policy changes that will benefit families and the society as a whole.

Study Questions

1. Match the characteristics listed with one of these family types: (1) regenerative, (2) resilient, (3) rhythmic.
   a. Flexibility is a strength
   b. Values family time
   c. Family hardiness
   d. Emotional closeness within the family
   e. Views illness as a challenge
   f. Routines provide sense of security
2. What are the five characteristics of an illness according to John Rolland, the author of *Families, Illness, and Disability?*
3. List three characteristics of a family that indicate a shared religious core.
4. Identify a family policy currently being debated in the state where you live.
5. The United States Constitution provides a guideline for establishing the rights of the family within society.
   a. True
   b. False
6. Legal definitions of the family have been challenged as family structures have changed over the past two decades.
   a. True
   b. False
7. The principle of beneficence supports the decision to ignore signs of neglect until physical abuse has occurred.
   a. True
   b. False

References

Aldous, J., & Dumon, W. (1990). Family policy in the 1980s: Controversy and consensus. *Journal of Marriage and the Family,* 52:1136–1151.

Allport, G.W., & Ross, J.M. (1967). Personal religious orientation and prejudice. *Journal of Personality and Social Psychology,* 5:432–443.

Anderson, C., Reiss, D., & Hogarty, B. (1986). *Schizophrenia and the Family.* New York: Guilford Press.

Basolo-Kunzer, M. (1964). Caring for families of psychiatric patients. *Mental Health Nursing,* 28:73–79.

Beauchamp, T.L., & Childress, J.F. (1983). *Principles of Biomedical Ethics,* ed 2. New York: Oxford University Press.

Belsky, J., et al. (1985). Stability and change in marriage across the transition to parenthood: A second study. *Journal of Marriage and the Family,* 47:855–865.

Belsky, J., et al. (1983). Stability and change in marriage across the transition to parenthood. *Journal of Marriage and the Family,* 45:567–577.

Bird, C.E. (1997). Gender differences in the social and economic burdens of parenting and psychological distress. *Journal of Marriage and the Family,* 59:809–823.

Brigman, K. (1992). Religion and family strengths: Implications for mental health professionals. *Topics in Family Psychology and Counseling,* 1:39–52.

Burman, B., & Margolin, G. (1992). Analyses of the association between marital relationships and health problems: An interactional perspective. *Psychological Bulletin,* 112:39–63.

Butzlaff, R.L., & Hooley, (1998). Expressed emotion and psychiatric relapse: A meta-analysis. *Archives of General Psychiatry,* 55:547–552.

Campbell, T. (1986). Family's impact on health: A critical review. *Family Systems Medicine,* 4:135–327.

Childress, J. (1997). The normative principles of medical ethics. In R.M. Veatch (Eds.), *Medical Ethics,* ed 2, pp. 29–56. Sudbury, MA: Jones & Bartlett.

Covinsky, L. E., et al. (1994). The impact of serious illness on patient's families. *Journal of the American Medical Association,* 272:1839–1844.

Curran, D. (1983). *Traits of a Healthy Family.* San Francisco: Harper & Row.

Curran, D. (1985). *Stress and the Healthy Family.* San Francisco: Harper & Row.

DeFrain, J., & Stinnett, N. (1992). Building on the inherent strengths of families: A positive approach for family psychologists and counselors. *Topics in Family Psychology and Counseling,* 1:15–26.

Dixon, R.B., & Weitzman, L.J. (1980). Evaluating the impact of no-fault divorce in California. *Family Relations,* 29:297–307.

Doane, J., et al. (1981). Parental communication deviance and affective style: Predictors of subsequent schizophrenia spectrum disorders in vulnerable adolescents. *Archives of General Psychiatry,* 38:679–685.

Doherty, W., & Campbell, T. (1988). *Families and Health.* Newbury Park, CA: Sage.

Dombeck, M.B. (1995). Dream-telling: A means of spiritual awareness. *Holistic Nursing Practice,* 9:37–47.

Douglas, M.R. (1997). Ethics and nursing practice. In N.J. Brent (Ed.). *Nurses and the Law: A Guide to Principles and Applications,* pp.187–210. Philadelphia: W.B. Saunders.

Dyson, J., et al. (1997). The meaning of spirituality: A literature review. *Journal of Advanced Nursing,* 26:1183–1188.

Emblen, J.D. (1992). Religion and spirituality defined according to current use in nursing literature. *Journal of Professional Nursing,* 8:41–47.

Fehring, R.J., et al. (1997). Spiritual well-being, religiosity, hope, depression, and other mood states in elderly people coping with cancer. *Oncology Nursing Forum,* 24:663–671.

Fichter, M.M., et al. (1997). Family climate and expressed emotion in the course of alcoholism. *Family Process,* 36:203–222.

Fisher, L., et al. (1993). The California Health Project: VII. Summary and integration of findings. *Family Process,* 32:69–86.

Foshee, V., & Bauman, K. (1992). Parental and peer characteristics as modifiers of the bond-behavior relationship: An elaboration of control theory. *Journal of Health Behavior,* 33:66.

Frank, M., & Zigler, E.F. (1996). Family leave: A developmental perspective. In E. Zigler, S.L. Kagan, & N.W. Hall (Eds.) *Children, Families and Government,* pp. 117–131. New York: Cambridge University Press.

Friedman, M., et al. (1998). Family stress and coping processes: Family adaptation. In M. Friedman (Ed.). *Family Nursing: Research, Theory, and Practice,* ed 4, pp. 435–478. Stamford, CN: Appleton & Lange.

From-Reichman, F. (1948). Notes on the development and treatment of schizophrenics by psychoanalytic-psychotherapy. *Psychiatry,* 11:263–273.

Gallop, G.H. (1993). *Religion in America: 1992–1993.* Princeton, NJ: The Gallop Organization.

Gerstel, N., et al. (1985). Explaining the symptomatology of separated and divorced women and men: The role of material conditions and social networks. *Social Forces,* 64:84–101.

Giron, M., & Gomez-Beneyto, M. (1998). Relationship between empathetic family attitude and relapse in schizophrenia: A two year follow-up prospective study. *Schizophrenia Bulletin,* 24:619–627.

Glaze, C.L. (1997). Combatting prenatal substance abuse: The state's current approach and the novel approach of court-ordered protective custody of the fetus. *Marquette Law Review,* 80:793.

Goldstein, M. (1985). Family factors that antedate the onset of schizophrenia and related disorders: The results of a 15 year prospective longitudinal study. *Acta Psychiatrica Scandinavia,* 319 (suppl):7–18.

Goldstein, M., & Strachan, A. (1987). The family and schizophrenia. In T. Jacob (Ed.), *Family interaction and psychopathology.* New York: Plenum Press.

Gove, W. (1984). Gender differences in mental and physical illness: The effects of fixed roles and nurturant role. *Social Science and Medicine,* 19:77–84.

Hartman, A. (1993). Challenges for family policy. In F. Walsh (Ed.). *Normal Family Processes,* ed 2, pp. 474–502. New York: Gilford Press.

Herth, K. (1993). Hope in the family caregiver of terminally ill people. *Journal of Advanced Nursing,* 18:538–548.

Hogarty, G.E., et al. (1991). Family psychoeducation, social skills training, and maintenance of chemotherapy in the aftercare treatment of schizophrenia: Two-year effects of a controlled study on relapse and adjustment. *Archives of General Psychiatry,* 48:340–347.

Hoge, D.R. (1972). A validated intrinsic religious motivation scale. *Journal for the Scientific Study of Religion,* 11:369–376.

Hooley, J., & Teasdale, J.D. (1989). Predictors of relapse in unipolar depression: Expressed emotion, marital quality, and perceived criticism. *Journal of Abnormal Psychology,* 98:229–235.

Irwin, M., et al. (1987). Impaired natural killer cell activity during bereavement. *Brain, Behavior, and Immunity,* 1:98–104.

Johnson, A., & Ooms, T. (1985). The pressures of government on families. In K. Powers (Ed.), *Lives of Families,* pp. 179–187. Atlanta: Humanics.

Kamerman, S.B. (1996). Child and family policies: An international overview. In E.F. Zigler, et al. (Eds.) *Children, Families, & Government.* New York: Cambridge University Press.

Kamerman, S.B., & Kahn, A.J. (1978). *Family Policy: Government and Families in Fourteen Countries.* New York: Columbia University Press.

Karon, B. P. & Widener, A.J. (1994). Is there really a schizophrenic parent? *Psychoanalytic Psychology,* 11:47–61.

Kaye, J., & Robinson, K.M. (1994). Spirituality among caregivers. *Image: Journal of Nursing Scholarship,* 26:218–221.

Kern, R.D. (1995). Family assessment and intervention. In P.M. Nicassio & T.W. Smith (Eds.), *Managing Chronic Illness: A Biopsychosocial Perspective,* pp. 207–244. Washington DC: American Psychological Association.

Kiecolt-Glaser, J.K., et al. (1991). Spousal caregivers of dementia victims: Longitudinal changes in immunity and health. *Psychosomatic Medicine,* 53:345–362.

Kiecolt-Glaser, J.K., & Glaser, R. (1991). Stress and immune function. In R. Ader, et al. (Eds.) *Psychoneuroimmunology,* ed 2. San Diego: Academic Press.

Kiecolt-Glaser, J.K., et al. (1988). Marital discord and immunity in males. *Psychosomatic Medicine,* 50:213–229.

Kitson, G., & Morgan, L. (1991). Consequences in divorce. In A. Booth (Ed.), *Contemporary Families: Looking Forward, Looking Back.* Minneapolis: National Council on Family Relations.

Kocsis, M.M. (1991). Pregnant women abusing drugs: A medical-legal dilemma. *Medical Trial Technique Quarterly,* 37:496–527.

Koenig, H.G. (1995). *Research in Religion and Aging.* Westport, CT: Greenwood Press.

Kruger, S.F., & Nichols, F.H. (1997). Family Dynamics. In F.H. Nichols & Zwelling, E. (Eds.), *Maternal-Newborn Nursing,* pp. 57–86. Philadelphia: W.B. Saunders.

Last, J.M. (1998). *Public Health and Human Ecology,* ed 2. Stamford, CN: Appleton and Lange.

Lewis, F.M., et al. (1993). The family's functioning with newly diagnosed breast cancer in the mother: The development of an explanatory model. *Journal of Behavioral Medicine,* 16:351–370.

Liss, L. (1987). Families and the law. In M. Sussman & S. Steinmetz. (Eds.) *Handbook of marriage and the family,* pp. 767–794. New York: Plenum.

McCubbin, M. (1991). CHIP-Coping health inventory for parents. In H. McCubbin & A. Thompson (Eds.), *Family Assessment Inventories for Research and Practice,* pp. 175–194. Madison: University of Wisconsin Press.

McCubbin, M. (1993). Predicting family adaptation following diagnosis of child's congenital heart disease. Paper presented at the Annual Meeting of the American Educational Research Association, Atlanta, Georgia.

McCubbin, M., & McCubbin, H. (1993). Families coping with illness: The Resiliency Model of Family Stress, Adjustment, and Adaptation. In C. Danielson, et al. (Eds.) *Families, Health, and Illness: Perspectives on Coping and Intervention,* pp. 21–63. St Louis: Mosby.

McCubbin, H.I., et al. (1996). *Family Assessment: Resiliency, Coping, and Adaptation: Inventories for Research and Practice.* Madison: University of Wisconsin Press.

McLanahan, S., & Adams, J. (1987). Parenthood and psychological well-being. *Annual Review of Sociology,* 13:237–257.

Meister, S. (1989). Health care financing, policy, and family practice nursing. In C. Gilliss, et al. (Eds.) *Toward a Science of Family Nursing,* pp. 146–155. Menlo Park, CA: Addison-Wesley.

Miller, M. (1995). Culture, spirituality, and women's health. *Journal of Obstetrics, Gynecology, and Neonatal Nursing,* March/April:257–263.

Mirowsky, J., & Ross, C. (1989). Social causes of psychological distress. New York: Aldine-de-Gruyter.

Moberg, D. (1974). Spiritual well-being in late life. In J. Gubrium (Ed.), *Late Life: Communities and Environmental Policy,* pp. 256–279. Springfield, IL: Charles C. Thomas.

Moore v. City of East Cleveland, Ohio, 431 U.S. 494 (1977).

Myers, J. (1992). *Legal issues in child abuse and neglect.* Newbury Park, CA: Sage.

Nelson, G. (1994). Emotional well-being of separated and married women: Long-term follow-up study. *American Journal of Orthopsychiatry,* 64:150–160.

Ojeda, S.H. (1996). *Whitner v. State:* Expanding child abuse and endagerment laws to protect viable fetuses from prenatal substance abuse. 99 W. Va. L. Rev. 311 (Winter, 1996).

O'Farrell, T.J., et al. (1998). Expressed emotion and relapse in alcoholic patients. *Journal of Consulting and Clinical Psychology,* 66:744–752.

O'Neil, D.P., & Kenny, E.K. (1998). Spirituality and chronic illness. *Image: Journal of Nursing Scholarship,* 30:275–280.

Palo Alto Tenants Union v. Morgan, 321 F.Supp. 908. 1970, N.D.Cal. aff'd 487 F.2d 883 (9th Cir. 1973).

Parker, G., & Hadzi-Pavlovic, D. (1990). Expressed emotion as a predictor of schizophrenic relapse: An analysis of aggregated data. *Psychological Medicine,* 20:961–965.

Rabins, P.V., et al. (1990). Emotional adaptation over time in care-givers for chronically ill elderly people. *Age and Aging,* 19:185–190.

Raschke, H.J. (1987). Divorce. In M.B. Sussman & S.K. Steinmetz. (Eds.) *Handbook of Marriage and the Family,* pp. 597–624. New York: Plenum.

Reed, P. (1992). An paradigm for the investigation of spirituality in nursing. *Research in Nursing & Health,* 15:349–357.

Reiss, D., et al. (1986). Family process, chronic illness, and death: On the weakness of strong bonds. *Archives of General Psychiatry,* 43:795–804.

Rhodes, A.M. (1992). Criminal penalties for maternal substance abuse. *Maternal Child Nursing,* 18:311.

Rolland, J. (1994). *Families, Illness, and Disability: An Integrative Treatment Model.* New York: Basic Books.

Ross, C., & Huber, J. (1985). Hardship and depression. *Journal of Health and Social Behavior,* 26:312–327.

Ross, C., et al. (1990). The impact of the family on health: The decade in review. *Journal of Marriage and the Family,* 52:1059–1078.

Rushton, C.H., & Infante, M.C. (1995). Keeping secrets: The ethical and legal challenges. *Pediatric Nursing,* 21:479–482.

Saayman, G., & Saayman, R. (1988/1989). The adversarial legal process and divorce: Negative effects upon the psychological adjustment of children. *Journal of Divorce,* 12:329–348.

Schor, E.L. (1995). The influence of families on child health: Family behaviors and child outcomes. *Pediatric Clinics of North America,* 42:89–102.

Schor, E.L., et al. (1987). Family health: Utilization and effects of family membership. *Medical Care,* 25:616–626.

Schwartzberg, A. (1981). Divorce, children, and adolescents: An overview. *Adolescent Psychiatry,* 9:119–132.

Shafranske, E., & Maloney, H. (1990). Clinical psychologists' religious and spiritual orientations and their practice of psychotherapy. *Psychotherapy,* 27:72–78.

Stinnet, N. (1979). Strengthening families. *Family Perspective,* 13:3–9.

Strong, B., & DeVault, C. (1993). *Essentials of the Marriage and Family Experience,* pp. 349–368. St Paul: West Publishing.

Thiroux, J. (1986). *Ethics Theory and Practice.* New York: MacMillan.

Thomas, D., & Henry, G. (1984). The religion and family connection: Increasing dialogue in the social sciences. *Journal of Marriage and the Family,* 47:369–379.

Tseng, W., & Hsu, I. (1991). *Culture and Family: Problems and Therapy*. New York: Haworth Press.

Umberson, D. (1989). Relationships with children: Explaining parents psychological well-being. *Journal of Marriage and the Family,* 51:999–1012.

Umberson, D., & Gove, W.R. (1989). Parenthood and psychological well-being: Theory, measurement, and stage in the family life course. *Journal of Family Issues,* 10:440–462.

Vaughn, C., et al. (1984). Family factors in schizophrenia relapse: Replication in California of British research on expressed emotion. *Archives of General Psychiatry,* 41:1169–1177.

Vaughn, F. (1986). *The Inward Arc: Healing and Wholeness in Psychotherapy and Spirituality*. Boston: New Science Library.

Veatch, R.M. (1997). *Medical Ethics,* ed 2. Boston: Jones & Bartlett.

Venters, M. (1986). Family life and cardiovascular risk: Implications for the prevention of chronic disease. *Social Science and Medicine,* 22:1067–1074.

Walker, T. (1992). Family law in the fifty states: An overview. *Family Law Quarterly,* 25:417–515.

Weaver, A.J., et al. (1998). An analysis of research on religious and spiritual variables in three major mental health nursing journals. *Issues in Mental Health Nursing,* 19:263–276.

Weitzman, L.J., & Dixon, R.B. (1989). The transformation of legal marriage through no-fault divorce. In A.S. Skolnick and J.H. Skolnick (Eds.), *Family in Transition,* ed 6, pp. 315–327. Glenview, IL: Scott, Foresman.

White, L., et al. (1986). Children and marital happiness: Why the negative correlations? *Journal of Family Issues,* 7:131–147.

Wood, A., et al. (1997). The downward spiral of postpartum depression. *Maternal Child Nursing,* 22:308–317.

Wright, L., Watson, W.L., & Bell, J.M. (1996). *Beliefs: The Heart of Healing in Families and Illness*. New York: Basic Books.

Yorker, B.C. (1993). Family law. In C.S. Fawcett (Ed.), *Family Psychiatric Nursing*. St Louis: Mosby.

Zimmerman, S. (1988). *Understanding Family Policy: Theoretical Approaches*. Newbury Park, CA: Sage.

Zimmerman, S. (1992). *Family Policies and Family Well-Being: The Role of Political Culture*. Newbury Park, CA: Sage.

Focus On

NURSING PROCESS AND FAMILY HEALTH CARE

You have heard about nursing process since you began your nursing education and are probably asking, "Why more of it?" At this point in your education, you are familiar with the use of the problem-solving process with individual clients. This chapter builds on your previous learning and challenges you to expand your understanding of nursing process and its application to the family as client.

Nurses work with different family members, ancillary caregivers, and new technologies in a rapidly changing health care delivery system. They must be prepared to offer support, information, and direct care services to families. The professional nurse's use of a logical, systematic approach to the family client is essential if care is to be appropriate. Nursing process provides that approach.

This chapter describes the five-step nursing process: assessment, analysis, planning, implementation, and evaluation and how to apply the nursing process in family situations.

Following this brief review, the complex role of the professional nurse with families is explored, and each step of the nursing process with the family is comprehensively addressed. The student is encouraged to use increasingly sophisticated assessment instruments in providing professional nursing care to family clients. In the analysis section, both the NANDA diagnostic framework and the Omaha classification system are described. Students are referred to resources for additional details of these methods of labeling family problems that are amenable to nursing intervention.

The importance of working in partnership with the family is emphasized in the section dealing with implementing family health care. Here, too, the need for culturally sensitive interventions is discussed, as is the evaluation of family nursing care based on criteria jointly determined by the family and the nurse. Finally, a case study of the Jones family provides nursing students with a clinical example of the cyclic and dynamic application of the nursing process.

Chapter 7

NURSING PROCESS AND FAMILY HEALTH CARE

Beverly J. Ross

OUTLINE

Critical Thinking

Creative Thinking

Overview of the Nursing Process
Assessment
Analysis
Nursing Diagnosis
Planning
Implementation
Evaluation

Family Nursing Process
Family Assessment
Analysis of Family Assessment Data
Family Care Planning
Implementation of Family Health Care
Evaluating Family Nursing Care

Case Study: The Jones Family

OBJECTIVES

On completion of this chapter, the reader will be able to:

- Define the nursing process.
- Describe the five steps of the nursing process.
- Discuss the application of the nursing process to the care of families.
- Contrast the application of the nursing process to the care of families with its application in the care of individuals.
- Describe the importance of family involvement in each step of the family process.

Florence Nightingale (1969) wrote, in the conclusion to her *Notes on Nursing,* "nothing but observation and experience will teach us the ways to maintain or to bring back the state of health" (p. 133). The importance of that statement has not diminished over time. Nurses have continued to make every effort to improve their ability to observe, analyze, and understand how best to meet the needs of clients. The nursing process, developed to enhance these essential skills, is a problem-solving approach based on the scientific method. Nursing process can be used by any nurse in any setting and can be applied to the care of individuals, families, groups, or communities.

CRITICAL THINKING

It is imperative in any discussion of nursing process that critical thinking be recognized as an essential underlying element. Facione and Facione (1996) describe critical thinking as increasingly recognized as the "cognitive engine" driving the process of professional judgment. Paul (1993) cited the National Council for Excellence in Critical Thinking as stating that critical thinking is the "intellectually disciplined process of actively and skillfully conceptualizing, applying, synthesizing, or evaluating information gathered from, or generated by, observation, experience, reflection, or communication, as a guide to belief or action" (p. 110). Paul and Heaslip (1995), in their discussion of critical thinking and nursing, stated that the demonstration of expertise in nursing practice entails the ability to use appropriate nursing knowledge and skilled judgments and that the nurse must be a "thinker" who can reason things through. The expert nurse is able to direct the intellectual process in a way that is disciplined and effective in the recognition of and subsequent solving of client problems. Each "comprehension" of client care needs, and the required nursing interventions, must be adjusted to the unique case.

Each step of the nursing process, whether applied to the individual within the family as context or to the family as client, requires thoughtful decision-making. The nurse must decide what data to collect and how, when, and where that data is collected. The relevance of each new piece of information and how it fits into the accumulating database must be decided. The nurse must decide whether sufficient information has been obtained to allow moving forward in terms of problem and strength identification or whether gaps exist that require additional data gathering. Each situation evolves as it is analyzed, and each item of new information must be judged in terms of accuracy, clarity, and relevance. This is especially true when working with the family as client. As Hanslik (1998) stated, "Nursing does involve task oriented practices, but it also encompasses reflective, reasonable, thought processes" (p. 442).

CREATIVE THINKING

Nurses and clients exist as "unique" individuals and groups in "unique" worlds that reflect varying family and sociocultural situations. Each person reacts to physiologic change in their own way, requiring health practitioners to recognize that illness will not manifest in the same way in each person. The same is true when you view the variety of responses to life changes, social disruption, or catastrophic events. Just as critical reflection is essential to appropriate application of nursing process, creative thinking is also essential. The nurse must always be aware that the "common" interpretation of the data may not be the "correct" interpretation in a given situation, and the commonly expected signs and symptoms or cues may not appear in every case or in the same configuration. The ability to be open to the unexpected, to be alert to the unusual or different response may be key to the identification of an underlying problem or concern or the best approach to meeting the expressed need of a client. As each new nurse-client interaction begins, creative thinking allows access to any or all the possibilities. Webster's New World Dictionary (1987) defined "to be creative" as to be inventive. The creative person is visionary, productive, and able to see that which is not obvious or clearly drawn. Used in the context of nursing process, the creative thinker must be open to the universe of possibilities in any given situation, able to recognize the new and the unusual, decipher unique and complex situations, and be inventive and imaginative in designing approaches to problem solving.

Bell (1998) underscored the importance of the desire to learn about families and the ability to be open to hearing what families are trying to tell us. The author described her experience at the "Family Nursing Unit" at the University of Calgary. The unit was designed to provide assistance, support, and guidance to families dealing with the stress of serious illness. Both master's and doctoral degree students were assigned to the unit for clinical experience. According to Bell, one characteristic distinguished an excellent family clinician: Those who were most effective had an "insatiable curiosity" which allowed them to continuously look for and offer different explanations and descriptions-other ways of seeing family members' beliefs, behaviors, and problems which might generate new perspectives and offer more options" (p. 125). One must understand that each individual sees the world differently. Our experiences shape our ideas of who we are, how we make sense of our world, and what is true for us. Rubenfeld and Sheffer (1999) described a type of thinking they label "New Ideas and Creativity," a type of thinking that these authors believed went beyond the usual textbook ideas and allowed one to see and address unique needs. This type of thinking allows the individual to reconfigure the norm. The approach is not limited to the way things have always been or have always been done; instead, it allows one to try a new way of doing something or to interpret presenting information in a new way. Such thinking is essential in effective use of the nursing process, and the nursing process is an essential component in the delivery of comprehensive care to all clients, including families. The reader is urged to "think family" as the following overview of the nursing process is presented. The remainder of the chapter is devoted to the application of the nursing process to the family as client, or the family nursing process.

OVERVIEW OF THE NURSING PROCESS

Yura and Walsh (1988) initially defined *nursing process* using four steps: assessment, planning, implementation, and evaluation. Ross and Cobb (1990) delineated a five-step process that included analysis as the second step. Gordon (1982, 1987, 1994) described a six-step process: assessment, analysis, outcome projection, planning, implementation, and evaluation. The five-step process seems to be the most commonly used at this time. The key concern is that, regardless of the number of steps, the process should embody a systematic approach to identify needs and concerns, to take appropriate action to assist the client in problem resolution, and to assess the degree to which those needs and concerns are met. The following is a brief review of each step of the five-step process.

Assessment

Assessment is the first step in the nursing process and is possibly the most critical (Shaw, 1993). Yura and Walsh (1988) describe "assessing" as the act of reviewing a human situation to obtain data about the client for the purpose of affirming an illness state, obtaining a client's diagnosis, and determining the strengths and health promotion needs of the client. Data collection involves both subjective and objective data, that is, data verbally shared with the nurse by the client and data obtained by direct observation and examination or in consultation with other health care providers.

Many sources may be used, and physical assessment is an essential element to validate history and identify areas in need of further exploration (Chitty, 1997). There are many guidelines available to assist the nurse in data collection and to help organize that information. It is extremely important that assessment instruments be selected with care. Instruments must be appropriate for the purpose for which they are intended. For instance, an assessment instrument designed to facilitate the identification of medical problems gathers medical data. Such an instrument does not necessarily uncover concerns and problems amenable to nursing intervention. Thus, care must be taken to select an instrument with an underlying conceptual framework that guides assessment activities toward the identification of nursing phenomena.

Analysis

Chitty (1993, 1997) described analysis, the second step in the nursing process, as using knowledge from the biological and social sciences, as well as nursing, to analyze the data collected; that is, to note and cluster together those pieces of information that attest to a particular problem or concern. Yura and Walsh (1988) stress the importance of noting gaps in information or contradictory information and of seeking out additional data as needed to ensure accuracy. The nurse must recognize that the problem presented by the client may not be the underlying or basic need or issue that must be addressed. Critical and creative thinking are essential to this analytical process. The desired outcome of the analysis step is the identification of client concerns for which some intervention is needed. In any given situation, a client may have concerns that are medical in nature and require referral. There may be needs that require collaboration and cooperative action by the nurse and another health care professional. In such instances, the nurse works with the involved discipline to solve the identified problem. Those problems that are amenable to nursing intervention, independently of other health care disciplines, are nursing diagnoses. It is the nursing diagnoses that form the foundation for the nursing care plan.

Nursing Diagnosis

Gordon (1982, 1987, 1994) believes that nursing diagnosis goes back to the founding of modern nursing. Although nursing diagnosis as a term is relatively new, Florence Nightingale and her colleagues diagnosed nutritional deficits as they cared for Crimean War casualties. This "nursing diagnosis" led to interventions designed to correct the system of care in military hospitals to improve nutrition. Gordon described nursing diagnosis as creating the link between collecting information and care planning.

Box 7–1 contains the current list of nursing diagnosis labels accepted for clinical testing by NANDA. During the proceedings of the Ninth National Conference, NANDA adopted the following definition of nursing diagnosis:

> A nursing diagnosis is a clinical judgment about individual, family, or community responses to actual or potential health problems [or] life processes. Nursing diagnosis provides the basis for selection of nursing interventions to achieve outcomes for which the nurse is accountable (NANDA, Nursing Diagnosis: Definitions and Classification 1992–1993, 1999).

Gordon used the NANDA nursing diagnoses in much of her work with nursing process, nursing diagnosis, and care planning. Gordon stated (1976, 1982, 1987, 1994) that there are three essential components in a nursing diagnosis. These three components are the problem (P); the etiology, or cause (E); and the defining cluster of signs and symptoms (S). They are often referred to as the PES format.

The problem statement describes a problem or health state of the client, who might be an individual, a family, or a community. An example of a problem statement for a family might be noncompliance with immunization requirements for their school-aged children. The problem statement represents a concise term for a cluster of signs or symptoms indicating a specific concern or health need. The NANDA labels accepted for clinical use and testing may be used as problem statements. In many instances, greater specificity is required. A number of labels are followed by the term "specify" in parentheses. In instances where that particular label is used (Box 7–1, e.g. decisional conflict or knowledge deficit), the specific area in which the problem has occurred must be included. In the previous example, the family was noncompliant with the school district immunization requirements. The term "noncompliant" alone is not sufficiently clear to communicate the problem.

The probable cause is the second component of any given nursing diagnosis statement. It identifies the factors that are believed to be causing or maintaining the health problem. The cause may involve the environment, client behaviors, interactions between client and environment, or external factors. The family described above may be noncompliant with immunization requirements because of lack of understanding of the importance and availability of immunizations. Another family might have home maintenance deficits because they lack the money to obtain proper equipment for home upkeep. A category label can be used to communicate or describe the cause. The term used in the cause statement summarizes the cluster of cues or data that indicate the particular phenomenon sustaining or causing the identified problem. The problem itself, and the factors believed to be the primary cause or sustaining factors for the problem, taken together, become the diagnostic statement (Figure 7-1).

Finally, Gordon describes the third component of the nursing diagnosis as the cluster of signs and symptoms supporting the diagnoses. Each diagnostic label or title has a set of signs and symptoms that permit discrimination between health problems. When the client receiving care manifests the signs and symptoms that indicate the presence of a particular diagnostic label or title, the use of that label to define the presenting problem is appropriate. Evaluation of client outcomes as care progresses may be based on ascertaining to what degree these presenting signs and symptoms have been relieved or improved.

Planning

Planning is the third step of the nursing process. Ross and Cobb (1990) discuss the planning step as the "the process by which objectives are determined, interventions selected or designed, and the care plan written. . . . " (p. 134). A clear plan of action is essential to the accomplishment of a complex task. The higher the degree of difficulty, the more important it is to plan carefully. Thus, the nurse must consider a number of elements in the task at hand. Priorities must be set; multiple concerns may

Box 7-1

NANDA-APPROVED NURSING DIAGNOSES FOR CLINICAL USE AND TESTING

Pattern 1: Exchanging

Nutrition, altered, risk for more than body requirements
Nutrition, altered, risk for less than body requirements
Nutrition, altered, potential for more than body requirements
Infection, risk for
Body temperature, risk for altered
Hypothermia
Hyperthermia
Ineffective thermoregulation
Dysreflexia
Automatic Dysreflexia, risk for
⋆Constipation
Constipation, perceived
Constipation, risk for
⋆Diarrhea
⋆Bowel Incontinence
Urinary Elimination, altered
Incontinence, stress
Incontinence, reflex
Incontinence, urge
Incontinence, functional
Incontinence, total
Urinary Urge Retention, risk for
Urinary Retention
⋆Tissue Perfusion, altered (specific type) renal, cerebral, cardiopulmonary, gastrointestinal, peripheral)
Fluid Volume, imbalance, risk for
Fluid Volume Excess
Fluid Volume Deficit
Fluid Volume Deficit, risk for
⋆Cardiac Output, decreased
Gas Exchange, impaired
Airway Clearance, ineffective
Breathing Pattern, ineffective
#Spontaneous Ventilation, inability to sustain
#Ventilatory Weaning, dysfunctional response (DVWR)
Injury, risk for
Suffocation, risk for
Poisoning, risk for
Trauma, risk for
Aspiration, risk for
Disuse Syndrome, risk for
Latex Allergy Response

continued

Box 7-1

Latex Allergy Response, risk for
Altered Protection
Impaired Tissue Integrity
*Oral Mucous Membrane, altered
Impaired Skin Integrity
Dentition, Altered
Decreased Adaptive Capacity: Intercranial
Energy Field Disturbance

Pattern 2: Communicating

Verbal communication, impaired

Pattern 3: Relating

Social Interaction, impaired
Social Isolation
Loneliness, risk for
*Role Performance, altered
Parenting, altered
Parenting, altered, risk for
Parent/Infant/Child Attachment, altered, risk for
Sexual Dysfunction
Family Processes, altered
*Caregiver Role Strain
#Caregiver Role Strain, risk for
Family Process, altered: alcoholism
Parental Role Conflict
Sexuality Patterns, altered

Pattern 4: Valuing

Spiritual Distress (distress of the human spirit)
Spiritual Distress, risk for
Spiritual Well-Being, enhanced, potential for

Pattern 5: Choosing

Individual Coping, ineffective
Adjustment, impaired
Defensive Coping
Denial, ineffective
Family Coping, ineffective: disabling
Family Coping, ineffective: compromised
Family Coping, potential for: Growth
Enhanced Community Coping, potential for
Community Coping, ineffective
Management of Therapeutic Regimen, ineffective: individuals
Noncompliance (Specify)
Management of Therapeutic Regimen, ineffective: families

continued

Box 7-1

Management of Therapeutic Regimen, ineffective: community
Management of Therapeutic Regimen, effective: individual
Decisional Conflict (Specify)
Health-Seeking Behaviors (Specify)

Pattern 6: Moving

Physical Mobility, impaired
#Peripheral Neurovascular Dysfunction, risk for
Perioperative Positioning Injury, risk for
*Infant Behavior, disorganized
Organized Infant Behavior, potential for, enhanced
Transfer Ability, impaired
Bed mobility, impaired
Activity Intolerance
Fatigue
Activity Intolerance, risk for
Sleep Pattern Disturbance
Sleep Deprivation
Diversional Activity Deficit
Home Maintenance Management, impaired
Health Maintenance, altered
Surgical Recovery, delayed
Adult Failure to Thrive
*Feeding Self-Care Deficit
Swallowing, impaired
Breastfeeding, ineffective
#Breastfeeding, interrupted
Breastfeeding, effective
#Infant Feeding Pattern, ineffective
*Self-Care Deficit: bathing/hygiene
*Self-Care Deficit: dressing/grooming
*Self-Care Deficit: toileting
Growth and Development, altered
Development, altered, risk for
Altered Growth, risk for
Relocation Stress Syndrome
Disorganized Infant Behavior, risk for
*Disorganized Infant Behavior
Organized Infant Behavior, potential for, enhanced

Pattern 7: Perceiving

*Body Image Disturbance
*Self-Esteem Disturbance
Low Self-Esteem: chronic
Low Self-Esteem: situational
*Personal Identity Disturbance
Sensory/Perceptual Alterations (Specify) (visual, auditory, kinesthetic, gustatory, tactile, olfactory)

continued

Box 7-1

Unilateral Neglect
Hopelessness
Powerlessness

Pattern 8: Knowing

Knowledge Deficit (specify)
Environmental Interpretation Syndrome, impaired
Confusion, acute
Confusion, chronic
Thought Processes, altered
Memory, impaired

Pattern 9: Feeling

*Pain
Pain, chronic
Nausea
Grieving, dysfunctional
Grieving, anticipatory
Sorrow, chronic
Violence, risk for: directed at others
Self-Mutilation, risk for
Violence, risk for: self-directed
Posttrauma Response
Rape Trauma Syndrome
Rape Trauma Syndrome: compound reaction
Rape Trauma Syndrome: silent reaction
Posttrauma Syndrome, risk for
Anxiety
Death Anxiety
Fear

*Revised diagnosis submitted and approved in 1998.
#Diagnosis revised by small work groups at the 1996 Biennial Conference on the Classification of Nursing Diagnosis, changes approved and added in 1998.
Source: NANDA Nursing Diagnoses: Definitions and Classifications, 1999–2000. North American Nursing Diagnosis Association, 1999.

need to be addressed. Those concerns, considered most crucial at a given point in time, must be dealt with first, and ascertaining what is important to the client is vital to successful planning. If the nurse and client do not agree on which concerns are primary, little headway is made. Moreover, as conditions change, priorities may change.

Because the availability of resources, including time, support systems, and financial resources, influence priority setting and the types of interventions selected, resources must be identified as a part of the planning process. "Although one might like to think finances need not be considered . . . in reality the lack of finances is one of the major reasons families neglect to follow through with mutually agreed upon plans of care" (Ross & Cobb, 1990, p. 135). Thus, it is essential to guard against recommending activities, equip-

Nursing Diagnosis Format

__________ Related to __________

Problem or Title — Cause

Sample Nursing Diagnosis Statement

Deficit, home maintenance/management Related to *Limited financial resources and knowledge deficit of available community resources*

Problem or Title — Cause

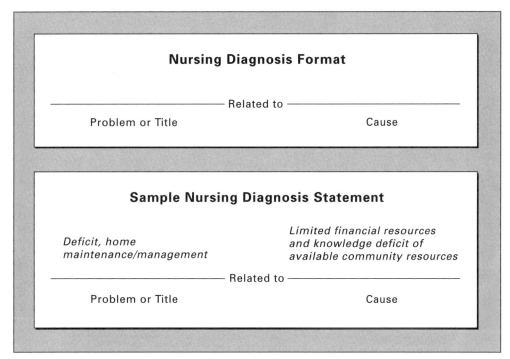

FIGURE 7-1
Nursing diagnosis and sample diagnosis statement.

ment, and placements that clients cannot afford, and if the client is not personally able to pay for the interventions being suggested and financial assistance cannot be found, another option must be sought.

Outcome Determination

Planning involves the determination of possible outcomes for the defined nursing diagnosis. To establish realistic, attainable objectives, the nurse must determine both the probable outcome and the best possible recovery or state of health, given optimal care in light of the presenting circumstances. A time frame for achievement must also be determined. How much time is required to achieve the identified objective? As indicated previously, conditions do change. Clients may progress more quickly or slowly than expected or achieve at levels of ability above or below that anticipated. Nevertheless, identifying potential outcomes increases the possibility of establishing achievable goals or objectives (Ross & Cobb, 1990).

Writing the Plan of Care

An essential and often neglected part of the planning process is writing the plan of care. It is this portion of the planning process that provides the means of communicating the care plan for this particular client to all those involved in care delivery. The written plan should include the specific concerns or nursing diagnoses being addressed. To ensure ongoing evaluation of progress, the specific objectives to be achieved by the care provided should be written in clear, measurable terms, with time frames for the achievement of the projected outcomes. Finally, the plan should include the nursing interventions selected or designed to assist this client in moving toward achievement of the mutually defined goals and objectives. The written nursing interventions direct the care providers to initiate or carry out specific actions or activities, and specify, how, when, and where these activities are to be completed. Yura and Walsh (1988) described the care plan as "the blue print for action, providing the direction for implementing the plan and providing the framework for an evaluation" (p. 39).

Implementation

The fourth step of the nursing process is implementation. Implementation is the process of initiating or putting into effect the plan of care and completing the actions necessary to accomplish the defined objectives. The implementation phase of the process involves critical and creative thinking, strong interpersonal skills, and technical expertise. As Yura and Walsh summarized, "Decision making, observation, and communication are significant skills. These skills are utilized with the client, the nurse, the nursing team members, and health team members" (Yura & Walsh, 1988, p. 154). Throughout the implementation phase, the nurse must work interdependently with others to encourage and support the client and significant others; to assist, guide, and support ancillary workers; and to keep other health team members informed of the type or degree of progress. The nurse must make decisions as to which interventions can or should be delegated to others and how to incorporate other persons into care delivery.

Throughout the implementation process, data gathering continues. New information is obtained with each contact with the client and this additional information must be incorporated into the current data base; it must be analyzed for relevance and importance; and decisions must be made as to whether to proceed as originally planned or to modify the plan of care. As indicated previously, nursing process is not static. In practice, there is a constant flow among the components. The cycle continues as long as interaction with the client occurs.

Evaluation

The fifth step of the nursing process is evaluation, which requires that the nurse determine to what degree the client has achieved the expected outcomes. It is concerned with the ongoing assessment of progress, as well as the degree to which the plan of care has been effective in solving the identified problem. As care is delivered, changes occur in the ability of clients to retain and use information, perform tasks, and assume necessary roles or adopt required behaviors. As knowledge and behaviors change, status changes. The status of the client involves the current physical, emotional, social, and economic conditions and how that client's circumstance has improved, remained the same, or deteriorated. The evaluation component has been the most neglected part of the nursing process and it may be perceived as the most difficult. It remains true, however, that "identification of the degree of progress made toward achievement of a specific standard is an essential element in health care delivery" (Martin & Scheet, 1992, p. 174).

FAMILY NURSING PROCESS

The nursing process that has been presented is a systematic approach to the design and delivery of nursing care to clients. Family nursing process assists the nurse in developing a care plan that will enhance the well-being of families. Healthy families have the ability to provide the "nurturing" needed to produce healthy individuals and are essential to a healthy society.

Nurses must be prepared to work with caregivers and family members to offer support and information and to direct care services. According to Berkley and Hanson (1991), the family is an essential focus of "nursing process." These authors described a comprehensive approach to the family nursing process in which family is seen as an open system interacting in a larger society. The family, as the nurturing place for its members, has specific functions and roles and must be viewed in terms of function, role, and needs. The comprehensive approach demands that the whole family and each of its members be assessed simultaneously. In this context, the "family" may be broader than just those persons identified as residing together in a particular household. Significant others may include not only friends and relatives who are located in close proximity to the household unit but also those who reside some distance away.

Family nursing process is a very complex undertaking. The nurse is dealing with many individuals rather than a single person and with the multiple relationships that exist among family members. According to Friedman (1998), "comprehensive family nursing is a complex process, making it necessary to have a logical systematic approach for working with families and individual family members. This approach is the nursing process" (p. 49). Family structure, family development, and family dynamics are only a few of the concepts essential to understanding families. The family nursing process entails the assessment of the family's strengths and limitations in meeting its needs and the needs of each of its members. A pattern of open communications between nurse and family and a willingness to share and validate information are crucial to determining the types of concerns and health care needs that the family is experiencing and evaluating which of these are amenable to nursing interventions. Figure 7-2 depicts the ongoing process of bidirectional communication in the family-nurse interaction, which is fundamental to effective family nursing care. The five steps in the family nursing process described in the following pages-assessment, analysis, planning, implementation, and evaluation-are the basic steps of the nursing process. Each step is discussed in terms of its application to the family as client.

Family Assessment

The establishment of a solid foundation on which to build or design the plan of care is essential if comprehensive, effective care is to be provided for any client. This is especially true in caring for families. Successful data gathering is predicated on the establishment of a relationship with the client family that facilitates an exchange of often sensitive information in as comfortable a manner as possible. As Martinson and Widmer (1989) stated, "A state exists prior to assessment during which the nurse establishes rapport with and gains the trust of the patient. This is the necessary beginning of ongoing mutual respect and cooperation essential to the success of any intervention" (p. 50).

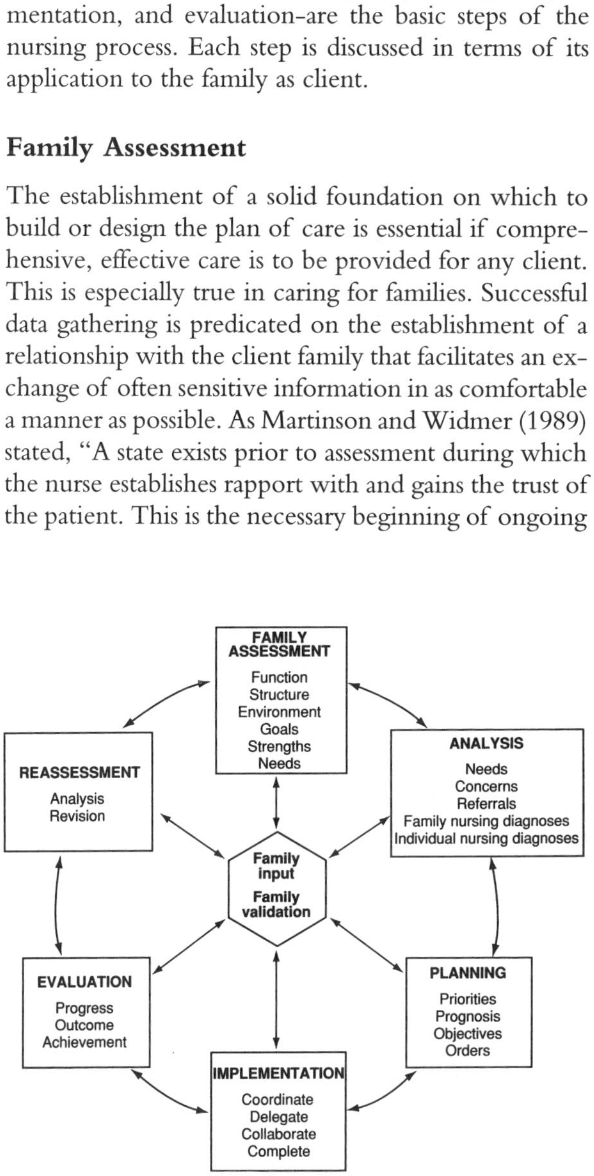

FIGURE 7-2
Family nursing process.

Providing holistic care carries with it the expectation that nurses consider the patients' family, because the family is a system in which change in one member affects all the other members. The alteration in family function that can result from illness may result in feelings of anger and guilt. Nurses need to recognize the importance of assessment, both "how the family is influencing the patient, and how they are influenced by the member who is ill" (Chitty, 1997, p. 373). In situations where family demands exceed coping resources, where family cooperation is unsteady or falters, where individuals express hurt feelings and pain in their interpersonal struggles, family nursing is always needed. Friedeman (1989) states that family health is a "state" that is dynamically balanced. It involves a process of weighing family togetherness and commitment to the family unit against individual achievement and the striving of individual family members to develop to their own personal potential. Assessing the family unit involves determining the ability of the family to function effectively in meeting the needs of its members.

Wasik, Bryant, and Lyons (1990) emphasized the importance of individualized approaches to family care needs. These authors recognized that today considerable diversity exists among families. This is true even among families of similar sociocultural backgrounds. The recognition of this diversity should lead to an acknowledgment of the importance of assessing each family's needs and priorities individually. Cantor (1991) described the American family as undergoing transformation. As the population ages, the ability to care for the elderly members of families will be challenged as a result of a number of factors. For example, individual family units are smaller; kin networks are multigenerational, but narrow, in the sense that there are fewer children, uncles, aunts, and cousins. As more elderly persons need care, there are fewer siblings, aunts, and uncles to share the responsibilities of care (Cantor, 1991). Allen (1991) discussed research results that indicated that there was considerable aging not only of the general population but also of the most prominent caregivers of the elderly. The families showed considerable amounts of pain. There was evidence that there was "family feeling" existing beyond the actual caregiving situation but that distance made it difficult for families to mobilize. As Allen saw it, the family was not organized to bear all burdens. It remains rather small and fragile in structure, yet it continues to be expected, at least in this country at this time, to care for all its members.

A variety of approaches are recommended in the assessment of the family, depending on the conceptual framework of the nurse. Christensen and Kenney (1995) discussed the use of family nursing models as unique perspectives or ways of understanding families. Which model is to be selected for use in a particular situation is decided during the initial contact with the family. As the nurse gathers initial data about the family, the unique and common patterns of interaction are identified and the nurse decides which model would best represent that family and best facilitate the identification of strengths, needs, and the delivery of care. The nurse must determine whether care needs indicate an approach that involves the individual client within the family as context, or whether the focus of care is the family as client.

A variety of family models exist and each may be used alone or used in combination with a nursing model. Lapp, Diemert, and Enestvedt (1990) describe the development of assessment guidelines based on a number of theoretical perspectives. Their guidelines emphasized the importance of "thinking" family and working with "the family as a partner" in making health care decisions. The guidelines do not prescribe questions, but allow an "exploratory and interactional experience in which the content and pace is mutually set" (p. 24). Many of these assessment techniques have been developed from family therapy and have been used in initial assessment by health care professionals. These include genograms and ecomaps.

The genogram is a modified "family tree" diagram. It allows the health care professional to organize a large amount of information in a way that allows intergenerational patterns in families to be more clearly visible. The ecomap is a diagram of a family's current connections with each other and with the environment, including the extended family. The diagram indicates strengths and weaknesses in a family's social support system (Paquin & Bushum, 1991). Genograms and ecomaps were described as allowing holistic and integrative analysis of behavior by the practitioner and the client. The activity was described as often positive for clients. The "drawing a picture" of life situations was enlightening and helpful (Mattaini, 1990). Genograms and ecomaps are discussed in greater detail in Chapter 8.

As the nurse gathers data by the variety of means available, information must be analyzed, sorted, and compared with the nurse's view of family health and those factors that influence family health. Finally, the question must be asked, what are the health care issues of concern to this family, and what are the strengths and limitations of this family? How can nursing best assist this family and these family members in achieving their goals? (Christensen & Kenney, 1995). These questions involve analysis, the second step of the nursing process.

Analysis of Family Assessment Data

In the care of families as units, analysis involves clarifying and validating information to make accurate diagnoses that provide a focus for nursing interventions. Donnelly (1990) described this analytical process as diagnostic reasoning. Many health care professionals make judgments about the needs of clients, and many use the term "diagnosis." The physician, social worker, nutritionist, or professional nurse diagnose within their specific discipline or area of specialization.

The Diagnostic Process

Nursing is defined by the American Nurses Association as "the diagnosis and treatment of human responses to actual or potential health problems" (A Social Policy Statement, 1980). Donnelly sees the term "diagnosis" as significant to this definition. Nurses have always made judgments about client care needs, but the concept that diagnosis is an integral part of the definition of nursing is relatively new. Only recently has nursing begun the process of developing a classification system of nomenclature to facilitate its diagnosis and treatment of the phenomena unique to nursing. Donnelly saw diagnosis as a critical aspect of the field.

Donnelly (1990) described the diagnostic reasoning process as a logical sequence that involves describing phenomena. The nurse is an observer of phenomena and describes those phenomena to identify signs and symptoms that might indicate problems or concerns. The family health care practitioner must then review the situation to identify the probable cause(s) for the identified problem(s). Practitioners working with families determine what information is significant, and assign meaning to the data, on the basis of their knowledge of baseline data and of established ranges of normal physical and emotional states. The conceptual perspective on the family as client and on nursing goals and outcomes strongly influences what kinds of information the nurse gathers. The nurse must develop a capacity to consider health as an effect and to reason out probable causes. Family nursing diagnoses are written to facilitate the achievement or maintenance of optimum health as it is defined by the family model or nursing model selected for use. They may be stated as functional, structural, or developmental or may reflect a particular diagnosis framework, such as the North American Nursing Diagnosis Association (NANDA) or Omaha system. A family nursing diagnosis may also speak to high-risk health concerns or promoting and maintaining family health (Christensen & Kenney, 1995). The question is: How can family health be enhanced?

The NANDA System

At the current state of development, the nurse may find the NANDA framework of nursing diagnosis shaping professional judgment. In view of the fact that a large part of the practice of community health nursing involves family health care, Donnelly (1990) expressed some concern that only seven of the approved diagnostic labels address family situations: (1) family coping, potential for growth; (2) family coping, ineffective: compromised; (3) family coping, ineffective: disabling; (4) family processes, altered; (5) parenting, altered; (6) parenting, altered, risk for; and (7) parental role conflict. Of particular concern is the fact that only one of the diagnoses identified—family coping, potential for growth—implies health promotion concepts. Donnelly strongly supported the importance of diagnosis as an essential step in the nursing process and as quite useful in the care of families. However, she saw the NANDA system as heavily weighted toward the individual.

Thomas, Barnard, and Sumner (1993) described the use of the work done by NANDA as a framework for family assessment and diagnosis. These authors note five areas of family functioning that they believed were appropriate. The areas identified were (1) family process, (2) family coping, (3) parenting, (4) health maintenance and (5) management, and home maintenance and management. These authors saw these areas as derived from the field of nursing but having relevance across health care disciplines. There are significant gaps in the current classification system, and an effort must be made to move forward more rapidly in the full development of a comprehensive set of family diagnostic categories. Vaughn-Cole and colleagues (1998) challenged those in the field of family nursing to assume the responsibility to explicate and refine nursing diagnoses that are applicable to the family as a unit of care.

Ross and Cobb (1990) discussed the use of the NANDA classification system in working with families. These authors identified 25 NANDA diagnostic labels that might be relevant to family nursing. Box 7–2 presents NANDA diagnoses relevant to family nursing that incorporate the previously identified 25 and an additional 11 diagnostic tables accepted at the 1998 conference. It might have been helpful if each NANDA category and title had been originally developed to address application to three kinds of clients–individuals, families, or communities. Progress in the development of nursing diagnoses specific to types of client is apparent, especially in the 1998 additions to the NANDA classifications. Common family nursing diagnoses were presented in table form by Ross and Cobb (1990) and are included to illustrate one approach to the use of the NANDA system (Table 7-1). Possible nursing diagnosis titles that are relevant to families are listed on the left in Table 7-1. The unique situation of each family requires that the nurse consider that the cause or sustaining factor varies. Possible causes are listed on the right.

The Omaha System

The Omaha system was designed to meet the challenge of describing the nursing needs of families. It was developed over a period of 20 years and is based on the results of several major research projects. The Visiting Nurse Association (VNA) of Omaha, Nebraska initiated this effort in 1970. The need to effectively document community health nursing practice, particularly the care of families, was a major concern. Implemented in 1986, the system consists of three components: the Problem Classification Schema, the Intervention Schema, and the Problem Rating Scale. The Problem Classification Schema "is a taxonomy of nursing diagnosis, that provides a consistent language for collecting, sorting, classifying, documenting, and analyzing data about client concerns" (Martin & Scheet, 1992, pp. 19–20). It consists of 40 problems organized in four domains. Each problem may be made more specific by the use of modifiers. Of special note is the provision of a modifier that specifies a family focus. The definitions of the modifiers and the four domains, together with a sample problem, are presented in Table 7-2. Martin and Norris (1996) reported a significant increase in the number of agencies that are using this system. Among the users described are home health care agencies and a family-nursing center. Merrill and asso-

Box 7-2

NANDA NURSING DIAGNOSES RELEVANT TO FAMILY NURSING

Family Processes, altered
Family Processes, altered: alcoholism
Health maintenance, altered
Nutrition, altered: Less than body requirements
Nutrition, altered: more than body requirements
Nutrition, altered: potential for more or potential for less than body requirements
Parenting, altered
Parenting, altered, risk for
Attachment, parent/infant/child altered, risk for
Patterns of Elimination altered: inadequate sanitary disposal conditions
Role Performance, altered
Sexuality Patterns, altered
Caregiver Role Strain, risk for
Decisional Conflict (Specify)
Defensive coping
Family Coping, growth, potential for
Health-Seeking Behavior
Denial, ineffective
Family Coping, ineffective: compromised
Family Coping, ineffective: disabling
Adjustment, impaired
Home Maintenance Management, impaired
Social Interaction, impaired
Management of Therapeutic Regimen, ineffective: family
Knowledge Deficit (Specify)
Noncompliance
Parental Role Conflict
Parenting, potential, altered
Spiritual Well-Being, enhanced, potential for
Trauma (Injury), potential for
Violence, potential for
Powerlessness
Social Isolation
Spiritual distress
Spiritual Distress, risk for

Source: Family Nursing: A Nursing Process Approach. B. Ross & K. L. Cobb, 1990, Redwood City, CA: Addison-Wesley.

TABLE 7-1
Common Nursing Diagnoses and Their Causes in Families

Nursing Diagnosis	Possible Causes
Inability to manage home care activities secondary to	1. Lack of knowledge of time-management techniques. 2. Lack of information related to community resources 3. Lack of support systems 4. Uncompensated physical limitations of family members
Ineffective parenting secondary to	1. Lack of knowledge of normal infant development and implications for care 2. Lack of available financial resources 3. Reactive depression (mother), perceived inadequacy after divorce
Altered nutritional intake, less than requirements (family) secondary to	1. Lack of knowledge of appropriate food intake 2. Financial limitations and lack of knowledge of available resources 3. Limited availability of culturally preferred foods
Alteration in family processes: inability to provide physical and emotional support to family member secondary to	1. Lack of knowledge of techniques of care delivery 2. Perception of self as incapable of learning complex tasks 3. Lack of available finances for needed equipment
Health management deficit: lack of immunizations (children) secondary to	1. Lack of knowledge of importance of immunizations 2. Value belief conflicts or religious beliefs deny injections 3. Lack of access to financial resources or available well–child care
Potential for injury secondary to	1. Uncontrolled refuse dumping and inadequate trash removal 2. Lack of awareness of lead paint present in housing units, local refuse used as fuel (e.g., lead batteries burned for heat) 3. Lack of knowledge of techniques to "toddler-proof" home environment 4. Inappropriate disposal of toxic waste materials

Source: Family Nursing: A Nursing Process Approach. B. Ross & K. L. Cobb, 1990. Redwood City, CA: Addison-Wesley. Copyright 1990 by Addison-Wesley. Reprinted with permission.

ciates (1998) described the use of the Omaha System as the organizing framework for their baccalaureate nursing curriculum. The reader is referred to the comprehensive text by Martin and Scheet (1992) for a very thorough description of this unique system. Once decisions have been made in regard to which specific problems will be addressed and resources and limitations have been identified, the next step is planning.

Family Care Planning

Establishing Priorities

As was mentioned previously, the unique aspect of caring for families is the importance of including all members of the family in the unit of care. Once assessment and analysis are complete, the health problems identified should be listed in order of priority, according to the preferences of the family. As Friedman (1998) stated so well, there may exist a difference of opinion between how the professional views the family's needs and how the family or family members see their needs. Unless each family member is heard and the nurse and family together determine the direction of care, interventions have little hope for success. Although there are certainly situations when families find it necessary to step back and allow others to provide care or even to make certain decisions, the essence of "healthy" family implies movement toward self-care. Family health care planning should encourage movement in the direction of independence (Martinson & Widmer, 1989).

Establishing Outcomes

Planning care for families involves the statement of outcomes. What does the family expect to achieve as the end result of their participation in the treatment

TABLE 7-2
The OMAHA System: Definitions of Modifiers and Domains and a Sample Problem

Modifier	Domain of the Problem Classification Scheme
Health Promotion. Client interest in increasing knowledge, behavior, and health expectations as well as developing resources that maintain or enhance well-being in the absence of risk factors, signs, or symptoms.	*The Environmental Domain* is defined as the material resources, physical surroundings, and substances both internal and external to the client, home, neighborhood, and broader community.
Potential Deficit or Impairment. Client status characterized by the absence of signs or symptoms and the presence of certain health patterns, practices, behaviors, or risk factors that may preclude optimal health.	*The Psychosocial Domain* is defined as patterns of behavior, communication, relationships, and development. The effects of situational and developmental crisis or stress are evident in the psychosocial domain.
Deficit or Impairment, Actual. Client status characterized by one or more existing signs or symptoms that may preclude optimal health.	*The Psychosocial Domain* is defined as activities that maintain or promote wellness and recovery or maximize rehabilitation.
Family. A social unit or related group of individuals who live together and who experience a health-related problem.	*The Health-Related Behaviors Domain* is defined as functional status of processes that maintain life.
Individual. A person who lives alone or a single family member who experiences a health-related problem.	
SAMPLE PROBLEM FROM THE ENVIRONMENTAL DOMAIN	
Problem 03.	
Residence. Place where individual or family lives	
Modifier	
Health Promotion	Family
Potential Deficit	Individual
Deficit	
Signs/Symptoms	
01. structurally unsound	
02. inadequate heating or cooling	
03. steep stairs	
04. inadequate or obstructed exits or entries	
05. cluttered living space	
06. unsafe storage of dangerous objects or substances	
07. unsafe mats or throw rugs	
08. inadequate safety devices	
09. presence of lead-based paint	
• unsafe gas or electric appliances	
• inadequate or crowded living space	
• homelessness	
• other	

Source: The Omaha System: Applications for Community Health Nursing. K.S. Martin & N.J. Scheet, Philadelphia: W.B. Saunders. Copyright 1992 by W.B. Saunders. Reprinted with permission.

activity? Outcomes guide decisions about interventions. Personal goals and values are important for all clients. Therefore, it is essential that planning for care be a collaborative process between the family and the nurse. The family best knows their needs as a family system and an interactive unit. The professional nurse, in contrast, brings an objective viewpoint that can be useful to clients. All those involved in the care situation must agree on what is to be accomplished and on what basis an objective can be judged to be achieved. Outcomes should be stated in clear terms. Criteria of success should be recognizable by any of those involved in the family care situation; for example, if the nursing diagnosis involves a health care management deficit regarding lack of immunizations and appropriate health supervision of minor children, the outcome would be that immunizations are up to date and regular health visits to the neighborhood health clinic are validated via written report. If a family's concern involves ineffective coping with psychiatric episodes of a young adult child and the care responsibilities of an elderly grandparent, a positive outcome might be effective family dynamics, which have led to decisions regarding care or placement needs and reports of a positive outlook for family coping. Gordon (1994) described this process as converting the nursing diagnosis problem statement into the desired health state and incorporating indicators by which nurse and client family know that the desired state has been achieved.

Designing Nursing Interventions

Reaching the desired health state established as the goal in collaboration with the family as client requires the design or selection of actions to assist the family in moving toward that state. Interventions are designed to modify the factors in the situation that are supporting or sustaining the unhealthy state. If the family is having difficulty caring for the health of a family member, the reasons may include limited financial resources or equipment, a lack of knowledge of the importance of treatments and how to carry out specific treatments, or insufficient assistance as a result of the complex nature of the care. The nursing interventions are directed toward identification of available financial assistance, obtaining equipment, providing or making arrangements for appropriate teaching, and seeking out community or family sources of support for family caregivers.

Robinson and Wright (1995) described interventions as happening from the time of the first interview to termination with the family, although the intervention stage of family nursing process is the defined core of treatment. These authors described two stages of therapeutic change process, (1) creating the circumstances for change, and (2) moving beyond, and overcoming the problems. The setting up of interviews, interactions which fostered comfort and trust, eliciting information which allowed distinguishing, verbally identifying and supporting positive responses, and supplying guidance in exploring options or assisting in clarifying beliefs, were all seen as nursing interventions. Nursing interventions were not just tools or tactics but also anything the nurse says or does with families that influences the family system.

Planning should encourage the family to make choices to ensure that the types of interventions implemented are accepted, supported, and carried out. When clients have difficulty making choices, it is the nurse's role to help the family identify alternatives, understand consequences, and make the decision as to which options are most acceptable to them. It is a basic premise of family nursing that families have both the right and the responsibility to make their own health care decisions. If we believe this to be true, there will be situations when families who have been fully informed of potential outcomes choose options with which the nurse may personally and professionally disagree. The nurse must be able to accept that choice (Friedman, 1998). Effective implementation of the plan of care requires client family acceptance and participation.

Implementation of Family Health Care

Working with the Family

In implementation, the family and nurse work together to carry out the interventions designed to achieve the identified goals (Ross & Cobb, 1990). Interventions are outlined in the plan of care; actions are taken by designated team members to assist in moving the client from a current state of health to a desired state of health; and the nurse supports, guides, and advocates for the family during the implementation of the plan of care. In the course of intervention it may be necessary to seek assistance from other caregivers, family members, or community agencies; and throughout the process, the nurse must evaluate progress in problem resolution and be alert for the emergence of new concerns with which the family must cope.

Smith, Smith, and Toseland (1991) worked extensively with family caregivers and found a number of concerns. As the process of providing care for their elderly relative continued, family members requested assistance with such concerns as improving coping skills, learning to meet the needs of their dependent elder relative, and dealing with issues surrounding spouses and siblings, the need for formal and informal support, feelings of inadequacy and guilt, and the necessary planning for their elderly relative's future. Two major themes seem to run through the comments of these family members: the need to maintain control and the onus of increasing responsibility (Smith, et al, 1991).

Whitlatch, Zarit, and Von Eye (1991) found that brief psychoeducational interventions may be more beneficial in working with family caregivers than previously thought and suggested that a program of individual and family counseling can have particular benefits in relieving stress. Wilson's experience with the families of hospice patients and their needs for assistance and support from hospice staff was especially helpful in describing the nature of support that families found helpful (Wilson, 1992). The hospice staff enabled families to fulfill their roles as caregivers in several ways. Staffers were extremely important in explaining to the caregivers the role they were undertaking and were available around-the-clock to families. Moreover, they made a conscious effort to give families recognition for the work they did as caregivers, and if family members were unable to continue the caregiving role, the hospice staff assisted families in making alternate arrangements.

Adaptation to the Family

The great value of family involvement in health behavior interventions was documented by Nader and colleagues (1992), who conducted a year-long study of a family-based cardiovascular disease risk reduction intervention that was to be used with Mexican-American and Anglo-American fifth and sixth graders and their parents. Cultural adaptations were made in the education sessions, which involved both parents and children and targeted dietary habits and physical activity. Follow-up, 3 years after the study, showed significant persistent changes in exercise and eating habits, even though there had been no additional education and no environmental changes. These authors reported that families participated and that the outcomes were positive.

The significance of adaptation to meet the special needs of the family was well-illustrated by the experience of Stephany (1990), a hospice nurse, who found herself caring for a 6-foot, 3-inch "biker" who was dying of colon cancer. He was frequently a problem patient, not cooperative with care, and finally refused to return to the hospital. Stephany found herself trying to assist this terminally ill patient at home in a tiny, less than well-equipped house, with only his alcoholic mother and a physically handicapped brother to provide care. After deterioration at home and continued refusal to return to the hospital, Stephany contacted her patient's "biker family," called a meeting, and taught his friends how to provide the needed care, including administering medication. The concern and carefulness of these caregivers and the gratefulness of her patient led her to believe she had mobilized this patient's unique community and family. He died a short time later, holding Stephany's hand.

Implementation must involve the family, however defined, and the nurse working together to carry out the plan of care to achieve the mutually established goals. One must always be alert to new information that may dictate adjustment or change of plans. Finally, the nurse must evaluate the effectiveness of the care given.

Evaluating Family Nursing Care

Achievement of Objectives

Evaluation of family nursing care is carried out in accordance with established objectives, outcomes, and identified criteria. The care provided is monitored from the initial implementation of the care plan through achievement of the final outcome and discharge of the client family from the facility or release from agency care. The written care plan with its specific nursing diagnoses and family care objectives, outcomes, and criteria provides the measures of success. Outcome evaluation refers to long-term individual client-centered goals in the situation involving an ill family member and also the maintenance of the family's health. Quality care is delivered to the extent that predefined goals and outcomes of care are met and family maintenance and growth are sustained (Keating & Kelman, 1988). Evaluation is an ongoing process that continues throughout care delivery and ends only when a final assessment by client and nurse determines that goals have been successfully met.

Termination with the Family

Termination of the therapeutic relationship is the final step. In the course of evaluating care delivery, the question of how and when to terminate with the family client does arise. Determining when the client family no longer is in need of the services of the nurse is part of evaluating outcomes. Fortune, Pearling, and Rochelle (1991) interviewed a number of practitioners about their reasoning in the decision to terminate family care. The practitioners identified the most important criteria as improvement in the family dynamics and family functioning and meeting the specified treatment goals. They also reported that the family's wish to terminate was important. There was, in many instances, a change in the therapeutic content that signaled a readiness to end. Generally, "practitioners waited for success before terminating and used both improved behavior and intrapsychic functioning to determine success" (Fortune, et al, 1991, p. 369). Bor, Mallander, and Vetere (1998) reported the results of an extensive study of family therapists in the United Kingdom, which revealed similar criteria for termination of the client family and nurse relationship. In most instances, the therapists indicated termination was initiated on the basis of client self-report of the effectiveness of the therapeutic interventions. Most therapists also reported the observation of positive change in family functioning and the ability to meet the needs of members. A limited number of family therapists reported the use of questionnaires or other types of standardized measures. Robinson and Wright (1995) spoke to the importance of this stage of problem resolution and family growth.

> The most rewarding aspect of the nursing of families is to observe family healing from emotion and/or physical suffering . . . when healing occurs in collaboration with nurses, it is because families and nurses co-evolve useful solutions to particular health problems" (p. 327).

Self-sufficiency is the preferred final outcome, and termination of the therapeutic relationship should follow. The case study illustrates the family nursing process with a childbearing family.

Case Study

THE JONES FAMILY

Family Assessment The Jones family is composed of Sarah and John Jones, ages 36 and 42, and their children: John, Jr., age 11; Tony, age 8; and a new infant girl, Susan. Susan was born at 35 weeks' gestation, weighing 4 pounds, 11 ounces. The public health nurse, whose initial visit revealed a caring, supportive family with limited financial resources, automatically follows all infants under the birth weight of 5 pounds. The family lives in a four-bedroom white frame house, which they are buying. Sarah is a teacher's assistant and plans to return to work. John, Sr., works in construction. They are of Italian and French ancestry and attend the Lutheran church regularly. Sarah's parents live in the area and visit often. She reports her father to be in good health at age 61. Her mother is 59 years old, with well-controlled adult-onset diabetes. Sarah is an only child. John, Sr., recently lost his father who was age 69 as a result of a heart attack. His mother, age 67, has arthritis, hypertension, and adult-onset diabetes. She will be coming to live with her son and his family within the month.

John, Sr., has three siblings, but they all live out of state. Sarah has primary responsibility for the household; John helps and participates in child care. Sarah describes herself as a "great cook." Family menus include both Italian favorites and "the best" French pastries. The family's activity together is largely sedentary and consists of watching television, going to movies, and attending their sons' sports events.

Both parents describe the family's health as "good." They go to a local clinic for checkups and immunizations. Sarah received prenatal care at the clinic of the community hospital. The family expressed several health concerns. Sarah worries about her weight gain during pregnancy. She reports a prenatal weight of 170 pounds, weight gain of 40 pounds during pregnancy, and a loss of 20 pounds since Susan's birth. John sees himself as "healthy," although "a little overweight." Both parents describe the children as in good health, but are concerned about giving proper care to the new baby ("she's pretty small") and see busy times ahead with the active older children and having to care for John's mother.

Analysis Issues that might be of concern include the following. The Jones family is a strong, supportive family with limited financial resources. There is expressed concern regarding weight gain, a history of diabetes and cardiovascular disease, and potential stress resulting from the dual responsibilities of caring for an older parent with health problems and a new baby with a history of prematurity. The family also must cope with active school-aged children, one of whom is entering adolescence. Possible diagnostic statements might include:

1. Potential ineffective family process related to ineffective coping, with multiple care responsibilities of elderly parent, new infant (premature), and school-aged children and limited financial resources.
2. Alteration in nutrition; excess caloric intake related to lack of knowledge of appropriate dietary adjustments and cooking techniques to reduce caloric intake.
3. High risk for diabetes mellitus and cardiovascular disease, related to lack of knowledge of risk factors and methods to reduce risk.
4. Family coping; potential for growth related to strong family support and readiness to seek assistance.

Planning The goals for the Jones family might include:

1. The family will report the ability to carry out multiple roles with minimal difficulty by second clinic visit and will demonstrate healthy interaction as evidenced by consistent weight gain and developmental progress of their newborn, positive school reports of children, and ability to involve grandparent in family life and in outside activity. Assess each visit.
2. Both parents will report commitment to a healthy eating and lifestyle program by third clinic visit and demonstrate positive results by minimum weight loss of 2 pounds.

Interventions for the Jones family might include:

1. Initial visit. Review infant development and follow-up needs and respond to questions and concerns related to prematurity. Reinforce positive expectations.
2. Initial visit. Review with Sarah diet history and possible alternatives to reduce calorie count, including food selection and cooking techniques. Pay particular attention to retaining favorite ethnic foods. (Review and provide written material on "healthy" ethnic or cultural foods; consider referral to nutritionist.)
3. Second visit. Discuss possible activities of interest to family that will increase physical exercise. Identify availability in neighborhood, participation of children, and availability of child care for infant.
4. Second visit. Review available activities for older adults and transportation options. Discuss needed adjustments to family routines; offer assistance and guidance as requested.
5. Arrange periodic contact with family, as acceptable and possible, to continue support and assistance. Identify preference for telephone contact or home visit and best time for approach of choice.

Implementation The plan of care for this family must involve facilitating their contact with available resources and following through as needed. It is essential to identify and deal with problems and concerns as they arise, including access issues, financial need, and the stress of dealing with change. Continuing contact with the family is needed to assess their ability to use the information given or the resources available, and their effectiveness in solving identified problems.

Evaluation Both formative and summative approaches are required. As plans are implemented, to what degree are positive results beginning to appear? As contacts with the family are made, the nurse must monitor infant development, family dynamics, and parental weight gain and loss. Time frames established when the goals are agreed on with the family become the point at which summative evaluation occurs. To what degree have the goals been achieved? Is the family satisfied with the level of achievement? Do new goals or plans need to be devised? Is the family comfortable with the current level of function and ready to assume a totally independent role and to terminate contact?

SUMMARY

Family nursing process is a systematic approach to identifying problems and initiating appropriate activities designed to meet the specified needs or concerns of the client family. It is an open approach that is dynamic and cyclic in nature and is ongoing throughout the time the family receives care. The family is a partner in care design and delivery, and family input and family validation are essential. Nurses have the unique role of diagnosing and guiding human responses to life's changes. In this role, the nurse is assisted by the nursing process, which provides the decision-making framework for the delivery of comprehensive care to families.

Study Questions

1. In what way is the use of the nursing process unique in providing care for the family as client?
2. Describe two diagnostic classification systems that might be used in interpreting data and identifying the specific health care needs of families.
3. What are the limitations of the NANDA system in the defining of family health care needs?
4. What is an ecomap?
5. Discuss how family health care might be evaluated.

References

Allen, C.V. (1991). *Comprehending the Nursing Process in Workbook Approach.* Norwalk, CT: Appleton & Lange.

Bell, F.M. (1998). Rx for certainty in clinical work with families: Insatiable curiosity. *Journal of Family Nursing, 4*(2): 123–126.

Berkley, K.M., & Hanson, S.M.H. (1991). *Pocket guide to family assessment in intervention.* St. Louis, MO: C.V. Mosby.

Bor, R., Mallander, I., & Vetere, A. (1998). What we say we do: Results of the 1997 UK Association of Family Therapy Members Survey. *Journal of Family Therapy, 20*:333–351.

Cantor, M.H. (1991). Family and community: Changing roles in an aging society. *Gerontologist, 31*:337–346.

Chitty, K.K. (1997). *Professional Nursing Concepts and Challenges.* Philadelphia: W. B. Saunders.

Christensen, P.J. & Kenney, J.W. (1995). *Nursing Process: Application of Conceptual Models,* ed 4. St. Louis, MO: Mosby.

Donnelly, E. (1990). Health promotion, families, and the diagnostic process. *Family and Community Health, 12*:12–20.

Facione, N., & Facione, P. (1996). Externalizing the critical thinking in knowledge development and clinical judgment. *Nursing Outlook, 44*(3):129–136.

Fortune, A.E., Pearling, B., & Rochelle, C.D. (1991). Criteria for terminating treatment. Families in Society: *The Journal of Contemporary Human Services, 72*:366–370.

Friedeman, M.L. (1989). Closing the gap between grand theory and mental health practice with families, part I. The framework of systematic organization for nursing of families and family members. *Archives of Psychiatric Nursing, 3*:10–19.

Friedman, M.M. (1998). *Family nursing: Theory and practice,* ed 3. Norwalk, CT: Appleton & Lange.

Gordon, M. (1976). Nursing diagnosis and the diagnostic process. *American Journal of Nursing, 76*:1276–1300.

Gordon, M. (1982). *Nursing Diagnosis: Process and Application.* New York: McGraw-Hill.

Gordon, M. (1994). *Nursing Diagnosis: Process and Application,* ed 2. New York: McGraw-Hill.

Guralink, D.B., editor-in-chief. (1987). *Webster's New World Dictionary of the American Language.* New York: Warner Books.

Hanslik, T. (1998). Critical thinking: An essential element. *Journal of Advanced Nursing, 27*(2):442–443.

Keating, S.B., & Kelman, G.B. (1988). *Home Health.* Philadelphia: J.B. Lippincott.

Lapp, C.A., et al. (1990). Family-based practice: Discussion of a tool merging assessment with intervention. *Family and Community Health, 12*:21–28.

Martin, K.S. & Norris, F. (1996). The Omaha system: A model of describing practice. *Holistic Nursing Practice, 10*(3):15–22.

Martin, K.S., & Scheet, N.J. (1992). *The Omaha System: Applications for Community Health Nursing.* Philadelphia: W.B. Saunders.

Martinson, L.M., & Widmer, A. (1989). *Home health care nursing.* Philadelphia. W.B. Saunders.

Mattaini, M.A. (1990). Contextual behavior analysis in the assessment process. *Family in Society: The Journal of Contemporary Human Services,* 71:236–245.

Merrill, A.S., et al. (1998). Curriculum restructuring using the practice-based Omaha system. *Nurse Educators, 23*(3):41–44.

Nader, P.R., et al. (1992). Family-based cardiovascular risk reduction education among Mexican and Anglo-Americans. *Family and Community Health, 15*:57–74.

NANDA nursing diagnosis: Definitions and classification 1999–2000. (1999). Philadelphia: North American Nursing Diagnosis Association.

Nightingale, F. (1969). Notes on Nursing. (Unabridged republication of original text published by Appleton-Century Crofts, 1860). New York: Dover Publications.

Paquin, G.W., & Bushum, R.J. (1991). Family treatment assessment for novices. *Family in Society: The Journal of Contemporary Human Services,* 72:353–359.

Paul, R., (1993). *Critical Thinking.* Foundation for Critical Thinking, Santa Rosa, CA.

Paul, R., & Heaslip, P. (1995). Critical thinking and intuitive nursing practice. *Journal of Advanced Nursing, 22*(1):40–47.

Robinson, C.A., & Wright, L.M. (1995). Family nursing interventions: What families say makes a difference. *Journal of Family Nursing, 1*(3):327–345.

Rosen, A. (1992). Facilitating clinical decision making and

evaluation. *Families in Society: The Journal of Contemporary Human Services*, *73*:522–532.

Ross, B., & Cobb, K.L. (1990). *Family Nursing: A Nursing Process Approach*. Redwood City, CA: Addison-Wesley.

Rubenfeld, M.G., & Scheffer, B.K. (1999). *Critical Thinking in Nursing: An Interactive Approach*. Philadelphia, PA: J.B. Lippincott.

Shaw, M. (1993). (Senior Ed.). *Nursing Progress in Clinical Practice*. Springhouse, PA: Springhouse.

Smith, G.C., et al. (1991). Problems identified by family caregivers in counseling. *Gerontologist*, *31*:15–22.

Stephany, T.M. (1990). A death in the family. *American Journal of Nursing*, *90*:54–56.

Thomas, R.B., et al. (1993). Family nursing diagnosis as a framework for family assessment. In S. L. Fuetham, et al. (Eds.) *The Nursing of Families: Theory, Research, Education, Practice*. Newbury Park, CA: Sage.

Vaughan-Cole, B., et al. (1998). *Family Nursing Practice*. Philadelphia: W.B. Saunders.

Wasik, B.H., et al. (1990). *Home Visiting: Procedures for Helping Families*. Newbury Park, CA: Sage.

Whitlatch, C.J., Zarit, S.H., & Von Eye, A. (1991). Efficacy of interventions with caregivers: A reanalysis. *Gerontologist*, *31*:9–14.

Wilson, S.A. (1992). The family as caregivers: Hospice home care. *Family and Community Health*, *15*:71–80.

Yura, H., & Walsh, M.B. (1988). *The nursing process*, ed 5. Norwalk, CT: Appleton & Lange.

Additional Bibliography

Alexander, M.K., & Giguere, B. (1996). Critical thinking in clinical learning: A holistic perspective. *Holistic Nursing Practice*, *10*(3):15–22.

Baum, M., & Page, M. (1991). Caregiving and multigenerational families. *Gerontologist*, *31*:762–769.

Clements, S.D. (1992). When family caregivers grieve for the Alzheimer's patient. *Geriatric Nursing*, *13*:305–309.

Davidhizar, R. (1992). Understanding powerlessness in family member caregivers of the chronically ill. *Geriatric Nursing*, *13*:66–69.

deMontigny, F., et al. (1997). Teaching family nursing based on conceptual models of nursing. *Journal of Family Nursing*, *3*(3):367–379.

Ernst, L. (1990). Value differences in families of differing socioeconomic status: Implications for family education. *Family Perspective*, *24*:401–410.

Feetham, S.L., et al. (Eds.) (1993). *The Nursing of Families*. Newbury Park, CA: Sage.

Ferris, M. (1992). Nursing interventions for families of nursing home residents. *Geriatric Nursing*, *13*:37–40.

Fisher, L.F., et al. (1990). Advancing a family perspective in health research: Models and methods. *Family Process*, *29*:177–189.

Glasser, M., et al. (1992). The role of the family in medical care seeking decisions of older adults. *Family and Community*, *15*:59–70.

Gillis, C.L. (1991). Family nursing research, theory, and practice. *Image: Journal of Nursing Scholarship*, *23*:19–22.

Hanson, S., et al. (1992). Education for family health care professionals: Nursing as a paradigm. *Family Relations*, *41*:49–53.

Heiney, S.P. (1988). Assessing and intervening with dysfunctional families. *Oncology Nursing Forum*, *15*:585–590. Reprinted in G.D. Wegner & R.J. Alexander (Eds.). (1993). *Readings in Family Nursing*, pp. 357–367. Philadelphia: J.B. Lippincott.

Johnson, M.A., et al. (1992). The transition to a nursing home: Meeting the family's needs. *Geriatric Nursing*, *13*:299–302.

Klee, M.A.E. (1989). Family influences on home care. In L.M. Martinson & A. Widmer, *Home Health Care Nursing*, pp. 151–162. Philadelphia: W.B. Saunders.

Kneeshaw, M.F., & Lunney, M. (1989). Nursing diagnosis: Not for individuals only. *Geriatric Nursing*, *10*:246–247.

Lemer, H., & Byme, M.W. (1991). Helping nursing students communicate with high-risk families. *Nursing and Health Care*, *12*:98–101.

Levin, L., & Trost, I. (1992). Understanding the concept of family. *Family Relations*, *41*:348–351.

Lynn-McHale, D.J., & Smith, A. (1991). Comprehensive assessment of families of the critically ill. *Critical Care Nurse*, *2*:195–209. Reprinted in R.J. Alexander & G.D. Wegner. (1993). *Readings in Family Nursing*, pp. 309–321. Philadelphia: J.B. Lippincott.

Martin, K.S., & Scheet, J.J. (1989). Nursing diagnosis in home health: The Omaha system. In L.M. Martinson & H. Widmer. (1992). *Home Health Care Nursing*, pp. 67–72. Philadelphia: W.B. Saunders.

Mason, G., & Attrer, M. (1997). The relationship between research and the nursing process in clinical practice. *Journal of Advanced Nursing*, *26*(5):1045–1049.

Moos, R.H. (1990). Conceptual and empirical approach to developing family-based assessment procedures: Resolving the case of the family environment scale. *Family Process*, *29*:199–208.

Novak, M., & Guest, C. (1989). Application of a multidimensional caregiver burden inventory. *Gerontologist*, *29*:798–803.

Richard, H. (1997). Nursing diagnosis and classification systems: A position paper. *Journal of Advanced Nursing, 26*(3):496–500.

St. John, W., & Rolls, C. (1996). Teaching family nursing: Strategies and experiences. *Journal of Advanced Nursing, 23*(1):91–96.

Silvia, L.Y., & Liepman, M.R. (1991). Family behavior loop mapping enhances treatment of alcoholism. *Family and Community Health, 13*:72–83.

Whyte, D.A. (1997). *Explorations in Family Nursing*. New York & London: Routledge.

Focus On

FAMILY ASSESSMENT AND INTERVENTION

In previous nursing courses, the assessment of individual clients was emphasized; this chapter focuses on the accurate assessment of families as a whole. It is essential for students preparing for professional practice with families to be thoroughly conversant with the sophisticated assessment models in use today. In this chapter, students are provided with a comprehensive overview of family assessment models and their importance to professional practice in family nursing and are exposed to the intricacies of systematic family assessment. While you may find this material particularly challenging, a careful reading of previous chapters provides a comprehensive foundation for understanding family assessment.

As discussed in Chapter 1, the family may be viewed as a context for individual development, as client, as system, and as a unit of society. Each view has a different philosophical base and a different set of operational assumptions that direct the assessment approach. An understanding of these views and their philosophical foundations will assist nursing students in selection of assessment models for use in practice.

The practice of family nursing requires that nurses use a systematic approach to assessment of the family as client. Comprehensive family assessment is the initial phase of the nursing process, which progresses into diagnosis, planning, intervention, and evaluation. The purpose of this chapter is to discuss family assessment and intervention using three different approaches derived from the nursing literature. These models and approaches are the Family Assessment and Intervention Model, Family Systems Stressor-Strength Inventory (FS^3I), Friedman's Family Assessment Model and Short Form, and Calgary Family Assessment Model (CFAM).

Assessment versus measurement and qualitative versus quantitative approaches are defined and differentiated. The use of genograms and ecomaps in conducting family assessment is summarized. The current status of measurement and instrumentation for family nursing is presented. Finally, a case study is presented to demonstrate the different kinds of data that can be collected with the three models and approaches, including a sample of a family genogram and ecomap. Assessment of the whole family is challenging and is the practice of tomorrow.

Chapter 8

FAMILY ASSESSMENT AND INTERVENTION

Shirley May Harmon Hanson

OUTLINE

OBJECTIVES

On completion of this chapter, the reader will be able to:

- Explain how family assessment and intervention fit into the nursing process.
- Distinguish between family assessment and family measurement.
- Differentiate between qualitative and quantitative approaches in family measurement.
- Summarize the current status of instrumentation for family nursing.
- Compare three different models and approaches that can be used for family assessment and intervention.
- Explain one assessment model and approach in detail.
- Describe other resources for assessment techniques and instruments.

Comprehensive family nursing requires that nurses use a logical, systematic approach when working with families. This approach is called the family nursing process, which consists of five steps in problem solving (all of which were discussed in some detail in Chapter 7): assessment (data collection), diagnosis, planning, intervention or treatment, and evaluation. The overall purpose of this chapter is to discuss in more detail the assessment and intervention phases of the family nursing process.

First, the client is explained in relation to family nursing. Second, assessment versus measurement and qualitative versus quantitative approaches are clarified. Third, three major assessment models are presented along with their approaches, guidelines, and instruments. Fourth, the use of genograms and ecomaps in conducting family assessment is summarized. Fifth, a case example is presented to demonstrate the different kinds of data that can be collected with each approach. Finally, the current status of measurement and instrumentation for family nursing is summarized. Resources for future reference are provided.

FAMILY ASSESSMENT AND MEASUREMENT APPROACHES

One must distinguish between assessment and measurement and between qualitative and quantitative assessment strategies. Assessment is a continuously evolving process of data collection, whereby the assessor, by drawing on the past and the present, is able to plan and predict for the future (Berkey & Hanson, 1991, p. 226). In contrast to assessment, measurement is defined as "the process of using a rule to assign numbers to objects or events which represent the amount and/or kind of specified attribute possessed" (Waltz, et al, 1991, p. 62). Measurement requires a formal instrument that gives numerical values to, or *quantifies,* the traits being measured and that gives a quantitative result when a particular attribute is examined. Measurement is often considered a narrower aspect of assessment that focuses on more specific concepts or traits.

Assessment is the first step in the family nursing process, and the data it yields are often qualitative or descriptive in nature. Clinical assessment often involves the use of a qualitative interview guide; in contrast, measurement often involves the administration of scales and other instruments that yield quantitative data. During family assessment, data about the family are systematically collected, using predetermined guidelines or questions, and then classified and analyzed according to their meaning.

In clinical practice, assessment involves collecting the information necessary to diagnose and treat presenting problems and evaluate the success of the intervention (Hanson, 1996). The initial assessment is often cursory. The assessment is then conducted in more detail, during which potential problem areas are identified, and is continued throughout the period of provision of health care services to the family. The amount of detail is determined by the client, the clinician, the time available, and the instrument or guidelines used. Data can come from many sources: family members, referrals, and community agencies working with the family. Structured and unstructured interview guidelines are generally used during the assessment process, but more structured quantitative instruments can also be used. In this book, the term "assessment" includes the use of measurement instruments and qualitative and quantitative data-gathering strategies and techniques.

FAMILY NURSING ASSESSMENT MODELS

Three family assessment models and approaches have been developed by family nurses: the Family Assessment and Intervention Model and the Family Systems Stressor-Strength Inventory (FS³I), the Friedman Family Assessment Model and Form, and the Calgary Family Assessment Model (CFAM). Nurses are encouraged to learn each of the three approaches and to select the model that best fits their philosophy and practice. The following discussion of each model assists in that process.

The Family Assessment and Intervention Model and the FS³I

The Family Assessment and Intervention Model diagrammed in Figure 8-1 is based on Betty Neuman's health care systems model (Berkey & Hanson, 1991; Hanson, 1996; Hanson & Mischke, 1996; Neuman, 1995; Reed, 1993). Neuman's theoretical constructs were extended by Berkey and Hanson to focus on the family rather than the individual.

According to the family assessment and intervention model, families are subject to tensions when stressors, in the form of problems, penetrate their defense system. The family's reaction depends on how deeply the stressor penetrates the family unit and how capable

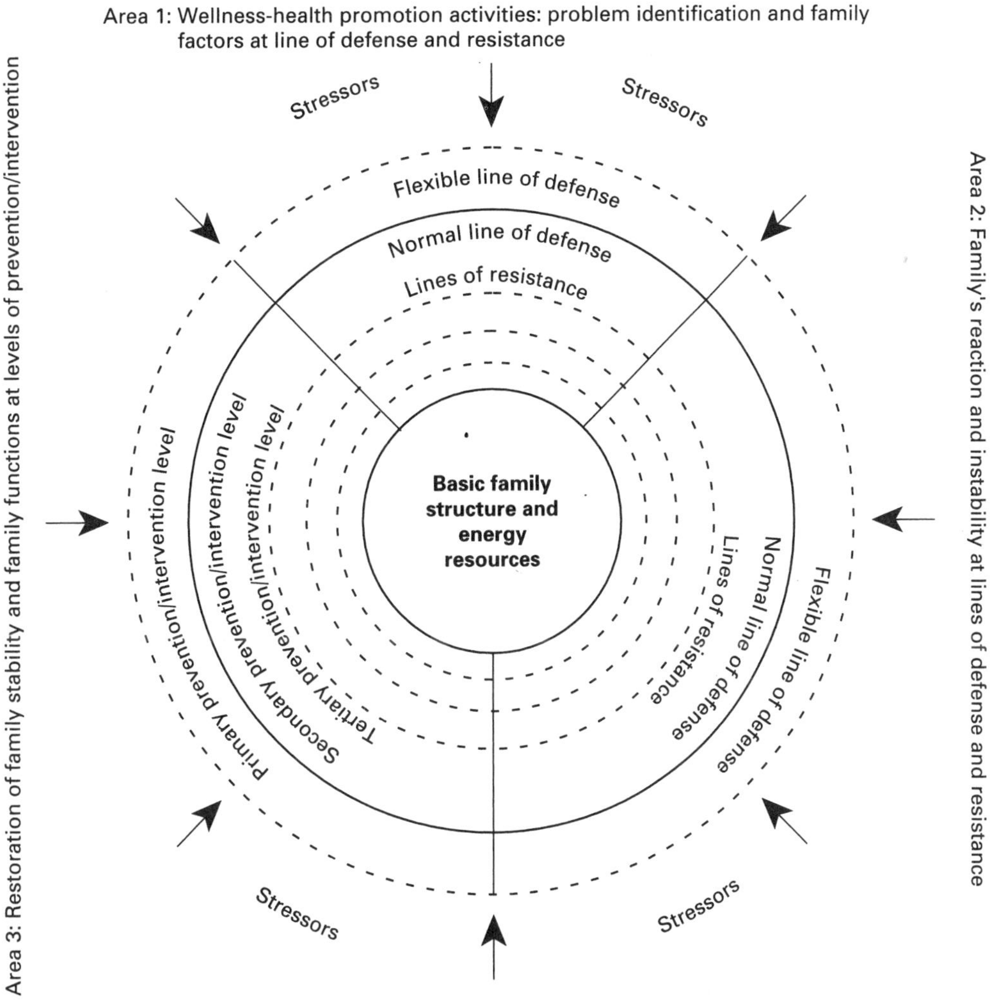

FIGURE 8-1
Family assessment intervention model. (From Hanson, S.M.H. (1996): *Family Nursing assessment and intervention.* In Hanson, S.M.H. and Boyd, S.T. (Eds.) *Family Health Care Nursing: Theory, Practice, and Research.* Philadelphia: F.A. Davis.

the family is in adapting to maintain its stability. The lines of resistance protect the family's basic structure, which includes the family's functions and energy resources. The core contains the patterns of family interactions and unit strengths. The basic structure must be protected at all costs, or the family ceases to exist. Reconstitution or adaptation is the work the family undertakes to preserve or restore family stability after stressors penetrate the family lines of defense, altering usual family functions. The model addresses three areas: (1) health promotion, wellness activities, problem identification, and family factors at lines of defense and resistance; (2) family reaction and instability at lines of defense and resistance; and (3) restoration of family stability and family functioning at levels of prevention and intervention. The basic assumptions of this family-focused model are listed in Box 8–1.

An assessment instrument based on this model is called the FS^{3}I (Berkey & Hanson, 1991; Hanson & Mischke, 1996; Hanson & Kaakinen, 1996). (Appendix C contains an updated copy of the instrument with instructions for administration and a scoring guide.) The FS^{3}I elicits both qualitative and quantitative information about family health, particularly about family

Box 8-1

BASIC ASSUMPTIONS FOR FAMILY ASSESSMENT AND INTERVENTION MODEL

- Though each family as a family system is unique, each system is a composite of common, known factors or innate characteristics within a normal given range of response contained within a basic structure.
- Many known, unknown, and universal environmental stressors exist. Each differs in its potential for disturbing a family's usual stability level, or normal line of defense. The particular interrelationships of family variables—physiological, psychological, sociocultural, developmental, and spiritual—at any time can affect the degree to which a family is protected by the flexible line of defense against possible reaction to one or more stressors.
- Over time, each family or family system has evolved a normal range of response to the environment, referred to as a "normal line of defense," or usual wellness or stability state.
- When the cushioning, accordion-like effect of the flexible line of defense is no longer capable of protecting the family or family system against an environmental stressor, the stressor breaks through the normal line of defense. The interrelationships of variables—physiological, psychological, sociocultural, developmental, and spiritual—determine the nature and degree of the system reaction or possible reaction to the stressor.
- The family, whether in a state of wellness or illness, is a dynamic composite of the interrelationships of variables—physiological, psychological, sociocultural, developmental, and spiritual. Wellness is on a continuum of available energy to support the system in its optimal state.
- Implicit within each family system is a set of internal resistance factors, known as "lines of resistance," which function to stabilize and return the family to the usual wellness state (normal line of defense) or possibly to a higher level of stability after an environmental stressor reaction.
- *Primary prevention* is general knowledge that is applied in family assessment and intervention for identification and mitigation of risk factors associated with environmental stressors to prevent possible reaction.
- *Secondary prevention* is symptomatology following reaction to stressors appropriate ranking of intervention priorities, and treatment to reduce their noxious effects.
- *Tertiary prevention* is the adjustive processes taking place as reconstitution begins and maintenance factors move the client back in a circular manner toward primary prevention.
- The family is in dynamic, constant energy exchange with the environment.

Source: Hanson, S.M.H. (1996) Family Nursing Assessment and Intervention. In Hanson, S.M.H. and Boyd, S.T. (Eds.) *Family Health Care Nursing: Theory, Practice, and Research*. Philadelphia: F.A. Davis.

stressors and strengths. The instrument provides direction for nurses (and other clinicians) in planning interventions to enhance or restore family functioning and growth. The FS^{3}I is simple to administer and interpret, is used to collect both qualitative and quantitative data, focuses on individuals and the family simultaneously, and identifies both family strengths and stressors.

The FS^{3}I is intended for use with multiple family members, who may be assessed collectively or individually, and it helps to identify both stressful situations that occur in families and the strengths families use to maintain healthy functioning, despite their problems. The FS^{3}I is divided into three sections: (1) family systems stressors: general, (2) family stressors: specific, and (3) family system strengths. Family members are asked to complete the instrument before an interview with the clinician. Questions can be read to members unable to read. Individual members can complete the FS^{3}I or the entire family can sit together and complete the assessment. Both types of data are useful.

The interview with the clinician clarifies perceived general stressors, specific stressors, and family strengths as identified by family members. The clinician evaluates family members on their stressors and strengths and overall family functioning and stability.

Family stability is assessed by gathering information on family stressors (Curran, 1985) and strengths (Curran, 1983). The assessment of general, overall stressors is followed by an assessment of specific problems. Family strengths are identified to give an indication of the potential and actual problem-solving abilities of the family system and of the strengths the family uses to deal with their problems. Nurses have a history of asking people about their problems (stressors), but often nurses have not identified the strengths and resources of the family for dealing with their problems.

The clinician records family members' scores on the quantitative summary; a different color code may be used for each individual member. The graph on the quantitative summary sheet (Appendix C) gives a visual representation of family health, and variations in how individuals or the clinician view the situation. The clinician also completes the qualitative summary (Appendix C), synthesizing the information gleaned from all participants. A family care plan summarizes intervention strategies (Appendix C).

The quantitative and qualitative data help determine the level of prevention and intervention needed: primary, secondary, or tertiary (Pender, et al, 1992). Primary prevention focuses on moving the individual and family toward a state of improved health or toward health promotion activities. Primary interventions include providing families with information about their strengths, supporting their coping and functioning capabilities, and encouraging movement toward health through family education. Secondary prevention is designed to attain system stability after stressors or problems have invaded the family system. Secondary interventions include helping the family to handle their problems, helping them find and use appropriate treatment, and intervening in crises. Tertiary prevention is designed to maintain system stability through intervention strategies that are initiated after treatment has been completed and may include, for example, coordination of care after discharge from the hospital or rehabilitation services.

Data on family stressors and family strengths are used to complete the family care plan. This plan requires the clinician to prioritize diagnoses; set goals; develop primary, secondary, or tertiary intervention activities; and evaluate outcomes (refer to Case Study for examples).

In summary, the Family Assessment and Intervention Model extends the Neuman Health Care Systems Model to focus on the family as client. The FS^{3}I was developed as one way of assessing families using this model. This approach focuses on family stressors and strengths and provides the nurse with data useful for nursing interventions.

The Friedman Family Assessment Model and Form

The Friedman Family Assessment Model and Form (Friedman, 1998) draw heavily on the structural-functional framework and developmental and systems theory. This model takes a macroscopic approach to family assessment (as compared with the microscopic approach of the FS^{3}I), viewing families as subsystems of the wider society. That is, the family is viewed as just one of the basic units of society, along with the institutions devoted to religion, education, and health, for example. This model views the family as an open social system and focuses on the family's structure (organization), functions (activities and purposes), and relationships with other social systems. This framework is commonly used when the family in community is the setting for care (e.g., in community and public health nursing). This approach enables family nurses to assess the family system as a whole, as a subunit of the society, and as an interactional system. The general assumptions of this model are delineated in Box 8–2 (Friedman, 1998, p. 100).

Structure refers to how a family is organized and how the parts relate to each other. The four basic structural dimensions are role systems, value systems, communication networks, and power structure (Friedman, 1998). These dimensions are interrelated and interactive, and they may differ in single-parent and two-parent families. For example, a single mother may be the head of the family, but she may not necessarily take on the authoritarian role that a traditional man might in a two-parent family. In turn, the value systems, communication networks, and power structures may be quite different in the single-parent and two-parent families as a result of these structural differences.

Function refers to how families go about meeting the needs of individuals and meeting the purposes of the broader society. In other words, family functions are what a family does (Friedman, 1998, p. 102). The

Box 8-2

ASSUMPTIONS UNDERLYING THE STRUCTURAL FUNCTIONAL THEORY IN FRIEDMAN'S FAMILY ASSESSMENT MODEL

- A family is a social system with functional requirements.
- A family is a small group possessing certain generic features common to all small groups.
- The family as a social system accomplishes functions that serve the individual and society.
- Individuals act in accordance with a set of internalized norms and values that are learned primarily through socialization.

Source: Friedman, M. M. (1998). *Family Nursing: Research, Theory and Practice,* ed 4. Norwalk, CT: Appleton & Lange, p. 100.

functions of the family have historically been to (see Chapter 1):

- Pass on culture (e.g., religion, ethnicity)
- Socialize young people for the next generation (e.g., to be good citizens, to be able to cope in society through education)
- Exist for sexual satisfaction and reproduction
- Provide economic security
- Serve as a protective mechanism for family members against outside forces
- Provide closer human contact and relations

The Friedman Family Assessment Model consists of six broad categories of interview questions: (1) identification data, (2) developmental stage and history of the family, (3) environmental data, (4) family structure (i.e., role structure, family values, communication patterns, and power structure), (5) family functions (i.e., affective functions, socialization functions, health care functions), and (6) family stress and coping. Each category has several subcategories. Friedman's family assessment guide exists in both a long form and a short form. The short form in Appendix D simply outlines the types of questions the nurse can ask. The long form is quite extensive, providing 13 pages of questions, and can be found in Friedman's book (Friedman, 1998, pp. 568–578).

Friedman's assessment model was developed to provide guidelines for family nurses who are interviewing a family. The guidelines list categories of information about which the interviewer asks questions to gain an overall view, in descriptive terms, of what is going on in the family. The list is quite extensive, and it may not be possible to collect all of the data in one visit. Also, all the categories of information listed in the guidelines may not be pertinent for every family. One problem with this approach is that it can generate large quantities of data with no clear direction as to how to use all this information in diagnosis, planning, and intervention. Like other approaches, this model has its strengths and weaknesses; it is one of many tools in the armamentarium of the family nurse.

The Calgary Family Assessment Model

The Calgary Family Assessment Model, developed for nursing by Wright and Leahey (2000), blends nursing and family therapy concepts and is grounded in systems theory, cybernetics, communication theory, change theory, and a biology of recognition. Wright and Leahey (2000, pp. 38–44) set forth a number of concepts from general systems theory and family systems theory as a theoretical framework for the model:

- A family system is part of a larger suprasystem and is also composed of many subsystems.
- The family as a whole is greater than the sum of its parts.
- A change in one family member affects all family members.
- The family is able to create a balance between change and stability.
- Family members' behaviors are best understood from a perspective of circular rather than linear causality.

A second theoretical foundation used in the model is cybernetics, or the science of communication and control theory. Cybernetics differs from systems theory.

Systems theory helps change the focus of our conceptual lens from parts to wholes; in contrast, cybernetics changes the focus from substance to form. Wright and Leahey (2000, p. 45) present two useful concepts from cybernetics theory:

1. Families possess self-regulating ability.
2. Feedback processes can simultaneously occur at several system levels with families.

A third theoretical foundation for the model is communication theory, based on the work of Watzlawick, et al (1967). Communication is how individuals interact with one another, so concepts derived from communication theory are used in the Calgary Family Assessment Model (Wright & Leahey, 2000, pp. 46–49). For example:

- All nonverbal communication is meaningful.
- All communication has two major channels for transmission: digital (verbal) and analogical (nonverbal).
- A dyadic relationship has varying degrees of symmetry and complementarity.
- All communication has two levels: content and relationship.

Because helping families to change is at the very core of family nursing interventions, change is also an important concept in this assessment model. Families need a balance between change and stability: Change is required to make things better, and stability is required to maintain some semblance of order. Watzlawick, et al (1974) support the notion that persistence (stability) and change have to be considered concurrently despite their opposing natures. A number of concepts from change theory are important to family nursing (Wright & Leahey, 2000, pp. 49–59):

- Change is dependent on the perception of the problem.
- Change is determined by structure.
- Change is dependent on context.
- Change is dependent on coevolving goals for treatment.
- Understanding alone does not lead to change.
- Change does not necessarily occur equally in all family members.
- Facilitating change is the nurse's responsibility.
- Change occurs by means of a "fit" or meshing between the therapeutic offerings (interventions of the nurse) and the biopsychosocial-spiritual structures of family members.
- Change can be the result of a myriad of causes.

Biology of Cognition

Maturana and Varela (1992) offered the notion that humans bring forth different views of their understanding of events and experiences in their lives. As humans, our ideas are not new but much more radical; they are based on biology and physiology. Thus a nurse adopts a particular view of reality that they bring to how they view individuals and families as they provide care. Wright and Leahey (2000) adopt two concepts from this source into their model:

1. Two possible avenues for explaining our world are objectivity and objectivity-in-parentheses.
2. We bring forth our realities through interacting with the world, ourselves, and others through language.

In sum, the world we see is not the "real" world but rather a world that we bring forth with others (Maturana & Varela, 1992).

Figure 8-2 shows the branching diagram of the Calgary Family Assessment Model (Wright & Leahey, 2000, p. 68). The assessment questions that accompany the model are organized in three major categories: (1) structural, (2) developmental, and (3) functional. Nurses examine a family's structural components to answer these questions: Who is in the family? What is the connection among family members? What is the family's context? Structure has internal, external, and contextual aspects. The internal aspects include family composition, gender, sexual orientation, rank order, subsystems, and the boundaries of the family system. The external structure refers to the extended family and larger systems. Strategies recommended to assess external structure include the genogram and the ecomap, which will be discussed later in this chapter.

The second major assessment category is family development, which includes assessment of family stages, tasks, and attachments. For example, nurses may ask, "Where is the family in the family life cycle?" Understanding the stage of the family enables nurses to assess and intervene in a more purposeful, specific, and meaningful way. There are no specific tools for assessing development, but developmental tasks can be used as guidelines. There have been many alterations to the traditional family life cycle as a result of modern trends such as divorce, remarriage, single-parent or unmarried-parent families, and childless families. Many families no longer fit the traditional family life cycle. Carter and McGoldrick (1988) discuss various "dislocations"

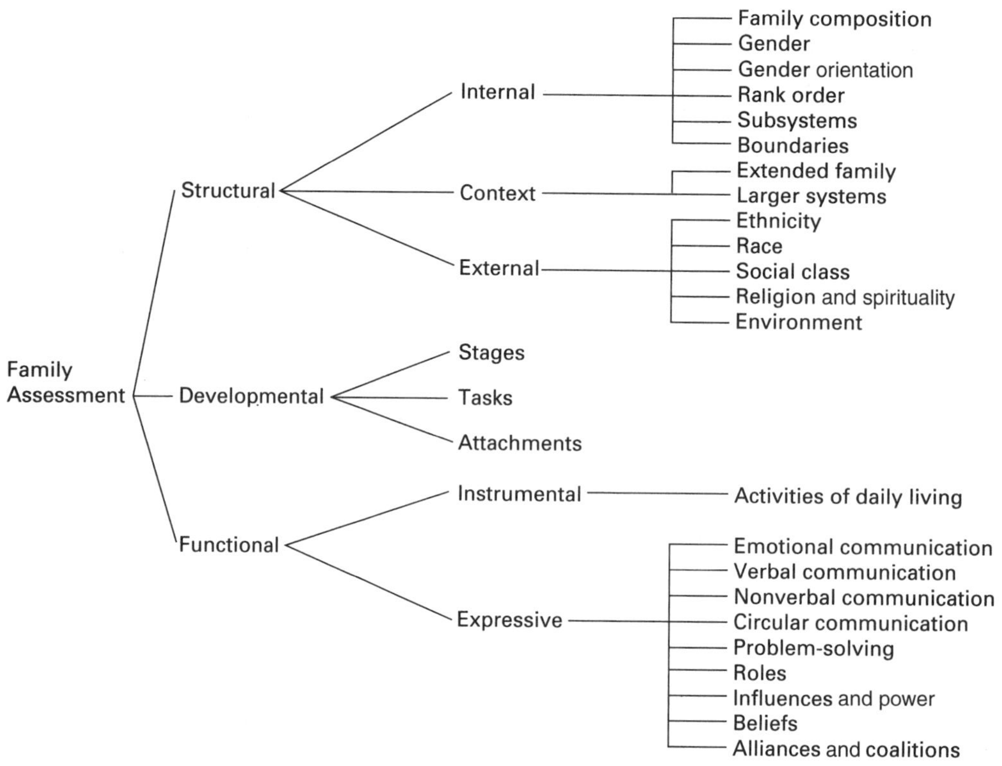

FIGURE 8-2
Branching diagram of the Calgary Family Assessment Model (CFAM). (From Wright, L.M., & Leahey, M. (2000): *Nurses and Families: A Guide to Family Assessment and Intervention ed. 2*. Philadelphia: F.A. Davis, p. 68, with permission.)

of the family life cycle, which require additional steps to restabilize and proceed developmentally.

The third area for assessment in the CFAM model is family functioning, which includes both instrumental and expressive aspects. Family functioning reflects how individuals actually behave in relation to one another, or the "here-and-now aspect of a family's life" (Wright & Leahey, 2000, p. 128). Instrumental aspects of family functioning are activities of daily life, such as eating, sleeping, meal preparation, and health care. Expressive aspects of family functioning are emotional communication, verbal and nonverbal communication, circular communication, problem solving, roles, influence and power, beliefs, and alliances and coalitions. Wright and Leahey indicate that nurses may assess in all three areas (i.e., structural, developmental, functional) for a macroview of the family or they can use any part of the approach for a microassessment.

Wright and Leahey also have developed a companion model to the CFAM, the Calgary Family Intervention Model (CFIM) (2000). This intervention model provides concrete strategies by which nurses can promote, improve, and sustain effective family functioning in the cognitive, affective, and behavioral domains. More detail about this assessment model and intervention is available in Wright and Leahey's book *Nurses and Families: A Guide to Family Assessment and Intervention* (2000).

Summary of Approaches

Each of these three family approaches is unique, and each creates a different database on which to plan interventions. The Hanson and Mischke Family Assessment and Intervention Model and the FS^3I are used to measure specific family dimensions. The FS^3I yields both qualitative and quantitative data.

Friedman's Family Assessment Model and Short Form is broader, more general, and particularly useful for viewing families in the context of their community. An interview guide (detailed in the long form) that lists specific categories for assessment enhances this approach.

Wright and Leahey's CFAM and CFIM provide an

approach for both assessment and intervention, though it is less specific than the other two approaches. The CFAM is broad in perspective, although it focuses on internal relations within the family rather than the interface between the family and community.

Finally, all three approaches can be used alone or in some combination. For example, the FS^{3}I can be used for specific assessment, while either the Friedman Family Assessment Short or Long Form or the CFAM model is used for more global assessment.

GENOGRAMS AND ECOMAPS

The genogram and ecomap are essential components of any family assessment. They should be used concurrently with all three models and approaches previously described.

Genograms

The genogram is a format for drawing a family tree that records information about family members and their relationships over at least three generations (McGoldrick & Gerson, 1985; McGoldrick et al, 1999). The genogram is a diagram, a skeleton, and a constellation showing the structure of intergenerational relationships. Genograms have been commonly used in both genealogy and genetic charts and are now being used in family therapy and in health care settings. They are a rich source of information for planning intervention strategies because they display the family visually and graphically in a way that provides a quick overview of family complexities.

The genogram was developed primarily out of the family systems theory of Murray Bowen (Bowen, 1985; Bowen & Kerr, 1988). According to Bowen, people are organized in family systems by generation, age, sex, and similar variables. How a person fits into the family structure influences the person's functioning, relational patterns, and type of family he or she will form in the next generation. Bowen incorporated Toman's (1976) ideas about the importance of sex and birth order in shaping sibling relationships and characteristics. According to Bowen (1985), families repeat themselves over generations in a phenomenon called the transmission of family patterns. What happens in one generation repeats itself in the next, so the same issues are played out from generation to generation. These include both psychosocial and health issues.

Figure 8-3 provides a basic genogram form from which the nurse can start plotting family members over the first, second, and third generations (McGoldrick & Gerson, 1985, p. 156).

Figure 8-4 shows symbols provided by McGoldrick and Gerson (1985, pp. 154–155) to describe basic family membership and structure, family interaction patterns, and other family information of particular importance, such as ethnic background, religion, education,

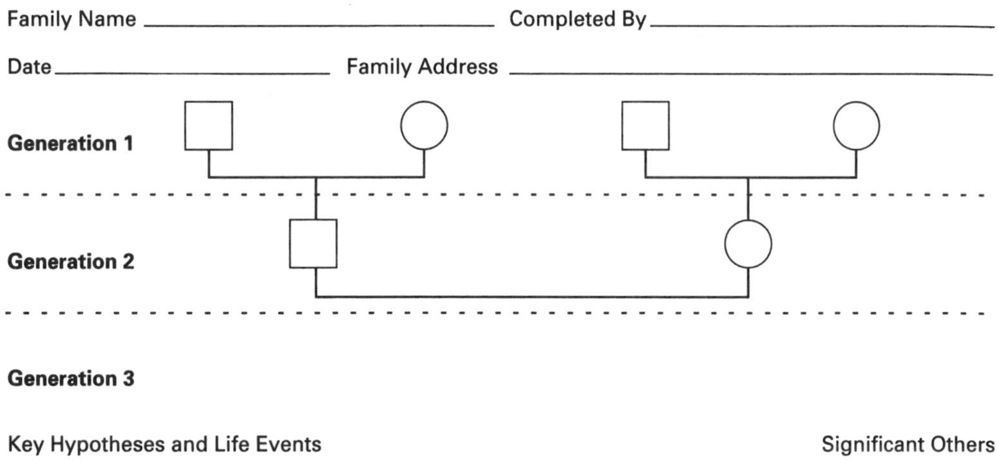

FIGURE 8-3
Genogram form. (Adapted from McGoldrick, M., & Gerson, R. (1985): *Genograms in Family Assessment*. New York: W.W. Norton, p. 156, with permission.)

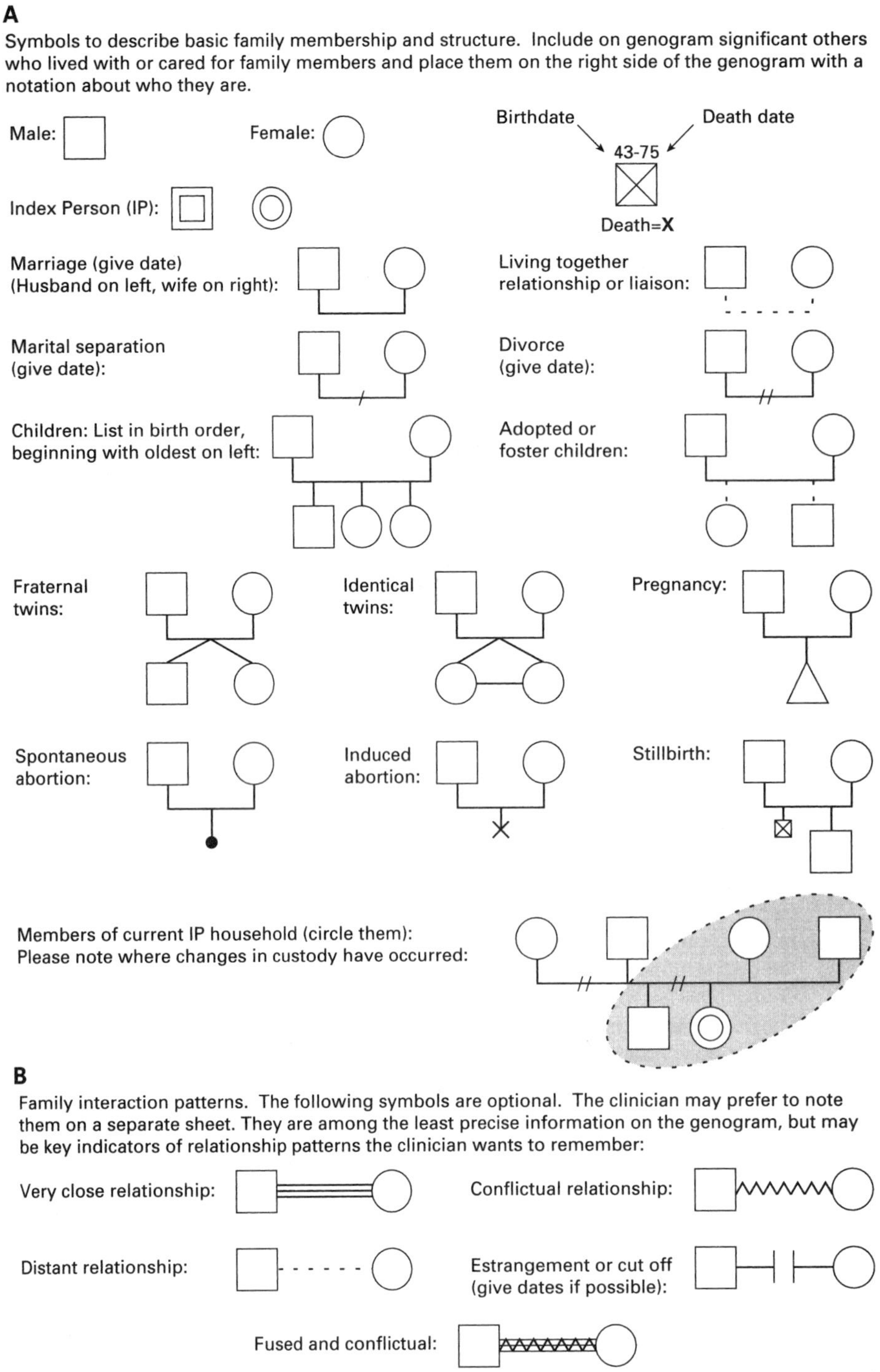

FIGURE 8-4

Genogram format. (From McGoldrick, M. and Gerson, R. (1985): *Genograms in family assessment.* New York: W.W. Norton, pp. 154–155, with permission.)

C

Medical history. Because the genogram is meant to be an orienting map of the family, there is room to indicate only the most important factors. Thus, list only major or chronic illnesses and problems. Include dates in parentheses where feasible or applicable. Use DSM-IIIR categories or recognized abbreviations where available (e.g., cancer: CA; stroke: CVA).

D

Other family information of special importance may also be noted on the genogram:

1. Ethnic background and migration date
2. Religion or religious change
3. Education
4. Occupation or unemployment
5. Military service
6. Retirement
7. Trouble with law
8. Physical abuse or incest
9. Obesity
10. Smoking
11. Dates when family members left home: LH '74
12. Current location of family members

It is useful to have a space at the bottom of the genogram for notes on *other key information.* This would include critical events, changes in the family structure since the genogram was made, hypotheses, and other notations of major family issues or changes. These notations should always be dated and kept to a minimum, since every extra piece of information on a genogram complicates it and therefore diminishes its readability.

FIGURE 8-4
Genogram format. (From McGoldrick, M., & Gerson, R. (1985): *Genograms in Family Assessment.* New York: W.W. Norton, pp. 154–155, with permission.)

health, drug and alcohol use, occupation, military service, and nodal events, such as retirement, trouble with the law, and family relocations.

The health history of all family members (e.g., morbidity, mortality, and onset of illness) is very important information for family nurses and can be the focus of analysis of the family genogram. An example of a family genogram developed from one interview is contained in the case study and is shown in Figure 8-5.

During the assessment interview, the nurse asks the family for background information and then completes the genogram together with the family; it is a joint nurse and family endeavor. An outline for a brief genogram interview is given in Box 8–3, and genogram interpretive categories are contained in Box 8–4 (McGoldrick & Gerson, 1985, pp. 157–160). Most families are cooperative and interested in completing their genogram, which becomes a part of the ongoing health care record. The genogram does not have to be completed at one sitting. As the same or a different nurse continues to work with the family, data can be added to the genogram over time in a continuing process.

Ecomaps

Another useful approach in assessing families is the ecologic map, or ecomap. Ecology is a branch of science concerned with the interrelationships of organisms to each other in the environment. The ecomap is a visual representation of the family unit in relation to the community; it shows the nature of the relationships among family members and between family members and the world around them. The ecomap is thus "an overview of the family in their situation, picturing both the important nurturant and stress-producing connections between the family and the world" (Ross & Cobb, 1990, p. 176).

The blank ecomap consists of a large circle with smaller circles around it (see Figure 8-6). To complete the ecomap, the genogram of the family is placed in the center of the large circle. This circle marks the boundary between the household and its external environment. The smaller outer circles represent "significant people, agencies, or institutions in the family's context" (Wright & Leahey, 1994, p. 56). Lines are drawn be-

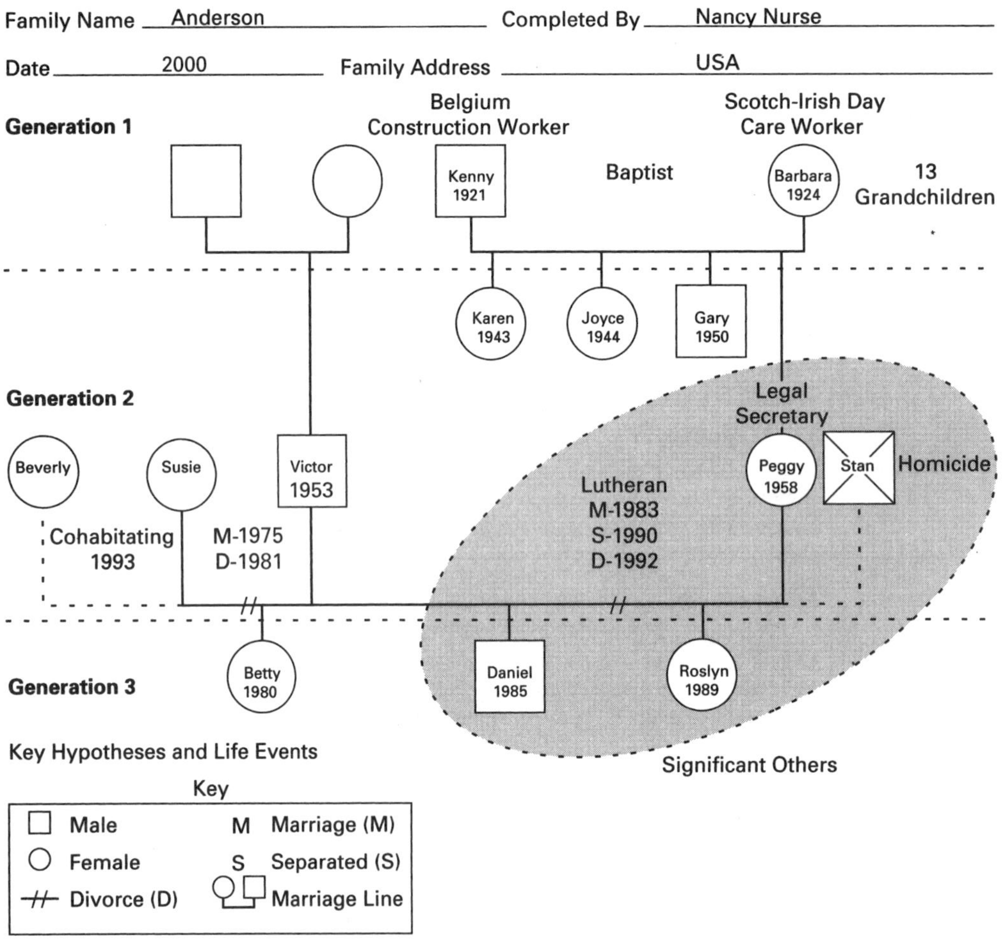

FIGURE 8-5
Example genogram of the Anderson family.

tween the circles and the family members to depict the nature and quality of the relationships and to show what kinds of resources are going in and coming out of the family. Straight lines show strong or close relationships; the more pronounced the line, the stronger the relationship. Straight lines with slashes denote stressful relationships and broken lines show tenuous or distant relationships. Arrows show the direction of the flow of energy and resources between individuals and between the family and the environment. Figure 8-7 gives an example of a completed family ecomap.

The ecomap is a tool for organizing a great deal of factual information to give the nurse a more integrated perception of the family situation. Ecomaps not only portray the present but also can be used to set goals, for example, to increase connections and exchanges with individuals and agencies in the community. More detailed discussions of ecomapping can be found in Hartman and Laird (1983), McGoldrick and Gerson (1985), Ross and Cobb (1990), Friedman (1998), and Hanson and Boyd (1996).

Clinical Uses

A key should be drawn on both the genogram and the ecomap, because the data become a part of the official family health record and other professionals need to be able to interpret the meaning at another time. Families find it stimulating to help develop the genogram and ecomap that depict their family and

Box 8-3

OUTLINE FOR A BRIEF GENOGRAM INTERVIEW

Index Person, Children, and Spouses

Name? Date of birth? Occupation? Are they married? If so, give names of spouses, and the name and sex of children with each spouse. Include all miscarriages, stillbirths and adopted and foster children. Include dates of marriages, separations, and divorces. Also include birth and death dates, cause of death, occupations, and education of the above family members. Who lives in the household now?

Family of Origin

Mother's name? Father's name? They were which of how many children? Given name and sex of each sibling. Include all miscarriages, stillbirths, and adopted and foster siblings. Include dates of the parents' marriages, separations, and divorces. Also, include birth and death dates, cause of death, occupations, and education of the above family members. Who lived in the household when they were growing up?

Mother's Family

The names of the mother's parents? The mother was which of how many children? Give name and sex of each of her siblings. Include all miscarriages, stillbirths, and adopted and foster siblings. Include dates of grandparents' marriages, separations, and divorces. Also include birth and death dates, cause of death, occupations, and education of the above family members.

Father's Family

The names of the father's parents? The father was which of how many children? Give name and sex of each of his siblings. Include all miscarriages, stillbirths, and adopted and foster siblings. Include dates of grandparents' marriages, separations, and divorces. Also include birth and death dates, cause of death, occupations, and education of the above family members.

Ethnicity

What are the ethnic and religious backgrounds of family members and the languages they speak, if not English?

Major Moves

Tell about major family relocations and migrations.

Significant Others

Add others who lived with or were important to the family.

For All Those Listed, Note Any of the Following

Serious medical, behavioral, or emotional problems
- Job problems
- Drug or alcohol problems
- Serious problems with the law

continued

Box 8-3 *(continued)*

For All Those Listed, Indicate Any Who Were

Especially close
- Distant or conflictual
- Cut off from each other
- Overly dependent on each other

Source: McGoldrick, M., & Gerson, R. (1985) *Genograms in Family Assessment.* New York: W. W. Norton, pp. 157–158. Reprinted with permission.

their situation, and the process helps build a full family-nurse partnership because everyone's voice is heard. Development of the genogram and ecomap are interventions in and of themselves and can also serve as useful teaching tools. Kissman and Allen (1993) describe a process that professionals can follow in ecomapping a single-parent family and using the information in therapeutic interventions. The case study at the end of the chapter illustrates the use of a genogram and an ecomap.

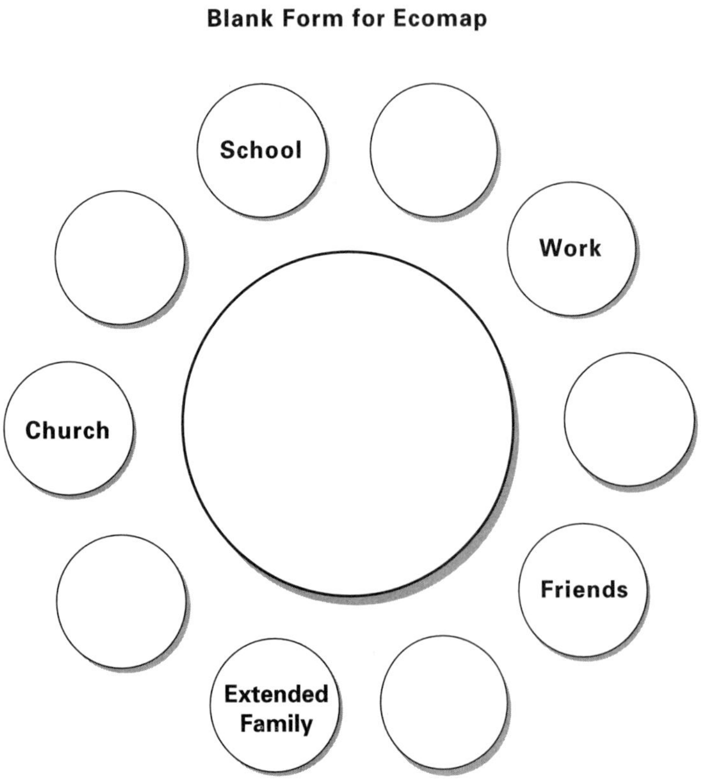

FIGURE 8-6
Blank ecomap form. (Adapted from Friedman, M.M. (1998). *Family Nursing: Research, Theory & Practice*, ed. 4. Norwalk, Conn: Appleton & Lange, p. 198.)

Box 8-4

GENOGRAM INTERPRETATIVE CATEGORIES

Category 1: Family Structure

A. Household composition
  1. Intact nuclear household
  2. Single-parent household
  3. Remarried family household
  4. Three-generational household
  5. Household including extended family members

B. Sibling constellation
  1. Birth order
  2. Siblings' gender
  3. Age differences among siblings
  4. Other factors influencing sibling constellation
     a. Timing of each child's birth in family history
     b. Child's characteristics
     c. Family's "program" for the child
     d. Parental attitudes and biases regarding sex differences
     e. Child's sibling position in relation to that of parent

C. Unusual family configurations

Category 2: Life Cycle Fit

Category 3: Pattern Repetition Across Generations

A. Patterns of functioning
B. Patterns of relationship
C. Structural patterns

Category 4: Life Events and Family Functioning

A. Coincidences of life events
B. The impact of life changes, transitions, and traumas
C. Anniversary reactions
D. Social, economic, and political events

Category 5: Relational Patterns and Triangles

A. Triangles
  1. Parent-child triangles
  2. Common couple triangles
  3. Divorced and remarried family triangles
  4. Triangles in families with foster or adopted children
  5. Multigenerational triangles

B. Relationships outside the family

continued

Box 8-4 (continued)

Category 6: Family Balance and Imbalance

A. Family structure
B. Roles
C. Level and style of functioning
D. Resources

Source: Adapted from McGoldrick, M., & Gerson, R. (1985). *Genograms in Family Assessment.* New York: W. W. Norton, pp. 159–160. Reprinted with permission.

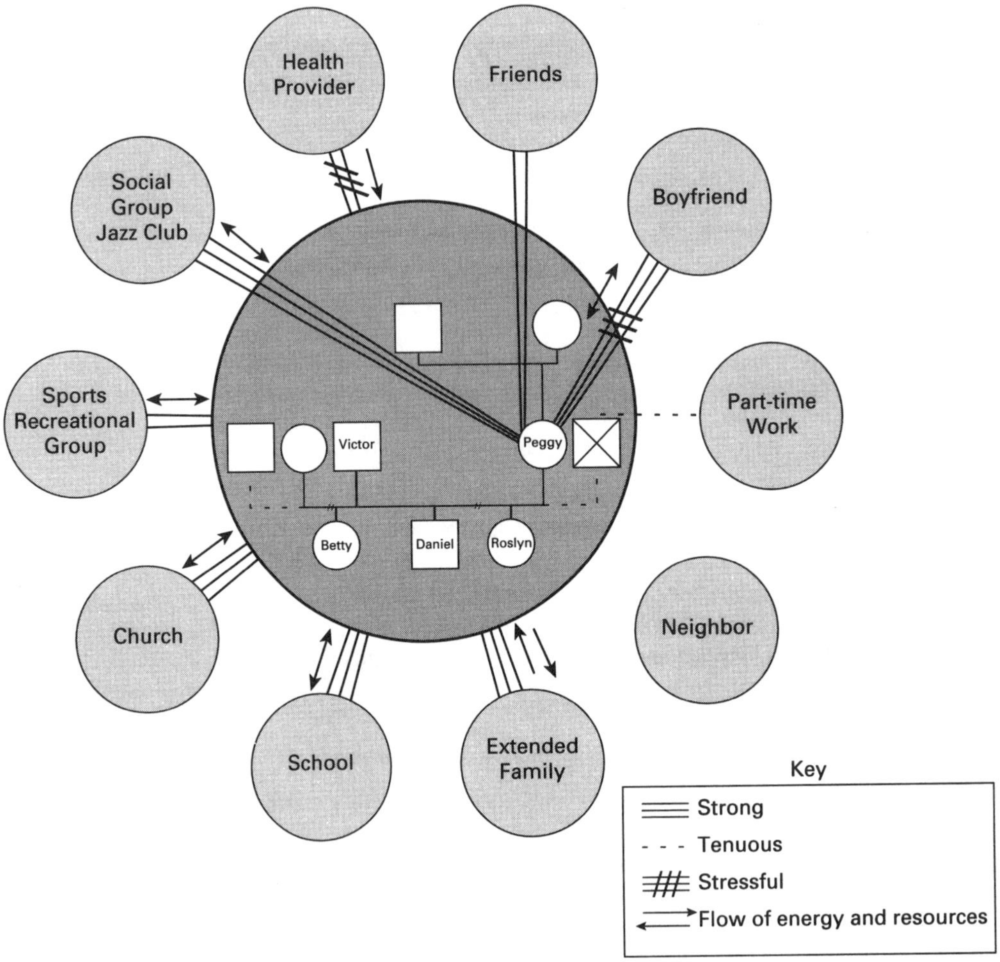

FIGURE 8-7
Example ecomap of the Anderson family.

Case Study

THE ANDERSONS

The Anderson family came to the attention of the nursing staff when Mrs. Anderson (Peggy) was hospitalized with a gunshot wound. The nurses cared for her first in the intensive care unit and then on the step-down trauma unit. This middle-class family consisted of Peggy (mother, age 42), Victor (father, age 47), Betty (daughter, age 20), Daniel (son, age 15), and Roslyn (daughter, age 11). (The family genogram, Figure 8-5, and ecomap, Figure 8-7, accompany this case study.)

Victor was originally married to Susie (in 1972), but they were divorced in 1975, after the birth of Betty, and Victor became the custodial parent for Betty. In 1983, Peggy and Victor were married and had two biological children, Daniel and Roslyn. Although Peggy was stepmother to Betty, she raised Betty as her own child, and they maintained a good relationship over the years. Victor graduated from law school and took his first job as an attorney after he and Peggy got married. The family relocated frequently (17 times), with Peggy serving as homemaker and legal secretary in various places, while Victor pursued his dream of a perfect job (i.e., being an attorney) in a perfect location.

As the children grew up, Peggy and Victor "grew apart" and the relationship ceased to be mutually supportive. Peggy neglected her personal needs for growth and adult development, and Victor sought sexual alliances outside of the marriage. Over time, their relationship became stormy, and they made a decision to separate in 1990. The court-mandated reconciliation counseling was merely a cursory review of the relationship difficulties, and they were divorced in 1992, after 9 years of marriage.

Peggy received legal custody of the two younger children and Victor got the customary visiting privileges (every other weekend and every Wednesday), an arrangement made to everyone's satisfaction. Victor was ordered to pay child support until the two younger children were 18 years of age and spousal support to Peggy for 2 years following the divorce. By the time of the divorce, Betty (Victor's daughter by his first marriage) had left home to go to college. Following his divorce from Peggy, Victor moved in with his new girlfriend, Beverly. This event was a source of considerable pain for Peggy and worsened her low self-esteem. Victor continued to have almost weekly contact with his children.

After the divorce, Peggy went to work and tried to get her life back together. For financial reasons, she and the children moved to a smaller house. She soon met Stan, a charming, socially adept, and seemingly supportive man with whom she became quickly infatuated. He moved into the family house with Peggy and the children soon after they met and initially brought an element of excitement and security to the home. As the realities of sharing a household emerged, Peggy noted some disturbing features about Stan: he became obsessive and possessive of her and the children. Peggy became extremely upset and decided she had moved too fast. She asked Stan to move out. Stan was furious; he became even more obsessed with Peggy and became hostile to her and the children after she asked him to leave.

Stan refused to leave and Peggy had to obtain a court order to remove him from the house. She was soon frightened to discover that Stan had been following her and asked for police support to enforce the restraining order. One afternoon Stan took Peggy hostage at gunpoint at the door of her house. The neighbors called the police and within a couple of hours, a violent confrontation took place. During the shootout, Stan shot Peggy in the shoulder, and the police killed Stan.

Peggy was hospitalized for multiple lacerations and a gunshot wound through the shoulder, which resulted in nerve damage to her right arm. Peggy's parents came from out of town and moved into the house to take care of the children and support their daughter. The first hospitalization lasted 10 days and consisted primarily of surgery and wound care. Peggy was sent home with minimal discharge planning, and when she got home, she experienced intractable pain in her arm, hand, and shoulder. Peggy's parents took her back to the hospital, where she was admitted to the psychiatric unit for pain management, physical therapy, and treatment of posttraumatic stress disorder. The hospital course was uneventful, and Peggy was discharged again after a month. By now, her pain was under control and she had regained some use of her injured arm.

Getting back to "normal," or system stability, was the goal of the family members. Within a year, the Anderson family had gone through divorce, relocation, and a violent episode. The initial family assessment involved the use of all three approaches described previously in this chapter and of course the genogram and ecomap. The findings from this assessment follow.

Family Systems Stressor-Strength Inventory The FS^3I was deemed the most suitable instrument to look at problems and the resources that the family had to cope with these problems. Peggy and her children were interviewed together by the nurse, but each person completed the FS^3I separately. Each person's score was tallied using the scoring guide for the FS^3I. Figure 8–8 summarizes the stressors and strengths perceived by the family members and the nurse.

The general stressors were viewed differently by different family members, and they were also assessed as more serious by the nurse than by the family. Everyone considered the general stress level as high, however, which was consistent with the family experiences. In addition, the family members viewed their strengths as fairly good, as did the nurse.

The qualitative summary in Figure 8-9 served as the guide for the family care plan in Figure 8-10. Figure 8-9 summarizes general stressors, specific stressors, and family strengths, as well as the overall physical and mental health of the family. The nurse completed this summary using both verbal input and written data from the FS^3I.

The family members and the nurse viewed the divorce, shooting, posttraumatic stress syndrome, and trauma surgery as general stressors. The family reported the specific stressors to be communication among the mother, children, and the noncustodial father; finances; and lack of fun time. The nurse listed the specific stressors as the aftermath of the divorce, single parenthood, and resource depletion. The strengths of the family were seen to be communication between the mother and children, religious faith, the social support network, and good physical and mental health before the events.

Overall, the family members had similar perceptions of their stressors and strengths and the nurse concurred with their perceptions; however, the nurse rated both stressors and strengths higher than the family members did. The nurse concluded that they had the strengths they needed to deal with the stressors. The ecomap shows that the family was supported well by community resources, an important factor in coping with stress, and that they used their resources to achieve a more positive health status than they had had in the beginning.

Friedman Family Assessment Form Friedman's Family Assessment Short Form was also used with this family and was particularly helpful in planning for Peggy Anderson's discharge. This assessment provided data on the developmental stage and history of the family; the environment; the family structure; family functions, including health care; and family stress and coping.

Developmental Stage and History of the Family The family was in the developmental stage of rearing a family of adolescents. Betty was a college student and Daniel and Roslyn were teenagers. The children were age-appropriate in terms of their developmental tasks at the time of the divorce, but the divorce and shooting created some regressive behavior in Roslyn and some parent-like behavior in Daniel.

Environmental Data The family lived in an upper-middle-class urban neighborhood at the time of the divorce. Afterwards, they were forced for economic reasons to move to a smaller three-bedroom house in a middle-class neighborhood. They were close to schools, church, and shopping areas, and the neighborhood was clean and safe. The family had a good network in the community, as the ecomap shows. The children were active in school, sports, and church activities. Victor lived in another part of the city with his new partner, Beverly. The children were transported back and forth between their parents because their dad had visitation every other weekend. There were also frequent telephone calls between father and children.

Family Structure The communication patterns in the family worked well, and the relationships between children and mother and children and father were good, although the relationship between the two parents was tense at times. Peggy was quite verbal and expressive about her life and needs, which encouraged open and honest communication.

Peggy had always made the decisions around the home, even before she was divorced from Victor. Some of this power focus changed, however, as the children got older and participated more in decision making. The role structure in this single-parent family could also be considered binuclear, because the mother was in charge in one setting most of the time, but the father was the head of his own household when the children were with him.

Family Values The mother, Peggy, was very clear about passing along her values to her children. The values she articulated included Christian philosophy and action, a work ethic, open communication, learning, family cohesion, and trust in one another.

Family Functions: Affective Function This single-parent family household was cohesive and close. Peggy was a responsive mother to her children and a child-centered parent in a healthy sense. She also stayed in contact with her extended family, and her parents were a great support to her and their grandchildren.

Family Functions: Socialization The parents assumed the major role in socializing their children. Peggy in particular was involved in child rearing and was very involved with her children's friends as well. The children were doing well in school, at home, and at church in terms of performance, friendships, and adjustment.

Family Functions: Health Care The family was connected with a primary physician and a major health center. They had good medical and dental care before the divorce and the shooting, and the care continued. Their physical and mental health appeared to be good, in part because of their dietary practices, sleeping and resting habits, exercise and recreation, and other self-care practices. Peggy received tertiary care at a major medical cen-

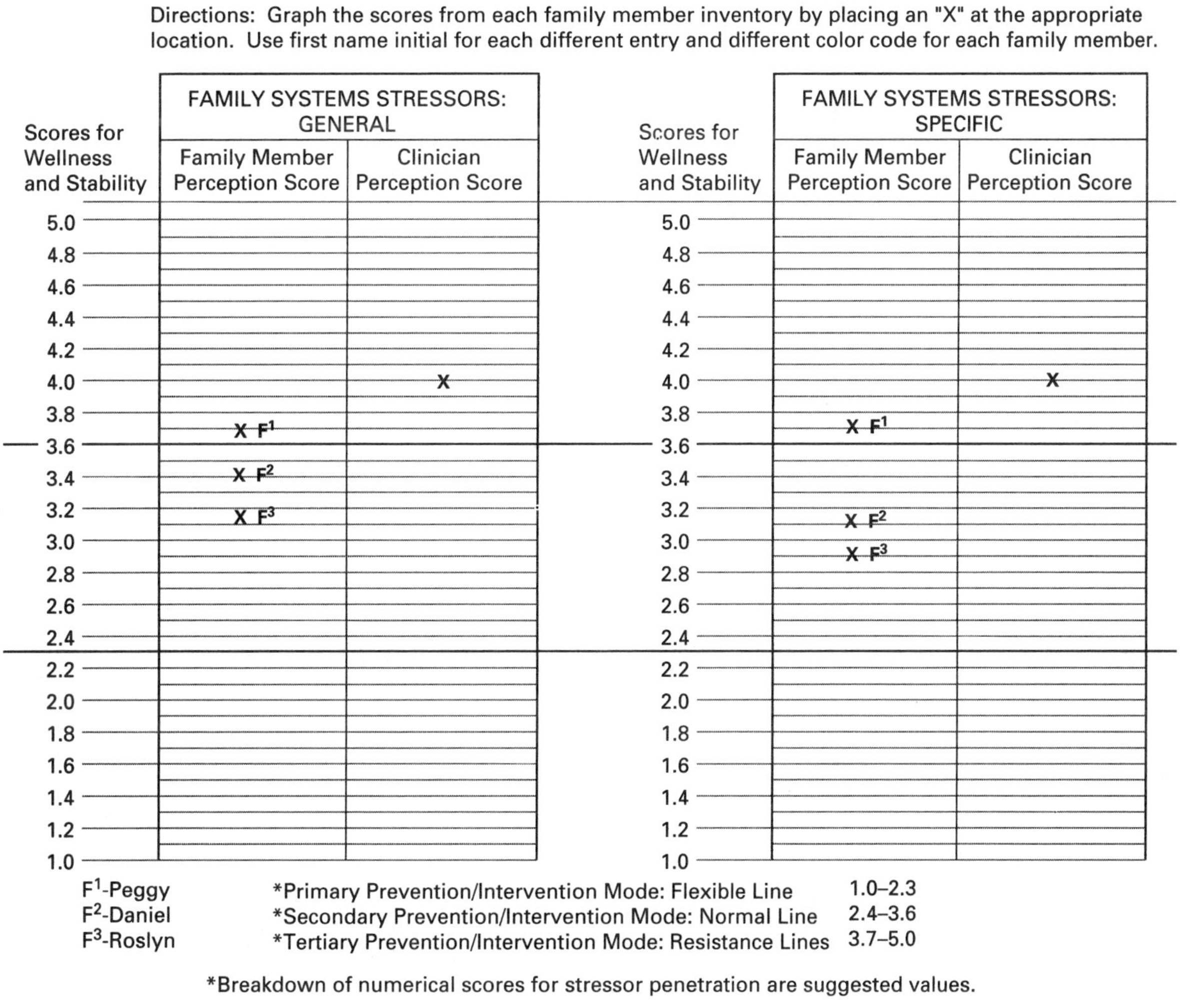

FIGURE 8-8
Example of the Anderson family Family Systems Stressor Strength Inventory (FS³I) quantitative summary of general and specific family systems stressors, including family and clinician perception scores. (*continued*)

Directions: Graph the scores from the inventory by placing an "X" at the appropriate location and connect with a line. Use first name initial for each different entry and different color code for each family member.

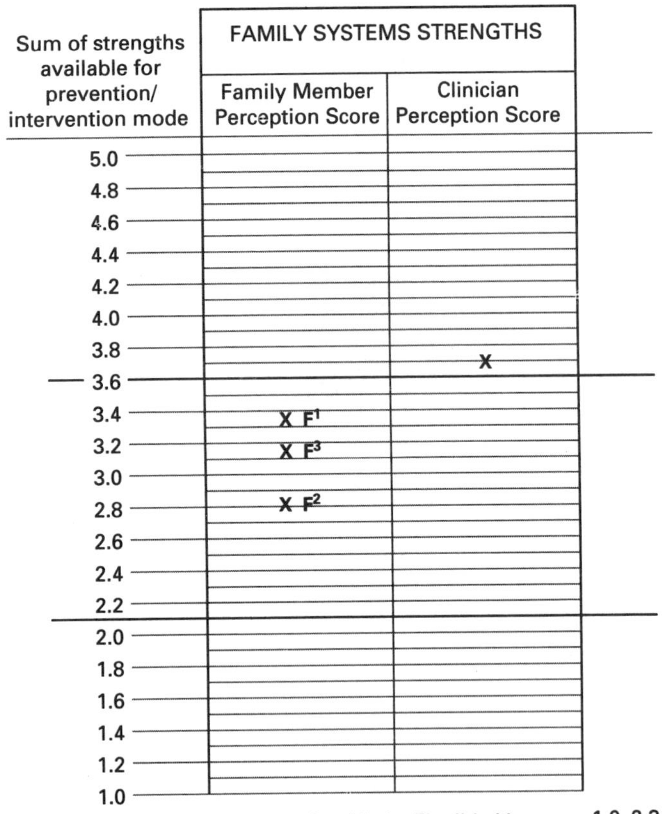

*Primary Prevention/Intervention Mode: Flexible Line 1.0–2.3
*Secondary Prevention/Intervention Mode: Normal Line 2.4–3.6
*Tertiary Prevention/Intervention Mode: Resistance Lines 3.7–5.0

*Breakdown of numerical scores for stressor penetration are suggested values.

F[1]-Peggy
F[2]-Daniel
F[3]-Roslyn

FIGURE 8-8, CONTINUED
Example of the Anderson family Family Systems Stressor Strength Inventory (FS^{3}I) quantitative summary of family systems, strengths, including family and clinician perception scores.

ter when she was hospitalized for the gunshot wound and posttraumatic stress syndrome. She continued to receive health care that included periodic counseling through the outpatient department of the medical center.

Family Stress and Coping This family was seen shortly after the shooting, hospitalization, and discharge. At that time, they were coping remarkably well with familial stressors. They had some experience in dealing with crises in the past, which enabled them to hold together during this crisis. This effective coping was the result, in part, of their financial stability, access to good health care resources, extended network and family support systems, and a past history of good physical and mental health.

Calgary Family Assessment Model The Calgary Family Assessment Model (CFAM) was also used to assess the Anderson family, along with the FS^{3}I and Friedman's family assessment form. The data obtained from the CFAM model on the structural, developmental, and functional components of the family were

Part I: Family Systems Stressors: General

Summarize general stressors and remarks of family and clinician. Prioritize stressors according to importance to family members.

Divorce (visitation, custody, and child support issues)

Homicide of family friend. Post-traumatic Stress Syndrome

Post-trauma/surgery rehabilitation

Part II: Family Systems Stressors: Specific

A. Summarize specific stressor and remarks of family and clinician.

Family: Communication between divorced parents, economics, time for fun

Clinician: Divorce issues, single parenthood, resource depletion.

B. Summarize differences (if discrepancies exist) between how family members and clinician view effects of stressful situation on family.

Family and clinician see stressors about the same. Clinician views general and specific stressors higher than family. Clinician sees more family strengths than family members see in themselves.

C. Summarize overall family functioning.

Functioning quite well given recent traumatizing events and single parent structure. Physical health average and mental health good. Good social networks. Family adaptable.

D. Summarize overall significant physical health status for family members.

Physical health status of family members is good. Peggy is still recovering from nerve damage to arm and shoulder. Receiving physical therapy.

E. Summarize overall significant mental health status for family members.

Mental health appears fairly good at this time. Family well adjusted. Open and sharing feelings. Mother receiving counseling once a month.

Part III: Family Systems Strengths

Summarize family systems strengths and family and clinician remarks that facilitate family health and stability.

Family has been cohesive in time of trauma. Good communication patterns established earlier in family history helped family during this time. Religion and social support play important role in getting family through crisis.

FIGURE 8-9
Example of the Anderson family Family Systems Stressor Strength Inventory (FS^{3}I) qualitative summary, including family and clinician remarks.

in many ways similar to the data obtained using Friedman's guidelines. However, the CFAM has a more expressive focus, and when the expressive segment of the CFAM tool was used with the Anderson family, more detailed information was obtained about emotional communication; verbal, nonverbal, and circular communication; and family alliances and coalitions. For example, the verbal and nonverbal communications between Peggy and her children were congruent. The expressive nature of the family becomes more visible when more time is spent interviewing the family.

Summary of Case Study In summary, there is some overlap in the kind of information the nurse can glean using the three assessment models and approaches, especially because all three use the genogram and ecomap concurrently. Whatever approach the nurse

Diagnosis General and Specific Family System Stressors	Family System Strengths Supporting Family Care Plan	Goals Family and Clinician	Prevention/Intervention Mode		Outcomes Evaluation and Replanning
			Primary, Secondary, or Tertiary	Prevention/Intervention Activities	
Divorce (custody, visitation, and child support) DX: Altered family processes	Religious faith Extended family support	Restoration of stability	Support family changes Children of divorce support group	Mother receive counseling	
Homicide of boyfriend Post-traumatic stress syndrome DX: Grieving, fear, powerlessness	Basic trust in one another Admit to and seek help with problems	Management of PTSD Healthy grieving process	Grief counseling Victim support group	Counseling Mother return to productive job that empowers her and strengthens her self-esteem	
Post-trauma surgery to arms and shoulders DX: Sensory-perceptual alterations	Seek help with problems Support one another Trust in family Trust health care professionals	Full arm and shoulder function without pain	Rehabilitation Physical therapy	Pain management	

FIGURE 8-10
Family Systems and Stressor Strength Inventory (FS[3]I) Family Care Plan. It is important to prioritize the three most significant diagnoses.

uses, it must be consistent and systematic. Each approach may lead to different intervention strategies, although there may be commonalities. Redundant information is less of a problem than missing information.

CURRENT STATUS OF FAMILY MEASUREMENT

The increasing sophistication of family nursing over the past decade has increased awareness of the need for more and better assessment and measurement strategies. While general family assessment guidelines have appeared in a number of nursing textbooks in the past decade, the development of family measurement instruments has only recently received major attention (Touliatos et al, 1990; Waltz, Strickland, & Lenz, 1991). Other professionals, such as psychologists, social workers, and family social scientists, developed most instruments in the family literature. "There is a paucity of material that speaks specifically to family nursing measurement" (Berkey and Hanson, 1991, p. 228). Thus, most family instruments are "non-nursing" and may or may not be relevant to phenomena of interest to family nurses.

Recently, some nurse academicians have developed qualitative assessment guidelines. Four family nursing textbooks discuss family focuses, assessment models, and approaches, and three have been presented in this chapter (Berkey & Hanson, 1991; Hanson & Mischke, 1996; Friedman, 1998; Wright & Leahey, 2000). Only Berkey and Hanson (1991) and Hanson and Mischke (1996), however, can be used both for assessment and measurement and for practice and research. Other nurse researches have developed instruments primarily for quantitative measurement purposes, such as in research (Feetham, 1983; Hanson, 1985, 1986; McCubbin & McCubbin, 1993; Waltz, Strickland, & Lenz, 1991).

Five major problems confront the developer of family nursing assessment and measurement instruments.

1. There is a lack of conceptual frameworks, particularly from nursing models, for existing instruments.
2. Instruments that have been developed by nurses

tend to be time-consuming to administer and to provide overwhelming amounts of information, which nurses must then summarize to set priorities for interventions.

3. Instruments have not demonstrated a clear link between assessment and intervention strategies nor can they be used for both assessment and measurement purposes.
4. Instruments have largely focused on problems that families experience, rather than on family strengths, on which nursing interventions can be built.
5. The psychometric properties (reliability and validity) of family instruments are largely untested.

The FS^{3}I was designed to address these areas of concern. However, much work still needs to be done by nurses to develop appropriate strategies and instruments to assess and measure families.

SUMMARY

There are many approaches, techniques, and models that can be used to collect data on families for assessment and intervention. This chapter presents three of the major models and approaches that appear in the literature on family nursing assessment. None of the existing models or approaches fulfills all the needs of families and clinicians in every circumstance. The benefit of learning and adopting one particular model and approach is that it provides a framework for each nurse to gain expertise in systematically collecting data on this complex client that we call "the family." The genogram and ecomap are tools that all nurses should use no matter what model they choose.

Much work is left to be done in refining the techniques and strategies that are available, and even more work must be done to make them efficient and effective in clinical settings. Bridging the gap between assessment data and intervention strategies is one of the main challenges. Existing family and family nursing measurement instruments must be developed and standardized. Nurses have become more involved in the development of these instruments during the last 10 years. Assessment of the family as client is a challenging but rewarding part of nursing practice today and represents the practice of tomorrow.

Study Questions

1. Family assessment and family measurement mean the same thing.
   a. True
   b. False
2. Once the nurse assesses the family, they have all the information needed to develop a comprehensive care plan.
   a. True
   b. False
3. Match the following terms:

a. Measurement	i. Systematic collection of data
b. Assessment	ii. Assigning numbers to an attribute
c. Qualitative	iii. Data that describe family characteristics
d. Quantitative	iv Data that compare, measure, or count family properties

4. The Family Systems Stressor-Strength Inventory is a measurement instrument that evolved out of the model of the nursing theorist
   a. Sister Callista Roy
   b. Dorthea Orem
   c. Madelaine Leininger
   d. Betty Neuman
5. Family stability is the goal of which model?
   a. Friedman's Family Assessment Model
   b. Calgary Family Assessment Model
   c. Family Assessment and Intervention Model
6. Friedman's model and the CFAM model yield substantially different kinds of information
   a. True
   b. False
7. Friedman's model is based on which of the following theoretical frameworks?
   a. Structural-functional theory
   b. Systems theory
   c. Developmental theory
   d. All of the above
8. Wright and Leahey's model is based on which of the following theoretical frameworks?
   a. Structural theory
   b. Systems theory
   c. Developmental theory

d. Communications theory
e. Functional theory

9. Genograms and ecomaps should only be used with families if you are working with the whole group.
a. True
b. False

10. Nursing instrumentation is at an early stage of development.
a. True
b. False

11. How does family assessment fit into what we call the nursing process?
12. How is family assessment different from individual assessment?
13. Give some examples of how qualitative measurement is used in your daily life. Do the same for quantitative measurement.
14. Compare measurement and assessment.
15. Discuss the current status of the development of family measurement.
16. Summarize the key parts of each family assessment model and discuss how they are different or overlap.

References

American Nurses Association. (1980). Social policy statement. Kansas City, MO: ANA.

Berkey, K. M., & Hanson, S. M. H. (1991). *Pocket Guide to Family Assessment and Intervention.* St. Louis, MO: Mosby Year Book.

Bomar, P.J. (1996). *Nurses and Family Health Promotion: Concepts, Assessment, and Interventions,* ed 2. Philadelphia: W.B. Saunders.

Bowen, M. (1985). *Family Therapy in Clinical Practice.* Norvale, NJ: Jason Aronson.

Bowen, M., & Kerr, M. (1988). *Family Evaluation: An Approach Based on Bowen's Theory.* New York: W.W. Norton.

Carlson, C. L. (1989). Criteria for family assessment in research and intervention contexts. *Journal of Family Psychology, 3*:158–176.

Carter, B., & McGoldrick, M. (Eds). (1988). *The Changing Family Life Cycle: A Framework for Family Therapy,* ed 2. NY: Gardner Press.

Carter, E., & McGoldrick, M. (1980). The family life cycle and family therapy: An overview. In E. Carter & M. McGoldrick (Eds.), *The Family Life Cycle: A Framework for Family Therapy,* pp. 3–28. New York: Gardner Press.

Curran, D. (1983). *Traits and the Healthy Family.* Minneapolis, MN: Winston Press.

Curran, D. (1985). *Stress and the Healthy Family.* Minneapolis, MN: Winston Press.

Feetham, S. (1983). Feetham Family Functioning Survey. Available from Suzanne Feetham, National Center for Nursing Research, Office of Planning Analysis Evaluation, Building 31, Room 5BO9, Rockville Pike, Bethesda, MD 20882.

Friedman, M. M. (1998). *Family Nursing: Research, Theory and Practice,* ed 4. Norwalk, CT: Appleton & Lange.

Grotevant, H. D. (1989). The role of theory in guiding family assessment. *Journal of Family Psychology, 3*:104–117.

Hanson, S. M. H. (1985). Family health inventory: A measurement. Paper presented at the National Council of Family Relations, Dallas, TX.

Hanson, S. M. H. (1986). Healthy Single Parent Families. *Family Relations, 35*:125–132.

Hanson, S.M.H. (1996). Family nursing assessment and intervention. In S.M.H. Hanson & S.T. Boyd, (Eds). *Family Health Care Nursing: Theory, Practice, and Research.* Philadelphia: F.A. Davis.

Hanson, S.M.H. & Boyd, S.T. (1996). *Family Health Care Nursing: Theory, Practice, and Research.* Philadelphia: F.A. Davis.

Hanson, S.M.H, & Kaakinen, J. (1996). Family assessment. In M. Stanhope & J. Lancaster (Eds.) *Community Health Nursing: Process and Practice for Promoting Health.* St. Louis: Mosby.

Hanson, S.M.H., & Mischke, K.M. (1996). Family health assessment and intervention. In P.J. Bomar (Ed) (1996) *Nurses and Family Health Promotion: Concepts, Assessment and Interventions,* ed 2, chapter 12, pp. 165–202. Philadelphia: W.B. Saunders.

Hartman, A., & Laird, J. (1983). *Family-Centered Social Work Practice.* New York: Free Press.

Kissman, K., & Allen, J. A. (1993). *Single-parent families.* Newbury Park, CA: Sage.

Maturana, H. & Varela, F. (1992). *The Tree of Knowledge: The Biological Roots of Human Understanding.* Boston: Sambhala Publications, Inc.

McCubbin, M. A., & McCubbin, H. L. (1993). Families coping with illness: The resiliency model of family stress, adjustment, and adaptation. In C. B. Danielson, et al. (Eds.) *Families, Health, and Illness: Perspectives on Coping and Intervention,* pp. 21–64. St. Louis: Mosby.

McGoldrick, M., & Gerson, R. (1985). *Genograms in Family Assessment.* New York: W. W. Norton.

McGoldrick, M., et al. (1999). *Genograms: Assessment and Intervention,* ed 2. NY: W.W. Norton & Company.

Mischke-Berkey, K., et al. (1989). Family health assessment and intervention. In P. J. Bomar (Ed.) *Nurses and Family Health Promotion: Concepts, Assessment, and Interventions* (pp. 115–154). Baltimore: Williams & Wilkins.

Neuman, B. (1995). The Neuman systems model. In B. Neuman (Ed.), *The Neuman Systems Model*, ed 3. Norwalk, CT: Appleton & Lange.

Nurse, A.R. (1999). *Family Assessment: Effective Uses of Personality Tests with Couples and Families.* NY: John Wiley & Sons.

Pender, N., et al. (1992). Health promotion and disease prevention: Toward excellence in nursing practice and education. *Nursing Outlook, 40*:106–109.

Reed, K. S. (1993). Betty Neuman: *The Neuman Systems Model.* Newbury Park, CA: Sage.

Ross, B., & Cobb, K. L. (1990). *Family Nursing: A Nursing Process Approach.* Redwood City, CA: Addison-Wesley.

Toman, W. (1976). *Family Constellation: Its Effect on Personality and Social Behavior*, ed 3. NY: Springer.

Touliatos, J., et al. (Eds.) (1990). *Handbook of Family Measurement Techniques.* Newbury Park, CA: Sage.

von Bertalanffy, L. (1972). The history and status of general systems theory. In G. Klir (Ed.), *Trends in General Systems Theory.* New York: John Wiley & Sons.

von Bertalanffy, L. (1974). General systems theory. In S. Arieti (Ed.) *American Handbook of Psychiatry*, pp. 1095–1117. New York: Basic Books.

Waltz, C.E., Strickland, D.L. & Lenz, E.R. (1991). *Measurement in Nursing Research*, ed. 2. Philadelphia: F.A. Davis.

Watzlawick, P., et al. (1967). *Pragmatics of Human Communication.* New York: W. W. Norton.

Watzlawick, P., et al. (1974). *Change: Principles of Problem Formulation and Problem Resolution.* New York: W. W. Norton.

Wright, L. M., & Leahey, M. (2000). *Nurses and Families: A Guide to Family Assessment and Intervention,* ed 3. Philadelphia: F. A. Davis.

Bibliography

Bowen, M. (1994). *Family Therapy in Clinical Practice.* New York: John Wiley & Sons.

Broome, M.E., et al. (1998). *Children and Families in Health and Illness.* Thousand Oaks, CA: Sage.

Carter, B., & McGoldrick, M. (1999). *The Expanded Family Life Cycle: Individual, Family, and Social Perspectives,* ed 3. Boston: Allyn & Bacon.

Clemen-Stone, S., et al. (1991). *Comprehensive Family Community Health Nursing,* ed 3. St. Louis: C. V. Mosby.

Danielson, C. B., et al. (Eds.) (1993). *Families, Health and Illness: Perspectives on Coping and Intervention.* St. Louis: Mosby.

Feetham, S. L., et al. (Eds.). (1993). *The Nursing of Families: Theory, Research, Education, Practice.* Newbury Park, CA: Sage.

Freeman, R. B., & Heinrich, J. (1981). *Community Health Nursing Practice,* ed 2. Philadelphia: W. B. Saunders.

Friedman, M.L. (1991). *The Framework of Systemic Organization: A Conceptual Approach to Families and Nursing.* Thousand Oaks, CA: Sage.

Gilliss, C. L., et al. (Eds.). (1989). *Toward a Science of Family Nursing.* Menlo Park, CA: Addison-Wesley.

Hanson, S. M. H. (1987). Family nursing and chronic illness. In M. Leahey & L. Wright (Eds.) *Families and Chronic Illness,* pp. 2–32. Springhouse, PA: Springhouse.

Holt, S., & Robinson, T. (1979). The school nurse's assessment tool. *American Journal of Nursing,* 79:950–953.

Leslie, G. F., & Korman, S. K. (1989). *The Family in Social Context,* ed 7. New York: Oxford University Press.

Nettle, C., et al. (1993). Family as client: Using Gordon's health pattern typology. *Journal of Community Health Nursing,* 10:53–61.

Parsons, T., & Bales, R. F. (1955). *Family Socialization and Interaction Process.* New York: Free Press.

Pearson, A., & Vaughan, B. (1986). *Nursing Models for Practice.* Rockville, MD: Aspen.

Stanhope, M., & Lancaster, J. (1992). *Community Health Nursing: Process and Practice for Promoting Health,* ed 3. St. Louis: Mosby.

Tomm, K., & Sanders, G. (1983). Family assessment in a problem-oriented record. In J. C. Hansen & B. F., Keeney (Eds.), *Diagnosis and Assessment in Family Therapy,* pp. 101–122. London: Aspen.

Vaughan-Cole, B., et al. (1998). *Family Nursing Practice.* Philadelphia: W.B. Saunders.

von Bertalanffy, L. (1968). *General Systems Theory: Foundations, Development, Applications.* New York: George Braziller.

Walsh, F. (1993). *Normal Family Processes,* ed 2. NY: The Guiford Press.

Wegner, G. B., & Alexander, R. J. (Eds.). (1993). *Readings in Family Nursing.* Philadelphia: J. B. Lippincott. Foundations of Family Health Care Nursing Family Assessment and Intervention.

Wright, L.M., et al. (1996). *Beliefs: The Heart of Healing in Families and Illness.* New York: Basic Books.

Focus On

FAMILY HEALTH PROMOTION

The education of nurses generally focuses on illness of individuals and how nurses manage human responses to illness. The concept of family health promotion provides an additional critical element in the conceptual foundation of professional nursing practice with individuals and their families.

This chapter begins with a brief overview of the history of health promotion and its historical relevance to family nursing in the United States. The discussion of family health and family health promotion will provide you with a clear understanding of these terms, their conceptual origins, and their contemporary applications. Models of both family health and family health promotion will assist you in distinguishing them in practice.

External and internal ecosystem variables influencing family health promotion are carefully described and will add to your understanding of sociocultural influences on families. You are urged to consider the influence of these factors on the roles of family nurses as described in Chapter 7. The discussion of nursing process for family health promotion uses health promotion as an organizing framework on which to base nursing actions with family clients. A discussion of the importance of family health promotion to family nursing practice, education, family policy, and research conclude the chapter.

Chapter 9

FAMILY HEALTH PROMOTION

Perri J. Bomar • Pammela Baker-Word

OUTLINE

OBJECTIVES

On completion of this chapter, the reader will be able to:

- Define family health and family health promotion.
- Understand the concept of family health promotion as distinct from but interrelated with individual health promotion.
- Trace the historical development of family health promotion.
- Describe selected models of family health.
- Explain variables influencing family health promotion.
- Describe the nursing interventions that facilitate family health promotion.

- Examine the role of the nurse in family health promotion in nursing practice, education, policy, and research.

Although the majority of health care professionals continue to focus their activities on prevention and treatment of illness in individuals and dysfunctional families, key social forces, including the wellness and self-care movement of the past 30 years, continue to stimulate the nursing profession to focus on health promotion for families. The 1980 White House Conference on Families pointed out the need to improve family functioning and encourage healthy family lifestyles. The conference brought to light the importance of disease prevention and health promotion for improving the quality of family life in the United States. Three documents from the U.S. Department of Health and Human Services: *Healthy People: The Surgeon General's Report on Health Promotion and Disease Prevention* (1979); *Promoting Health/Preventing Disease: Objectives for the Nation* (1980); and *Healthy People 2000: National Health Promotion and Disease Prevention Objectives* (1990) provided overall goals for the nation regarding health promotion for individuals and families. Although there are many improvements in the health status of the nation as a whole, the newest document *Healthy People 2010* (1998) builds on the lessons learned from the three previous documents. The goals for the year 2010 are to eliminate health disparities and to increase the quality and years of life. Major objectives for the new millennium include promoting healthy behaviors, promoting healthy and safe communities, improving systems for personal and public health, and preventing and reducing diseases and disorders. Box 9–1 lists target health behaviors for each objective.

An example of a targeted objective that can be facilitated by family health promotion is reducing violent and abusive behavior. Family communication patterns, power issues, decision making, and excessive punitive discipline contribute to violent behaviors. Negative expression of anger, poor media role models, and inadequate conflict resolution also influence the likelihood of violent or abusive behaviors within the family. Teaching individuals and families strategies to prevent abusive or violent incidents will enhance a family unit's quality of health.

Since the first report by the Surgeon General in 1979 and the continued national interest on health promotion the 1990s, health professionals, family scientists, sociologists, psychologists, religious leaders, and social workers have made considerable strides in understanding and intervening to improve the quality of family life. For example, the National Council of Family Relations (NCFR) established a section on family health in 1984. Members include health professionals with special interest in the health and illness of families across the lifespan. Another example of this continuing national interest in health promotion is the increasing use of parish nurses, who provide health care and health promotion to individuals and families in faith communities (Solari-Twadell, et al., 1999). "Health for All" is also a priority of the World Health Organization (WHO) for the twenty-first century; WHO will use the strategies recommended by *Healthy People 2010* as a framework for improving the quality of life for the world population.

FAMILY HEALTH AND FAMILY HEALTH PROMOTION

Fostering the health of the family unit as a whole and encouraging families to value and incorporate health promotion into their lifestyles are essential components of family nursing practice. Health promotion is learned within families, in which beliefs, values, and patterns of health behaviors are formed and passed on to future generations. The family is primarily responsible for providing health and illness care, being a role model, teaching self-care and wellness behaviors, providing for care for members across their lifespan and during varied family transitions, and supporting each other during health-promoting activities and acute and chronic illnesses. A major task of the family is to teach health maintenance and promotion. Individual members and the family as a whole must be taught health promotion, regardless of age. The case study at the end of the chapter describes a family scenario in which lifestyle changes would improve the mother's and the whole family's health. The role of the nurse is to help families attain, maintain, and regain the highest level of family health possible.

Definitions

The terms "family health" and "family health promotion" are not interchangeable. The term *family health* is a holistic term, which refers to both functional and dysfunctional families. The term further encompasses the biological, psychological, sociological, spiritual, and cultural aspects of family life (see Chapter 1 for a discussion of other definitions). *Family health promotion* is defined as achieving family well-being.

Box 9-1

HEALTHY PEOPLE 2010 OBJECTIVES

A. Goals

1. Increase quality and years of healthy life
2. Eliminate health disparities

B. Objectives

Promote Healthy Behaviors

1. Physical activity and fitness
2. Nutrition
3. Eliminate tobacco use

Promote Healthy and Safe Communities

4. Educational and community-based programs
5. Environmental health
6. Foot safety
7. Injury and violence prevention
    a. Injuries that cut across intent
    b. Unintentional injuries
    c. Violence and abuse
8. Occupational safety and health
9. Oral health

Improve Systems for Personal and Public Health

10. Access to quality health services
    a. Preventive care
    b. Primary care
    c. Emergency services
    d. Long-term care and rehabilitative services
11. Family planning
12. Maternal, infant, and child health
13. Medical product safety
14. Public health infrastructure
15. Health communication

Prevent and Reduce Diseases and Disorders

16. Arthritis, osteoporosis, and chronic back conditions
17. Cancer
18. Diabetes
19. Disability and secondary conditions
20. Heart disease and stroke
21. HIV infection
22. Immunization and infectious diseases
23. Mental health and mental disorders
24. Respiratory diseases
25. Sexually transmitted diseases
26. Substance abuse

US Department of Health and Human Services (1998). Healthy People 2010: National Health Promotion and Disease Prevention Objectives. (Department of Health and Human Services, Office of Public Health and Science). Washington, DC: US Government Printing Office.

Family Health

As discussed in Chapter 1, definitions of family health have evolved from anthropological, biopsychosocial, developmental, family science, religious, cultural, and nursing paradigms. They vary depending on their origin (Anderson & Tomlinson, 1992; Bomar & McNeeley, 1996; Doherty & Campbell, 1988). Family scientists define healthy families as resilient (McCubbin & McCubbin, 1993) and possessing a balance of cohesion and adaptability that is facilitated by good communication (Olson, et al., 1989). Family therapy definitions often emphasize optimal family functioning and freedom from psychopathology (Bradshaw, 1988). Within the developmental framework, healthy families complete developmental tasks at appropriate times (Duval & Miller, 1985). Taking a sociological view, Pratt (1976) describes a healthy family as an *energized family:* a family that responds to the needs and interests of all its members, copes effectively with life transitions and problems, is flexible and egalitarian in distribution of power, interacts regularly among its members and with the community, and encompasses a health-promoting lifestyle of individual members and the family unit.

Other definitions include the totality, or *gestalt,* of the family's existence and include the internal and external environment of the family. A holistic definition of family health encompasses all the aspects of family life, including interaction and the health care functions. The family health care function includes family nutrition, recreation, communication, sleep and rest patterns, problem solving, sexuality, use of time and space, coping with stress, hygiene and safety, spirituality, illness care, health promotion and protection, and emotional health of family members (Bomar, 1996; Friedman, 1998). A healthy family has a sense of well-being and is free from dysfunction (see Chapter 1). In summary, *family health* is a dynamic and complex state. In a healthy family, there is a sense of belonging and connectedness in family interactions; the family is flexible and adapts easily; and they work together to maintain the unit. Family health is more than the absence of disease in an individual family member or absence of dysfunction in family dynamics; rather, it is a state of family well-being.

The *characteristics of a healthy family* have been described by a number of authors (Curran, 1983; DeFrain & Stinnett, 1992; McCubbin & McCubbin, 1993; Olson & DeFrain, 1994). Table 9-1 summarizes the characteristics of healthy families described in the literature.

Models

Building on Smith's (1983) models of health, Loveland-Cherry (1986) suggests that there are four views of family health:

1. The *clinical model.* Examined from this perspective, a family is healthy if its members are free of physical, mental, and social dysfunction.
2. The *role-performance model.* This view of family health is based on the idea that family health is the ability of family members to perform their routine roles and achieve developmental tasks.
3. The *adaptive model.* In this model, families are adaptive if they have the ability to change and grow and possess the capacity to rebound quickly after a crisis.
4. The *eudaimonistic model.* Professionals who use this model as their philosophy of practice focus on efforts to maximize the family's well-being and to support the entire family and individual members in reaching their highest potential.

According to Loveland-Cherry, these family health models are useful in three ways: (1) they provide frameworks for understanding the level of health that families are experiencing; (2) they may be useful in designing interventions to assist families in maintaining or regaining good health or in coping with illness; (3) they may facilitate organization of the family nursing literature and serve as a focus for family research. There are numerous models that incorporate the stages of wellness and illness and explain the impact of illness on individuals and families.

Family Cycle of Health and Illness

Danielson, Hamel-Bissell, and Winstead-Fry (1993) synthesize the previous work of Doherty and McCubbin (1985) and of Coe (1970) in their model of the family cycle of health and illness. Table 9-2 outlines this model, which depicts the dynamic movement between the phases of illness and wellness. Families do not always progress sequentially from one phase to another; some phases may be bypassed. For example, if an illness is transitory and brief (such as influenza), the family rapidly passes from a healthy state to experiencing symptoms, the sick role, medical consultation, adaptation, and then back to a healthy state. In transitory illness, the process takes about 10 days. On the other hand, in the case of a chronic disease, the stages are longer and require more permanent family adjust-

TABLE 9-1
Traits of a Healthy Family

Unity	
Commitment	• Develops a sense of trust • Teaches respect for others • Exhibits a sense of shared responsibility
Time Together	• Shares family rituals and traditions • Enjoys each other's company • Shares leisure time • Shares simple and quality time
Flexibility	
Ability to Deal with Stress	• Displays adaptability • Sees crises as a challenge and opportunity • Shows openness to change • Grows together in crisis • Seeks help with problems
Spiritual Well-being	• Encourages hope • Shares faith • Teaches compassion for others • Teaches ethical values • Respects the privacy of one another
Communication	
Positive Communication	• Communicates and listens effectively • Fosters family table time and conversation • Shares feelings • Displays nonblaming attitudes • Is able to compromise and disagree • Agrees to disagree
Appreciation and Affection	• Cares for each other • Exhibits a sense of humor • Maintains friendship • Respects individuality • Has a spirit of playfulness

Source: Curran, D. (1983). *Traits of a Healthy Family.* Minneapolis, MN: Winston Press. (pp. 23–24). Olson, D., & DeFrain, J. (1994). *Marriage and the Family: Diversity and Strengths.* Mountain View, CA: Mayfield.

ments and adaptations. During each phase, the family and its members engage in activities to foster family health and attain optimal levels of functioning.

Phases of the Cycle

Family health promotion and risk reduction is the first phase of the cycle. During this phase, the family engages in a variety of activities to improve and maintain the health of individual members and promote family functioning. For example, one health-promoting behavior is spending an evening together as a family.

The second phase in the health and illness cycle is the *family vulnerability and symptom experience phase,* when the family perceives that its members are vulnerable and takes action to reduce the risk of illness of a member or the risk of family dysfunction. Examples of risk reduction behaviors include routine breast self-examination, keeping up with recommended immunizations, and regularly scheduled family meetings to solve problems related to family risk reduction. During this phase, some families may use folk and home remedies for illnesses and consult their social network for advice.

If symptoms persist or adequate resources are not available, the family may then decide to make contact with a health professional. This decision initiates the third phase assumption of the *family illness appraisal and sick role.* During the third phase, the family accepts the sick role of the family member, evaluates potential threats or loss from the illness and their resources, and makes adjustments in family activities and the family lifestyle to accommodate the illness (Danielson, et al., 1993).

In the fourth phase, the family *consults the health care system for diagnosis* of the illness and to assist the family in understanding the health problem. The level of family communication contributes significantly to family understanding and negotiating in this phase.

After the diagnosis is obtained, the family begins the fifth phase, which is called the *family acute response.* The illness may progress to become acute or chronic, or it may result in death. If the ill member is cured and gives up the sick role, the family returns to the first phase: family health promotion and risk reduction. If the illness continues, the family becomes a family with a chronically ill family member.

The sixth phase is the period of *recovery and rehabilitation,* in which the major tasks are relinquishment of the sick role, establishment of new patterns of family life, and return to the first phase. Long-term chronic diseases or severe disabilities bring about the seventh phase: *chronic adjustment adaptation.* The family's ability to cope with the illness is influenced by their resources and their ability to adapt during crisis (McCubbin & McCubbin, 1993).

TABLE 9-2
Phases of the Family Cycle of Health and Illness

Phase	Description
Family Health Promotion and Risk Reduction	The family develops and instills beliefs, values, and patterns that promote a healthy lifestyle and reduce the risk of disease or family dysfunction.
Family Vulnerability and Symptoms of Illness	Members are vulnerable to disease or the family unit vulnerable to dysfunction, stress, or crisis, and are aware that illness or dysfunction is present.
Family Illness Appraisal and Assumption of Sick Role	The family gives meaning to the illness or situation. This phase includes initial role changes that give evidence of illness.
Contact with the Health Care System and Diagnosis of the Problem or Illness	Family seeks to make the sick role or problem legitimate. Family acceptance of the diagnosis or solution.
Family Acute Response	The family makes adjustments in response to an illness or situation. This includes making arrangements in the family to care for the ill member, temporary role changes, and financial management.
Family Adaptation to Illness and Recovery	Incorporation of the illness or event into the family lifestyle while attempting to return to normalcy in family roles, structures, functions, and interactions.
Death of a Family Member and Recovery	Family adjustments and adaptations to the death of a member. This includes the period of grief and the role adjustments involved in recovery as a healthy family of a different type.

Source: Doherty, W.J. & Campbell, T.L. (1988). *Families and Health.* Newbury Park: Sage. Danielson, C., Hamel-Bissel, B. & Winstead-Fry, P. (1993) *Families in Health and Illness* (pp. 65–91). St. Louis: Mosby.

After the death of a family member, the family enters the eighth phase, *death and family reorganization,* which includes the stressful processes of family grieving and reorganization of both family and extrafamilial roles and functions. After completing reorganization, the family unit returns to the first phase of the cycle.

Family Health Promotion

Family health promotion occurs in the first phase of the family health and illness cycle. As described in Chapter 1, there is a lack of agreement on the definition of family health promotion. Bomar (1996) defines *family health promotion* as behaviors of the family that are undertaken to increase the family's well-being or quality of life. According to Pender (1996), family health promotion denotes family activities directed toward increasing their level of well-being and actualizing their potential. It involves the family's lifelong efforts to nurture its members, to maintain family cohesion, and to reach the family's highest potential in all aspects of health. In the past, most of the attention of health professionals has focused on individuals and family subsystems (marital and parent-child dyads) and community health problems. There is a great need to encourage health promotion of the whole family unit, because health behaviors, values, and patterns are learned within a family context. Family health promotion activities are crucial during both wellness and illness of a family member. For example, if one member is ill, the family may work together to provide for the physical needs of the sick person. At the same time, they must provide respite for the primary caregiver, so that this family member has time for health-promoting and health-protecting activities. Examples of family health promotion are planning to have mealtimes together and nurturing the needs of all family members during an illness.

Family health promotion refers to activities families engage in to strengthen the family as a unit. The goal of these activities is to attain, retain, or regain the emotional and physical health of all family members. For example, in the Budd family, health promotion can be enhanced through planning consistent family time. (For the Budd family story, see the case study at the end of the chapter.)

Family recreation and leisure time spent together promote family cohesion, unity, and bonding. For the Budds, participation in family time and sharing of responsibilities could serve to reduce Eleanor's stress. During interactions, the family may think of ways for each member to assist in maintaining the family routines, chores, and activities.

Models

Most models of health promotion focus on the individual. Adapting Pender's (1996) health promotion model, Loveland-Cherry (1996) suggests a family health promotion model.

In this model, the probability of a family engaging in health promotion behaviors is influenced by the following factors relating to general health and specific behaviors:

General factors
Family systems patterns
Demographics
Biological characteristics

Health-related factors
Family health socialization patterns
Family definition of health
Perceived family health status

Behavior-specific factors
Perceived barriers to health-promoting behavior
Perceived benefits to health-promoting behavior
Previous related behavior
Family norms
Intersystem support for behavior
Situational influences
Internal family cues

Pearsall (1990) offers a lay model for family health promotion in his book *Power of the Family: Strength, Comfort, and Healing*. He encourages families to use their inner resources to strengthen, comfort, and heal family relationships. The major focus is on lifelong family unity and caring, using 10 strategies that he calls the "Rx For a Health Family" (Box 9-2). Nurses could encourage families to work together and use these strategies to promote health in family life.

In the past decade, family health promotion has received considerable emphasis in nursing and related fields. However, reports on the effectiveness of family-focused health promotion interventions are limited. In a study of parents' health-promoting lifestyles, Bomar (1991) noted significant changes in lifestyles 6 months after a family contracted with a family nurse to make one change in lifestyle patterns. There is a need for more research on the effectiveness of interventions to promote family health.

ECOSYSTEM FACTORS

Family health promotion is the by-product of interactions with both external ecosystems and internal family processes (Bomar, 1996). External ecosystem factors include such things as the national economy, family and health policy, societal and cultural norms, media, and environmental hazards (e.g., noise, air, and soil pollution; overcrowding; chemical wastes). Internal ecosystem factors include family type, family lifestyle patterns, family processes, the personalities of family members, power structure, family role models, coping strategies and processes, resilience, and culture.

External Factors

National Economy

The national economy directly affects the family's economic health. The availability of jobs to meet the family's basic and health promotion needs directly affects the quality of a family's lifestyle. In addition, the availability of goods and services (e.g., food, clothing, shelter, medical care, insurance, transportation, and recreation) is basic to survival. In the past, the primary targets for health promotion programs were the workplace, some schools, and the middle class. Emphasis has been placed on preventing heart disease by cessation of smoking, improved nutrition, and moderate exercise. Until the mid-1980s, little attention was given to the health of minorities, people of low income, and elderly people (U.S. Department of Health and Human Services [USDHHS], 1985). With the adoption of *Healthy People 2000* and *Healthy People 2010,* the focus has moved more toward alleviating health disparities in the total population with health promotion and disease prevention as priorities (USDHHS, 1990; USDHHS, 1998).

Family Economic Resources

When a family has economic health, they have the resources needed for family health promotion. Adequate family income contributes to emotional well-being and supplies resources for family recreation and leisure. Socioeconomic class is a crucial ingredient in family health promotion. Middle- and upper-class families are more likely than low-income families to engage in health-promoting and preventive activities. The cost of buying recreational and exercise equipment and apparel or paying for recreational activities is often beyond the means of low-income families. The activities

Box 9-2

RX FOR A HEALTHY FAMILY

Families are encouraged to consider the following strategies to promote family health:

- **Family *Rituals*** are the receptive behaviors or activities between two or more family members that occur with regularity in day-to-day activities. Examples are a hug when a member leaves or returns, saying grace at meals, bedtime stories for children, and so forth. Rituals provide security and attachment to oneness (unity) of the family system.
- **Family *Rhythm*** is learning to do things together. This is a calm moving together in harmony during the family activities of daily living.
- **Family *Reason*** is being reasonable during irrational times. Is there fairness and effort on everyone's part to reduce conflict? Recognition that family health is created not by being an actor but rather by interaction with others.
- **Family *Remembrance*** is keeping of the family heritage, respect for family history, and learning from the conflicts of members from the previous generation.
- **Family *Resilience*** is the process of staying together through the stresses of life, to tolerate and grow as a unit with family spirit.
- **Family *Resonance*** is making good family "vibes." It is a sense of the family as a unit of energy, rather than a group of individuals. Family members are free to self-actualize as well as work together for family unity.
- **Family *Reconciliation*** is the process of getting back together again after conflict. This includes always forgiving, tolerating, and loving, no matter what the family problem. Not allowing anything to destroy the family because lack of forgiveness leads to a life of regret.
- **Family *Reverence*** is protecting the dignity of the family unit by concern for "us." It means having a pride and respect for the uniqueness of the family unit and an "enduring commitment to the eternal unity of the family."
- **Family *Revival*** is quick recovery from family conflicts, arguments, and feuds.
- **Family *Reunion*** is the process of assembling the family for the purpose of celebrating life together, maintaining family cohesion, comforting one another, learning from each other, and loving.

Source: Pearsall, P. (1990). *The Power of the Family: Strength, Comfort, and Healing.* New York: Doubleday, with permission.

of low-income families are often directed toward meeting basic needs; providing for food, shelter, and safety; and curing acute illness, rather than prevention or health promotion. Achieving better health for vulnerable and low-income families in adverse family circumstances should be a goal for health professionals (Aday, 1993).

Family Policies

The United States does not have a specific national family policy. Historically, policy has focused on individuals rather than families. Even though there was a White House Conference on Families in 1980, there are still only a few policies specific to families. Debates on family policies are often highly politicized, and there is great disagreement about the need to provide family housing, universal access to health care, intergenerational supports, and consideration for family diversity (Wisensale, 1993). The recent overhaul of the nation's welfare program (titled "Temporary Assistance to Needy Families") shifted the primary administrative burden from the federal government to the state and local governments. The effects of this legislation could lead to increased stressors on impoverished, underserved families (Hagen, 1999). (For additional information on the impact of national social policies on family life, see Chapter 16.)

Health Policies

Health policies at state, county, and city levels also affect the quality of family health. Local communities provide water and monitor its quality, maintain sanitation, develop and maintain parks for recreation, and provide health services to low-income and elder families. Such local services enhance the health of individuals and enhance family health. At the state level, services include assistance with medical care through Medicaid, the maintenance of state recreational areas and parks, health promotion and prevention programs, and economic assistance for low-income families. Additional federal-level policies and fiscal support are needed to improve the quality of family health; in particular, there is a need for:

- Primary care for individuals across the life span
- Child care policy
- Agencies that monitor and develop legislation and implement health policies
- Economic support for vulnerable families
- More national parks and recreation areas
- Research on families and family health

Many of the objectives in *Healthy People 2000* and *Healthy People 2010* are couched in terms of individuals; however, many of these objectives can only be attained by providing access to health care for families and changing family health lifestyles (Shi & Singh, 1998). In a nation of culturally diverse individuals and families (because of the number of different government agencies involved in health care and family issues), there is a need for collaboration among these policy-making bodies (Aday, 1993). Gebby, in Chapter 16, discusses policies related to caregiving, child care, education, and welfare in more detail.

Environment

Family nurses must be aware of environmental issues that affect health. According to Wiley (1996), the family living environment (visible and invisible) is crucial. The family and its members are exposed to public, occupational, and residential hazards. All environmental hazards are not consistently monitored. It is imperative to teach families to prevent, remove, or develop methods for coping with environmental hazards, such as noise, air, soil, and chemical pollution (Garman, 1995).

Media

The visual and print media are another influence on family health. Many advertisements advocate consumption of foods high in sugar, salt, and alcoholic beverages, as well as the use of tobacco products. Health promotion advertisements have generally targeted the more health-conscious middle-class person, rather than the vulnerable and underserved person, who is often the target for alcohol and tobacco advertising campaigns. Recent tobacco legislation, which was widely covered by the media, is a small step in the right direction toward promoting healthier families.

Science and Technology

Advances in science and technology have increased the life span of Americans, decreased the length of hospital stays, and contributed to our understanding of how to prevent, reduce, and treat disease. The development of more effective medications and advanced medical equipment technology has greatly increased the feasibility of home health care for chronically ill family members of all ages. Families are often the caregivers for ill members, and they provide the majority of care for older adults. There are now many valuable sources of information on health promotion for families and individuals. The Internet and the World Wide Web are a forum that is fast becoming important in family life education and health promotion (Elliot, 1999).

Internal Factors

Family Type and Development

The family type (e.g., vulnerable, secure, durable, or regenerative) affects the health and well-being of its members (McCubbin & McCubbin, 1993). Families who are flexible and able to adjust to change are more likely to be involved in health-promoting activities. Vulnerable families are often coping with a pileup of stressors and may be unable to focus on activities to enhance health (Hertz & Ferguson, 1997). When families experience transitions, changes in their health-promoting lifestyles are often required (Faux, 1998). Thus, when a family member becomes ill, the health-promoting activities of the caretakers are generally curtailed. Often, the well-being of the family and caregiver is compromised, beginning with the third phase of the family health and illness cycle and continuing to the end of the eighth phase (i.e., from the sick role and family appraisal to the chronic illness phase or death and reorganization phase). The stages of family development, including childbearing, school-age launching, retirement, and the accomplishment of developmental tasks, also significantly influence a family's health (Grove, 1996). For example, in the case study, Eleanor's ability to reach her potential is influenced by the fact that her children are of school age and that she and her husband are a dual-career couple.

Family Structure

Families in the 1990s, and into the new millennium, are quite different from the families of the 1970s. Family structures are more diverse; there are more dual-career, dual-earner families; blended families; and single-parent families. Vulnerable families have also increased: low-income traditional and migrant families, homeless families, and low-income older adults. Included in the vulnerable population are low-income, single-parent families and single-parent teen families. Health promotion for these different types of family presents various challenges (Pender, 1996). For example, a single, working parent may lack parent-child time, experience role stress, or have poor lifestyle patterns and poor life satisfaction (Hanson, 1996; Loveland-Cherry, 1986; Wijnberg & Weinger, 1998). Low-income families may focus less on health promotion and more on the basic needs of obtaining shelter, adequate food, and health care.

Family Processes

Family processes are continual actions, or series of changes, that take place in the family experience. Essential processes of a healthy family include functional communication (Miller et al., 1991) and family interaction. Through both verbal and nonverbal communication, parents teach behavior, share feelings and values, and make decisions about family health practices. It is through communication that families adapt to transitions and develop cohesiveness (Olson, et al., 1989). Positive, reinforcing interaction between family members leads to a healthier family lifestyle. For optimal health promotion to take place, families must use their natural support systems (McGoldrick & Giordano, 1996). Social support networks (Roth, 1996) likewise enhance family health.

Culture

The influences of culture on family beliefs, attitudes, lifestyle patterns, and health behaviors are discussed in Chapter 4. Often, different cultures define and value health, health promotion, and disease prevention differently (Huff & Kline, 1999). There is a mounting trend toward a global society with ever-increasing diversity among the populations. An expanded world view is necessary for health care students and providers (Purnell and Paulanka, 1998). Clients may not respond to the family nurse's suggestions for health promotion because the suggestions conflict with their health beliefs and values. Hence, it is crucial to assess and understand the family culture and health beliefs before suggesting changes in health behavior (Lipson, 1998).

Family Lifestyle Patterns

Lifestyle patterns affect family health. In America, there are hundreds of thousands of unnecessary fatalities each year that can be directly attributed to unhealthy lifestyles (Friedman, 1998). These deaths can be traced back to heart disease, hypertension, cancer, cirrhosis of the liver, diabetes, suicide, and homicide. When family members engage often in leisure activities, recreation, and exercise, they are better able to cope with day-to-day problems (McCown, 1996). In addition, time together often promotes family closeness. In families with children, parents teach health practices and beliefs. Moreover, healthy lifestyle practices, such as good eating habits (James, 1996), good sleep patterns (Kick, 1996), proper hygiene, and positive approaches to stress management (McCubbin & McCubbin, 1993), are passed from one generation to another. Also, when one family member initiates a health behavior change, other family members often make a change too. For example, when an individual family member changes eating patterns, perhaps by going on a diet, other family members often change their eating pattern. Moreno (1975) calls this process "vertical diffusion."

Family Role Models

Family members provide both negative and positive role models (Friedman, 1992, 1998). For example, smoking, use of drugs and alcohol, poor nutrition, and inactivity are often intergenerational patterns (Crooks et al., 1987; Loveland-Cherry, 1996). Stress management, exercise, and communication are learned from parents, siblings, and extended family members, such as grandparents (Duffy, 1986). This patterning of behavior, be it positive or negative, is integral to the overall family health and well-being (Anderson, 1992). Health professionals can promote positive family role modeling by teaching health in the community, the churches, and the workplace.

Religion and Spirituality

Other factors that influence family health promotion include religion and spirituality (Warner, 1996). A review of the research on religion and family health by Thomas and Cornwall (1990) suggests there is a significant positive relationship between religion and marital well-being and satisfaction. In a study of 225 families in California, on a nine-item religiousness scale, family religiousness was positively related to general well-being and social relations (Ranson et al., 1992). Further, in a study of the health of 42 single-parent families, Hanson (1986) found a significant positive relationship between religiousness and a child's mental and physical health. Religion is a significant factor in family health (Solari-Twadell, 1999). Religion shapes family health values, practices, and beliefs and may be a positive force in family life because it:

- Provides a source of social support and belonging
- Encourages family togetherness through family activities and recreation
- Provides a sense of meaning in family life
- Promotes love, hope, faith, trust, forgiveness, forbearance, goodness, self-control, morality, justice, and peace
- Encourages the use of divine assistance during times of family stress and crisis
- Teaches reverence for family life (Abbott et al., 1990; Brigman, 1992; Warner, 1996)

The social support of religion and the clergy is particularly helpful during family transitions (Warner, 1996). Many churches have support groups and are a valuable resource for single parents, stepfamilies, single adults, bereaved persons, widows and widowers, unemployed workers, and parents of young children. To meet spiritual needs, many congregations hire pastors for a family life ministry, healing ministries (emotional healing and health promotion), ministry to youth and single adults, and senior ministry.

Religion aids in family coping responses (Friedman, 1998). To provide holistic care, the nurse needs to assess a family's spiritual health, support the family's spiritual beliefs, assist families to meet their spiritual needs, provide spiritual resources for family transitions and lifestyle changes, and assist families to find meaning in their circumstances (Carson, 1989; Warner, 1996; Brigman, 1992; Solari-Twadell & McDermott, 1999). Such activity is validated by findings that families are spiritually strengthened by togetherness, making the family a priority, honor and respect for each family member, support of the needs of individuation, commitment to the family, daily prayer, dedication, renewal, honesty, and integrity (Friedemann, 1995; Warner, 1996).

THE NURSING PROCESS FOR HEALTH PROMOTION

Family nurses have a crucial role in facilitating health promotion and wellness in all stages of family development. Enhancing the well-being of the family unit is essential during periods of wellness, as well as during illness, recovery, and stress. Holistic wellness is a lifestyle that provides a family with an opportunity to reach its highest potential (Ma & Wenk, 1997). A primary goal of nursing care for families is empowering family members to work together to attain and maintain family health. Family nursing that focuses on health promotion should be logical and systematic and include the clients. The family nursing process for health promotion includes: family assessment; intervention for health promotion, which includes contracting and goal setting, empowerment, encouraging family confluence, anticipatory guidance, and health teaching; evaluation; and follow-up. The reader is encouraged to consult Chapters 7 and 8 for additional discussion of aspects of the family nursing process and family assessment. Also, for specific measures of family health promotion, see Bomar's *Nurses and Family Health Promotion* (1996).

According to Pender (1996), there are four phases in the nurse-client relationship: the initial phase, the transition phase, the working phase, and the step-down and follow-up phase.

During the initial *contact phase,* the nurse identifies the need for health care. This is followed by the *transition phase,* in which the client decides whether to continue the nurse-client relationship. Commitment to do so may be demonstrated by signing a contract.

In the *working phase,* the energies of both the nurse and client are expended to meet the stated goals. This is a process requiring that the nurse and client collaboratively devise a plan for reaching these goals. During the working phase, for the family's health goal to be met, it is essential that the client and nurse meet periodically to review progress and that the nurse provides feedback and reinforcement. This periodic review process requires commitment on the part of both the nurse and family. A final *evaluation* of progress and provisions for *follow-up* comprise the terminal phase of the nurse-client relationship.

When working with families in the realm of health promotion, the nurse often makes assumptions about families and self-responsibility for their health. According to Bomar (1996), the following assumptions are a useful guide for family health promotion and nursing practice:

- Families are ultimately responsible for their own health.
- Families have the capacity to change in constructive as well as destructive directions.
- Families have a right to health information to make informed decisions about behaviors and lifestyle choices.
- The health-seeking process occurs in the context of interpersonal and social relationships.
- Families use only health behaviors that they find relevant and compatible with their family lifestyle and structure.
- Families have the potential for improvement in their health, and this can be enhanced by a nurse who is caring and culturally competent.

Family health promotion needs and interventions, which differ for each family, are influenced by the nurse's assumptions.

Assessment

As discussed in Chapter 8, nurses are encouraged to base family assessment on scientific models of family health developed by family scientists or family nurses. As explained in Chapter 2, models that nurses use to assess family health vary. A holistic nursing model for family health promotion includes components of the family system that are structural and functional and promote and protect health. The purpose of assessment is to determine a family's health status by thorough examination of family interaction, development, coping, health processes, and integrity (Anderson & Tomlinson, 1992).

Assessment helps the nurse to identify family strengths that foster health promotion and stressors that impede health promotion (Pender, 1996). Integration of the family perspective into assessment and planning facilitates more effective plans for health promotion (Papenfus and Bryan, 1998). It also assists the nurse in identifying areas for intervention. Such interventions may include empowerment, education, promotion of family integrity, maintenance of family process, exercise promotion, environmental management, mutual goal setting, and parent education (Hulme, 1999). The assessment of the Budd Family in the case study provides an example in which there are many areas for growth in health promotion and lifestyle.

Interventions

Interventions and factors that facilitate family health promotion include family contracting, empowerment, and confluence and anticipatory guidance and teaching.

Family Contracting

Contracting with a family to change or initiate an activity to strengthen family health increases the likelihood of attaining desired goals (Hill & Smith, 1990; Gray, 1996; Pender, 1996).

A health *contract* is based on a set of goals mutually agreed on by a health care provider and an individual or family (Hill & Smith, 1990; Friedman, 1998). A contract may be oral or written. There are three types of contracts. The first is a *nurse-client contract,* which is an agreement between the nurse and client (family) to work together to attain goals that are determined by the client. The second type is a *contingency contract.* This type of contract includes the process of setting a goal and identifying costs and rewards of goal attainment with a health professional or other support person. The purpose of the contingency contract is to reinforce the behaviors needed to reach a goal. The third type of contract is the *self-care contract.* The client develops this type of contract independently. The contract is between two individuals for the purpose of improving a health behavior.

Contracts are useful for making lifestyle changes, reframing attitudes, and modifying unhealthy interaction patterns. Family-centered nurses are encouraged to use health promotion diagnoses when contracting with families (Loveland-Cherry, 1996). They are most effective when the components are negotiated and signed by all family members. The disadvantages of contracts are that they are time-consuming to develop and that they require commitment by the health professional and all family members involved. In addition, periodic reevaluation and renegotiations may be necessary.

The health of the Budd family in the case study might be improved by contracting to work as a family on such activities as increasing family time and recreation, providing personal time for Eleanor, sharing household tasks, and revising the family calendar. The family could be advised to contract as a unit to reduce each of the identified stressors. There are few reports on the success rate of family contracting. However, Swain and Steckle (1981) reported improvement in health-promoting behaviors in clients with hypertension, diabetes, and arthritis who followed their contracts. Detailed discussions of contracting can be found in Hill and Smith's *Self-Care Nursing Promoting Health* (1990) and Pender's *Health Promotion in Nursing Practice* (1996). These authors also suggest strategies to facilitate attaining, regaining, or maintaining a health-promoting lifestyle.

Family Empowerment

Trust building is a prelude to the working phase. Reciprocal trust is a cornerstone for effective family nursing care (Robinson, 1998). In the working phase, the family and the nurse collaborate to make changes in the family's lifestyle that will enhance the family's health. The nurse collaborates with the family and provides information, encouragement, and strategies to help the family make lifestyle changes. This process is termed *empowerment.*

According to Hulme (1999) empowerment can be viewed as a process (becoming empowered), an outcome (being empowered), and an intervention (empowering others). To be most effective in empowering a family, the nurse should have not only the theoretical knowledge but educational and training opportunities in empowerment as well (Valentine, 1998). A family's goal may be to reframe a situation, strengthen behaviors that enhance coping with stress or crisis, or incorporate health-promoting activities in family behavior patterns. A family in which a member is dying of AIDS can be empowered by teaching them how to cope with feelings of isolation and how to obtain resources and social support in the family and the community. The primary emphasis in family empowerment is on involving the family in goal setting and planning, not on having the nurse do this for the family (Gray, 1996).

Often, contemporary families focus on individual family members while the family unit seems to be overlooked. For example, the Budd family spent little time together as a family. The parents provided food, shelter, safety, health care, and education for their family, but there was little time for family bonding and closeness. Antibiotics cured Eleanor's inner ear infection; however, getting rid of her extreme fatigue might require changes involving the entire family. After an assessment of the Budd family's strengths and stressors, nursing interventions might include: (1) evaluation of the family and individual calendars and schedules; (2) discussion of strategies to provide rest and personal time for James and Eleanor; (3) discussion of the significance of family togetherness; and (4) encouragement to plan for more couple time and parental time with each of their sons.

A key role of nurses is to help the family members to value their "oneness," to appreciate family togetherness (Friedemann, 1995; Bradshaw, 1988), and to plan activities to foster their unity. One way to enhance family bonding among the Budds would be to share meals together, when possible. Because Eleanor has extreme fatigue, other family members could help with meal preparation. This would give them an opportunity to be together, enhance communication, and reduce role strain for Eleanor. This family could also negotiate a family contract for scheduled weekly family time. Each member would make that family time a priority and let no other activity interfere with it. The nurse could help by consulting local newspapers, family magazines, and community agencies for activities that might interest the entire family and, afterwards, by encouraging them to continue this themselves.

During their life course, families inevitably experience crises and stress. The family's resilience, unity, and resources influence how they cope with crisis and stress (McCubbin & McCubbin, 1993; Pearsall, 1990). The goal of the family nurse is to facilitate family adaptation by empowering the family to promote resilience, reduce the pileup of stressors, make use of resources, and negotiate necessary changes to enhance the family's ability to rebound from stressful events or crises. The nurse can teach families to anticipate life changes, make the necessary adjustments in family routines, evaluate roles and relationships, and cognitively reframe events. For example, in military families, changes occur in family decision making, roles, responsibilities, communication patterns, and power when the military member is deployed. Anticipatory guidance by health professionals could help military families plan to anticipate economic changes, maintain the household, maintain communication, and parent the children when one adult is a long distance away.

Families may need help in meeting both the needs of the family as a whole and individually. To find a balance, each family member should have time alone to develop a sense of self and to focus on spiritual growth.

Friedemann calls this "individuation." The family also needs to plan "family time," when the sense of belonging and "oneness" or "togetherness" can be experienced. Healthy families have both kinds of time (Olson & DeFrain, 1994; Friedemann, 1995).

Families may need to be reminded of the importance of togetherness, a sense of which can help them cope with life stressors and crises more effectively. Family unity often improves as a result of family celebrations, rituals, and routine family activities. Instruments, such as the family times and routines inventory (McCubbin & McCubbin, 1993), can help the professional to identify family routines, and the APGAR (Smilkstein, 1978) can be used to determine the level of family satisfaction.

Family Confluence

Confluence, or the process of combining activities to promote togetherness, fosters family unity and closeness (Friedemann, 1995). The use of confluence by the Budd family in the case study would give them more time for family interaction and reduce the workload for Eleanor. For example, James and Eleanor could work side by side doing household chores on Saturday, everyone could alternate in assisting Eleanor with meal preparation and cleanup, the boys could do their homework in the same room while their parents graded papers, and everyone could be assigned a task so that they could work together to complete the weekend household upkeep. Pearsall (1990) suggests that planning to routinely eat most meals as a unit, having regularly scheduled family time, and going to bed and waking up at the same time fosters family togetherness.

Intervention Strategies

Once the nurse and family have identified family strengths and areas for growth or change, the family should prioritize their goals. The commitment of all family members to achieving a goal is crucial to the family's success in reaching it. Negotiating contracts, which often include agreements to change family interaction, behavior, or lifestyle patterns, can encourage goal attainment. The nurse can help to negotiate and implement contracts and can also serve as health teacher, resource finder, and evaluator of the family's health promotion plan. Pender (1996) provides in-depth information on developing a plan for health protection and promotion.

An example of an activity to promote family unity is an African-American family's desire to start an annual celebration of Kwanza (Mgeni, 1992). Supporting traditional ceremonies and customs such as the Hispanic "quincenera" (Perez, 1999) may also promote family unity. To be successful, the specifics of rituals, time, supplies, and activities must be learned and negotiated by each family member. The primary role of the nurse is health teaching about the goal and strategies to reach this goal, including information about community resources. The family's primary activity is to agree on family system changes and to evaluate their progress. Periodic discussions are needed to determine the effectiveness of the activities.

Areas in which the nurse can provide family support, anticipatory guidance, family education, and family enrichment include:

- Family transitions, such as births, acute and chronic illnesses, separations, launching of children, divorce, death, and retirement.
- Family and individual dietary patterns.
- Family and individual recreation and exercise.
- Family sexuality.
- Family sleep and rest patterns.
- Family environmental practices.
- Transition from illness to wellness.
- Socialization and rearing of children.
- Risk reduction and socialization in health care practices (prevention and promotion).
- Encouragement of a balance between togetherness and individuation.
- Provision for family systems and household maintenance.
- Encouragement of family spirituality (Bomar, 1996; Friedman, 1998; Friedemann, 1995; Warner, 1996).

Although beginning family nurses may not be skilled in all these areas, they can seek out community resources, such as websites on family recreation, classes on parenting, communication, understanding family dynamics, and health promotion for well families and individual members (Table 9-3).

Family needs and nursing interventions differ with varying family structures and depend on stage in the family life course. For example, in a nuclear family, health promotion includes promotion of a healthy marriage as well as health of each individual. In such a family, the family nurse can suggest that the family:

TABLE 9-3
Selected Websites for Family and Family Member Health Promotion

Topic	Website Address
Federal Health Related Sites	
Healthy People 2010	http://www.health.gov/healthypeople
Centers for Disease Control and Prevention	http://www.cdc.gov
Office of Disease Prevention and Health Promotion, Office of Public Health and Science, US Department of Health and Human Services	http://odphp.osophs.dhhs.gov/
National Health Information Center	http://nhic-nt.health.org/
Health Promotion and Disease Prevention for Individuals and Families	
Lay health information in English and Spanish	http://www.healthfinder.gov/
Men's Health	http://menshealthnetwork.org/library
Women's Health	http://www.4women.org
Adolescent Health	http://www.healthyteens.com
Child and Youth Health	http://www.cyh.sa.gov.au
Children's Health	http://www.kidshealth.org
National Clearinghouse on Families and Youth	http://www.ncfy.com
Marriage and Parenting	http://www.drheller.com/parenting.html
Marital Health	http://www.healthyway.hypermart.net/marriag8.htm
Smoking Cessation	http://www.smokefree.gov/
Nutrition: American Dietetic Association	http://www.eatright.org/nuresources.html
Food and Drug Administration	http://fda.gov
Physical Fitness and Recreation	
Elders	http://www.aoa.dhhs.gov/elderpage.html#ea
Across the Life Span	http://www.americanheart.org/catalog/health_catpage9.html
Shape-up America	http://www.shapeup.org/general/
American Alliance of Health, Physical Exercise, Recreation and Dance	http://www.aahperd.org
National Park and Recreation Association	http://www.nrpa.org
Parenting	
Fatherhood	http://aspe.hhs.gov/fathers/fhoodini.htm
Motherhood Web Directory	http://hometown.aol.com/Solhouse5/index.html
Parenting	http://www.kidshealth.org/parent/index/html

- Make the marriage a priority.
- Communicate regularly.
- Practice encouragement.
- Schedule meetings about family maintenance and couple issues.
- Set up rules for negotiations and conflict resolution.
- Plan regularly for activities to have fun (Carlson, et al., 1992).

Family legacy is a living tradition that is developed through dialogue between families of origin and past generations. It is reshaped over time and influenced by family, culture, and society. According to Plager (1999), exploring and acknowledging family legacy recognizes a rich part of family life. This can enhance the nurse's and the family's understanding of family health, related practices, activities, and habits.

A major force in the development of a healthy family is commitment to family unity and shared negotiation of family goals. A vital aspect of family nursing practice is provision of anticipatory guidance to adult family members to help them understand and value individual, dyad, parent-child, and family development issues and transitions.

Health Teaching and Anticipatory Guidance

Nurses working with well families can teach family awareness, encourage family enrichment, and provide information on community agencies and websites (Table 9-3) that are resources for strengthening and enriching families. One example of a community resource is a family wellness program founded in 1980 in San Jose, California (Doub & Scott, 1992). A class in the program, called "Survival Skills for Healthy Families" is taught to families in schools, churches, community centers, and hospitals and is also a component of drug, alcohol, and spouse and child abuse prevention programs. A contract can be made with the family to attend or find out more about such a program. In some cases, the nurse may need to call or visit and observe an agency in action to determine its appropriateness.

The beginning family nurse is prepared to intervene by teaching about healthy processes (e.g., basic nutrition, exercise routines, hygiene, preventive health practice, and awareness of family). Advanced family nursing interventions such as family life education, family enrichment, and marriage enrichment are more appropriate for graduate nurses, family life educators, marriage and family counselors, and therapists.

Some communities have family enrichment programs for well families. Recently, "ministers of health" have been appointed in churches, parishes, and synagogues. In the early 1980s, a national multidisciplinary organization called the Health Ministries Association was formed with the goal of promoting a healthy body, mind, and spirit for all persons in religious congregations. Members include pastors, health educators, health professionals, and concerned congregation members. With the development of such health ministries, many nurses are assuming positions as *parish nurses,* in which the role of the community or family nurse is combined with spiritual counseling from a holistic perspective. The number of universities that provide graduate specialty degrees in parish nursing increases annually. According to the National Parish Nurse Resource Center there are over 60 educational programs for parish nursing (Solari-Twadell, et al., 1999).

Activities of a health ministry program often include:

- Education on health promotion, wellness, disease prevention, and other topics for families and individuals across the life span.
- Coordination of volunteers to provide social and network support to members with lifestyle and health problems.
- Personal counseling.
- Monitoring and screening for health promotion, disease prevention, and treatment of chronic diseases.
- Parenting and fatherhood classes.
- Service as a health resource and referral agent.
- Support groups for single parents, older adults, and remarried families.
- Promotion of the integration of faith and health.

For further information concerning the Parish Nurse Resource Center and selected educational programs, please refer to *Parish Nursing: Promoting Whole Person Health within Faith Communities* (Solari-Twadell, et al., 1999).

Many communities provide resources such as couple communication workshops, family retreats, family magazines, parenting classes for young and adolescent families, support for stepfamilies, and lesbian and gay support groups. A list of selected family agencies and resources appears in the aforementioned parish nursing book.

Preparation for Termination

As the individual or family approaches their goal, the nurse sees the client less frequently (Wright & Leahey, 2000). Pender (1996) calls this the step-down phase. During this phase, the family takes on more responsibility for planned activities and becomes more self-reliant in problem solving and evaluating their progress toward goals. When the goal is met, the nurse and client negotiate the time for termination of the relationship. Throughout the nursing process, regular, frequent reviews of goals and progress may eliminate problems with termination (Friedman, 1998).

Evaluation and Follow-Up

The evaluation and follow-up to include modification (Friedman, 1998) is the last phase of nursing intervention. During this phase, the progress of the client family toward the health promotion goals is reviewed, and if the goals are not met, other options are discussed and planned. After the desired change has been incorporated into the family lifestyle, the nurse discontinues family appointments; however, an opportunity is provided for families to follow-up with the nurse by appointments, calls, or periodic visits. The client is taught problem solving, how to contract as a family, and provided with resources in regard to other areas of family health promotion and protection.

HEALTH PROMOTION AND FAMILY NURSING

Nursing Practice

As resources change in the future and individuals and families are encouraged to assume more responsibility for their care, supporting families in the area of health promotion will be essential. Major tasks of nursing with families are:

- Use the nursing process in partnership with families.
- Partner with families to find ways to achieve their lifestyle and health care goals.
- Illuminate the importance of family health promotion.
- Serve as a family advocate.
- Be an expert in family health promotion matters.

The goals are for families to attain, maintain, or regain the highest possible level of family health. The following discussion concerns the importance of health promotion to the future of family nursing.

In the next decade, the settings where nurses encounter families will change. There is a continuing shift in health care from hospital to community settings, so that nurses will have more direct interactions with families in ambulatory health care settings and homes, and strategies will be needed to provide health promotion and protection in all of these settings.

A comprehensive family assessment may facilitate the development of a holistic health plan for those who are ill. And because more ill family members will receive care in their homes, the impact on family wellness will also need evaluation. Basic and advanced roles of family nurses are discussed in Chapter 1. At all stages of the family health and illness cycle, the goal is to return the family, as a whole, to their highest health potential. In community settings, such as churches and work sites, the nurse can provide programs for family health promotion. Selected topics include parenting from infancy to old age; role changes during family and individual transitions, such as retirement, birth of a new baby, or bereavement; and coping with individual and family stressors. Single-parent and blended families often need anticipatory guidance, family enrichment activities, and parenting and stepparenting education. The nurse can encourage all family members to monitor their family for its unity, strengths, and a sense of belonging. In any setting, nurses can advocate for families by writing and voting on family issues, supporting a philosophy of practice that encourages family nursing, volunteering in community activities for families, and supporting family programs.

Nursing Education

In addition to traditional content on family theoretical frameworks, illness, stress and coping, and crisis, curricula at the undergraduate and graduate level should include content on family health promotion. At the present time, however, few students are prepared in family health promotion. The emphasis in most curricula continues to focus primarily on acute and chronic physical illness, psychosocial problems, and community nursing; the primary focus is on the individual in the context of the family. Limited attention is paid to groups of families in the community and to healthy families.

If nurses are to be a part of the efforts to meet the national health goals for the year 2010, undergraduate and graduate curricula in schools of nursing must include content on the family as the unit of care and on family health promotion and disease prevention. Schools of nursing should use learning-service community partnership models and create innovative sites for clinical practice, where students can provide nursing care to well families (Kataoka-Yahiro, et al., 1998). Such sites might include a nursing clinic in a low-income housing project, a senior center, a family exercise center, a faith community, work site, rural health clinic, or a school or nursing clinic.

Family Policy

The document *Healthy People 2010* and the current emphasis eliminating disparities in health care for all citizens, will help to shape local, state, and national policies geared toward improving family health. The passage of the 1993 Family Leave Policy marked a beginning in the effort to implement policies to improve the quality of family

RESEARCH BRIEF

Although the research about individual health promotion is voluminous, research on the topic of family health promotion is sparse. It has been documented that health promotion and self-care education improves the quality of well-being and health status. Family health promotion is a critical component of family health; however, little documentation of its effectiveness is reported. Considerations for family health promotion research include the following.

- Development of additional family health promotion models. Two family health promotion models are noted in the literature (Loveland-Cherry, 1996; Ma & Wenk, 1997).
- Field-testing of family promotion models with the varied family forms across the lifespan and from diverse cultures.
- Field-testing instruments to measure specific aspects of family health promotion, such as recreation, nutrition, sleep, spirituality, and communication with families from diverse cultures.
- Further testing of measures of family stress, coping, and social support with families from diverse cultures and types.
- Testing of ways to teach and evaluate family health promotion with diverse families.
- Teaching nursing students the concept of family health promotion and the family nursing process with a focus on family health promotion. It is crucial that, in addition to a focus on individual health and families during illness, students are taught family nursing research to support well families.

health. To reach the goals for the nation by the year 2010, families must be empowered to assume more responsibilities in the realm of health promotion and disease prevention for family members. Family issues most frequently reviewed by policy makers include marriage, divorce, family violence, abortion, childcare, child health care, and family health insurance coverage.

Based on an in-depth review of the literature, Zimmerman, (1992) concluded that the well-being of individuals and families is better in states where the government meets the needs of the citizens through policies to improve the quality of life. According to Wisensale (1993), family health policy should include:

- A national family policy agenda.
- Universal access to health care.
- Housing for low- and middle-income families.
- Intergenerational family issues.
- Work and family issues.

Further, policy should reflect the diversity in family structure (Wisendale, 1993, pp. 249–250). The family nurse should be aware of and support policies advancing family health throughout the family life course. Nurses can support family policy legislation by keeping informed about issues, voting, communicating with policy makers, giving expert testimony, maintaining membership in and supporting professional nursing organizations, and financially supporting the political advocacy activities of health professional organizations.

Family Nursing Research

Many regional and national nursing research societies and organizations sponsor family research interest groups; however, research on family health promotion continues to be needed. The creation of the National Institute of Nursing Research (NINR) in 1993 provided a focus for family nursing research. The NINR agenda for nursing research includes developing and testing community-based programs to promote family health using nursing models and assessing the effectiveness of nursing intervention for families during the chronic illness of a family member. Although in the past most family research was actually research on individuals in the family context, the research agenda set by NINR will provide significant knowledge about approaches to improving the quality of family life. See the Research Brief above for recommendations for family health promotion research.

SUMMARY

As resources change in the new millennium and families are encouraged to assume more responsibility for their health care and prevention of disease, supporting families in health promotion will be a vital responsibility for nurses providing care to families. This chapter has presented definitions and models, influencing factors, and nursing process issues related to health promotion with families. Knowledge of the importance of family health promotion and empowering families to attain, maintain, or regain the highest level of family health are among the crucial components of family nursing practice.

Case Study

THE BUDD FAMILY

James (age 38) and Eleanor (age 36) have two sons, Derek (age 8) and Dustin (age 10). James is a full-time engineer who teaches part-time at a community college. Eleanor has a full-time position as a professor of education and her classes are scheduled in the evenings two nights a week. James teaches Monday and Wednesday evenings, and Eleanor teaches Tuesday and Thursday evenings.

On the weekends and the other evenings, the couple are either doing household chores, preparing for classes, or grading papers. Meals are usually rushed and often in front of the television, and the family rarely eats meals together. While their parents are reading, working, or grading papers, the boys either watch television, play video games, or do their homework.

Except for family vacations and holidays, the Budds rarely spent time together enjoying each other's company. Eleanor was seen by a nurse in the family practice clinic for complaints of fatigue, lingering fluid and pain in her ears, vertigo, and nausea for 2 months. She was given antibiotics and nasal cortisone for her ear infection, after which her ear condition improved gradually. However, her complaint of extreme fatigue lingered. Laboratory tests revealed no physiological reason for the continuing fatigue.

A nursing assessment of the family and of Eleanor was completed using Pender's (1996) framework for individual health assessment and the FS^3I by Berkey and Hanson (1996). The results follow.

Major Family Stressors Family stressors include insufficient "me" time, Eleanor's illness, decreased housekeeping standards, insufficient couple and family play time, too much television, inadequate time with the children, over-scheduled family calendar, and lack of shared responsibility.

Family Strengths Family strengths include a shared religious core, respect for the privacy of one another, and the fact that work satisfaction, financial security, encouragement of individualism, affirmation and support of one another, and trust between members are all valued.

Lifestyle Changes Indicated Lifestyle changes needed are increased individual time for parents, improved family recreation and couple time, revision of family calendar, and increased sharing of household tasks.

Study Questions

1. Many factors help determine whether a family is involved in health promotion. Which of the following factors may influence promotion of a family's health?
   a. Type of family
   b. Quality of family interaction
   c. Developmental level of family
   d. Quality of family housing
   e. All of the above

Questions 2 through 6 are based on the following vignette:
The Jones family has four members: Tyrone, the father, age 39; Marcia, the mother, age 30; Barbara, age 8; and James, age 15. James has hemophilia and AIDS, which he contracted from a blood transfusion about 3 years ago. He began to

show symptoms 1 year ago, an experimental drug was prescribed, and he is currently asymptomatic. He attends high school daily but tires easily. The parents come in to the HIV clinic with James for a routine checkup. They say that he does not have much to say and stays in his room a lot after school; in fact, all the family members stay in their own rooms most of the time. Meals are usually eaten separately. James says he eats dinner in his room most evenings and complains about feeling lonely and avoided. The parents, in turn, feel that James is avoiding them at meals.

2. What stage of the family health and illness cycle is this family experiencing?
   a. The vulnerability and symptom-experiencing cycle
   b. The health phase
   c. Chronic adjustment/adaptation phase
   d. Rehabilitation
3. Family process influences how a person adapts to a family health issue. Which of the following processes would be most helpful in improving the quality of this family's life?
   a. Insist that James eat with family.
   b. Ignore the problem, it will take care of itself.
   c. Schedule a family meeting in which each family member talks about how he or she feels about James' health.
   d. Schedule a family meeting and explain that the family is grieving and decide not to worry about it.
4. Which of the following best describes key traits of a healthy family that this family does *not* appear to have?
   a. Resiliency, shared time together, and positive communication
   b. Resiliency, shared time together, and adaptability
   c. Happiness, financial security, shared vacations together
   d. Flexibility, sense of humor, positive communication
5. An internal family factor that is influencing the level of this family's well-being is:
   a. James' disease
   b. Reaction of peers to AIDS
   c. Community fear of the family with AIDS
   d. Poor family communication
6. To empower this family to resolve the crisis so that James does not feel alone and the rest of the family does not feel avoided, the nurse would:
   a. Teach them exactly what to do to resolve the problem.
   b. Encourage James to eat once a week with the family.
   c. Teach them family communication and problem solving.
   d. Allow them to work the issue out by themselves.

References

Abbott, D.A., Berry, N.I., & Meredith, W.H. (1990). Religious belief and practice: A potential asset in helping families. *Family Relations, 39*:443–448.

Aday, L. (1993). *At Risk in America.* San Francisco: Jossey-Bass.

American Nurses' Association. (1995). *Nursing: A Social Policy Statement.* Kansas City, MO.

Anderson, K.H., & Tomlinson, P.S. (1992). The family health system as an emerging paradigmatic view for nursing. *Image: Journal of Nursing Scholarship 24*:57–63.

Berkey, K.M., & Hanson, S.M.H. (1991). *Pocket Guide to Family Assessment and Intervention.* St. Louis: C.V. Mosby.

Bomar, P.J. (Ed.). (1996). *Nurses and Family Health Promotion: Concepts, Assessment and Intervention.* Philadelphia: W. B. Saunders.

Bomar, P.J. (1991). Health-promoting lifestyles of childbearing parents. Proceedings of the Second International Family Nursing Conference. Oregon Health Sciences University School of Nursing: Portland, OR.

Bomar, P.J., & McNeeley, G. (1996). Family health nursing role: Past, present, and future. In P.J. Bomar (Ed.), *Nurses and Family Health Promotion: Concepts, Assessment and Intervention*, ed 2. Philadelphia: W.B. Saunders.

Bradshaw, J. (1988). *Bradshaw on Family.* Deerfield Beach, FL: Heath Communications.

Brigman, K. (1992). Religion and family strengths: Implications for mental health professionals. *Topics in Family Psychology and Counseling, 1*:39–52.

Broome, M.E., et al. (Eds.). (1998). *Children and Families in Health and Illness.* Thousand Oaks: Sage Publications.

Burr, W.R., Day, R.D., & Bahr, K.S. (1993). *Family Science.* Pacific Grove, CA: Brooks/Cole.

Burr, W.R., & Klein, S.R. (1994). *Reexamining Family*

Stress: New Theory and Research. Thousand Oaks, CA: Sage Publications.

Carlson, J., et al. (1992). Marriage maintenance: How to stay healthy. *Topics in Family Psychology and Counseling, 1*:84–90.

Carson, V. (1989). *Spiritual Dimensions of Nursing Practice*. Philadelphia: W. B. Saunders.

Chandler, R. (1991, June 19). Nurses: Ministers of health. Los Angeles: Los Angeles Times, p. Al.

Clark, C. (1998). Wellness self-care by healthy older adults. *Image: Journal of Nursing Scholarship, 30*(4):351–355.

Coe, R. (1970). *Sociology of Medicine*. New York: McGraw-Hill.

Crooks, C., et al. (1987). The family's role in health promotion. *Health Values, 2*:7–12.

Curan, D. (1983). *Traits of a Health Family*. Minneapolis, MN: Winston Press.

Danielson, C.B., et al. (1993). *Families in Health and Illness*. St. Louis, MO: Mosby.

DeFrain, J., & Stinnett, N. (1992). Building on the inherent strengths of families: A positive approach for family psychologists and counselors. *Topics in Family Psychology and Counseling, 1*:15–26.

Doherty, W., & Campbell, T. (1988). *Families and Health*. Newbury Park, CA: Sage Publications.

Doherty, W., & McCubbin, H.I. (1985). Families and health care: An emerging arena of theory, research, and clinical interventions. *Family Relations, 34*:5–10.

Doub, G., & Scott, V. (1992). Family wellness: An enrichment model for teaching skills that build healthy families. *Topics in Family Psychology and Counseling, 1*:72–83.

Duffy, M. E. (1986). Primary prevention behaviors: The female-headed, one-parent family. *Research in Nursing and Health, 9*:115–122.

Duffy, M.E. (1988). Health promotion in the family: Current findings and directives for nursing research. *Journal of Advanced Nursing, 13*:109–17.

Duval, E.M., & Miller, B.C. (1985). *Marriage and Family Development*, ed 6. New York: Harper & Row.

Elliot, M. (1999). Classifying family life education on the World Wide Web. *Family Relations, 48*:7–13.

Faux, S. (1998). Historical overview of responses of children and their families to chronic illness. In Knafl, K. (Ed.), *Children and Families in Health and Illness* (pp. 179–195). Thousand Oaks: Sage Publications.

Friedemann, M.L. (1989). Closing the gap between grand theory and mental health practice with families: Part 1. The framework of systematic organization for nursing of families and family members. *Archives of Psychiatric Nursing, 3*:10–19.

Friedeman, M.L. (1995). *The Framework of Systemic Organization: A Conceptual Approach to Families and Nursing*. Thousand Oaks: Sage Publications.

Friedman, M.M. (1992). *Family Nursing Theory and Assessment*, ed 3. Norwalk, CT: Appleton & Lange.

Friedman, M.M. (1998). *Family Nursing: Research, Theory and Practice*, ed 4. Norwalk, CT: Appleton & Lange.

Garman, C. (1995). The nurse and the environment: How one thinks globally and acts locally. *Holistic Nursing Practice, 9*(2):58–65.

Gillis, C. (1991). Family nursing research, theory, and practice. *Image: Journal of Nursing Scholarship, 22*:19–22.

Gillis, C.L., & Davis, L.L. (1992). Family nursing research: Precepts from paragons and peccadillos. *Journal of Advanced Nursing, 17*:28–33.

Gillis, C.L., et al. (1989). *Toward a Science in Family Nursing*. Reading, MA: Addison-Wesley.

Gray, R. (1996). Family self-care. In P.J. Bomar, (Ed.). *Nurses and Family Health Promotion: Concepts, Assessment, and Intervention*, ed 2. Philadelphia: W. B. Saunders.

Grove, K.A. (1996). The American family: History and development. In P.J. Bomar (Ed.), *Nurses and Family Health Promotion: Concepts, Assessment, and Intervention*, (pp. 36–45). Philadelphia: W.B. Saunders.

Hagen, J.L. (1999). Public welfare and human services: New directions under TANF? *Families in Society: The Journal of Contemporary Human Services, 80*:1.

Hanson, S.M.H. (1986). Healthy single parent families. *Family Relations, 35*:125–132.

Hanson, S.M.H., & Heims, M. (1992). Family nursing curricula in U.S. schools of nursing. *Journal of Nursing Education, 31*:303–308.

Hanson, S.M.H., et al. (1992). Education for family health care professionals: Nursing as a paradigm. *Family Relations*, 41:4952.

Hanson, S.M.H., & Mischke, K. (1996). Family health assessment and intervention. In P.J. Bomar (Ed.). *Nurses and Family Health Promotion: Concepts, Assessment, and Intervention*. Philadelphia: W.B. Saunders.

Heinrich, K. (1996). Family sexuality. In P.J. Bomar (Ed.). *Nurses and Family Health Promotion: Concepts, Assessment and Intervention*, ed 2. Philadelphia: W. B. Saunders.

Hertz, R., & Ferguson, I.T. (1997). Kinship strategies and self-sufficiency among single mothers by choice: Postmodern family ties. *Qualitative Sociology, 20*(2):187–208.

Hill, L., & Smith, N. (1990). *Self-Care Nursing Promoting Health*. Englewood Cliffs, NJ: Prentice-Hall.

Hoffer, J. (1996). Family communication. In P.J. Bomar (Ed.). *Nurses and Family Health Promotion: Concepts, Assessment, and Intervention*, ed 2. Philadelphia: W. B. Saunders.

Huff, R. M., & Kline, M.V. (1999). *Promoting Health in Multicultural Populations*. Thousand Oaks: Sage.

Hulme, P.A. (1999). Family Empowerment: A nursing intervention with suggested outcomes for families of children with a chronic health condition. *Journal of Family Nursing, 5*(1), 35–50.

Iowa Intervention Project. McClosky, J.C., & Bulechek, G.M., (Eds.) (1992). Nursing Interventions Classification (NIC). St. Louis: Mosby Year Book.

James, K. (1996). Family nutrition. In P.J. Bomar, (Ed.) *Nurses and Family Health Promotion: Concepts, Assessment and Intervention*, ed 2. Philadelphia: W. B. Saunders.

Kataoka-Yahiro, M., et al. (1998). A learning-service community partnership model. *Nursing and Heath Care Perspectives*, *19*:274–277.

Kick, E. (1996). Sleep and the family. In P.J. Bomar, (Ed.). *Nurses and Family Health Promotion: Concepts, Assessment and Intervention*, ed 2. Philadelphia: W. B. Saunders.

King, I.M. (1983). King's theory of nursing. In I.W. Clements & F.B. Roberts, (Eds.). *Family Health: A Theoretical Approach to Nursing Care*, (pp. 177–188). New York: John Wiley & Sons.

Labun, E. (1988). Spiritual care: An element in nursing care planning. *Journal of Advanced Nursing*, *13*:314–320.

Lipson, J.G. (1998). Iranians. In L.D. Purnell & B.J. Paulanka, (Eds.). *Transcultural Health Care: A Culturally Competent Approach*. Philadelphia: F.A. Davis.

Loveland-Cherry, C.J. (1986). Personal health practices of single-parent and two-parent families. *Family Relations*, *35*:133–139.

Loveland-Cherry, C.J. (1996). Family health promotion and protection. In P.J. Bomar, (Ed.). *Nurses and Family Health Promotion: Concepts, Assessment and Interventions*, ed 2. Philadelphia: W.B. Saunders.

Ma, G.X., & Wenk, D. (1997). A holistic family wellness program focusing on family strengths. *Practicing Anthropology*, 19:30–34.

McCown, D. (1996). Family recreation and exercise. In P.J. Bomar, (Ed.) *Nurses and Family Health Promotion: Concepts, Assessment and Intervention*, ed 2. Philadelphia: W.B. Saunders.

McCubbin, M.A., & McCubbin, H.I. (1993). Families coping with illness: The resilience model of family stress adjustment and adaptation. In Danielson, C.B., et al. (Eds.). *Families in Health and Illness*, (pp. 21–63). St. Louis: Mosby.

McGoldrick, M., & Giordano, J. (1996). Overview: Ethnicity and family therapy. In M. McGoldrick, et al. (Eds.) *Ethnicity and Family Therapy*, (pp. 1–30). New York: Guilford Press.

Melson, G.F. (1980). *Family and Environment: An Eco-Systems Perspective*. Minneapolis: Burgess.

Mgeni, Y. (1992, December 17). Kwanza holidays celebrate black principles, unity. Minneapolis: Minneapolis Star Tribune, p. 4.

Miller, S., et al. (1991). *Talking and Listening Together*. Littleton, CO: Interpersonal Communication Programs.

Mischke, K.B., & Hanson, S.M.H. (1996). Family health assessment and intervention. In P.J. Bomar, (Ed.) *Nurses in Family Health Promotion: Concepts, Assessment and Interventions*, ed 2. Philadelphia: W.B. Saunders.

Moreno, P.R. (1975). Vertical diffusion effects within black and Mexican-American families participating in the Florida parent education model. *Dissertation Abstracts International*, 36:1358.

Murphy, S. (1986). Family study and family science. *Image: Journal of Nursing Scholarship*, *18*:170–174.

National Institute of Nursing Research. (1999). Research directions: capsule descriptions of selected studies. Retrieved March 26, 1999 from the World Wide Web: http://www.nih.gov/ninr/ResDir.htm.

Neuman, B. (1983). Family intervention using the Betty Neuman health care system model. In Clements, I.W. & Roberts, F.B., (Eds.) *Family Health: A Theoretical Approach to Nursing Care*, (pp. 239–254). New York: John Wiley & Sons.

Newman, M.A. (1986). *Health As Expanding Consciousness*. St. Louis: C.V. Mosby.

Nursing Outreach. (Fall, 1993). Bethesda, MD: National Institute of Nursing Research.

Olson, D.H., & DeFrain, J. (1994). *Marriage and the Family: Diversity and Strengths*. Mountain View, CA: Mayfield.

Olson, D.H., et al. (1989). *Families: What Makes Them Work*, ed 2. Beverly Hills, CA: Sage Publications.

Papenfus, H., & Bryan, A.A. (1998). Nurses' involvement in interdisciplinary team evaluations: Incorporating the family perspective. *Journal of School Health*, *68*(5):184–195.

Pearsall, P. (1990). *The Power of the Family: Strength, Comfort, and Healing*. New York: Doubleday.

Pender, N.J. (1996). *Health Promotion in Nursing Practice*, ed 3. Norwalk, CT: Appleton & Lange.

Perez, M. (1999). Quincenera. *New Moon*, *6*(3): 184–195.

Plager, K. (1999). Understanding family legacy in family health concerns. *Journal of Family Nursing*, *5*(1):51–71.

Pratt, L. (1976). *Family Structure and Effective Health Behavior and the Energized Family*. Boston: Houghton Mifflin.

Purnell, L.D., & Paulanka, B.J. (1998). *Transcultural Health Care: A Culturally Competent Approach*. Philadelphia: F.A. Davis.

Ranson, D.D., et al. (1992). The California Health Project: II. Family world view and adult health. *Family Process*, *31*:251–267.

Robinson, C. (1998). Women, families, chronic illness and nursing interventions: from burden to balance. *Journal of Family Nursing*, *4*(3):271–291.

Roth, P. (1996). Family social support. In P.J. Bomar, (Ed.) *Nurses and Family Health Promotion: Concepts, Assessment, and Intervention*, ed 2. Philadelphia: W.B. Saunders.

Shi, L., & Singh, D.A. (1998). *Delivering Health Care in America: A Systems Approach*. Baerrien Springs, MI: Aspen.

Smilkstein, G. (1978). The family APGAR: A proposal for family function test and its use by physicians. *Family Practice*, *6*:1231–1239.

Smith, J. (1983). *The Idea of Health: Implications for the Nursing Profession*. New York: Teachers College Press.

Solari-Twadell, P.A., et al. (1999). Educational preparation. In P.A. Solari-Twadell & M. McDermott, (Eds.) *Parish Nursing: Promoting Whole Person Health within Faith Communities*. Thousand Oaks: Sage Publications.

Solari-Twadell, P.A. (1999). The community as clients: Assessment of assets and the needs of the faith community and the parish nurse. In P.A. Solari-Twadell & M. McDermott, (Eds.) *Parish Nursing: Promoting Whole Person Health Within Faith Communities*, (pp. 83–92). Thousand Oaks: Sage Publications.

Steieger, N.J., & Lipson, J.G. (1985). *Self-Care Nursing: Theory and Practice*. Bowie, MD: Brady.

Swain, M.S., & Steckle, S. (1981). Contracting with patients to improve compliance. *Hospitals*, *51*:81–84.

Thomas, D.L., & Cornwall, M. (1990). Religion and families in the 1980s: Discovery and development. *Journal of Marriage and the Family*, *52*:983–992.

US Department of Health and Human Services (1998). *Healthy People 2010: National Health Promotion and Disease Prevention Objectives*. (Department of Health and Human Services, Office of Public Health and Science). Washington, DC: US Government Printing Office.

US Department of Health and Human Services (1990). *Healthy People 2000: National Health Promotion and Disease Prevention Objectives* (Department of Health and Human Services, Publication No. PHS 91–50213). Washington, DC: US Government Printing Office.

US Department of Health and Human Services (1986). *The 1990 Health Objectives: A Midcourse Review*. Rockville, MD: Office of Disease and Health Promotion, Public Health Service. Washington, DC: US Government Printing Office.

US Department of Health and Human Services (1985). *Report of the Secretary's Task Force on Black and Minority*. Washington, DC: US Government Printing Office.

US Department of Health and Human Services (1980). *Promoting Health/Preventing Disease: Objectives for the Nation*. Washington, DC: US Government Printing Office.

US Department of Health and Human Services. (1979). *Healthy People: The Surgeon General's Report on Health Promotion and Disease Prevention*. (U.S. Public Health Service, Pub. No. PHS 79–55071) US Department of Health, Education, and Welfare. Washington, DC: US Government Printing Office.

US Department of Health and Human Services (1996). *Report of Final Natality Statistics*. Retrieved February 17, 1999 from the World Wide Web: http://www.hhs.gov.

Valentine, F. (1998). Empowerment: Family-centered care. *Pediatric Nursing*, *10*:24–27.

Warner, C.G. (1996). Family spirituality. In P.J. Bomar (Ed.), *Nurses and Family Health Promotion: Concepts, Assessment, and Intervention*, ed 2. Philadelphia: W.B. Saunders.

Whall, A.L., & Fawcett, J. (1991). The family as a focal phenomenon in nursing. In A.L. Whall & J. Fawcett, (Eds.) *Family Theory Development in Nursing: State of the Science and Art*, (pp. 7–29). Philadelphia: F.A. Davis.

White House Conference on Families (1980). Listening to America's Families: Action for the 1980s. Washington, DC: US Government Printing Office.

Wijnberg, M., & Weinger, S. (1998). When dreams wither and resources fail: the social support system of poor single mothers. *Families in Society: The Journal of Contemporary Human Services*, *79*(2):212–219.

Wiley, D. (1996). Family environmental health. In P.J. Bomar, (Ed.) *Nurses and Family Health Promotion: Concepts, Assessment, and Interventions*, ed 2, (pp. 339–364). Philadelphia: W.B. Saunders.

Wisensale, S.K. (1993). State and federal initiatives in family policy. In T.H. Brubaker, (Ed.) *Family Relations: Challenges for the Future*, (pp. 229–250). Newbury Park, CA: Sage Publications.

Wright, L. (1997). Suffering and spirituality: The soul of clinical work with families. *Journal of Family Nursing*, 3:3–14.

Wright, L., et al. (1990). The family nursing unit: A unique integration of research, education, and clinical practice. In J. Bell, et al. (Eds.) *The Cutting Edge of Family Nursing*. Calgary, AL: Family Nursing Unit Publications.

Wright, L., & Leahey, M. (1984). *Nurses and Families: A Guide to Interviewing Families*. Philadelphia: F.A. Davis.

Wright, L. & Leahey, M. (2000). *Nurses and Families: A Guide to Family Assessment and Intervention*, ed. 3. Philadelphia: F.A. Davis.

Zimmermann, S.L. (1992). *Family Policies and Family Well-Being*. Newbury Park, CA: Sage.

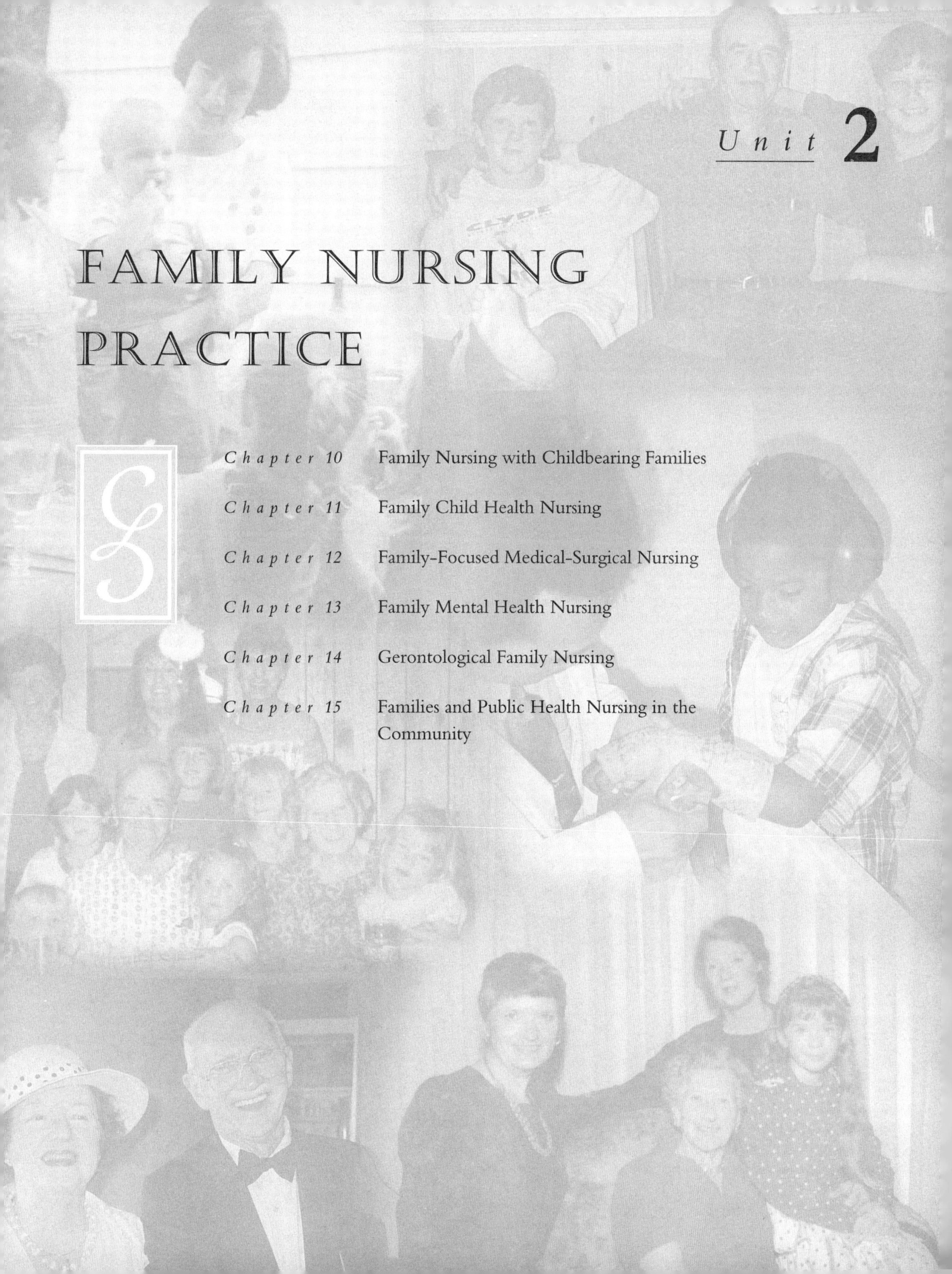

Unit **2**

FAMILY NURSING PRACTICE

Focus On

FAMILY NURSING WITH CHILDBEARING FAMILIES

Family nursing can make a difference in the health of childbearing families. While giving direct physical care, teaching patients, or performing other traditional modes of nursing care, childbearing family nurses focus on family relationships and the health of all members of a childbearing family. Childbearing family nursing is more complex than maternity nursing because of the inclusion of the family in all aspects of the nursing process. This chapter includes a brief history of family nursing and discusses the use of theory to guide the childbearing family nursing process, health promotion, threats to health, and implications for education, research, and policy. The emphasis is on health promotion in relation to developmental tasks of childbearing families. A case study of a family experiencing a preterm birth illustrates the effect of threats to health on childbearing families. Throughout the chapter, nursing interventions are emphasized. The chapter concludes with implications for education, research, and policy development.

Chapter 10

FAMILY NURSING WITH CHILDBEARING FAMILIES

Louise K. Martell

OUTLINE

OBJECTIVES

On completion of this chapter, the reader will be able to:

- Differentiate between childbearing family nursing and maternity nursing.

- Discuss the history of childbearing family nursing.
- Understand the use of selected theories to guide nursing actions with childbearing families.
- Analyze the impact of developmental tasks of the childbearing stage of the family life cycle on family health.
- Use the childbearing family stage developmental tasks to guide family health promotion.
- Determine when childbearing families should be referred to other family health care providers.
- Analyze how threats to health during childbearing affect a family.
- Discuss childbearing family nursing care for families with threats to health.
- Describe implications of childbearing family nursing for education, research, and policy development.

WHAT IS CHILDBEARING FAMILY NURSING?

Today, more and more, health care providers for women are including families in their care, as knowledge increases about the impact of reproductive events on all family members. Consequently, family nursing concepts are being integrated into traditional care of women.

Family nursing with childbearing families covers the period before conception and pregnancy, labor, birth, and the postpartum period. Childbearing family nursing traditionally begins when families are considering whether to start having children and continues until parents have achieved a degree of relative comfort in their roles as parents of infants and have ceased adding babies to their families. Often family nursing expands to include the periods between pregnancies and other aspects of reproduction, such as family planning and sexuality. Decisions and changes surrounding physical bearing of children vary for families according to their cultural and psychological needs and social customs; the beginning and end point of the reproductive cycle may be different for each family.

Childbearing family nursing is not synonymous with obstetric nursing. Rather, it considers the family as a unit of care or as context for the care of its members. It focuses on health and wellness rather than on procedures and medical treatment.

Family functioning, family structure, and life events have been shown to relate to pregnancy outcomes (Ramsey et al, 1986). For example, women living with their spouses or other family members were more likely to have healthy full-term babies than women living alone. Women living with families who were sources of stress, rather than protectors from stress, had smaller babies. Mercer and Ferketich (1990) found that antenatal hospitalization was stressful to women and their partners and that negative (or stressful) life events had a negative impact on family functioning.

In childbearing family nursing, nurses use family concepts and theories as part of assessment, diagnosis, planning, interventions, and evaluation. At any one time, family members may have related, but different, family health needs. In particular, family nursing process addresses relationships, the essence of families. Thus, childbearing family nursing practice uses all the traditional components of nursing, such as direct physical care, patient teaching, and referral to other health care providers; these components are oriented to the entire family.

In this chapter, childbearing family nursing is explored. The history of childbearing family nursing will give the reader the context for present-day practice. The theoretical perspectives are the basis for the rest of the chapter. Most of the chapter focuses on health promotion for the childbearing family with consideration of threats to health that are akin to "acute" and "chronic" illness. The chapter ends with implications for education, research, and policy.

HISTORY

Before the onset of professional nursing in North America, during the late nineteenth century, care givers for childbearing were primarily female networks of midwives, neighbors, friends, servants, and relatives (Wertz & Wertz, 1989). Most caregiving activities were carried out in the family home during the birth and postpartum periods. Care was not solely for births but included maintaining the functions of the household, tending to new babies and the other children in the family, and providing postpartum physical care.

After industrialization, many families moved to

more urban areas, and household size and functions diminished. The traditional networks of women were not always available, and mothers needed to replace care previously carried out in the home. At the same time, with the development of anesthesia and surgical obstetrics, care for childbirth shifted from networks of women to male physicians. Even with the rise of physician-attended births in the late nineteenth and early twentieth centuries, childbearing still occurred at home for many middle-class families (Leavitt, 1986; Wertz & Wertz, 1989).

During the first third of the twentieth century, physicians began to centralize their services in hospitals. Thus, the hospital became the place for labor, birth, and early postpartum recovery.

Although more middle-class families had hospital births tended by physicians, many immigrant and working-class urban families continued to have babies at home with their traditional female care providers. An impetus to the development of public health nursing was concern for the health of these urban mothers and babies. These early public health nurses were the predecessors of childbearing family nurses. When these nurses made home visits, their attention often expanded to other family members. For example, while on a home visit to a new mother, a nurse may have found out that the unemployed father had experienced a job-related illness and that the children were undernourished. Realizing that the health needs of all the family members were intertwined, early public health nurses made families, not individuals, their clients. The concerns for families laid the foundation for maternity care reforms, such as the family planning movement and prenatal and postnatal home visits by nurses.

From the 1930s through the "Baby Boom" of the 1950s, there was a dramatic shift of births to hospitals and family involvement with childbearing diminished (Leavitt, 1986). Women were heavily sedated and anesthetized for labor and birth. Births became "deliveries," which were more like surgery than a life event. Concerns about infection control contributed to separation of family members. Family members and other companions were forbidden to be with women in labor. Young children were barred from visiting their mothers during the postpartum period. Babies were segregated into nurseries and brought out to their mothers only for brief feeding sessions. The nurses' contribution was the smooth operation of postpartum wards and nurseries through the use of routine and orderliness. Nursing care was inflexible. Despite the inflexibility of these conditions, families tolerated them because of the prevailing belief that hospital births were safer for mothers and babies.

In the late 1950s and 1960s, some women and a few physicians began to question the need for heavy sedation and analgesia for childbearing and embraced natural childbirth, a change that was also taking place in Europe and the Soviet Union. A feature of natural childbirth was the close relationship between the laboring woman and a supportive person who served as a coach. In North America, husbands assumed this supportive role for women who wanted natural childbirth (Wertz & Wertz, 1989).

In the 1970s, many families wanted involvement by fathers not only in labor and birth but throughout childbearing experience, and families went to classes to prepare them for their birth experiences. Expectant parents actively sought out physicians and hospitals that would best meet their expectations, and the control over childbearing began to shift from health care professionals to families.

Nurses responded in different ways to the shift in the role of families in childbearing health care. Some were skeptical about the changes families demanded. Others were enthusiastic about increased family participation. They conducted childbirth classes, taught parents to be assertive with their physicians, and lobbied hospital policy makers to allow fathers in delivery rooms. In line with these changes, many hospital-based maternity nurses began to consider themselves to be mother-baby nurses rather than nursery or postpartum nurses, and labor and delivery nurses often collaborated with family members in helping women cope with the discomforts of labor.

The research conducted by Klaus and Kennell (1976) on mother-infant bonding supported the idea that contact between a mother and her baby soon after birth has a positive impact on their relationship. This finding served as the impetus for the growth of family-centered care (American College of Obstetricians and Gynecologists, 1978). Today the maintenance or promotion of family contact is a hallmark of childbearing care. Many hospitals have renamed their obstetrical services, using names such as "family birth center" to convey the importance of family members in childbearing health care even though obstetrical care is becoming more dependent on technologic developments such as electronic fetal monitoring.

Economic issues and the complexity of technology now demands foremost attention from contemporary health care providers. Family-centered care may not be a reality for many childbearing families, as hospital-based nurses grapple with diminished resources of time and personnel while attempting to meet basic needs of patients. With the trend for shorter hospital stays after birth, postpartum care is becoming family-based with nursing guidance. As history points out, the partnership of families and nurses in the childbearing experience is constantly evolving.

THEORIES

A number of theories, especially those from family social science contribute to nurses' understanding of how families grow, develop, function, and change during childbearing. Application of theory to family health situations during childbearing can guide family nurses in making more complete assessments and planning interventions that are congruent with the predictable consequences of family events during childbearing. The theories presented in Chapter 2 that are especially applicable to childbearing families include general systems theory, change (transition), and developmental theory. A brief summary of their application follows.

General Systems Theory

Even though much of the classic work on general systems theory for childbearing families was done more than a decade ago, this theory still applies to childbearing family nursing. General systems theory focuses on both family process and outcomes. The central idea of general systems theory is that a family functions in such a way as to maintain homeostasis. Homeostasis is maintained or regained through adaptation. Because a family is considered to be an open system, it is affected by exchanges with its environment. The degree of openness is regulated by the family boundary that may impede or facilitate a family's interaction with social systems outside itself (Broderick, 1993; Mercer, 1989). Individuals within a family are interdependent on one another, which contributes to a family's ability to adapt and maintain homeostasis even when responding to stress and strains from both inside and outside the family.

Becoming parents or adding a child brings more stress to families that challenge homeostasis. Disequilibrium occurs while adjustments are still needed and new roles are being learned. Families with greater flexibility in role expectations and behaviors tend to weather these periods of disequilibrium with less discomfort. The greater the flexibility of family members' coping and ability to engage in various family roles, the more effective a family's response will be to both internal strains and external stress associated with childbearing.

The stress of pregnancy and birth influence not only nuclear and extended family systems but also the individual members and subsystems of the family. Changes in the family occur in response to changes in individual family members and family subsystems (Miller & Winstead-Fry, 1982). As new subsystems are created or modified by pregnancy and childbirth, there is a sense of disequilibrium until a family adapts to its new member. For example, changes in the husband-wife subsystem occur as a response to development of the parent-child subsystems.

Research regarding social support, stress, and disequilibrium in childbearing women suggests that general systems theory is relevant for childbearing families (Norbeck & Tilden, 1983; Tilden, 1983). External stresses may be important in predicting disequilibrium in pregnant women, and nurses should assess the effect of stress on family homeostasis.

The general systems theory is especially effective for childbearing family nurses when they consider that a family, while in a state of change and readjustment, is often engaged in more than usual interactions with health care and social systems outside the family. When families respond to changes inherent in childbearing, they are more open to both positive and negative influences from the environment. This openness of family boundaries allows health care providers, particularly family nurses, greater access to the family for health promotion. Families become more receptive to interventions, such as health teaching, than they may be at other times in the family life cycle.

Very closed or enmeshed families are at greater risk for poor childbearing outcomes than are more open families (Ramsey et al, 1986). They have closed, nonpermeable boundaries and reject influences from the environment. Another disadvantage of closed boundaries is that these families do not allow stress or energy to diffuse out from the family, and consequently, they do not obtain the help they need. These families may be far less readily accessible or responsive to family nurses.

Transition Concepts

The concept of transition is similar to change theory, discussed in Chapter 2, but it differs in that it focuses on the processes involved with second-order change as families move from nonchildbearing to childbearing. Inherent in transition is a period of upheaval as the family moves from one state to another. Historically, "transition to parenthood" has been studied extensively by family researchers and has framed how nurses think about childbearing families. For example, the notion that having a first child is a crisis for families came out of the work of LeMasters (1957) in the 1950s. Whether the transition to parenthood is a "crisis" for families was supported or refuted by several early investigators (Steffensmeier, 1982). This debate is not studied any more; more recent work focuses on the processes associated with change in families.

In a more contemporary approach, transition to parenthood has been defined as a long-term process that results in qualitative reorganization of both inner life and external behavior (Cowan, 1991). Reorganization occurs in three phases. First, there is disbelief in the reality of the change. Second, there is frustration over not being able to cope in the old ways. Third, there is accommodation, when the new identity as parents is claimed and role expectations consistent with being parents are learned.

Developmental Theories

Developmental theories focus on predictable changes and growth that occur during a person's and a family's life. Changes occur in stages, during which there is upheaval while adjustments are being made. What occurs during these stages are generally referred to as developmental tasks. Duvall's (Duvall & Miller, 1986) family life cycle theory describes tasks and processes for different stages. In this theory, the family childbearing stage is defined as the period from the beginning of the first pregnancy until the oldest child is 18 months old. The tasks during the childbearing stage are explained in more detail with the section on health promotion in this chapter. Some of these tasks recur as other children are added during a family's life cycle, although others are more salient for first children. This developmental theory can guide childbearing family nurses in assessment of family achievement of developmental tasks and interaction aspects, such as roles and relationships. However, family nurses must consider that the family life cycle theory was developed decades ago and that many present-day families do not precisely fit into the stages and tasks. Examples are a family in which one or both partners have children from previous relationships, unmarried and single parents, same-sex couples, and childbearing in "later life."

An Eclectic Use of Theories

None of the theories in Chapter 2 is entirely satisfactory for guiding childbearing family nursing. General systems theory emphasizes the need to maintain balance and counteract change. With childbearing, change is inevitable and may be in conflict with homeostasis, which is the goal of a family system. The concept of change or transition may imply a negative response to a new situation, which may not be the case with childbearing. The family developmental theory is rooted in change, but it has been criticized for not being applicable to many contemporary family situations because it was based on the typical experiences of mainstream American families in the middle of the twentieth century. However, the idea of change and development being both normal and yet potentially unsettling events can help nurses assess and manage the impact of predictable and unpredictable events on a family during childbearing.

The following concepts, which are derived from general systems, transition, and family development theories, are highly relevant for childbearing family nursing.

- Changes occur in a family during the childbearing cycle.
- Changes that occur during childbearing are not necessarily negative.
- Change in one member or one aspect of a childbearing family induces changes in other members and aspects of a family.
- Families are usually more open to influence of the environment during the childbearing cycle.
- Environmental influences, such as social support and family nursing, can have a positive impact on a childbearing family.
- Developmental tasks for pregnancy and childbearing families are predictable and lead to new ways of functioning for individuals and families.

Family nurses use these concepts with childbearing families. For example, the nursing interventions of patient teaching, anticipatory guidance, and direct physical care are environmental influences that may reduce or prevent stress or promote development.

Nurses come into contact with members of childbearing families in health care providers' offices, clinics, classes, hospitals, family homes, and other community settings. While some nurses may have only mothers and infants as identified patients, actions of family nurses affect the entire family, because families are systems. Likewise, nursing care directed toward an entire family will affect its individual members.

HEALTH PROMOTION

The developmental tasks of the childbearing family mentioned with the family life cycle theory (Duvall & Miller, 1986) can be used to guide health promotion. This theory is helpful because it addresses the pattern of adaptation to parenthood that is typical for many families of Western cultures. Family nurses will find that many of these tasks are similar for families of different configurations and cultures and may adapt the tasks accordingly. The developmental tasks, with appropriate nursing actions, are discussed below.

Arranging Space (Territory) for a Child

Typically, during the third trimester of pregnancy, families make material and space preparations for their babies. Often, families move to a new residence, during pregnancy or the first year after birth, to obtain more space, or they modify their living quarters and furnishings to accommodate new babies.

Family nurses are not usually involved in actually arranging or providing space for childbearing families; however, family concerns about space are of interest to family nurses. By simply asking during the third trimester about the living space and physical preparation for the baby, nurses can assess whether these developmental tasks are being met. If a family has not made physical preparations for the baby, nurses should investigate the reasons why.

Busy families may inadvertently delay preparations. A nurse's inquiries about spatial and physical preparation for the baby may prompt parents to arrange space. Lack of spatial preparation may have other causes. Families who fear or have actually experienced perinatal loss often delay preparations. These families may fear that their babies will not live and do not wish to go through the heartbreak of dismantling nurseries that will not be used. Nurses can help these families explore and manage their fear about survival of the baby. By recognizing and managing fears, a family's development can be mobilized. Lack of space preparation may be due to the fact that the parents have not accepted the reality of the oncoming baby, perhaps because stress has diverted their attention.

Stress affecting childbearing families needs to be recognized and, if possible, dealt with promptly. Nurses should be concerned if adolescent parents have not made arrangements. It could be the result of denial of the pregnancy or fear about repercussions from their families if pregnancy is revealed. Nurses can help adolescents face issues about communicating with their families and making plans for the future of the baby *and* the adolescent parents. Nurses need to be aware of any family's cultural practices regarding preparation for the baby. For some cultural groups, preparation for a baby's material needs during pregnancy is not acceptable; it may mean bad luck or misfortune for the baby. A further difficulty may be inadequate, unsafe housing and homelessness, which may be real threats to the safety of some childbearing families. Nurses should refer these families to appropriate resources for obtaining safer housing or for further investigation of their living situations.

Financing Childbearing and Childrearing

Childbearing family nurses should recognize the importance of financing on family health. For example, health care providers may not accept patients who are not insured or cannot pay for obstetric services. The nurse's role is to help families seek out the necessary resources, such as nutrition programs and prenatal clinics, that fit with the financial resources of the family. A less obvious but equally important role is to help families overcome nonfinancial barriers for needed care. Such barriers to prenatal care often include lack of transportation and child care, hours of service that conflict with family employment, and cultural insensitivity of the prenatal setting.

For most present-day families, childbearing results in both additional expenses and lower family income because most employed women miss some work during childbearing. Even with legislation to protect women from loss of jobs during childbearing, maintaining earnings and opportunities for advancement may be difficult to realize for women returning to work after giving birth. This can be extremely stressful for mothers without partners or for those who provide the sole income for their families.

Families cope with threats to income in a variety of ways. It is not uncommon for new and expectant fathers to work more hours at their current jobs or to change jobs, which may be a source of more anxiety and stress for the family. Women tend to alter their employment situation to be more compatible with caring for a newborn. Families may use their savings, increase their debt, or alter their lifestyles to match changing levels of income. Adolescents are especially prone to financial difficulties. Childbearing may disrupt their education, which sets them up for future poverty if they are not able to obtain jobs that pay well enough to support a family.

Child care should be considered long before families need it. Last-minute scrambling to obtain safe and adequate child care can be extremely stressful for families and often results in less than satisfactory arrangements for both parents and babies. Nurses can direct families to information and resources to help them choose safe and appropriate child care and encourage them to make arrangements well in advance of need.

Assuming Mutual Responsibility for Child Care and Nurturing

In addition to increased expenses, the care and nurturing of infants bring sleep disruptions, demands on time and energy, additional household tasks, and personal discomfort for caretakers. Most people would not consider these aspects of parenting pleasant. Why then, do adults voluntarily assume responsibility for a helpless infant? Explanations range from the biological drive to reproduce, the expectation of producing a new generation, or fulfillment of personal expectations to social desirability and acceptance. The affectionate bonds of attachment that develop between parents and their children may be one of the driving forces for engaging in infant care and nurturing, even under difficult circumstances.

Interventions to promote parent-infant attachment at the time of birth are well described in up-to-date maternity nursing texts. Promotion of family integrity, feeding management, and risk identification for poor attachment are particularly important to family nurses whose goals are to enhance nurturing among all family members. The rest of this section focuses on these interventions.

Family Integrity Promotion

Throughout the childbearing cycle, nurses can assist families in understanding and responding to the effects of a new baby on the existing children. No matter what age siblings are, the addition of a new baby affects the position, role, and power of older children, which is stressful for both parents and children. Nurses can emphasize the positive aspects of adding a family member by focusing on sibling "relationships" rather than "rivalry." Parents may need help to recognize that *all* the children, not just the new baby, have needs. Parents may be concerned about whether they have enough energy, time, and love for additional children. Practical ideas for time and task management can alleviate some of their concerns.

Once a baby has been born, opportunities for children to visit their mothers and new siblings in perinatal health settings can enhance sibling relationships. Nurses can make older children feel special by expressing warmth and hospitality to them, recognizing their new roles as "big brother" or "big sister." Availability of age-appropriate toys, furnishings, and educational materials help children feel welcomed. Family nurses can use sibling visitation as an opportunity to explain older children's expected or unexpected behavior to parents. For example, crying by a 2-year-old may be the child's way of expressing stress over the strange environment rather than rejection of the new baby. Although parents may want to discourage children's visits because of crying, nurses can use the situation to discuss the needs of children in adapting to new siblings, including ongoing contact with their mothers.

In some settings, older siblings may be present at the birth. What is important for siblings at the time of birth, whether they are present or not, is that they be cared for and supported by a responsible adult who they trust. During pregnancy, nurses should remind the parents to consider the logistics of care for their other children at the time of birth and during the mother's hospital stay.

All family members experience household upheaval during the first few days to weeks that a new baby is in the home. Nurses must remind parents to be realistic in their expectations about themselves, each other, and their children. Such realistic expectations help families plan ahead to identify appropriate support resources, such as help with household chores.

Feeding Management

Feeding tends to be synonymous with love and nurturing, and the success of mothers in feeding their babies induces feelings of competency in themselves and love toward their babies. Feeding is such a powerful reinforcement of love and attachment that some fathers have expressed envy of their partner's ability to breastfeed (Jordan, 1986).

Even though breastfeeding is the recommended

mode of infant feeding, nurses must recognize that a family's comfort with its method of infant feeding is as crucial for physical, emotional, and social well-being of the infant as the food itself. Regardless of the choice of feeding method, nurses must emphasize the development of relationships between infant and parent through feeding. Being held during feeding enhances social development, whether a baby is being breastfed or bottle fed. Parents should take the time during feedings to enjoy interacting with their babies.

Nurses can promote paternal-infant attachment by encouraging breastfeeding women to involve fathers in the feeding experience. For example, the father can comfort the baby while the mother is getting ready to breastfeed, or burp the baby during and after feedings. Another way to involve fathers in feeding is to have them give the breastfed baby an occasional bottle of expressed breast milk or formula. Early involvement of fathers in feeding is especially beneficial later when infants are being weaned or mothers are preparing to return to employment.

Risk Identification

Risk identification involves identifying families and individuals who are likely to have difficulty with attachment. The difficulty may be related to the health of either the parents or the infant, or to parents' ability to carry out their role as parents. Unrealistic expectations about the baby may be another factor in difficulty with attachment. Examples are adolescents thinking that a baby will fulfill their needs for love and status, or parents feeling that a baby will strengthen a failing marriage.

Extreme stress, health-risk factors, and illness can interfere with the parent-newborn contact that is needed for the development of attachment. Stressful conditions that pull parents' energies and attention away from their newborns can also be detrimental to attachment. Family nurses can be instrumental in assuring contact between families and supportive networks in these situations. In extremely stressful family situations, such as drug dependency, childbearing family nurses may refer these families for appropriate therapy. Postpartum depression negatively affects mother's interactions with her baby (Beck, 1995; 1998b). Family nurses must be aware of the negative impact of postpartum depression. Early identification and referral for treatment of women with postpartum depression can reduce the risk of adverse parent-infant interactions.

In a family where a parent has suffered abuse, neglect, and abandonment there is a risk for poor attachment. Nurses need to help them gain a perspective on the poor parenting they experienced and make them aware that they can choose not to repeat these behaviors with their own children. Family nurses can convey to these families a sense of caring and concern that may have been missing in their own childhoods. Family nurses can also help parents develop new skills in caregiving and interacting with their babies, such as soothing a fussy baby. In these situations family nurses will often work with social workers, psychotherapists, and developmental specialists to help these parents care for and nurture their children.

Nurses often identify families at risk for poor attachment through observing parent behaviors. Behaviors that could be of concern include verbal expressions of dissatisfaction with the baby, comparison of the baby and disliked family members, failure to respond to the infant's crying, lack of spontaneity in touching the baby, and stiffness or discomfort in holding the baby after the first week. Isolated incidences of these behaviors are probably not detrimental to attachment. What is important are trends and patterns, that is, whether the parent-infant relationship is progressing positively. Love and enjoyment of children grow over time. If the parents' enjoyment of the baby as a unique individual and commitment to the baby are not progressing, the family needs continuing support, education, role-modeling, encouragement, and realistic appraisal. Childbearing family nurses may need to refer families who do not demonstrate these behaviors to other professionals who can provide more intensive intervention.

Facilitating Role Learning

Learning roles is particularly important for the childbearing family. For many couples, taking on the role of parents is a dramatic shift in their lives. Difficulty with adaptation to parenthood may be related to the stress of learning new roles as well as to role conflicts. Role learning involves expectations about the role, developing the ability to assume the role, and taking on the role.

Expectations about the Parent Role

Expectations about parent roles are part of the stress new parents experience during the transition to parenthood. Mothers compare their actual experiences with their expectations. Those whose actual experience was disappointing regarding the relationship with their spouse, physical well-being, maternal competence, and maternal satisfaction, have had more difficulty adjusting to parenthood (Imle, 1989; Kalmuss, et al, 1992). Expectations about the partner's role also influences the transition to parenthood. For example, men have often been regarded as helpmates, supporters, and bystanders during childbearing, rather than as parents. If women are regarded as the "real" parents, men are not encouraged to grasp the reality of fatherhood (Jordan, 1990). These expectations can keep men from believing that they have the knowledge, support, or skills to become involved parents.

In North America, societal expectations about the parent role, especially motherhood, are unrealistic and may set up parents to feel inadequate. The myth of motherhood is supported by the media, which are full of images of new mothers clad in luxurious lace while they feed glowing, contented babies in immaculate houses. The reality of early motherhood is that prepregnancy clothes do not fit, babies periodically become demanding malcontents, and houses are messy because family members are too exhausted to clean. Nursing and medical textbooks reinforce this myth of the mother role by implying that at 6 weeks after birth, when healing of the reproductive system is complete, women are ready to resume all their activities. In reality, it takes longer for women to resume their role. Studies of postpartum women showed that virtually no woman had regained full functioning 6 weeks after birth (Smith-Hanrahan & Deblois, 1995; Tulman, et al, 1990). Incongruence between the ideal and the reality of the parent role may result in frustration, turmoil, and loss of confidence. Unrealistic expectations about being parents and about children's development are often present in angry, abusive families (Johnson, 1986). Unrealistic expectations about the effects of a baby on an adolescent parent's life also affect the parent role.

Family nurses can help parents discuss and face their ideals and to bridge the gap between the idealized and actual roles. One way to start is to have expectant parents, before their baby's birth, describe what being parents will be like. From these responses, family nurses can assess their expectations and begin to educate parents about the realities of parenting. For example, nurses can help expectant parents see themselves in very real situations–with interrupted sleep and little free time. Nurses must present a realistic but balanced view of parenthood; having parents shift from a totally positive view to an entirely negative one may not help them assume the parent role. Encouraging contact with new parents who are in the process of assuming the role may be more effective than any description of parenting that nurses can give. Contact with other parents is especially helpful for parents who are isolated, adolescent, or culturally diverse and living apart from traditional networks,

Family nurses can also help pregnant couples explore their attitudes and expectations about the role of their partners. For instance, a woman may not realize that she is placing her mate in a role subordinate to her when she considers herself as the primary parent or the "expert." Nurses can encourage expectant women to bring their mates into their experience by sharing the physical sensations and emotions of being pregnant. Many men need to be encouraged to think about how they expect to enact their role as fathers. Being relegated to a subordinate role can be discouraging to men and ultimately they may become less involved in parenting. If women expect their mates to be fully involved parents, they need to provide opportunities for partners to become skilled infant caregivers. For example, when her mate assumes infant care responsibilities, women should not rush in to correct their mates' "mistakes," such as a loose diaper or a shirt that is backwards. Coincidentally, family nurses must consider cultural meanings attached to gender roles when they are addressing parenting roles.

Developing Abilities for the Parent Role

Family nurses in all childbearing care settings teach parenting skills. The content of and process of teaching these skills are well delineated in current textbooks and other sources on expectant parent education (Nichols, 1993; Peterson & Peterson, 1993; Starn, 1993). Expectant mothers and fathers develop parenting abilities and skills through their own childhood experiences and contact with other parents, friends, family members, and health care providers. When planning educational strategies for parents, nurses must consider expectant parents' past experiences and the range and diversity of their information sources.

The role of parent is a dynamic one, because children's needs change as they develop. Fortunately, parents' skills grow and change along with their children. Family nurses can continue to help families develop the abilities they need for the parent role beyond the childbearing stage. This is especially important for teen-aged parents and parents with limited experience with children.

Taking on the Role of Parent

Becoming parents requires not only learning to perform caretaking tasks but also developing the feelings associated with parenting and the ability to solve problems associated with being a parent. Family nurses can assist parents in taking on the parental role by praising parents in their early efforts and modeling the feelings associated with the role. Specific behaviors to model include displaying warmth toward the baby and expressing pleasure over care of the baby. This is especially important for parents who are not deriving pleasure from caring for their babies. Depressed parents often do not experience pleasure.

As parents take on their roles, they begin to use problem solving to modify these roles to suit their own life situations and needs (Drayden & Imle, 1991). As parents meet their baby's needs consistently and successfully under a variety of conditions, their positive feelings about being parents grow. Nurses can help families discuss how to perform parenting tasks in their own environment with their own equipment. This problem-solving process can be enhanced by helping parents to associate their baby's behavior with its meaning. While helping parents empathize with their baby, nurses should also help families understand what is developmentally appropriate behavior for their baby, so that parents do not misinterpret the infant's behavior. If parents are becoming skilled caregivers with warmth, concern, and affection for their babies in their own environments, then they are clearly taking on the parent role.

Parents who experience frustration in taking on the parent role tend to evaluate themselves negatively. Intensive work with these parents to help them understand and develop empathy for their baby and understand the parent problem-solving process is necessary. If the new parents do not display warmth and affection toward the baby, family nurses should be concerned. These parents may need interventions to develop attachment.

Adjusting Communication Patterns to Accommodate a Newborn

As parents and infants learn to interpret and respond to each other's communication cues, they develop effective communication patterns. However, infant cues may be so subtle that parents may not be sensitive to cues until a nurse points them out (Sumner, 1990). Because of differences in temperament, different infants respond in different ways, which may make it difficult for parents to interpret cues. Mothers who are depressed are less attuned to their infants, which can lead to poor cognition later in infants' lives (Murray, et al, 1996). Depressed mothers may withdraw socially from their infants and act like robots in their everyday activities with their babies (Beck, 1996). Many babies respond to being held by cuddling and nuzzling but others respond by back arching and stiffening. Parents may interpret the latter as rejecting responses, and these negative interpretations may adversely affect the parent-infant relationship. Family nurses should be aware of interaction styles of depressed mothers and take steps to improve the quality of parent-infant interaction through facilitating treatment of depression. Educating parents about different infant temperaments so that they can interpret their baby's unique style of communication is another way to promote better communication patterns (Brazelton, 1992).

A useful tool to help parents learn about their infant's interactive behavior is the Brazelton Neonatal Behavioral Assessment Scale (BNBAS) (Brazelton, 1995). By observing the baby's assessment, parents can learn about the interaction style of their infants. Learning to perform the BNBAS involves extensive training; however, for family nurses involved with parent-infant interaction issues, learning the BNBAS is definitely worthwhile.

Communication between parents changes with the transition to parenthood. During the years of childbearing many men and women devote considerable time to career development. The time demands of work may affect a couple's relationship. While taking on the everyday aspects of parenting, couples often do not give their relationships the attention needed to sustain them. Yet, families thrive with a strong, sustained couple relationship, and couples need to recognize this (Jordan, et al, 1999).

Couple communication should be incorporated into expectant parent education programs. Parents must communicate with each other long after they have used the labor coping skills that are the essence of traditional expectant-parent preparation programs. An innovative expectant-parent education program under investigation incorporates a communication program that uses the psychoeducational model of information, skills, and support, based on research (Jordan, P., personal communication, January 1999).

Planning for Subsequent Children

Some families with their first baby have definite, mutually agreed on plans for additional children, while others have definitely decided not to have more children. Families who have definite plans primarily need information about family planning options so they can carry out their plans.

Often, family nurses will encounter parents who are uncertain about having more children. In these situations nurses can help families clarify their values and decision making. However, when discussing childbearing decisions, family nurses must consider the power structure and locus of decisions in the family. Mutual decision making means that both persons in the couple have equal power and status, which is rarely the case. It would be counter-productive for nurses not to consider the male partner in families with male-dominated power structures. In such a family, the woman may acquiesce in her partner's decisions, even when she does not agree with him.

Realigning Intergenerational Patterns

With childbearing, family organization and networks across generations enlarge. Contact with members of the extended family and exchange of helping activities increase across generations for most families at the onset of childbearing and grandparenting (Belsky & Rovine, 1984). Patterns of past relationships and intergenerational family patterns are sometimes brought into conflict by change that accompanies the childbearing period. Past patterns of family relationships may be recalled by parents and grandparents, contributing to disagreement and a sense of nonresolution.

The first baby adds a new generation in the family lineage, which carries the family into the future. During their first pregnancy, expectant parents change from being the children of their own parents to becoming parents themselves (Bennet, et al, 1988). As they see themselves approaching the same status held by their own mothers and fathers, they begin to redefine themselves, to consider themselves as parents as well as adults (Imle, 1989). Parenthood brings prestige and a sense of their own power, as they see themselves becoming more like their parents. Childbearing may mean the onset of being an adult for adolescent parents and some cultural groups.

Childbearing changes relationships within the extended families of the parents. Their siblings become aunts and uncles, children from previous relationships become stepsiblings, and their own parents become grandparents. When the expected baby is the first grandchild, the parents of the expectant parents also experience a change in status and become grandparents (Hagestad & Lang, 1986). Nurses working with pregnant women can promote development of grandparent-parent relationships in several ways (Martell, 1990). Many women talk spontaneously about their mothers, but nurses may have to encourage discussion with a simple phrase, such as, "Tell me about how things are going between you and your mother." From the pregnant woman's response, nurses can assess the quality of the relationship and, when appropriate, consider interventions to enhance their relationship. For example, nurses may suggest that the pregnant woman ask her mother to tell her about her own pregnancy and birth experiences. Sharing these experiences can enhance the sense of continuity. If conflict exists, family nurses can help by teaching pregnant women some simple communication strategies to open discussion with their mothers and help resolve conflict. This is especially important for adolescents and their mothers.

Potential areas of conflict between generations include infant feeding methods, dealing with crying babies, and other aspects of childrearing. Current recommendations for infant care and feeding may not be the same as what grandparents did with their own children a generation ago. Consequently, new parents may receive conflicting information. If conflicts persist or if, out of sheer exhaustion, new parents take outmoded or unwanted advice, they can become resentful, and intergenerational bonds can break down. Even with the change in status, new parents may find it stressful to confront their parents on an adult-to-adult level, especially when their parents genuinely want to be helpful. Nurses can suggest tactful ways for expectant parents to confront their own parents, who may have outmoded advice and information. Ideally, conflict can be prevented through information sharing and open discussion about what would be helpful before the arrival of the baby. Nurses can educate new and expectant grandparents about recommendations by helping them compare their experiences with present-day practices, giving them tours of hospital facilities, and providing up-to-date reading materials (Starn, 1993).

Reliance on health care professionals for childbearing and childrearing guidance is primarily a middle-class phenomenon; for other socioeconomic and cultural groups, nurses may not be as esteemed as the older women in families on matters relating to childbearing. In these situations, nurses may feel frustrated when new parents more readily accept the advice of other family members, such as their own mothers, rather than the health care provider's recommendations. Such a reaction should not be allowed to interfere with the nurse's primary goal of enhancing family relationships.

Maintaining Motivation and Morale

The care, feeding, and comforting of infants demand time, energy, and personal resources. Women may be fatigued for months from the physical exertion and blood loss of birth compounded by the demands of infant care. Some women have little chance to be well rested before they are expected to return to their jobs (Killien, 1993). In addition, maternal exhaustion can contribute to postpartum depression, which is detrimental to women and their families. The demands of early parenting tend to draw mothers and fathers away from the couple relationship.

Family nurses can help family members to maintain motivation and morale and to avoid becoming overwhelmed by the transition to parenthood. Before new mothers are discharged from their nurse's care, both parents need to know about ways to promote rest and sleep. For example, helping new mothers with comfort measures for a sore perineum or uterine cramps makes it easier for them to rest and cope with fatigue, which improves morale. Families need to be realistic about infant sleep patterns; typically, babies need nighttime feedings for several months, no matter how parents modify the timing and content of feedings. Time-honored ways to promote rest while a baby needs nighttime feedings are to alternate who responds to the baby and to feed the baby in the parents' bed. Infant crying seems to be more irritating if parents are fatigued, and it can exacerbate sleep loss and fatigue. Thus helping parents cope with crying can help family morale. Being able to soothe a fussy baby can boost confidence for new parents and allow them to get additional sleep.

In present-day North American families, the postpartum period can be lonely. Many young families live in communities far distant from their extended families. They may have recently moved into a new neighborhood and not had a chance to establish friendships or community. Many ethnically diverse groups had special support and recognition of the postpartum period in their countries of origin, but in the United States and Canada, they may have no replacement for traditional postpartum care. Family nurses should counsel families realistically about the duration of postpartum recovery and how isolated they may feel during this time. Expectant parents should be encouraged to ask their support networks for help with meals and household tasks after birth.

Frequently, new parents can find such support from childbirth education groups and colleagues at work. When young families find that their parenting experiences are similar to those of others, their morale tends to improve. Morale is also boosted by nurses and other health professionals who give realistic and positive feedback. Often new parents who want to appear self-sufficient are reluctant to accept offers of help; they may be vague about their needs. In such cases, nurses can help them to articulate their needs and accept help.

Couples do need to be aware of potential changes in their sexual relationship with the arrival of a baby. Sensitive family nurses can counsel couples about changes in sexuality after birth and assist them to develop mutually satisfying sexual expression. Often couples need to be encouraged to take time for themselves apart from the baby. The actual separation from the baby is not as important in itself as the fact that it allows parents to interact with each other and enjoy each other's company outside of the parenting role. This can be done even in very brief periods of conversation and physical closeness when the baby is asleep.

Most parents also need activity, companionship, and interests beyond the family for improved quality of their lives. For example, a study on postpartum well-being showed that women who exercised vigorously had more confidence in the tasks of mothering, more satisfaction with motherhood and their partner's participation in child care, and a higher quality of relationship with their partners (Sampselle, et al, 1999). Family nurses need to recognize these needs and help families to develop strategies that maintain their activities, adult interests, and friendships.

Establishing Rituals and Routines

Rituals develop as children come into a family and become part of the uniqueness and identity of a family. Family rituals are bedtime and bathing routines; baby's special possessions, such as a treasured blanket; and nicknames for body functions. For some families, rituals have a special cultural meaning, which nurses must respect. When families are disrupted or separated during childbearing, nurses can help them deal with stress by encouraging them to carry out their usual routines and establish rituals related to their babies.

THREATS TO HEALTH DURING CHILDBEARING

For the majority of families, childbearing is a physically healthy experience. For some families, health during childbearing is threatened, and the childbearing experience becomes an illness experience. In such cases, concern for the physical health of the mother and the fetus tends to outweigh other aspects of pregnancy, and rather than eagerly anticipating the birth and baby, family members have fear and apprehension. Moreover the family's functioning as a system and accomplishment of developmental tasks are disrupted as they focus attention on the health of the mother and survival of the fetus or baby. The effect of threats to health during childbearing is illustrated in the case study of a family with a preterm birth at the end of this chapter.

Acute and Chronic Illness during Childbearing

Classifying threats to health during childbearing as "acute" or "chronic" is difficult because childbearing is not an "illness." For this chapter, "acute" is defined as health threats that come on suddenly and may have life-threatening implications. Examples are fetal distress during labor and pulmonary embolism for postpartum women. "Chronic" conditions occur during pregnancy and persist, linger, or must be controlled to avoid becoming acute. Examples are pregnancy-induced hypertension, gestational and pre-existing diabetes, and postpartum depression. Some threats to health vacillate between acute and chronic. Preterm labor can be acute and result in a preterm birth. However, if preterm labor contractions are suppressed, they become "chronic" because of the regimens to keep contractions from recurring.

At times, a mother or a newborn may be so ill that they are best cared for in intensive care units: this presents unique challenges to childbearing families. Astute critical care nurses can function as family nurses by increasing their sensitivity and minimizing the barriers to family development (Harvey, 1992).

The most extreme threats to health during childbearing are maternal death, miscarriage, stillbirth, or neonatal death. Family nurses help families manage their grief in many ways. The death must not be "glossed over" but acknowledged in a sensitive way. Nurses give families opportunities to express grief, facilitate funeral arrangements, and carry out culturally important rituals.

A Family's Experience with Threats to Health

The case study of the Johnson family at the end of this chapter illustrates the impact of threats to health during childbearing. Mary's gestational diabetes could be considered chronic in that it could be stabilized for the duration of her pregnancy. Her preterm labor vacillated between being acute and chronic. When she was transferred to the regional center, her preterm labor became acute. For baby Jason, being preterm could be considered acute. As he matured and became stable enough to be discharged, he no longer had acute threats to his health. Mary, his mother, showed signs of postpartum depression. Without treatment, this depression could become chronic and affect other family members. The research brief at the end of the chapter explores postpartum depression.

Even though gestational diabetes and suppression of preterm labor are often managed at home, these threats to childbearing health are disruptive for the family system. The health threat to a member of the childbearing family affects the other members. The functioning and structure of the family that keeps the system stable, or in homeostasis, is upset, and the family strives to regain balance, which is stressful on all the components of the system. The following are examples of systems issues faced by childbearing families with threats to health.

Other family members must assume household and family tasks so that the expectant mother or a sick baby can stay on prescribed regimens. As the description of the Johnson family shows, shifting of these tasks may be stressful and affect the family's functioning. Expectant fathers, especially, find that all their time and energy are consumed by employment and household management, which previously were shared with or done solely by their partners. Children's lives change when mothers have to limit activities. Toddlers do not understand why their mothers cannot pick them up or run after them. The resulting frustration for children can manifest itself in behavior changes, such as Jenny's tantrums and lapses in toilet training. The demands of families, on the other hand, may make bed rest a stressful experience for expectant mothers and fathers (Gupton et al, 1997; McCain & Deatrick, 1994). Certainly Mary's anxiety was, in part, a response to feeling unable to handle family demands, and her nagging and complaining were probably expressions of her anxiety. Because of their frustration and the burdens of family tasks, women may not be fully compliant with the regimens to control potential health problems (Josten, et al, 1995).

The at-risk pregnancy is stressful in terms of the family's financial situation and other resources. Loss of income may result from time away from work, and medical expenses may rise as a result of the need for increased care, including possible neonatal intensive care. Personal expenses may increase because of a need for changes in diet, medications, alterations in transportation, and help with household tasks. The cost in terms of family energy and emotional response cannot be measured as easily, but the impact is evident in a situation like Tom's, in which the demands of household management are added to those of his new job.

Because of the unpredictable nature of high-risk childbearing, planning for the future becomes more difficult. The family may have to cope with sudden hospitalization, and if there are other small children in the home, they may become extremely anxious over their mother's sudden departure if they have not been prepared for it, especially if they are unable to comprehend what is going on.

High-risk childbearing is especially stressful when a family has a limited social or family network to assume family tasks, such as meal preparation, child care, and household maintenance. Mary's premature labor occurred before the Johnson's had developed a social network in their new community. Had they had a supportive network, some of the burden of household management may have been eliminated. With adequate support, Mary may not have felt so lonely and perhaps someone could have taken Jenny out to play. In other families, both parents' jobs may be affected by unpredictability. With pending preterm birth, for example, parents, especially employed women, may not be able to accurately determine when to begin parental leave or when it will end.

Transfer to a distant perinatal center is not uncommon for families in remote rural areas. Such transfers can separate family members for days or weeks and make it difficult to maintain established relationships. In the case of Tom and Mary, being with their new son was difficult because each visit required a 200-mile round trip, Tom had a full-time job, and Mary cared for Jenny during the day. Even if the logistical problems are solved and a family can be together, coping with even basic tasks of living is a challenge in these high-tech settings. For instance, the family may not know where to stay, how to find reasonably priced meals, or even where to park the car.

Interventions for health promotion need to be modified for the family experiencing a high-risk pregnancy. For example, a family nurse managing Mary's care for preterm labor would see that the prescribed regimen of bed rest was disrupting family morale and plans to arrange space for the new baby, that Tom was suffering role overload, and that the mother-child relationship between Mary and Jenny was strained. Lacking a local social network, the Johnson family had little exchange with outsiders and, consequently, stress could not be diffused from this family. Family nurses might help a family identify and use resources such as home health agencies and parents' groups in the community for assistance with household management and morale. Nurses could help Tom and Mary discuss the frustration accompanying Mary's bed rest and diet changes, Tom's role overload, and how stress was affecting their relationship.

Information about the impact of change on a 2-year-old child could help Tom and Mary understand and better manage Jenny's behavior. When Jason needed to remain at the perinatal center, neonatal nurses with a family focus would recognize the impact on development of attachment to the baby, role learning, and family morale of having a preterm baby in a regional neonatal intensive care unit far from home. Interventions for the Johnson family would include creating ways for them to have contact with Jason through telephone updates on his condition and photographs when they could not be physically with him, allowing them to do normal infant care tasks for Jason when they were visiting him, and encouraging them to develop a support system with other parents of intensive care infants.

Parents' concerns about themselves may be overlooked after birth. Mary Johnson's postpartum recovery was long and difficult because of her bed rest during pregnancy. After bed rest during pregnancy, postpartum women have reduced muscle strength, leaving them weak and vulnerable (Maloni, 1993). Even though Jason was healthy, a preterm birth experience can be disappointing because of unmet expectations. Consequently, Mary developed symptoms of postpartum depression. Astute family nurses would continue care for the family after the birth. Families should be informed about the realities of a prolonged postpartum physical recovery after prolonged bed rest. Mary may have been able to breastfeed Jason through a program of breast pumping to stimulate lactation while she was separated from him and the support of nurses who are enthusiastic about and capable of helping women breastfeed their preterm babies. Mary could have been referred to a lactation consultant, a breastfeeding support group, and home nursing services. Nurses must counsel families about postpartum depression and the importance to the family of prompt, expert care for postpartum depression.

In situations of threat, the coping strategies of families may be inadequate or be exhausted in the face of extreme stress. Before experiencing an at-risk pregnancy, many young families have never had to face situations of threatened health, a drain on financial resources, or separation from loved ones. The family's coping strategies can be further compromised by the fact that families under stress often have unrealistic perceptions of their situation. In these situations, family nurses can help childbearing families develop appropriate coping strategies. Nurses can help them realistically appraise threats to health and identify their strengths and resources for coping. Strengths include positive ways they have coped with stressful situations in the past; resources include available helpful persons, financial assistance, and informational sources. Finally, nurses can assist families in the longer term by teaching them to solve problems and develop new resources and strategies for healthy, effective coping.

IMPLICATIONS FOR EDUCATION, RESEARCH, AND POLICY

The concerns of childbearing family nurses go beyond care of the individual family. These nurses are participants in guiding nursing education, developing and using research, and setting and implementing policy.

Education

Family nursing with childbearing families has developed, in part, as a response to the increasing emphasis in nursing education on families as the client or the context for nursing care. With the shift of health care into nonacute care settings and homes, some of the traditional care done by nurses now has to be done within families. On the other hand, health care for some childbearing families is becoming extremely technical and intensive. Examples are fertility treatments and obstetrical critical care units. Consequently, education about family nursing will become even more crucial for childbearing health care.

Research

Research on family nursing interventions and outcomes needs to be increased for development of evidence-based nursing practice. Evaluation of the effectiveness of family nursing interventions is especially critical when health care costs are under close scrutiny, and third-party payers need to be convinced that family nursing interventions result in improved outcomes of childbearing and that they are cost-effective (Cook, 1997).

Policy

Family-centered care is prevalent in North America. In a survey of 50 hospital obstetric units across the United States, 90% had implemented or were in the process of developing mother-and-baby care, while 10% still had separate postpartum and nursery units (Bajo, et al, 1998). The incorporation of the word "family" into the names of health care institutions may make nurses complacent about the state of family nursing practice in their settings. Serious examination of institutional policies could help nurses determine whether the word "family" is part of a catchy name for marketing purposes or betokens a strong influence on philosophy, policies, and nursing standards. Nurses may find barriers in their practice settings that interfere with promoting family development. For example, lack of privacy, complex machinery, and location of a neonatal intensive care unit may stifle interaction between family members and babies. Some suggestions for making family-centered care a reality are: (1) identifying physical, psychological, and nursing staff requirements for family-centered care; (2) developing a clear vision of family-centered care units; and (3) involving nurses in the planning and implementation of change.

Nurses must be aware of the impact of legislation on childbearing families. One example is family leave for childbirth, which can profoundly affect health and development of childbearing families. More recently in the United States, the Newborns and Mothers Health Protection Act of 1996 sets standards for minimal length of inpatient hospital stay for mothers and newborn infants. Many states now have legislation addressing postpartum care (Ferguson & Engelhard, 1997).

Family nurses need to be proactive in caring for families within the framework set by legislation.

SUMMARY

Childbearing family nursing is not synonymous with maternity nursing. Family nurses care for all members of the childbearing family and focus on families who are healthy as well as those who experience threats to health during the childbearing cycle. Although childbearing family nursing is not yet universally practiced in health care settings, it is evolving through education, research, and policy development. Various family theories, such as Duvall's family life cycle theory, help family nurses organize nursing assessments, plan interventions, and evaluate outcomes of nursing care with childbearing families. Through its impact on adaptation to parenthood, family nursing can make a major difference in family health during the childbearing years.

RESEARCH BRIEF

Postpartum Depression and the Family

Research on postpartum depression is especially important for family nurses because it affects all members of the family. Postpartum depression affects 10 to 15 percent of all childbearing women (Beck, 1995). Consequently, a large number of children and adults, especially fathers, are affected by postpartum depression.

Beck, a nurse-researcher, conducted a meta-analysis of 19 research studies on the effects of postpartum depression on mother-infant interaction. Depressed women and their babies show consistent patterns of maternal-infant interaction (Beck, 1995). Depressed mothers display less affectionate contact behavior, less responsiveness to infant cues, a flattened affect, and withdrawal or hostility toward their infants. Infants of depressed mothers behaved differently from infants of mentally healthy women. The infants were fussier, had more avoidant behaviors, and made fewer positive vocalizations and facial expressions. Statistically, the meta-analysis indicated that postpartum depression had a moderate to large effect on maternal-infant interaction during the infants' first year. The adverse effects of postpartum depression may have long-term effects on children's cognitive and emotional development (Beck, 1998a).

The impact of postpartum depression on women's partners is drawing more interest. A team of nurse-researchers (Meighan, et al, 1999) studied the experiences of eight men whose spouses had postpartum depression. These fathers' lives and relationships with their wives were disrupted. They felt fear, confusion, and concern for their spouses, yet they were frustrated by not being able to do anything to alleviate the depression. They made sacrifices to hold the family together and were uncertain about the future with their wives, who seemed very different after the birth.

Nurses, through recognizing postpartum depression and promptly referring women for treatment, not only help affected women and enhance the social and emotional environment for infants but also may promote the survival of family relationships.

Source: Beck, C. T. (1998). The effects of postpartum depression on child development: A meta-analysis. *Archives of Psychiatric Nursing, 12*:12–20; Beck, C. T. (1995). The effects of postpartum depression on maternal-infant interaction: A meta-analysis. *Nursing Research,* 44:298–304; Meighan, M., et al. (1999). Living with postpartum depression: The father's experience. *MCN: The American Journal of Maternal/Child Nursing, 24*:202–208.

Case Study

THE JOHNSONS: A FAMILY WITH A PRETERM NEWBORN

Tom and Mary Johnson's first child, Jenny, was born at full term. Mary had no health problems with the pregnancy. At the time, the Johnsons lived in a large city in the western part of the United States, near their parents, siblings, and childhood friends.

Two years later, the Johnsons moved to a small town 500 miles away from their friends and families to find better professional opportunities for Tom and more affordable housing. A month after the move, they discovered that Mary was about 3 months pregnant. Mary decided to postpone seeking employment as a secretary until after the birth and concentrate on fixing up their older two-story house.

Unexpectedly, Mary had health problems with this pregnancy. At 27 weeks of pregnancy, her obstetrician diagnosed gestational diabetes, and Mary had to modify her diet to keep her blood glucose under control. At 29 weeks, she began to experience preterm labor contractions. To stop the contractions, her physician insisted that Mary stay on bed rest around the clock, except for a very brief daily shower and use of the bathroom. Tom had to take over meal preparation, house cleaning, and caring for Jenny. He arranged the living room so that Mary could lie on the couch and Jenny could play near her mother while he was at work. Because he had not yet accrued vacation or sick time, Tom could not take off time from his job to help Mary and take care of Jenny without sacrificing wages.

Mary found it difficult to follow her diet and stay on bed rest. She was frustrated because she had to stop her house renovation and Tom's cooking and housecleaning were not up to her standards. She was tempted to run the vacuum cleaner, wash dishes, and eat sweets while Tom was at work. The medication to suppress contractions made her so anxious and tremulous that she could not amuse herself with crafts, sewing, or puzzles. She was lonely for her mother and friends, who were 500 miles away; she longed for companionship but found herself complaining and nagging Tom when he was home. Jenny frequently had tantrums because she could not play outside with her mother and began to have lapses in toilet training.

At 32 weeks of pregnancy, Mary's membranes ruptured, and her physician sent her to a perinatal center 100 miles away from home because it had better facilities to care for preterm babies. Jenny went with her parents to the perinatal center to wait until one of her grandmothers could come and take care of her. Jason was born 28 hours after the Johnsons arrived at the perinatal center hospital.

Mary was discharged from the perinatal center within 24 hours after birth. At home, she felt extremely weak and was overwhelmed by household tasks and caring for Jenny. She was disappointed that she was unable to breastfeed the baby. Two weeks later she was weeping frequently, felt very sad, had no appetite, and had difficulty sleeping. Jason, the new baby, remained at the perinatal center in the special care nursery until he was mature and stable enough to go home, 4 weeks later.

Study Questions

1. Early predecessors of childbearing family nurses were
   a. Childbirth educators.
   b. Nurse midwives.
   c. Nursery nurses.
   d. Public health nurses.
2. Currently the best theory to guide childbearing family nursing is
   a. Family systems.
   b. Structural-functional.
   c. Change theory.
   d. None of the above.
3. Families with closed boundaries are often not accessible to nursing interventions because
   a. These families do not have children.
   b. These are unstable families.
   c. Family members do not interact with each other.
   d. These families reject influences from the outside environment.
4. Childbearing family nurses may ask about a family's space arrangement for an expected baby to assess whether the family

a. Is meeting its basic needs.
b. Is accepting the reality of the expected baby.
c. Has fears about the survival of the baby.
d. All of the above.

5. The priority for research related to childbearing family nursing is
a. The effectiveness of family nursing interventions.
b. Development of theories that describe childbearing families.
c. The importance of immediate contact between newborn babies and their parents.
d. Explain how the "Baby Boom" of the 1950s influenced present-day childbearing family nursing.

6. Write a care plan to help the Johnson family, who are portrayed in the case study, develop a relationship with Jason while he is in the special care nursery.

References

American College of Obstetricians and Gynecologists (ACOG) and the Interprofessional Task Force on Health Care of Women and Children (1978). Joint statement on the development of family centered maternity/newborn care in hospitals. Chicago: ACOG.

Bajo, K., et al. (1998). Clinical focus: Keeping moms and babies together. *AWHONN Lifelines*, *2*(2):44–48.

Beck, C. T. (1998a). A checklist to identify women at risk for developing postpartum depression. *Journal of Obstetric, Gynecologic, and Neonatal Nursing*, *27*:39–46.

Beck, C. T. (1998b). The effects of postpartum depression on child development: A meta-analysis. *Archives of Psychiatric Nursing*, *12*, 12–20.

Beck, C. T. (1996). Postpartum depressed mothers' experiences interacting with their children. *Nursing Research*, *45*:98–104.

Beck, C. T. (1995). The effects of postpartum depression on maternal-infant interaction: A meta-analysis. *Nursing Research*, *44*:289–304.

Belsky, J., & Rovine, M. (1984). Social network contact, family support, and the transition to parenthood. *Journal of Marriage and the Family*, *46*:455–462.

Bennet, L. A., et al. (1988). Family identity, ritual and myth: A cultural perspective on life cycle transition. In C. J. Falico (Ed.), *Family Transitions*, (pp. 211–234). New York: Guilford Press.

Brazelton, T. B. (1995). *Neonatal behavioral assessment scale* (ed 3): Clinics in developmental medicine, 137. London: MacKeith Press.

Brazelton, T. B. (1992). *Touchpoints: Your Child's Emotional and Behavioral Development*. Reading, MA: Addison-Wesley.

Broderick, C. B. (1993). *Understanding Family Process*. Newbury Park, CA: Sage.

Cook, S. S. (1997). Configuring childbirth education to survive managed care. *Advanced Practice Nursing Quarterly*, *2*:22–26.

Cowan, P. A. (1991). The individual and family life transitions: A proposal for a new definition. In P. A. Cowan and M. Hetherington (Eds.). *Family Transitions* (pp. 3–30). Hinsdale, NJ: Laurence Erlbaum Assoc.

Drayden, T., & Imle, M. (1991, May). First-time parents' perspectives of family care needs during the postpartum period of transition to parenthood. Paper presented at the Second International Family Nursing Conference. Portland, OR.

Duvall, E. M., & Miller, B. C. (1986). *Marriage and Family Development*. New York: Harper & Row.

Ferguson, S. L., & Engelhard, C. L. (1997). Short stay: The art of legislating quality and economy. *AWHONN Lifelines*, *1*:16–23.

Gupton, A., Heaman, M., and Ashcroft, T. (1997). Bed rest from the perspective of the high-risk pregnant woman. *Journal of Obstetric, Gynecologic, and Neonatal Nursing*, *26*:423–430.

Hagestad, G. O., & Lang, M. E. (1986). The transition to grandparenthood. *Journal of Family Issues*, *7*:115–130.

Harvey, M. G. (1992). Promoting parenting: The obstetric patient in an intensive care unit. *Critical Care Nursing Clinics of North America*, *4*: 721–728.

Imle, M. A. (1989). Adjustment to parenthood: Model and scale development: Final report (1984–1988). (USDH Grant #5R23NU01181). Washington, DC: PHS Division of Nursing.

Johnson, S. H. (1986). *Nursing Assessments and Strategies for the Family at Risk: High-Risk Parenting*. Philadelphia: Lippincott.

Jordan, P. (1990). Laboring for relevance. *Nursing Research*, *13*:11–16.

Josten, L. E., et al. (1995). Bed rest compliance for women with pregnancy problems. *Birth*, *22*:1–14.

Kalmuss, D., et al. (1992). Parenting expectations, experiences, and adjustment to parenthood: A test of the violated expectations framework. *Journal of Marriage and the Family*, *54*:516–526.

Killien, M. G. (1993). Returning to work after childbirth: Considerations for health policy. *Nursing Outlook*, *41*:73–78.

Klaus, M. H., & Kennell, J. H. (1976). *Maternal-infant Bonding*. St. Louis: Mosby.

Leavitt, J. W. (1986). *Brought to Bed: Childbearing in America 1750–1950*. New York: Oxford University Press.

LeMasters, E. E. (1957). Parenthood as crisis. *Marriage and the Family, 31*:352–355.

Maloni, J. (1993). Bed rest during pregnancy: Implications for nursing. *Journal of Obstetric, Gynecologic, and Neonatal Nursing, 22*:422–426.

Martell, L. K. (1990). The mother-daughter relationship during daughter's first pregnancy: The transition experience. *Holistic Nursing Practice, 4*(3):47–55.

McCain, G. C., and Deatrick, J. A. (1994). The experience of high-risk pregnancy. *Journal of Obstetric, Gynecologic, and Neonatal Nursing, 23*:421–427.

Meighan, M., et al. (1999). Living with postpartum depression: The father's experience. *MCN: The American Journal of Maternal/Child Nursing, 24*:202–208.

Mercer, R. T. (1989). Theoretical perspectives on family. In C. L. Gillis, et al. (Eds.) *Toward a Science of Family Nursing* (pp. 9–36). Menlo Park, CA: Addison-Wesley.

Mercer, R. T., and Ferketich, S. L. (1990). Predictors of family functioning 8 weeks following birth. *Nursing Research, 39*:76–82.

Miller, S. R., & Winstead-Fry, P. (1982). Family systems theory in nursing practice. Reston, VA: Reston Publishing

Murray, L., et al. (1996). The impact of postpartum depression and associated adversity on early mother-infant interactions and later infant outcome. *Child Development, 67*:2512–2526.

Nichols, F. H., (Ed.) (1993). Perinatal education. *Clinical Issues in Perinatal and Women's Health Nursing, 4*:1–159.

Norbeck, J., & Tilden, V. P. (1983). Life stress, social support and emotional disequilibrium in complication of pregnancy: A prospective multivariate study. *Journal of Health and Social Behavior, 24*:30–46.

Peterson, K. J., & Peterson, F. L. (1993). Family-centered perinatal education. *Clinical Issues in Perinatal and Women's Health Nursing, 4*:1–4.

Ramsey, C. N., et al. (1986). The relationship between family functioning, life events, family structure, and the outcome of pregnancy. *Journal of Family Practice, 22*:521–527.

Sampselle, C. M., et al. (1999). Physical activity and postpartum well-being. *Journal of Obstetric, Gynecologic, and Neonatal Nursing, 28*:41–49.

Smith-Hanrahan, C., & Deblois, D. (1995). Postpartum early discharge: Impact on maternal fatigue and functional ability. *Clinical Nursing Research, 4*:50–66.

Starn, J. (1993). Strengthening family systems. *Clinical Issues in Perinatal and Women's Health Care Nursing, 4*:35–43.

Steffensmeier, T. H. (1982). A role model of the transition to parenthood. *Journal of Marriage and the Family, 44*:319–334.

Sumner, G. (1990). Keys to caregiving. Seattle: NCAST Publications.

Tilden, V. P. (1983). The relation of life stress and social support to emotional disequilibrium during pregnancy. *Research in Nursing and Health, 6*:167–174.

Tulman, L., et al. (1990). Changes in functional status after childbirth. *Nursing Research, 39*:70–75.

Wertz, R. W., & Wertz, D. C. (1989). *Lying-in: A history of childbirth in America*. New Haven, CT: Yale University Press.

Bibliography

Ainsworth, M. D. S. (1973) The development of infant-mother attachment. In B. M. Caldwell & H. N. Riccuiuti (Eds.). *Review of Infant Research*, vol 3. Chicago: University of Chicago Press.

Brazelton, T. B. (1989). *The Earliest Relationship: Parents, Infants, and the Drama of Early Attachment*. Reading, MA: Addison-Wesley.

Carter, E., & McGoldrick, M. (1980) *The Family Life Cycle: A Framework for Family Therapy*. New York: Gardner Press.

Cowan, C. P., & Cowan, P. A. (1992). *When Partners Become Parents: The Big Life Change for Couples*. New York: Basic Books.

House, J. S. (1981). *Work Stress and Social Support*. Reading, MA: Addison-Wesley.

Imle, M. A. (1990). Third trimester concerns of expectant parents in transition to parenthood. *Holistic Nursing Practice, 4*:25–36.

Martin-Arafeh, J. M., et al. (1999). Promoting family-centered care in high-risk pregnancy. *Journal of Perinatal and Neonatal Nursing, 13*:27–42.

Meleis, A. I., & Trangenstein, P. A. (1994) Facilitating transitions: Redefinition of the nursing mission. *Nursing Outlook, 42*: 255–259.

Mercer, R. T. (1990) *Parents at Risk*. New York: Springer.

Mercer, R. T., et al. (1989). *Transition in a Woman's Life: Major Life Events in Developmental Context*. New York: Springer.

Spero, D. (1993). Sibling preparation classes. *Clinical Issues in Perinatal and Women's Health Care Nursing, 4*:122–131.

Walker, L. O. (1992). *Parent-Infant Nursing Science: Paradigms, Phenomena, Methods*. Philadelphia: F. A. Davis.

Focus On

FAMILY CHILD HEALTH NURSING

This chapter provides a brief history of family-centered care of children and presents the family interactional model as a guide for nursing practice for families with children. The model uses three major concepts, family career, individual development, and patterns of health/disease/illness, to help explain and plan care in health promotion, acute illness, chronic illness, and life-threatening illness situations.

Health promotion and prevention are related to families' daily routines and occur through the daily activities of parenting, grandparenting, and child-care and after-school facilities. Physical health is promoted by hygiene, nutrition, exercise, and sleep. Mental and social health are promoted by helping children and adults reach developmentally appropriate landmarks in the family environment. Because the leading causes of morbidity and mortality among youth are substance use, sexual activity, and violence (both suicidal and homicidal), school failure, increased attention to health promotion and prevention are needed. Nurses can facilitate and teach health activities.

While members of American families experience health during 85 percent of their lifetime, they will experience illness for 15 percent of the time. Acute illness, chronic illness, and life-threatening illness present overlapping and distinct challenges for family nurses. The family interaction model can be used by the nurses to facilitate and teach healthful activities for growth in families. The chapter includes a case to illustrate use of the model.

Finally, implications for practice, research, education, and policy are discussed. After completing this chapter, students may find it helpful to think about their own family child nursing experiences or those they have read about and consider how the information contained in this chapter might have been used in those situations.

Chapter 11

FAMILY CHILD HEALTH NURSING

Vivian Gedaly-Duff • Marsha L. Heims

OUTLINE

OBJECTIVES

On completion of this chapter, the reader will be able to:

- Define and describe family child health nursing.
- Describe the components of the Family Interaction Model.
- Discuss the family theories used in the Family Interaction Model.
- Discuss how the concept of family career can guide the formulation of nursing actions for family child health.
- Discuss family transitions amenable to intervention by family child health nurses.
- Propose nursing interventions for families with children that reflect knowledge of patterns of health.

- Propose nursing interventions for families with children that reflect knowledge of patterns of illness.
- Describe health issues for families experiencing situational and developmental health transitions.
- Describe screening measures that family child health nurses use during family transitions.
- Propose health promotion interventions for families experiencing health transitions.
- Propose nursing strategies for situational and developmental family transitions.
- List health outcomes for a child and family using developmental and situational health events in a family career.
- List health outcomes for a child and family experiencing a health transition.
- List health outcomes for a child and family experiencing an illness transition during an acute illness, a chronic illness, and a life-threatening illness.
- Describe profiles of family needs for various types of families encountered by nurses.
- Describe social and community influences on family and child health.
- Describe social and legal policies that influence children, families and family child health nursing.
- Describe standards of care that family child health nurses use in practice.

A major task of families is to nurture children to become healthy, responsible, and creative adults. Parents, as primary caretakers of their children, are charged with keeping them healthy as well as caring for them during illness. Yet most mothers and fathers have little formal education for parenting. In fact, most parents learn the role "on the job," relying on memories of their childhood experiences in their families of origin to help them.

Family nurses help families promote health, prevent disease, and cope with illness. The importance of family life for children's health and illness is often invisible, because families' everyday routines are commonplace and lie below the level of conscious awareness. However, family life influences the promotion of health and the experience of illness in children.

Families are groups with unique features, including specific family memories and intergenerational relationships; family rules and routines; family aspirations and achievements; and ethnic or cultural patterns (Burr, et al, 1988). Family changes in structure and relationships interact with these family features.

Healthy outcomes for children—for example, tripling their birth weight by one year of age, or successfully completing high school if they have juvenile diabetes—are partially attributable to the intangible, invisible daily interactions among family members. Family features related to illness are often not discussed, but they are evident in daily activities. Nurses, in collaboration with families, examine how the features of families influence health.

Family child health nursing is about the relationships between family tasks and health care and their effects on family well-being and children's health. Nurses care for children within the context of their family, and they care for children by treating the family as a whole. (See Chapter 1 for approaches to family nursing.) In both approaches, families affect their children's health, while children's health affects their families.

This chapter provides a brief history of family-centered care of children and then presents a family interactional model that can be used to guide nursing practice with families with children. A case study is used to illustrate application of the model. Finally, implications for practice, research, education, and policy are discussed.

HISTORY OF FAMILY-CENTERED CARE OF CHILDREN

Family-centered care may be defined as the collaborative efforts of families and health care professionals to care for children's health. However, the family's role in the health care of children has often been debated. Besser (1977) reports that Dr. Armstrong, who opened the first Dispensary for the Infant Poor in 1769, argued that taking sick children from their parents would break their hearts, and said that the "air" of a crowded open room was contaminated. The poor survival rates of children in institutions supported his view. The Foundling Hospital in London admitted 14,934 infants between 1756 and 1760, but only 4400 lived to enter apprenticeships (Besser). In contrast, Dr. West, who founded Britain's Great Ormond Street Hospital in 1852, was convinced by his visits to families in "homes" that were dark, cold hovels that a hospital was essential for promoting children's health (Besser).

Nurses have always worked with families with children (Schultz & Meleis, 1988). Lillian Wald (1904), the founder of public health or community nursing, described a 2-year-old child ill with pneumonia:

> . . . Baby was found on a feather bed covered with feather pillows, with a temperature of 105°F. The nurse explained to the mother the desirability of cooler bedding and taught her how to arrange the crib properly. The front room was reserved for the sick baby and the mother was taught how to give the medicines, how to sponge the baby, and how to keep a record of the treatment. She devoted herself to the sick child, while her sister came to take care of the house and the two other children. The child's fever ran on for 4 days, and at the end subsided and the baby recovered (p. 605).

Faville (1925), depicted a nurse who visited a child's home after sending home a note explaining that the child had a communicable disease and could not return to school without a note from the doctor.

> The visiting nurse walked with Tony and Mike up the alley to their home. . . . The mother could not read English and so had attached small importance to the printed slip of paper brought from school. Two more children, Mary and the baby, were found to be scratching vigorously, and the father was sick in bed with a bad cold. . . . "All the time, he cough," the mother explained. "Now hot, now cold." "Did he spit blood?" "Yes, last week." The Italian doctor had been in and said that the man must go to the country at once. "But how can we? No place to go; no money and I must stay here to get Jimmie off to work each night." Jimmie being the pale-faced boy of 17 who was eating his supper preparatory to going on night shift at the mill (p. 14).

As these vignettes illustrate, nurses have historically gone to families to evaluate their condition, and striven to improve the health of children and their families. In this first instance, the nurse focused on the child and taught the mother how to care for the child's fever. In the second case, the nurse who started out assessing why the child came to school ill discovered a whole family who had health and social problems. To effectively treat the child, she needed to deal with other health and social family problems.

The effect of hospitalization on children and their families is a concern for nurses. In the past, parents and family had restricted visiting hours. Yet early studies of hospitalized children indicated that they suffered from a lack of family nurturance during long isolation periods. During and after World War II, Burlingham and Freud's work (1942) and Spitz's study (1945) demonstrated the negative effects of separating infants and children from their families. After reviewing this work on hospitalization, Goslin (1978), concluded that young children separated from families (particularly infants older than 6 months and children under 4 years) exhibited depression. Today, all nurses know that infants and toddlers show protest, despair, and detachment behaviors when separated from their families. Young children are profoundly affected by the health care environment and the people in it.

Hospitalization also causes stress and anxiety in the parents of sick children (Melnyk, 1998; Miles et al, 1989; Tiedeman, 1997) and their siblings (Morrison, 1997). Nurses who have cared for hospitalized children have found that the parents often needed care particularly when their children were undergoing unpleasant procedures (Callery, 1997a). Expert nurses now routinely include parents in their care of acutely or critically ill children (Gedaly-Duff et al, 1997; Hill & Gedaly-Duff, 1998). Nurses can reduce the stress for sick children, demystify the experience for their siblings, educate parents and grandparents about the children's disease, and support the family as a whole during hospitalization. Nursing research that began in the 1960s has now led to open visiting hours for all family members, parent rooming-in, family preparation for procedures, and hospital play (Thompson, 1986).

Infants and children may be hospitalized for hours as in day-surgery, for months as in neonatal intensive care units, or repeatedly as for chronic disease. Families desire to participate but do not know what to do, and they often feel left out of the decision-making about their children's health (Callery, 1997b). Often families are also unprepared for the emotional, physical, social, and financial burdens of home care.

Family-centered care is a system-wide approach to child health care based on the assumption that families are their children's primary source of strength and support (Harticker, 1998). "Family-centered care" has emerged in response to increasing family responsibilities for health care. The principles of family-centered care include: (1) recognizing families as "the constants" in children's lives, while the personnel in the health care system fluctuate; (2) openly sharing information about alternative treatments, ethical concerns, and uncertainties about health care treatments; (3) forming partnerships between families and health professionals to decide what is important for families; (4) respecting the racial, ethnic, cultural, and socioeconomic diversity of families and their ways of coping; and (5) supporting and strengthening families' abilities to grow and develop (Lash & Wertlieb, 1993). For example, families that live with the everyday routine of a child's chronic disease not only know the pattern of the disease, drugs, and other medical treatments, but they also know the responses of the child and family members to these factors. Many times health professionals fail to recognize the expertise that families acquire as they care for their children (Gedaly-Duff, et al, 2000).

As a result of their ongoing involvement, families learn that health professionals base decisions on theory, research, and clinical experience but do not know specifically how their child will respond until after the interventions are completed (Paget, 1982). Families acknowledge the uncertainty that surrounds their child's disease, but they want to be informed partners of the health team in decision-making. In an American society that respects family diversity, a health team that includes the family is preferable to a hierarchical team with physicians at the top, nurses in between, and families at the bottom. Family-centered care brings attention back to the importance of families in health care.

FAMILY INTERACTION MODEL

Family nurses need a theoretical model to describe, explain, predict, and prescribe child nursing care and address diverse family situations. (See Chapter 2 for theories in family nursing.) Nurses work with families when they are healthy and ill; they see families in homes, clinics, and hospitals; they know some families for a short time and with others have ongoing relationships. To be useful, a model for nurses caring for families with children must be applicable to all these situations. The *family interaction model* uses the concepts of *family career, individual development, and patterns of health, disease, and illness* to guide nursing practice of families with children (Gedaly-Duff & Heims, 1996).

The family interaction model is derived from *symbolic interaction theory* and *developmental theory*. (See Chapter 2 for theories on family nursing.) Based on the insights of social interactionist George Herbert Mead (1934), the model assumes that (1) meanings and responses to health, disease, and illness are created through interactions among family members and between the family and society, and (2) families' meanings and responses are partially influenced by family and individual development (Figure 11-1). Thus, not only do families shape their members, but members shape their families (Wallace, et al, 1999). Much of the time, the daily nature of family activities makes meanings implicit rather than explicit. When nurses understand that families and family members have unique perceptions and meanings for health or illness situations, they can help families redefine situations if necessary and create a shared family meaning. For example, a child diagnosed with sickle-cell anemia may be labeled by the family as a "son with a handicapping, painful disease." The nurse can help the family reframe the situation and create a new meaning for it by showing that children with this disease are suc-

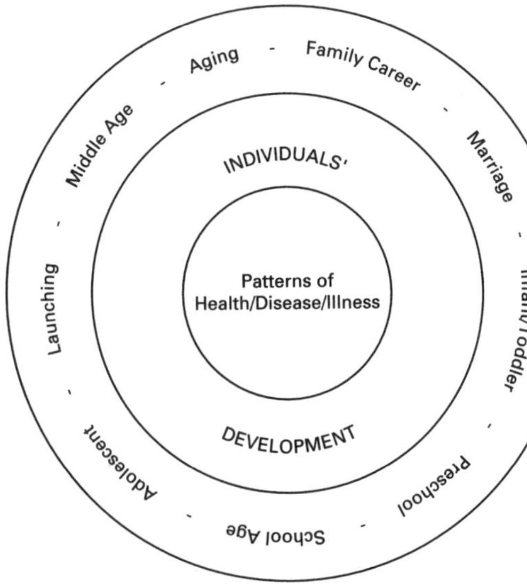

FIGURE 11-1
Family interaction model.

cessful in playing sports. The family may now label their son as "a boy who can grow and develop but who lives with an episodic, painful condition."

The *developmental perspective* suggests that families and individuals change over time. Families, which consist of adults and children, experience the various developmental stages of their members, and they also progress through a series of family developmental stages. Nurses, by comparing their observations of particular families to expected family and individual developmental stages, can plan appropriate care.

As noted above, the family interaction model uses three concepts to guide nursing care: (1) family career, which is the dynamic and unique developmental and situational experiences of a family's life time represented by family stages and family transitions; (2) individual development, which is the expected changes in each member associated with growth and development; and (3) patterns of health, disease, and illness, which are expected behaviors in these health situations. Knowledge of these three concepts and their interactions with each other can provide nurses with an understanding of the effects of health and illness on family interactions. These three concepts and their components are illustrated in Figure 11-1 and described in the next section.

Family Career

Family career is the dynamic process of change that occurs during the life span of the unique group called the family. Family career is similar to family life cycle and family development in that it takes into account family tasks and raising children. However, family development stages view the family in standard sequential steps and similarly, the family life cycle sees the family as progressing from the birth of the first child to raising and launching children, to experiencing the death of a parent figure in old age (Duvall & Miller, 1985). In contrast, family career takes into account the diverse experiences of American families (Aldous, 1996). Many types of families care for children, including single-parent, divorced custody co-parent, divorced non-custody co-parent, stepparent through a remarriage, and homosexual parent families. The family career includes both the expected developmental changes of the family life cycle, and the unexpected changes of situational crises such as divorce, remarriage, and death.

The notion of family career includes the many paths that families can take during their life span. Changes do not necessarily occur in a linear fashion. For example, while family development theory assumes that families raising more than one child have already experienced the stage of birthing and resulting family development tasks, a person may marry a partner who already has adolescent children and experience parenthood, but not the parenthood of young children. The research describes family career stages and developmental tasks in many types of families such as single-parent (Anderson, 1999), divorced (Ahrons, 1999; Carter & McGoldrick, 1999), remarried (McGoldrick & Carter, 1999), and homosexual families (Johnson & Colucci, 1999). The concept of family career is thus useful because it reminds us that families are dynamic. Nurses working with childrearing families need to be knowledgeable about family careers, which include both the stages of family development and family transition events that affect family health. Family stages and family transitions are presented in the next two sections, with examples from the literature.

Family Stages

Duvall's eight stages of family development, based on the oldest child, describe expected changes in families who are raising children (Duvall & Miller, 1985). Some family careers start with marriage without children, then proceed to childbearing, preschool children, school children, adolescents, the launching of young adults (first child gone to last child leaving home), middle age of parents (empty nest to retirement), and aging of family members (retirement to death of both parents). These *family stages* help nurses anticipate the family reorganization necessary to accommodate the growth and development of its members. For example, families with school-aged children expect children to be able to take care of their own hygiene, whereas families with infants expect to do all the hygiene care.

Across all family stages, there are basic *family tasks* that are essential to survival and continuity (Duvall & Miller, 1985): (1) to secure shelter, food, and clothing; (2) to develop emotionally healthy individuals who can manage crisis and experience nonmonetary achievement; (3) to assure each individual's socialization in school, work, spiritual, and community life; (4) to contribute to the next generation, by giving birth, adopting a child, or foster-caring a child; and (5) to promote the health of its members and care for them during illness.

The aim of the nurse is to help families develop appropriate ways to carry out the tasks necessary to prevent or restore illness and disease, and to promote health.

Family Transitions

Family transitions are a second component of the family career; They may be developmental or situational. *Family transitions* are events that signal a reorganization of family roles and tasks. Such transitions are central to nursing practice because they have profound health-related effects on people (Schumacher & Meleis, 1994). Developmental transitions are predictable changes that occur in an expected time line congruent with movement through the eight family stages. Because they are usual, developmental transitions are also called normative transitions. Thus, family members expect and learn to interact differently as children grow. Sometimes families may not make the transition to an expected family stage. For example, families with children with disabilities, who are not capable of independent living, have difficulty launching their children because of lack of residential living facilities and caregivers.

Situational transitions include changes in personal relationships, roles and status, the environment, physical and mental capabilities, and the loss of possessions (Rankin, 1989). Situational transitions are also called non-normative transitions. Not all families experience each situational transition. Further, they may occur irrespective of time or family developmental stages. For example, changes occur in personal relationships when a stepchild is integrated into the family group, or when one becomes a new stepparent after divorce and remarriage; changes in roles and status happen when an only child becomes a sibling after the family adopts a new child; changes in the familiar environment occur when working parents move to a new job and family members encounter a new house, school, friends, and community. Even greater changes occur when families immigrate to a new country, learn a new language and a new culture, and perhaps have to work at a lower-status job. Changes in physical and mental capabilities—for example, an illness that incapacitates a working parent—may shift caregiving activities to other members of the family and create uncertainty about skills needed (Schumacher & Meleis, 1994). A natural disaster may destroy family possessions and heirlooms, causing stress, fear, a sense of loss and problems with family members' ways of being and interacting (Schumacher & Meleis).

Family transitions may follow expected or unexpected time lines. For example, increased independence is expected in children as they grow older; but children are not expected to die before their parents. Nurses screen families for transition events because transitions (Schumacher & Meleis, 1994), both developmental and situational, are signals to nurses that families may be at risk for health problems. See the research brief on marital separation and children.

RESEARCH BRIEF

Marital Separation And Children

Divorce is a stressful multistage process that can have long-lasting negative outcomes for parents and children. Pediatric nurse practitioners are often the first health care professionals to be informed of family transitions. They must be knowledgeable of the impact of divorce on parents and children to be able to enhance coping outcomes in this population. This article discusses the effects of divorce on parents and children and identifies intervention strategies that can be used by nurse practitioners when dealing with separated families. Description of the Creating Opportunities for Parental Empowerment (COPE) Program, an intervention program recently implemented with parents and young children experiencing marital separation, is highlighted.

Source: Melnyk, B.M. (1997). Coping with marital situational separation: Smoothing the transition for parents and children. *Journal of Pediatric Health Care, 11*(4):165–174.

Individual Development

The second concept in the *family interaction model* is individual development. Families with children are complex groups of adults and children. Because no one perspective explains humans adequately, nurses must consider multiple dimensions of human development. Some family developmental stages are related to the growth of individual members and the differing needs of maturing human beings. Table 11-1, a schematic overview of human development, highlights the stages of individual experiences over time. Adult developmental aspects are included because adults' needs may complement or conflict with their children's, and because the focus is on the family.

Nurses need to review with families the individual family members' developmental stages that are occurring concurrently among children and adults and are affecting daily family interactions. Nurses can also assist families to accommodate to children's and adults' changing abilities. Table 11-1 presents three dimensions of individual development: social-emotional, cognitive, and physical. The table is meant to be a guide and is not all inclusive. Some items may not be representative of cultural or socioeconomic status. The table has 12 columns. The first and second columns, *period* and *age,* are orienting time lines: the period column identifies eight stages from infancy through late adulthood, and the age column is divided into chronological years from birth through 18 years, plus the adult years beyond. Column 3, *social-emotional stages,* represents Erikson's theory (1973), which views social-emotional development across the eight stages of human life. Column 4, the *radius of significant relations,* shows how the world of individuals expands as they move beyond their immediate families. Column 5, *stage-sensitive family developmental tasks,* provides the orientation of families as they raise and launch children (Duvall & Miller, 1985). Column 6, *human needs,* is a hierarchy of individual requirements ranging from basic physiological needs to the need for self-actualization (Maslow, 1970). Column 7, *values orientation,* reflects moral development from undifferentiated to complex stages (Kohlberg, 1984; Thomas, 1992). Individual family members have their own values, but their values also relate to the values of their family and community. Column 8 shows the *cognitive stages of development* (Piaget & Inhelder, 1969; Thomas, 1992).The *developmental landmarks* shown in column 9 are milestones that families use to measure their children's progress. Column 10, *physical maturation,* shows bodily changes as children grow. Column 11 lists the *developmental steps* that individuals experience. Column 12 outlines *developmental problems* associated with changes throughout the life span. Nurses can use this table to identify expected developmental progression and potential areas of concern for families.

Patterns of Health, Disease, and Illness

The third concept that comprises the *family interaction model* is patterns of health, disease, and illness. Families experience these patterns. Healthy behaviors promote optimal physical and social-emotional well-being. Disease is pathology. Illness represents the family activities associated with managing disease. Family interactions shape these patterns.

Health

In their daily activities, families create *health patterns,* which are the family's and family members' understandings and behaviors associated, not merely with the absence of disease and incapacitation, but with optimal physical, mental, and social well-being (Loveland-Cherry, 1996; Meister, 1991). Healthy behaviors in families include both promotional and protective actions. For example, parents may promote children's growth towards self-actualization through after-school programs that encourage school friendships and creativity. Parents prevent disease through childhood immunizations and they avoid injuries through poison prevention efforts. Families' normative behaviors are the healthy patterns they follow as they promote and protect the health of their children and the family as a whole.

Disease

Diseases and pathological conditions are abnormal patterns, of physical, social-emotional, or family processes. For example, an abnormal physical pattern is sickle cell anemia, a genetic disease characterized by periodic pain and bleeding into cellular tissues (Shapiro, 1993). Child abuse, an abnormal family pattern, is a pattern of inappropriate and non-nurturing parenting. Families learn to recognize symptoms and signs of disease in order to treat and care for their children's health. For example, parents will bring their child with a fever to the physician's office or clinic. Disease is culturally defined and families are influenced by the opinions of health professionals (Kleinman, 1988). This is evident to nurses who observe families of other cultures with their own

TABLE 11-1
Social-Emotional, Cognitive, and Physical Dimensions of Individual Development

Period	Age	Social-Emotional Stages	Significant Relations	Stage-Sensitive Family Development Tasks	Human Needs	Values Orientation
Infancy						
	Birth	Trust vs. mistrust (I am what I am given.)			Physiological: air, food, and shelter	
	3 mo		Primary parent	Having, adjusting to, and encouraging the development of infants Establishing a satisfying home for both parents and infant(s)		Undifferentiated
	6 mo					
	9 mo					
	1 yr	Autonomy vs. shame or doubt (I am what I "will.")	Parental persons		Safety/security	
Preschool-Age						
	2 yr					
	3 yr	Initiative vs. guilt (I am what I imagine I can be.)	Basic family	Adapting to the critical needs and interests of preschool children in stimulating, growth-promoting ways Coping with energy depletion and lack of privacy as parents	Belonging, rootedness, family, friends	Punishment and obedience
School-Age						
	4 yr					
	5 yr					
	6 yr	Industry vs. inferiority (I am what I learn.)	Neighborhood school	Fitting into the community of school-age families in constructive ways	Self-respect, self-esteem	

TABLE 11-1
Social-Emotional, Cognitive, and Physical Dimensions of Individual Development (cont.)

Cognitive Stages of Development	Developmental Landmarks	Physical Maturation	Developmental Steps	Developmental Problems
Sensory-Motor Infants move from neonatal reflex level of complete self-world undifferentiation to relatively coherent organization of sensory-motor actions. They learn that certain actions have specific effects on the environment. Minimal symbolic activity is involved. Recognition of the constancy of external objects and primitive internal representation of the world begins.	Gazes at complete patterns Social smile (2 mo) 180° visual pursuit (2 mo) Reaches for objects (4 mo) Rolls over (5 mo) Raking grasp (7 mo) Crude purposeful release (9 mo) Inferior pincer grasp Walks unassisted (10–14 mo) Words: 3–4 (13 mo) Builds tower of 2 cubes (15 mo) Scribbles with crayon (18 mo) Words: 10 (18 mo) Builds tower of 5–6 cubes (21 mo)	**Rapid (Skeletal)** Transitory reflexes present (3 mo) (i.e., moro, sucking, grasp, tonic neck reflex) Muscle constitutes 25% of total body weight Birth weight doubles (6 mo) Eruption of decidious central incisors (5–10 mo) Birth weight triples (1 yr) Anterior fontanel closes (10–14 mo) Transitory reflexes disappear (10 mo) Eruption of decidious first molars (11–18 mo)	Anticipation of feeding Symbiosis (4–18 mo) Stranger anxiety (6–10 mo) Separation anxiety (8–24 mo) Self feeding Oppositional behavior Messiness Exploratory behavior Parallel play Pleasure in looking at or being looked at	Birth defects Feeding disorders: colic, regurgitation, vomiting, failure to thrive, marasmus, feeding refusal, atopic eczema Stranger anxiety Physiologic failure to thrive Sleep disturbances resistance or response to over–stimulation Extreme separation anxiety Pica Teeth grinding Poisoning Temper tantrums, negativism
Preoperational Thought (Prelogical) Children make their first relatively unorganized and fumbling attempts to come to grips with the new and strange world of symbols. Thinking tends to be egocentric and intuitive. Conclusions are based on what they feel or what they would like to believe.	Uses 3-word sentences (30 mo) Names 6 body parts (30 mo) Uses appropriate personal pronouns, i.e., I, you, me (30 mo) Rides tricycle (36 mo) Copies circle (36 mo) Matches 4 colors (36 mo) Talks of self and others (42 mo)	Babinski reflex extinguished (18 mo) Bowel and bladder nerves myelinated (18 mo) Increase in lymphoid tissue	Beginning self-concept Orderliness Disgust Curiosity Masturbation Cooperative play Fantasy play Imaginary companions	Toilet training disturbances: constipation, diarrhea Excessive feeding Bedtime and toilet rituals Speech disorders: delayed, elective mutism, stuttering Physical injuries: falls Nightmares, night terrors Extreme separation anxiety
	Takes turns (42 mo) Tandem walks (42 mo) Uses 4-word sentences (48 mo) Copies cross (48 mo) Throws ball overhand (48 mo)	**Slower (Skeletal)** Weight gain 2 kg per year (12–36 mo)		Excessive thumb sucking Phobias and marked fears Developmental deviations: lags and accelerations in motor, sensory, and affective development
	Copies square (54 mo) Copies triangle (60 mo) Prints name Rides two-wheel bike Copies diamond	**Rapid (Skeletal)** Weight gain 2 kg per year (4–6 yr) Eruption of permanent teeth (5.5–8 yr) Body image solidifying	Task completion Rivalry with parents of same sex Games and rules Problem solving Achievement Voluntary hygiene	Food rituals and fads Sleep walking School phobias Developmental deviations: lags and accelerations in cognitive functions, psychosexual, and integrative development Self-destructive behaviors Enuresis, soiling, and excessive masturbation Physical injuries: fractures

Continued

TABLE 11-1
Social-Emotional, Cognitive, and Physical Dimensions of Individual Development (cont.)

Period	Age	Social-Emotional Stages	Significant Relations	Stage-Sensitive Family Development Tasks	Human Needs	Values Orientation
School-Age						
	7 yr			Encouraging child's educational achievement		Instrumental exchange: "If you scratch my back, I'll scratch yours."
	8 yr					
	9 yr					
	10 yr					
	11 yr	Identity vs. identity diffusion (I know who I am.)	Peer in-groups and out-groups Adult models of leadership	Balancing freedom with responsibility as teenagers mature and emancipate themselves Establishing postparental interests and careers as growing parents		
Adolescence						
	12 yr					
	13 yr					
	14 yr					
	15 yr					Conventional law and order: "They mean well."
	16 yr					
	17 yr					
	18 yr					
Early Adulthood						
		Intimacy vs. isolation	Partners in friendship, sex, completion	Releasing young adults into work, military service, college, marriage, and so on with appropriate rituals and assistance Maintaining a supportive home base		Principled social contract
Middle Adulthood						
		Generativity vs. self-absorption or stagnation	Divided labor and shared household	Refocusing on the marriage relationship Maintaining kin ties with older and younger generations	Self-actualization: doing what one is capable of	
Late Adulthood						
		Integrity vs. despair, disgust	"Humankind" "My kind"	Coping with bereavement and living alone Closing the family home in adapting to aging Adjusting to retirement		Universal ethical principles

TABLE 11-1
Social-Emotional, Cognitive, and Physical Dimensions of Individual Development

Cognitive Stages of Development	Developmental Landmarks	Physical Maturation	Developmental Steps	Developmental problems
Concrete Operational Thought Conceptual organization takes on stability and coherence. Children begin to seem rational and well organized in their adaptation. The fairly stable and orderly conceptual framework is systematically brought to bear on the world of objects around them. Physical quantities, such as weight and volume, are now viewed as constant, despite changes in shape and size.	Simple opposite analogies Can name days of week Repeats 5 digits forward Can define "brave," "nonsense" Knows seasons of the year Able to rhyme words Repeats 4 digits in reverse Understands pity, grief, surprise Knows where sun sets Can define "nitrogen," "microscope"	**Slowest (Skeletal)** Weight gain 2–4 kg per year (7–11 yr) Uterus begins to grow Budding of nipples in girls Increased vascularity of penis and scrotum Pubic hair appears in girls Menarche (9–16 yr) **Spurt (Skeletal)** (Girls 1.5 yrs ahead of boys) Pubic hair appears in boys Rapid growth of testes and penis Axillary hair starts to grow	Competes with partners Hobbies Ritualistic play Rational attitudes about food Companionship Invests in community leaders, teachers, impersonal ideals	Learning problems Psychophysiologic disorders Personality disorders: compulsive, anxious, overdependent, oppositional, overinhibited, overindependent, isolated, and mistrustful; tension discharge disorders, and sexual deviations Legal delinquency Anorexia nervosa Dysmenorrhea Sexual promiscuity Drug overdose Suicidal attempts Acute confusional state Motor vehicle accidents
Formal Operational Thought People can now deal effectively not only with the reality before them, but also with the world of the abstract and the world of possibility ("as if"). Cognition is of the adult type. Adolescents use deductive reasoning and have the ability to evaluate the logic and quality of their own thinking. Their increased abstract power provides them with the capacity to deal with laws and principles. Although egocentrism is still evident at times, important idealistic attitudes are developing in the late adolescent and young adult.	Knows why oil floats on water Can divide 72 by 4 without pencil or paper Understands "belfry" and "espionage" Can repeat 6 digits forward and 5 digits in reverse	Down on upper lip appears Voice changes Mature spermatozoa (11–17 yr) Acne may appear	"Revolt" Loosens tie to family Cliques Responsible independence Work habits solidifying Heterosexual interests Recreational activities	Schizophrenic disorders (adult type) Affective disorders; manic-depressive psychoses Involutional reactions: depression, suicide Senile disorders: chronic brain syndromes
		Cessation of skeletal growth Involution of lymphoid tissue Muscle constitutes 43% total body weight Permanent teeth calcified Eruption of permanent third molars (17–30 yr)	Preparation for occupational choice Occupational commitment Elaboration of recreational outlets Marriage readiness Parenthood readiness	

Adapted from D. Prugh (1983) in *The Psychological Aspects of Pediatrics,* Philadelphia: Lea & Febiger; R. Murray Thomas (1992) in *Comparing Theories of Child Development* (pp 166–167, 501) Belmont, CA: Wadsworth; E.M. Duvall and B.C. Miller (1985) in *Marriage and Family Development* (6th ed.) (p. 62), New York, Harper and Collins.

health beliefs treat their members' health problems using a mix of conventional and folk medicine (Mikhail, 1994; Spruhan, 1996).

Illness

In contrast to disease, which is a pathological condition, *illness patterns* are the processes families go through to manage a condition or disease and the medical treatments that become a part of their daily lives (Corbin & Strauss, 1988). Diseases may be classified as *acute, chronic,* or *life-threatening* (Rolland, 1999). Families reorganize themselves and have different illness tasks for each. They temporarily alter daily routines to deal with the crisis of acute diseases and injuries such as communicable diseases, bone fractures, and appendicitis. After disease treatment, however, families usually return to the family routines that were in place before the disease.

In contrast, families permanently reorganize their daily routines to accommodate ongoing, incurable diseases such as juvenile arthritis, diabetes, and asthma, as well as abnormal conditions such as cerebral palsy, seizures, or mental retardation. Family careers continue to unfold, and family tasks still need to be performed as siblings and affected children grow and develop. For example, siblings may be jealous of the attention that a chronically ill child receives from parents; and chronically ill adolescents often ignore treatments and aggravate their disease as they search for identity and try to avoid appearing different from their peers.

Families reorganize during life-threatening illness. They may experience the unexpectedly shortened life span of children due to sudden infant death syndrome, fatal ingestion of household poisons or medications by a toddler, cystic fibrosis, or childhood cancer. When death is inevitable, families grieve and mourn for their child. Rituals such as funerals help families remember and make the transition to ongoing life as they heal (McGoldrick & Walsh, 1999). All family members are affected and need to be included in the dying, mourning, and healing process.

In summary, as caretakers, families promote health and cope with acute, chronic, and life-threatening illnesses in their children. Health issues for families with children are influenced by the interacting dynamics of (1) family career, (2) individuals' development, and (3) patterns of health, disease, and illness. The family interaction model allows nurses to analyze the intersecting points of these three processes and develop interventions that will assist families to care for their children's health.

The next section addresses practice for family child health nurses in four areas: health promotion, acute illness, chronic illness, and life-threatening illness. A case study follows, to illustrate use of the *family interaction model.*

HEALTH PROMOTION

Families' daily routines influence their children's physical, mental, and social health, as well as the health of the family (Denham, 1995). Patterns of *family well-being* are facilitated by balancing the needs of individuals and the family with the resources and options available to meet these needs (Meister, 1991). Nurses help families integrate physical, social-emotional, and cognitive health promotion into family routines; in doing so, they also affirm positive patterns of health or provide alternative ones (Bomar, 1996). Thus nurses reduce the risk of illness by shaping the family environment to encourage optimally healthy behaviors (Doherty & McCubbin, 1985).

Because the leading causes of morbidity and mortality among youth are poor nutrition, substance use, school failure, sexual activity, accidental injury, and violence (both suicidal and homicidal) (Sells & Blum,1996; Weissberg & Kuster, 1997), increased attention to health promotion and prevention of unhealthy social-emotional behaviors among children and their families is needed. Data on the prevalence of risk behaviors among adolescents is collected by the Youth Risk Behavior Surveillance System (YRBS) (Kann et al, 1998), using a national probability sample of 9th to 12th graders, state and local school-based surveys, and a national household-based survey (Dryfoos, 1997).

The 1993 report showed that about one-third of all in-school adolescents currently smoked, one-half used alcohol, and one-fifth used marijuana within 30 days of the survey (Centers for Disease Control and Prevention, as cited in Dryfoos, 1997). More than half of high school students had had sexual intercourse. When students in the survey were asked whether they carried a weapon such as a gun or knife onto school property, one in four reported yes. Adolescent aggression may not be more violent than in previous generations, but violent behaviors are now more lethal (Murray et al, 1997). The use of guns over other weapons has increased the numbers of people killed and wounded. The YRBS survey revealed that one in four high school students had had serious thoughts about attempting suicide within the past year, 19 percent had had a suicide plan, and 9 percent actually attempted suicide. Youth susceptible to drug use, unhealthy sexual behaviors, violence/aggression, and suicide are often experiencing depression (Compas et al, 1997; Kalafat, 1997). The leading cause of death among children and youth is unintentional injuries. In 1997, the rate of death from injuries was 5376 per 100,000 children under the age of 15 (Hoyert et al, 1999). An additional 13,367 per 100,000 young people, ages 14 to 24, died from accidents of which 10,208 per 100,000 were motor vehicle accidents (Hoyert et al, 1999). Accidents among children and youth are not unpredictable twists of fates, but are "accidents waiting to happen" (Tuchfaber et al, 1997). Poor school performance is correlated with increased health risk behaviors. The YRBS did not include questions about school performance, but another longitudinal study that has tracked eighth graders since 1988 found that one in five students were not proficient at basic math, and 14 percent could not read adequately. By 10th grade, many low-performing students drop out (Hawkins, 1997). Family predictors of children at high risk for poor school performance include single-parent homes, family incomes of less than $15,000, older siblings who have dropped out, parents who did not finish high school, limited proficiency in English, and being at home for 2 hours a day or more without supervision (Dryfoos, 1997). Socioeconomic factors such as poverty, lack of education, little or no health insurance, and immigrant status are strongly related to poor health. In light of these statistics, nurses can screen for risk factors during health assessments, make appropriate referrals, and advocate for community health and social programs that target high-risk youth and their families.

Families sometimes experience conflict between family tasks and the needs of individual family members, and they must try to balance these. For example, working parents of an infant must decide if and when to place their child in child care. Working parents of school-age children and adolescents must decide if the children can be at home without adult supervision during the after-school period before parents return home from work. In both situations the family task is to provide economic resources for shelter and food, and the children's need is for a trusted caretaker and safe environment. Families settle these conflicts differently. Nurses can help families resolve the issues through anticipatory guidance, which involves providing information about what to expect in various situations and how to deal with unwanted developmental problems and life changes (Pridham, 1993). Family nurses in school-based health clinics can participate in health prevention programs directed at high risk behaviors leading to sexually transmitted disease and early pregnancy, depression, injuries, substance use, suicide, and violence (Falsetti & Kovel, 1994). Nurses need to be aware that families with limited financial resources and those who do not have health insurance have more difficulty with health promotion than families with insurance or other methods of payment. A recent study on access to health care in the U.S. reported that Hispanic children were more than twice as likely as white children to have no insurance. Black children were most likely to have public health care coverage (40.8 percent), followed by Hispanics (32.55) and whites (13.1 percent)(Kass et al, 1996).

Families are the major determinant of children's well-being. Nurses and other health professionals should collaborate with parents, not view parents as secondary to nurses (Pesznecker et al, 1989). Too often in the past, professionals decided what was best for children (Darbyshire, 1993). Today, nurses are exploring parents' perceptions and definitions of health to develop more relevant health care plans.

Health promotion for children occurs during parenting activities, and many American families are assisted in parenting by other child caretakers, including grandparents, and child-care and after-school facilities.

Parenting

Families with children promote health by practicing behaviors that advance their own physical, mental, and social well-being and that of their children. Everyday parenting activities nurture and socialize children to be healthy, responsible adults. However, parents sometimes are not aware of or do not use developmental principles. Sameroff and Feil (1985) found, for example, that parents whose socioeconomic status (SES) was higher explained their children's behavior with developmental understanding and were flexible in their parenting, but parents of lower SES used fewer explanations of development and expected their children to conform. Nurses might conclude that the parents with developmental understanding who are flexible in parenting are "better" parents; however, these parents are also often overanxious and worry about everything. Parents who expect conformity of their children often have themselves experienced an environment with few choices. Sameroff and Feil (1985) concluded that such parents are preparing their children to survive in a harsh environment.

Nurses need to learn more about Latino (Falicov, 1999) and African-American values and the effects of poverty and class on family life (Hines, 1999). Because parents' understandings of their roles and child development vary, it is important for nurses to explore parents' beliefs in order to tailor health promotion activities to families.

In 1993, over 1.5 million cases of child abuse and neglect occurred (23.1 cases per 1000 children) (Federal Interagency Forum on Child and Family Statistics, 1997). Extreme forms of inappropriate parenting are termed child abuse or neglect. "Abuse" is a comprehensive term that includes physical, emotional, and sexual harm. For example, a 2-year-old child is physically abused for a temper tantrum because the temper tantrum is perceived as disrespect of the parent rather than the toddler's struggle for autonomy. A teenager may be verbally and physically abused at home because the assertive behavior of the adolescent is perceived by the parent as disrespectful of social values. The parent does not see that the adolescent is struggling for a self-identity separate from family. Hitting a child hard enough to cause bruising is considered physical abuse and an inappropriate way to socialize a toddler to control his or her temper. An appropriate way to discipline the child is to use a "time out," or 5 minutes in a quiet place immediately after the tantrum (Howard, 1991).

Discipline involves establishing rules and guidelines so that children know what is expected of them. Parents may punish their children for disregarding the rules. In American culture, physical harm resulting from punishment is considered abuse. The difference between discipline and abuse may be uncertain because of different cultural traditions, but nurses must be alert to helping families learn appropriate discipline measures (American Academy of Pediatrics, 1998).

Nurses often assist parents with health promotion. They teach parenting classes for children of various ages and provide programs aimed at preventing the injuries associated with various ages, such as physical safety classes for school-age children with attention deficit hyperactivity disorder (ADHD) (Bentson-Royal, 1999, personal communication; Selekman & Snyder, 1996). In addition, nurses screen families for potentially harmful parenting situations such as child abuse and family violence, asking the following questions (Shelton & Gedaly-Duff, 1999):

- Right now, who is living at home with you and your child?
- Is everyone getting along well at home or is there a lot of stress, arguing or fighting?
- Anybody ever been hit or hurt, pushed or shoved in a fight or argument at your house?
- Anybody in the family in trouble with the police or in jail?
- Anybody worried that your children have been disciplined too harshly?
- Anybody worried that your children have been touched inappropriately or sexually abused?
- Anybody living with you or close to you who drinks a lot or uses drugs?
- Are there guns or knives or weapons at your house?
- Anything major (e.g., people dying, losing jobs, disasters or accidents) happened recently?
- What is the best part and the worst part of life for you right now?

Families that are stressed frequently will seek help if given the opportunity to tell about their situations. Using these screening questions, a nurse can assess the family and child for dangerous situations, teach safety, and make a referral as necessary.

Grandparenting

Grandparents also influence health promotion in childrearing families, though grandparenting is not fully acknowledged as a way to promote health in children (Kivett, 1991). Grandparents indirectly influence the values that parents bring to their parenting, because parenting values are derived in part from families of origin. In addition, grandparents provide continuity both for the nuclear family and for the extended family of aunts, uncles, and cousins. During illness, a grandparent can serve as a valued backup, watch dog, safety valve, and stabilizing force for children and their families. Nurses who understand the influence of grandparenting on childrearing families' health include them in their interventions. Grandparents may serve as child care providers for working families (Burton et al, 1995; Jendrek, 1993). Parents and grandparents must develop rules for childrearing that differ from those during grandparent visits since grandparents often indulge their grandchildren and are sometimes seen as "spoiling" the child. Grandparents may become major influences if, for instance, they raise a grandchild while a teenaged parent finishes high school. Or serve as primary parents to their grandchildren—for example, in the case of drug-addicted babies born to addicted parents (Minkler & Roe, 1993). In these situations, nurses must teach grandparents health promotion strategies for their grandchildren and also discuss strategies for reducing caregiver stress (Kelley et al, 1997; Pruchno, 1999).

Grandparents can also promote health during situational transitions such as divorce, when they can provide emotional and physical support to divorced parents and children. In some cases, however, grandparents may be completely separated from their grandchildren by divorce. Nurses may then need to help them with the complex issues of "grandparent visitation rights" (Purnell & Bagby, 1993).

Child Care and After-School Activities

One task of families is to nurture children. Families raise children without expectation of monetary reward, as a "gift" to society. Today, however, many families can no longer "give" all the work of childraising without turning to child-care and after-school facilities for assistance. In 1970, 29 percent of women with children under age 6 were in the labor force; by 1990, that figure was 52 percent (Bianchi, 1995). In the year 2000, it is projected that 75 percent of all mothers will return to work before their child's first birthday (Dawson & Cain, 1990). Nurses can help families review the types of child-care and after-school options available, select compatible philosophies for health promotion, and examine the site for health protection features. They can also participate on community boards that regulate these facilities.

Health promotion for school-age children in the home and at after-school facilities is gaining increasing attention. Between 2 and 5 million children, or 20 percent of all children between the ages of 5 and 13 years, are estimated to be "latchkey" children who are at home while parents work (Bianchi, 1990, p. 28). The situation of these children has raised concerns about loneliness, injuries, and violence. Nurses, parents, and teachers must develop before- and after-school programs at schools, and homework telephone services with teachers and teachers' aides.

In selecting daycare and after-school options, protection against injuries and infections is a key issue. Nurses can provide families with a series of questions to help them check safety precautions and see how a facility will handle their children's illnesses. For example, are indoor and outdoor activity areas safe for active children? Are there functioning toilets and wash sinks that children can reach? What is the policy for children who arrive ill or develop an illness during their stay?

Families composed of minority groups and families with children with disabilities require special consideration when choosing child-care and after-school options. Children with special health needs are integrated into federally supported child-care facilities such as Head Start (American Academy of Pediatrics, 1973). Children from families from minority backgrounds are more likely to live below the poverty line and live with parents who have limited educational and/or English proficiency levels, and thus they are at risk for health problems (Kirby et al, 1999).

Symbolic interaction theory (Klein & White, 1996) suggests that children learn meanings, responses to, and values about health through their interactions with their families and communities. Thus parents, grandparents, and childcare workers responses may shape children's experience and the childrearing done by parents, grandparents, and daycare and after-school caretakers is important in health promotion. Nurses can facilitate and teach health promotion activities.

ILLNESS

Although members of American families experience health during 85 percent of their lifetime, they will experience illness for 15 percent of the time (US Department of Health and Human Services, National Center for Health Statistics, 1993). Acute illness, chronic illness and life-threatening illness present overlapping though distinct challenges for family nurses.

Acute Illness

Families with children frequently experience acute illness and injury. In fact, injuries are the leading cause of morbidity (illness) and mortality (death) in children. The patterns of illness and injury in children are revealed by the following statistics. In 1997, 5376 per 100,000 children between the ages of 1 and 15 years died from accidents and injuries, while only 1619 died from cancer (Hoyert et al, 1999). Some 54 percent of ambulatory visits (74,108 per 100,000 children who are under 15 years) are for injuries and acute problems (Woodwell, 1999). Three million children experience surgery every year (Tyler, 1990). Families with children also experience respiratory infectious diseases, which account for approximately 50 percent of visits to health care settings and are a leading cause of mortality in children (Pillitteri, 1992).

Acute illness in children is characterized by the sudden onset of signs and symptoms; treatment can usually restore the children to the predisease state. Childhood acute illnesses include communicable infections such as chickenpox, conditions such as appendicitis, and injuries such as bone fractures.

The American health care system is encouraging more home care of acute and chronic conditions as well as more day procedures; thus families are managing their children's diseases and illnesses more than health professionals (Coyne, 1995). Typically, families whose children undergo a day procedure such as an adenoidectomy or tonsillectomy will care for their children at home after the first 4 to 8 hours following surgery. Gedaly-Duff and Ziebarth (2000), who studied mothers' experiences in identifying and managing their children's acute pain associated with surgery, found that mothers learned to manage the pain through trial and error. One mother was fearful of both overdosing and under-medicating for the pain. She said:

> I was concerned about giving him too much . . . and I went too long, he was extremely uncomfortable. After that I said, "It's not worth it" it took longer for the medication to get back into his system, so then I gave it every three hours, like the label said.

Families in that study also altered their daily routines. Parent work schedules were rearranged and most mothers took time off to care for their children. Mothers described apprehension about the lack of sleep in the household because of their acutely ill child's irritability. Siblings were attentive, anxious, or misbehaving at the extra attention given their ill sister or brother. Most families endured the misbehavior. In such situations parents want to protect siblings by not involving them and trying to keep life as usual; however, siblings know things have changed and do not know what to do. Nurses using anticipatory guidance can teach families to explain what is happening to the sick child and how the siblings can help.

To help families experiencing acute illness, nurses must first become aware of families' past experiences with and knowledge about acute illness. Second, nurses must alert families to potential disruptions among parents and siblings because of conflicts between family members' needs. Nurses can plan with families how to alter family routines to accommodate the temporary changes required by the acute illness and teach families how to assess the developmentally related reactions children have to acute illness-for example, how to use age-appropriate methods to assess pain (Gedaly-Duff, 1991). Nurses can also teach families to recognize the patterns and potential complications of acute illness. At the time of discharge families may not hear some discharge teaching because they are concerned about their child's recovery and arrangements for going home. Nurses can facilitate follow-up care to assess the children's status, and reteach what families need to learn when their child is at home. (See the research brief on parent empowerment.)

RESEARCH BRIEF

Parent Empowerment

Critically ill young children and their parents are subjected to multiple stressors during hospitalization, which may predispose them to short- and long-term negative outcomes. Nurses who care for children who are critically ill and their families during and following their intensive care unit stay must be knowledgeable of the impact of a child's critical illness on the family and factors influencing adjustment to the stressful experience. This knowledge is essential to plan effective intervention strategies to enhance coping outcomes in this population. This article (a) discusses how young children and their parents are affected by critical illness; (b) outlines major sources of stress for families; (c) identifies factors that influence coping outcomes; and (d) describes the COPE program, a newly devised early intervention program for critically ill young children and their parents.

Source: Melnyk, B.M.(1998). The COPE program: A strategy to improve outcomes of critically ill young children and their parents. Creating opportunities for parent empowerment. *Pediatric Nursing, 24*(6):521–527, 539–540.

Chronic Illness

Health conditions that limit children's daily activities such as playing and going to school, that are long term, and that are not curable or require special assistance in function are considered chronic (Federal Interagency Forum on Child and Family Statistics, 1997; Jackson, 1996). Depending on the definition of "chronic illness," which may include or exclude cancer and mental illness, the proportion of families with children experiencing chronic illness is estimated to be between 20 percent and 31 percent (Cioro et al, 1994; Newacheck et al, 1998). Fourteen percent (19,221 per 100,000 children under 15 years) of all primary care providers' office visits are for chronic problems (Woodwell, 1999). While most childrearing families experience acute illnesses and become familiar with managing these crises, families do not anticipate that their children may have chronic illness, and they are unprepared for the unknowns and uncertainties of the course of the disease, the effects on their child's development, and the effects on each family member and family life.

Chronic illnesses such as juvenile arthritis, diabetes, and asthma or long-term conditions, such as cerebral palsy, mental retardation, learning disability and behavioral problems require daily management (Cioro et al, 1994; Federal Interagency Forum on Child and Family Statistics, 1997). Families accommodate to the effects of chronic illness on their child and the family through a process called "reality negotiation" (Ersek, 1992). The meaning of an illness can change for a family over time (Patterson & Garwick, 1994). Initially, families may experience disbelief because they have assumed that children are healthy and grow up to be independent. Families hope the disease will resolve. Sometimes families have to experience the continuing signs and symptoms before they believe the disease is not going away. For example, juvenile rheumatoid arthritis (JRA) has a pattern of inflammation and remission. Parents experiencing the remission of the disease may believe the disease is gone and stop the medication and exercise treatments. When the inflammation in the joints recurs, they begin to believe that the disease is long-term. Families then find ways of consistently giving medications and doing exercise treatments for their child. Nurses who recognize this process can support families as they develop new understandings of their child's illness and adjust to the chronic illness (Gedaly-Duff and Ayres, unpublished). For example, the nurse can conduct family workshops on issues such as sibling responses and the burden of taking care of the ill child at home (Gedaly-Duff & Heims, 1996).

Families use a variety of strategies to normalize the disease experience and cope with chronic illness (Deatrick et al, 1999). Initially families may be unaware that they have made changes in daily routines to accommodate to their child's chronic disease (Gedaly-Duff & Heims, 1996). However, when asked, these families describe new routines for giving medicines, and new rituals such as stopping for a special hamburger after the monthly clinic visit. The nurse, by asking a family to describe how their family routines have changed, helps them to recognize their flexibility. The intervention is health promoting because the family discovers their resilience and strength.

Parents are flexible in their approach to the health care of their children and are concerned that their children develop to their fullest potential in spite of disease. For example, the mother of a 5-year-old girl with juvenile rheumatoid arthritis (JRA) once said:

> Sometimes I'll see her knee seems to be swollen, but I won't say anything. I won't ask her because I figure that if it's really bad, she'll let me know. I mean, she knows she can tell me that, and then we'll figure out what it is we should do. But I'm not going to plant the seed in her mind. . . . She might always have a little bit of pain. She's not going to be very productive as a human being if she props it up on a pillow.

Nurses and families can together create new routines to accommodate disease and continue with the family's life. For example, a 5-year-old's kindergarten class can be scheduled for the afternoon so that he can treat his JRA with a warm bath before he gets dressed in the morning. Or a motorized tricycle can be taken to Fourth of July picnics so that the 4-year-old with JRA can ride alongside his playmates. Grandparents can help organize a softball team to enable their grandson with JRA to play ball. A person from the community fireman squad can run for the boy with JRA (Gedaly-Duff, 1990). Researchers suggest that chronically ill adolescent children have better self-esteem when their families emphasize independence and participation in recreational activities (Hauser et al, 1985). With their knowledge of family and child development, nurses can collaborate with families with chronically ill children to help them achieve development landmarks. However, nurses need to know community resources in order to facilitate family health (Appendix A).

A chronic illness or condition affects all members of the family. Nurses can help families look at how each member (e.g., father, mother, sibling, grandparent, family friend, neighbor, or school) is affected, and discuss how to help each member of the family and the people in the community adjust to the child with a disability or chronic condition. For example, siblings may have the dilemma of telling their friends, or keeping it a secret that their sister or brother has mental retardation (Faux, 1993). Sharing a book with a sibling that tells the story of a similar situation can be a useful intervention (Ahmann, 1997). Other challenges to families whose children have disabilities and chronic conditions are listed in Table 11-2 (Gedaly-Duff et al, 2000).

Families are put in a difficult situation when their chronically ill children are hospitalized (Robinson, 1985). The families have been the primary caregivers at home, but now they are placed in a dependent role, as if they did not understand their child's illness pattern. Nurses who have worked with families of chronically ill children know that they are knowledgeable about how their children respond to disease and about their developmental capabilities. Thus it is important for nurses to collaborate with these families (Graves & Hayes, 1996). To help families care for their chronically ill children, the nurse can:

- Learn how the family's past experiences and expectations of disease and illness are affecting the current illness situation.
- Determine whether the family is responding to a diagnosis of a new condition or is experienced in caring for their child's chronic illness.
- Help families to promote health in spite of illness by meeting the continually evolving needs of family members.
- Help families accommodate to the child's developmental limitations related to the disease or condition.

In carrying out these tasks, the nurse must consider the specific characteristics and manifestations of the illness, the stage of family development, and the resulting demands on relationships (Rolland, 1999).

Life-Threatening Illness

Families know that chronic illness, like acute injuries and diseases, may be life-threatening; however, the death of a child is a rare and shocking experience for families. Even though children's deaths are often reported in television and newspaper media, the death is a distant event. Daily life in America focuses on a happy childhood and does not prepare families for the unlikely event of their children's death. Of children in the United States under the age of 14 years, 5.6 in 10,000 (56.6 per 100,000) died from all causes in 1997 (Hoyert et al, 1999); 5.6 per 100,000 under 14 years died from cancer (Hoyert et al, 1999).

A serious illness is characterized by hospitalization, life-threatening circumstances, and uncertainty. Much of the time a child's disease state can be cured as in acute illness, or the children can be restored to a previous functional level. At other times, a child's bodily functions continue to fail, and the child and family come to an end-of-life phase. Nurses can support and guide families through this traumatic experience.

Waechter's classic study (1971) demonstrated that children knew and worried about their illness. When children did not know exactly what was wrong, they speculated, and they sometimes thought they had done something wrong and were being punished by having the disease. Nurses can teach families how to talk to their children about their life-threatening illness (Doka, 1995). Children are aware of the seriousness of the illness from external cues such as relatives visiting from long distances, and conversations that cease when they enter a room. Internal cues come from their own pain and weakness. When they are hospitalized or come to the clinic, they realize what types of patients are being treated. Families need guidance on how to answer children's questions about "what is wrong," and "how will it affect me," and "what can be done?"

Doka (1995) provides the following guidelines for answering children's questions about illness:

- Begin on the children's level, starting with their past experiences, such as when Grandmother was ill.
- Let the children's questions guide the conversation because sometimes adults give too much overwhelming information.
- Listen for the underlying feelings behind a comment, such as "Are you worried that you have gotten worse since your last visit?"
- Allow for honest expression of anger, sadness, guilt, and ambivalence and validate these feelings by sharing your own feelings and ways to cope with them.
- Share your own faith or philosophy, not by pronouncements that end talking, such as "We must trust in God's will," but by showing the struggle to find answers by commenting that "it is so hard to understand why this is happening."

TABLE 11-2
Stages, Tasks, and Situational Needs of Families of Children with Disabilities and Chronic Conditions

Family Stage	Developmental Tasks	Situational Needs that Alter Transitions
1. Beginning family: Married couple without children.	a. Establish mutually satisfying relationship. b. Relate to kin network. c. Plan family.	a. Unprepared for birth of children with disabilities; prenatal testing or visible anomalies at birth begin the process. b. In the United States, parents usually want to know their infant's diagnosis as early as possible.
2. Early childbearing: First birth, up to developmental age of 30 mo.	a. Integrate new baby into family. b. Reconcile conflicting needs of various family members. c. Develop parental role. d. Accommodate to changes in marital couple. e. Expand relationships with extended family; add grandparent, aunt, and uncle roles.	a. Learn meaning of infant's behavior, symptoms, and treatments. b. Hampered parent role if children not able to respond to parents' efforts to interact with them (e.g., not smiling or returning sounds in response to parental cooing). c. Search for adequate health care. d. Establish early intervention programs (e.g., speech and physical therapy, special education).
3. Family with preschool children: First child at developmental age of 2 1/2–5 yr.	a. Foster development of children. b. Create parental privacy. c. Increase competence of child. d. Socialize children. e. Maintain couple relationship.	a. Formal education of disabled children begins at birth. Families may not find adequate programs until preschool years. b. Failure to achieve developmental milestones (e.g., toilet training, self-feeding, language) lead to chronic sorrow. c. Families try to establish routines for themselves and their children.
4. Family with school-age children: Oldest child at developmental age of 6–13 yr.	a. Let children go. b. Balance parental needs with children's needs. c. Promote school achievement.	a. Moving from family to community requires creating new routines and relationships. b. "Going public," explaining to others. c. Negotiating appropriate school services and curriculum. d. Behavioral problems may isolate families.
5. Family with adolescents: Oldest child at developmental age of 13 to age of leaving home.	a. Loosen family ties. b. Strengthen couple relationship. c. Emphasize parent-teen communication. d. Maintain family moral and ethical standards	a. Continued dependency may mean children never leave home. b. Family examines how to continue family life with increasing physical growth but ongoing dependence of children.
6. Launching center family: First through last child to leave home.	a. Promote independence of children while maintaining relationship. b. Build new life together. c. Deal with mid-life developmental crisis.	a. Financial costs do not decrease because child still must depend on care.
7. Families in middle years: Empty nest to retirement.	a. Redefine activities and goals b. Provide healthy environment. c. Develop meaningful relationships with aging parents. d. Strengthen couple relationship.	a. Relationships with grown children and child with special health care needs are redefined.
8. Retirement to old age: Retirement to death of both parents.	a. Deal with losses. b. Find living place. c. Adapt to role changes. d. Adjust to less income. e. Control chronic illness. f. Adjust to mate loss. g. Become aware of death. h. Review life.	a. "Living trust" is created for children with special health care needs. Planning begins for care of child after elderly parents and siblings become unable to care for adult member with special health care needs.

Gedaly-Duff, V., Stoeger, S., & Shelton, K. (2000). Working with families. In R. Nickel & L. W. Desch (Eds.), *The Physician's Guide to Caring for Children with Disabilities and Chronic Conditions.* Baltimore, MD: Paul Brooke.

- Ask children to tell you what they think they heard to clarify misunderstandings.
- Use other resources, such as books and films, to help with the conversation.
- Give children opportunities to express themselves in stories, games, art and music, since play is the natural form of children's expression.

Besides teaching families home care, including adequate pain management (Ferrell et al, 1998; Sirkia et al, 1998), nurses often find themselves helping parents, siblings, and grandparents work through life and death issues (Murray, 1999; Tilden, 1998). During the intense time of grieving over the child's shortened life span, finding ways to complete things in life that are important to the child and family can promote opportunities for family growth (Byock, 1999; McGoldrick & Walsh, 1999; McQuillan & Finlay, 1996). Guidance may also be needed to bring closure. Examples include recognizing the child's life through a journal kept in the room for all visitors to sign and comment, or collecting a hand print, drawings, or favorite stories.

Nurses can use the family interaction model to support families during life-threatening illnesses. First, nurses should assess families' past experiences with a child's death. Generally families have few models for learning how to cope with this situation. Second, nurses should help families learn how children understand and cope with life-threatening illnesses. Nurses can teach them strategies for comfort care (U.S. Department of Health and Human Services, Agency for Health Care Policy and Research, 1994), help them anticipate the signs and symptoms of body failure they will experience, and plan support for these families at the point of death of their child. Finally, nurses can facilitate families' grieving and mourning of the child's death through discussions about each person's needs and interpretations of the behaviors of family members (Kramer, 1989; Solari-Twadell Bunkers et al, 1995).

Although some acute illnesses are quickly resolved by medical and nursing treatments, others involve a longer interaction with health care providers and are more life-threatening. Cancer in children is a challenging illness that often involves acute, chronic and life-threatening phases. The case example below involves a young child with cancer and his family. Components of the family interaction model are incorporated in the analysis. (See the research brief on Hispanic practices at the end of the chapter.)

NURSING IMPLICATIONS

Family nurses interact with families and other health professionals and use a family perspective to guide (1) health care delivery, that is, practice; (2) education, both for families and for other health care providers; (3) research, to systematically explore family child health nursing; and (4) health policy proposals and evaluation.

The *family interaction model,* which incorporates relevant components of family life, family development and transitions, and family health issues, promotes a comprehensive and holistic approach to the nursing of families. Using this model, nurses are able to collaborate with families who are in the processes of health promotion, disease prevention, and illness management.

Practice

Family child health nursing must be practiced in collaboration and cooperation with families as well as other health professionals. In family-centered care, nurses work with families to promote health, prevent disease, and cope with acute, chronic, and life-threatening illnesses. Cooperation means talking "with" rather than "to" families about solving problems and attaining health goals, such as acquiring immunizations for family members. Collaboration with families requires an even more involved relationship wherein ideas, expertise, resources, values and ways of doing are considered by both nurse and family. Actions and solutions are initiated by both the nurse and the family, and they work together with this information to address the health needs of the family and its members. The family interaction model provides a framework through which nurses can construct and evaluate their approaches and interactions with families with children, and a framework for a collaborative approach that acknowledges and respects the individual family.

Families in America are diverse and nurses who work with them need to understand these differences in order to be effective in problem-solving and health promotion. For example, nurses find that many parents work outside the home, and much of their children's time is spent at child-care or after-school care facilities. In addition, families of school-age and adolescent children may focus on school and school-related activities. Igoe (1993), Igoe and Giordano (1992), and others are therefore recommending that more of child health care take place in this arena-as school-based and school-linked health care. For example, families could receive care for their school-enrolled child as well as other members of the family at school-based health clinics. It is clear that family child nurses must consider these diverse patterns of family life in order to achieve health outcomes.

The family interaction model also has implications for balancing health promotion. It is well known that anticipating health problems can prevent their occurrence or minimize their effects. With their close and often frequent contacts with families and their children, nurses are in a position to form a partnership with families for wellness promotion. Nurses can work collaboratively with clients to assist them in taking on self-care responsibilities appropriate to their abilities and developmental levels.

A recent report by the National Institute for Nursing Research (1993) indicates that most morbidity and mortality in children and adolescents are due to behavior and lifestyle and are therefore preventable. Nurses who are aware of these risk factors can intervene with children and families to help prevent or at least minimize situational and developmentally-related problems. For example, nurses can discuss immunizations for vaccine-preventable diseases and safety restraints in automobiles at every health visit or encounter, regardless of the primary reason for the health care encounter.

Nurses can identify health issues or risks for the family and its members by expanding assessment of children. Nurses who explore comprehensively the situation of the family will detect those individual members who are at risk. For example, in a family whose child has been newly diagnosed with a severe disease such as leukemia, a sibling may begin to fail at school due to family situation. The nurse who assesses the whole family can identify the new behavior and facilitate a family conference so that each child understands what is happening and has an opportunity to discuss the meanings of the events. This keeps the focus on the family. The family can then see that other family members need attention. The family child health nurse assists the family to construct their career towards more healthy outcomes for all members.

Research

Family nurses need to explore ways in which the family interactional approach can be implemented and evaluated. For example, a collaborative approach to anticipatory guidance, a commonly used yet underexplored interventional strategy, could be tested (Pridham, 1993), as could long-term interventions for achieving positive health outcomes for children living in poverty. Research could also identify risk factors for families, to assist nurses and other health care providers to focus their interactions with clients. One question might be: What is the impact of a child's developmental delay on a family with impaired parents? Family nurses could identify patterns that are cues for future problems and explore the efficacy of interventions. Using an interactional approach, family child health nurses could identify factors in family and child health that are not apparent when the individual is the focus. This comprehensive family-centered approach could facilitate early screening and interventions, which could produce efficient and cost-saving strategies.

Education

Use of the family interaction model must be based on thorough knowledge of family development and patterns of health, disease, and illness. Family-focused care that balances health promotion, disease prevention, and illness management needs to be emphasized in formal and informal settings, as well as in academic and community programs (Hanson et al, 1992). Educational curricula need to include opportunities for discussion and case analyses as nurses learn and/or reformulate their perspectives toward family-centered child health. Family child health nursing involves many areas of knowledge and expertise. Therefore, many educational interactions may be needed in order for changes in practice to develop. Practicing nurses as well as those receiving their initial nursing education need interactions in which to explore a comprehensive framework for constructing effective approaches to family child health.

Policy

Policies made at agency, institutional, regional, state, and national levels influence family health in multiple and diverse ways. For example, public policies often place single-parent families in conflicting circumstances (Bowen et al, 1995). A parent may find a job, but make too much money to qualify for state-assisted health insurance and not have enough to pay for other types of health insurance. Family nurses can influence the development of public policies through their professional organizations as well as their individual efforts. A professional organization such as the American Nurses' Association can develop standards of practice and provide position papers to public servants developing health policies and laws. Policy analysis is therefore the job of every nurse (Gilliss, 1991).

Family child health nurses practice in many settings;

therefore they need to be aware of policies that apply in and between these settings. For example, a family with a chronically ill child may interact with nurses in an agency, in a hospital, and in the home. At a public policy level, family nurses must advocate for not only "adequate" but "growth-promoting" child-care facilities for the American working family. Safe and health-promoting options are needed for families with children from infancy to adolescence. Another area in need of attention at the policy level is nutrition. Although Americans are slowly changing eating practices towards healthier diets, many gaps exist between the recommendations and actual practices. For example, iron deficiency among infants and young children is decreasing but still needs attention, and the two subgroups who are at greatest risk for nutrition-related problems are people of color and those with low-income. Family child health nurses are challenged to implement policies to protect and promote nutritional health for these and other populations of children and families (Story & Harnack, 1999). (See Chapter 16 for a discussion of family health policy.)

Family child health nurses can use the goals of current health care leaders and national recommendations on child health issues to guide their own policy evaluations and efforts for change. The Surgeon General, Dr. David Satcher, has stated his goals: Eliminate disparities in health care among all racial and ethnic groups, make all children's health a primary goal, and focus more resources on mental health (Pierce, 1998). *Healthy Children 2010: Enhancing Children's Wellness* (1997) is an example of a national guideline for family child health nurses to establish priorities of action.

SUMMARY

Key points to remember are that family child health nurses focus on the relationship of family life to children's health and illness, and they assist families and each of their members to achieve well-being. Through family-centered care, family child health nurses enhance family life and the development of their members to their fullest potential. The *family interaction model* incorporates relevant components of family life and interaction, family development and transitions, and family health and illness and helps nurses to take a comprehensive and collaborative approach to families. It also enables them to screen for potentially harmful situations, instruct families about health issues, and help families to cope with acute illness, chronic illness, and life-threatening conditions.

RESEARCH BRIEF

Hispanic Mothers and Children's Health Problems

The purpose of this study was to identify Hispanic mothers' initial sources of advice and help with children's illnesses; their beliefs about the cause and seriousness of certain illnesses, including fever, cough, diarrhea, vomiting, conjunctivitis, skin rash, minor wounds, and burns; and how they manage these children's health problems, including the use of home remedies. Interviews were conducted with 100 women of Hispanic origin who had at least one child who was age 5 or younger and who were attending a community clinic in a rural area of central California. Mothers' beliefs about causes of problems varied widely, revealing misconceptions, folk beliefs, and lack of knowledge. Only 32 percent of the mothers used or would use health professionals as the initial source of advice or help with children's problems. The majority of mothers (81 percent) used home remedies to manage children's problems; 17 percent sought the help of a folk healer. The various types of home remedies used by mothers included the ingestion or application of certain foods, fluids, herbal teas, or other materials and methods to eliminate the perceived causes of the problems. Eleven percent of the mothers had used *azarcon* (lead tetroxide) or *greta* (lead oxide), both substances contain lead as laxatives, for treating *empacho* (diarrhea) or other stomach problems in children. The need for culturally responsive and sensitive health care is also discussed.

Source: Mikhail, B.I. (1994). Hispanic mothers' beliefs and practices regarding selected children's health problems. *Western Journal of Nursing Research, 16*(6):623–638.

Study Questions

1. The family child health nurse determines the most *appropriate* health promotion activities in a family with young children through analysis of:
   a. Children's health practices.
   b. Patterns of parenting and family and child developmental tasks.
   c. Parents' and grandparents' health beliefs.
   d. Patterns of disease and illness reorganization task management.
2. Family child health nurses practice family-centered health care, which is most accurately characterized as:
   a. Fostering partnerships between members of different families
   b. Providing consistently high-quality care for all families
   c. Forming partnerships between families and nurses
   d. Viewing the nurse as the constant in family and child health
3. The family interaction model has three major concepts. Which one of the following is *not* one of these major concepts?
   a. Task development cycles
   b. Individual development
   c. Family career
   d. Patterns of health, disease, and illness
4. Which of these principles should family nurses incorporate in their care in order to help a family with a child who has diabetes?
   a. Patterns of illness are usually predictable in families
   b. Protection is paramount in each interaction
   c. Patterns of illness and disease differ in different families
   d. Reorganization of family routines is discouraged
5. Using the family interaction model, the family child health nurse knows that one of the more important assessments of families experiencing a chronic illness of their child is:
   a. Definition of the disease with which the child has been diagnosed
   b. How the family's past crises have altered their growth
   c. Definition of the limitations that the family is experiencing
   d. How the family's past experience with the illness affects the current situation
6. Why is it important for family child health nurses to explore a family's developmental tasks when analyzing the family's response to an illness event?
7. What principles of family-centered care would family child health nurses use with a hospitalized infant and family?

Discussion Questions

1. Discuss with your classmates your experiences with families. Compare your expectations as you think about the behaviors of the various types of children and families with whom you are familiar and those with whom you are less familiar.
2. Compare how you, a family child health nurse, would discuss health outcomes with a family in the following situations: a family with a chronically ill child, a family with an acutely ill child, and a family with a child with a life-threatening illness. Consider families with multiple children in which one has an illness or disease and the others do not.
3. Obtain a child and/or family health policy in your city, state, country, etc. Discuss the implications of that policy for families with a chronically ill child, and for a family who has few or limited financial resources, or has no health insurance.

Case Study

CAZO

Cazo was a 23-month-old boy born to Serrita, age 25, and Carlos, age 29, who were of Mexican-American heritage. Cazo was born at term, but he was slightly underweight for his gestational age. The family household consisted of the patient, Cazo, his father, his mother, his 4-year-old sister, Mona, and his paternal grandmother, Señora Serena. They resided in a rural farming area. The nearest neighbor was 10 miles distant. Cazo's father and mother both worked on farms in the area. Cazo and his sister were cared for by their grandmother. The family was generally healthy. No one in the family smoked tobacco, consumed drugs or used alcohol. They were Roman Catholic.

Seven months ago Cazo was diagnosed with acute lymphocytic leukemia. After that he received chemotherapy on an out-patient basis every few weeks. The family hoped for remission. Cazo ate the general diet of the family, although he consumed little. He played in the yard with his sister and their pet dog. While he got tired, a common side effect of chemotherapy, he seemed to recover between doses. His parents and grandmother constantly worried about other side effects such as easy bruising and infection. The adults and his sister talked about his hair loss, another side effect of chemotherapy, contrasting his shiny little head with his former thick dark hair.

Analysis The nurse assessed Cazo's family members for their experience, asking about patterns of health, illness, disease. The nurse used symbolic interaction theory to search for and build meaning in the illness event. The nurse explored for features that the family associated with this illness experience. The whole family, that is, parents, grandmother and sister were included in the assessment. Cazo was in the room but did not pay attention to the discussion. Developmentally this is appropriate 2-year-old behavior.

Families are a function of their history as well as their current context. Thus, opening questions about previous illness experiences with hospitals and sickness can elicit information this family was using to interpret the current situation. The grandmother related that when she was a young child she experienced the deaths of two of her siblings from pneumonia. Because of this, she was very concerned about fevers, breathing or exposure to cold, damp night air.

The nurse observed that the parents were eager to adhere to the details of the treatment regimen. Both of them had had positive and healing experiences with health care providers in American society, and trusted the nurse's and physician's judgment completely. However, the nurse noted that they had not had any hospitalization experiences prior to the very recent one with Cazo. They indicated that the in-patient period had gone smoothly, with one of them staying with him at all times. However, the nurse knew that stressors would occur. Furthermore, the nurse knew that trust in the relationship between providers and families is a major issue and often requires dealing with different points of view and priorities talking with the family about their experiences and beliefs would help the issues to become known and thus help to maintain trust (Burke et al, 1991). The nurse knew that families have their own cultural ways of treating illness; therefore, it was important to learn what meanings the family had. Therefore, the nurse asked: What are the main problems you have experienced that are related to your child's illness? For you as individuals and for the family as a whole? How severe do you consider your child's illness to be? What are the results you hope to receive from the treatments? What do you fear about this illness and the treatment? What family goals do you have in relation to your child's illness and the experience you are going through?

The nurse anticipated that the childrearing tasks of the family in the toddler-preschool stage would be disrupted. The nurse assessed the impact of repeated trips to the health care center for chemotherapy on family time and family members' needs. The nurse learned that Mona, who was less than 4 years old at the time of the diagnosis, had regressed in her toileting behaviors. In addition, Mona had separated easily from her parents and grandmother before Cazo's hospitalization, but now she clung to her parents and grandmother and whined. The nurse evaluated this data and concluded that Mona's behavior was expected at this stressful family time. The nurse planned to talk with the family about their interpretations of Mona's behavior and their responses to the child.

The nurse used knowledge of individual development and systems theory to examine family interactions. Realizing that this family was experiencing both developmental and situational family transitions, the nurse also assessed for reorganization of family roles and tasks.

At a subsequent visit, the nurse spoke with the family about the separations needed for the trips to the clinic for Cazo's treatments. The parents expressed concern over these separations, both for their daughter and for the grandmother left at home to manage the household and Mona. Using the collaborative approach, the nurse and family considered solutions to the separations created by the clinic appointments. Ideas about ways for the whole family to attend the treatment sessions arose in the discussion. The grandmother had been staying home with the daughter, thinking that would lessen the stress for her son and his wife and allow them to focus on Cazo during the treatments. The nurse's intervention was to encourage the family to consider how they did best: separating with part of the family staying home or all coming together. The nurse built on the family strength of mutual support in assisting them to plan to all come together. After this discussion, the whole family came to the clinic. Grandmother Serena felt a lot less upset. Family togetherness and support were things she valued and had experienced with her extended family in Mexico. Mona's behavior began to return to her former level and she interacted more in her usual patterns. The nurse recognized the importance of acute and chronic illness patterns for both Cazo and his sister, and the importance of grandparenting for the children. She kept the family as the focus of her intervention.

Another problem for this family arose during the clinic visits. Cazo was protesting the invasive diagnostic measures and chemotherapy treatment, which involved needles and various other equipment. Even though numbing measures were used for intravenous administration of medications, he would cry and writhe about and yell loudly at the nurses and doctors. The nurse interpreted this as normal developmental behavior for a 23-month-old child and an expected response to the illness and treatment. However, through observation and focused questioning, the nurse assessed that this behavior was troubling to Cazo's father. Carlos said that he thought the boy should be brave, withstand pain without crying and be fully cooperative with this important treatment. Carlos said that his daughter had been a quiet child and had received immunization injections, for example, without crying or protesting. Carlos said he realized that his daughter had not had to endure the same level and length of discomfort that Cazo was experiencing. The nurse's understanding of the value for Carlos's of Cazo being a strong boy-child allowed her to support the father and not attempt to change this value. The nurse was an active listener, understood the importance of gaining the father's trust, and allowed him to bring his own meaning to the situation.

The nurse acknowledged Carlos's expectations and reframed the situation, saying to the father that despite the fatigue that chemotherapy often produces, Cazo possessed the strength and energy to protest strongly. Carlos was encouraged by his son's strength and ability to fight the cancer, and the nurse encouraged Carlos to stay with his son during the painful procedures and coach him. He encouraged Cazo to use his strength to hold his arms or legs in a certain position. Carlos still wanted Cazo not to cry, but now he directed him to yell out to the cancer to "go away." The father stayed in a guiding and supportive role with this redirected focus for his actions. The nurse did not say to him that his expectations were wrong; instead, she provided information about the ability of 2-year-old children to change their behavior in the face of pain and restraints. Carlos and the nurse thus both contributed to the support of the child and of the parent-child unit. The father and son built a successful coping pattern for both of them, and the father's role was maintained. The nurse realized that the family and parents are the constants in a child's life, and that their solutions are likely to be most effective.

Nurses focus on the overall features of the individual and family, the environment or context, and the health of the persons involved. Within this framework, the nurse continually assessed, planned, acted and evaluated as she managed the health of Cazo and his family. The nurse's practice was guided and influenced by multiple perspectives, including contextual and transitional factors for the child and family at home and in the treatment setting. The nurse continually adjusted her approach to the family and individual responses, while simultaneously guiding through giving and interpreting information. This case illustrates use of the *family interaction model* to work with family strengths and capabilities to facilitate family well-being.

References

Ahrons, C. (1999). Divorce: An unscheduled family transition. In B. Carter & M. McGoldrick (Eds.) *The Expanded*

Family Life Cycle: Individual, Family and Social Perspectives, ed 3, (pp. 381–398). Boston: Allyn & Bacon.

Ahmann, E. (1997). Family matters. Books for siblings of children having illness or disability. *Pediatric Nursing*, *23*(5):500–502.

Aldous, J. (1996). *Family Careers: Rethinking the Developmental Perspective*. Thousand Oaks, CA: Sage.

American Academy of Pediatrics. (1998). Guidance for effective discipline. *Pediatrics*, *101*(4):723–728.

American Academy of Pediatrics, Committee on Children with Handicaps. (1973). Day care for handicapped children. *Pediatrics*, *51*:948.

Anderson, C. (1999). Single-parent families: Strengths, vulnerabilities, and interventions. In B. Carter & M. McGoldrick (Eds.) *The Expanded Family Life Cycle: Individual, Family, and Social Perspectives*, ed 3, (pp. 399–416). Boston: Allyn & Bacon.

Besser, F. (1977). Great Ormond Street anniversary. *Nursing Mirror*, *144*(6)(Feb 10):60–63.

Bianchi, S. M. (1990). America's children: Mixed prospects. *Population Bulletin*, *45*:1–43. Washington, DC: Population Reference Bureau.

Bianchi, S. M. (1995). The changing demographic and socioeconomic character of single-parent families. *Marriage and Family Review*, *20*:71–98.

Bomar, P. J. (1996). Family health promotion. In S.M.H. Hanson & S.T. Boyd. *Family Health Care Nursing. Theory, Practice and Research*, (pp. 175–199). Philadelphia: F.A. Davis.

Bowen, G. C., et al. (1995). Poverty and the single mother family: A macroeconomic perspective. *Marriage and Family Review*, *20*:115–142.

Burke, S.O., et al. (1991). Hazardous secrets and reluctantly taking charge: Parenting a child with repeated hospitalizations. *Image: Journal of Nursing Scholarship*, *23*(1): 39–45.

Burlingham, D., & Freud, A. (1942). *Young Children in War Time*. London: Allen & Unwin.

Burr, W. R., et al. (1988). Epistemologies that lead to primary explanations in family science. *Family Science Review*, *1*:185–210.

Burton, L. M., et al. (1995). Context and surrogate parenting among contemporary grandparents. In S.M.H. Hanson, et al. (Eds.), Single parent families: Diversity, myths, and realities: Part two, *Marriage & Family Review*, *20*(3/4):349–366.

Byock, I. R. (1999). Conceptual models and the outcomes of caring. *Journal of Pain and Symptom Management*, *17*(2):83–92.

Callery, P. (1997a). Caring for parents of hospitalized children: A hidden area of nursing work. *Journal of Advanced Nursing*, *26*(5):992–998.

Callery, P. (1997b). Paying to participate: Financial, social, and personal costs to parents of involvement in their children's care in hospital. *Journal of Advanced Nursing*, *26*(4):746–752.

Carter, B., & McGoldrick, M. (1999). Divorce: An unscheduled family transition. In B. Carter and M. McGoldrick (Eds.) *The Expanded Family Life Cycle: Individual, Family, and Social Perspectives*, ed 3, (pp. 373–380). Boston: Allyn & Bacon.

Cioro, M. J., et al. (1994). Health of our nation's children. National Center for Health Statistics. *Vital Health Stat*, *10*(191).Http://www.cdc.gov/nchswww/data/sr10191. pdf.

Compas, B., et al. (1997). Prevention of depression. In R. Weissberg, et al. (Eds) *Healthy Children 2010: Enhancing Children's Wellness*, (pp. 129–174). Thousand Oaks, CA: Sage.

Corbin, J. M., & Strauss, A..(1988). Illness trajectories. In *Unending Work and Care: Managing Chronic Illness at Home*, (pp. 33–48). San Francisco: Jossey-Bass.

Coyne, I.T. (1995). Partnership in care: parents' views of participation in their hospitalized child's care. *Journal of Clinical Nursing*, *4*(2):71–79.

Darbyshire, P. (1993). Parents, nurses and pediatric nursing: A critical review. *Journal of Advanced Nursing*, *18*:1670–1680.

Dawson, D.A., & Cain, V.S. (1990). Child care arrangements: Health of our nation's children, United States, 1988. Advance data from vital and health statistics, no. 187. Hyattsville, Maryland: National Center for Health Statistics.

Deatrick, J. A., et al. (1999). Clarifying the concept of normalization. *Image: Journal of Nursing Scholarship*, *31*(3) :209–214.

Denham, S. (1995). Family routines: A construct for considering family health. *Holistic Nursing Practice*, *9*(4):11–13.

Doherty, W., & McCubbin, H. (1985). Families and health care: An emerging arena of theory, research, and clinical intervention. *Family Relations*, *34*:5–11.

Doka, K. J. (1995). Talking to children about illness. In K. J. Doka (Ed.) *Children Mourning, Mourning Children*, (pp. 31–39). Washington, DC: Hospice Foundation of America.

Dryfoos, J. (1997). The prevalence of problem behaviors: Implications for programs. In R. Weissberg, et al. (Eds.) *Healthy Children 2010: Enhancing Children's Wellness*, (pp. 17–46). Thousand Oaks, CA: Sage.

Duvall, E.M., & Miller, B. C. (1985). Developmental tasks: Individual and family. In E. M. Duvall & B. C. Miller, *Marriage and Family Development*. New York: Harper & Row.

Erikson, E. H. (1973). *Childhood and Society*. New York: W.W. Norton.

Ersek, M. (1992). Examining the process and dilemmas of reality negotiation. *Image: The Journal of Nursing Scholarship*, *24*:19–25.

Falicov, C. (1999). The Latino family life cycle. In B. Carter and M. McGoldrick (Eds.) *The Expanded Family Life Cycle: Individual, Family and Social Perspectives*, ed 3, (pp. 141–152). Boston: Allyn & Bacon.

Falsetti, D., & Kovel, A. (1994). How one school-based clinic is meeting the challenge of adolescent health care. *Journal of the American Academy of Nurse Practitioners*, *6*(8):363–368.

Faux, S. (1993). Siblings of children with chronic physical and cognitive disabilities. *Journal of Pediatric Nursing*, *8*(5):305–317.

Faville, K. (1925). The nurse as counselor in troubled homes. *The Red Cross Courier*, *4*:14–15, 22.

Federal Interagency Forum on Child and Family Statistics. (1997). America's Children: Key National Indicators of Well-Being. National Maternal and Child Health Bureau Clearinghouse (703):356–1964. http://www.cdc.gov/nchswww/data/amchild.pdf.

Ferrell, B. R., et al. (1998). Integration of pain education in home care. *Journal of Palliative Care*, *14*(3):62–68.

Gedaly-Duff, V. (1990). Family management of childhood pain. Phase 2: Parents' experiences in care of their children's repeated pain episodes associated with chronic illness such as juvenile rheumatoid arthritis. Final Report for Robert Wood Johnson Clinical Nurse Scholars Program, 1998–1990, University of Pennsylvania, Philadelphia, PA.

Gedaly-Duff, V. (1991). Developmental issues: Preschool and school-age children. In J. P. Bush & S. W. Harkins (Eds.) *Children in Pain: Clinical and Research Issues from a Developmental Perspective*, (pp.195–230). New York: Springer-Verlag.

Gedaly-Duff, V., & Aryes, L. (Unpublished data). "Parenting children with chronic pain": Further analysis of the data from "Family Management of Childhood Pain. Phase 2: Families' Experiences in Care of their Children's Repeated Pain Episodes Associated with Chronic Illness such as Juvenile Rheumatoid Arthritis."

Gedaly-Duff, V. & Heims, M.L.(1996). Family child health nursing. In S.M.H. Hanson & S.T. Boyd. *Family Health Care Nursing. Theory, Practice and Research*, (pp. 239–265). Philadelphia: F.A. Davis.

Gedaly-Duff, V., et al. (November, 1997). Families, trust, and pain in children. In IV Conferencia Internacional de Enfermeria Familiar [Fourth International Family Nursing Conference], Program and Abstracts, (Salon Los Pioneros, 13 Novembre 1997). Valdivia, Chile.

Gedaly-Duff, V., et al. (2000). Working with families. In R. Nickel & L. W. Desch (Eds.), *Physician's Guide to the Care of Children with Disabilities and Chronic Conditions*. Baltimore, MD: Paul Brooke.

Gedaly-Duff, V., & Ziebarth, D. (2000). Mothers' management of 4- to 8-year-olds' adenoid-tonsillectomy pain: A preliminary study. *Pain*, *57*:293–299.

Gilliss, C. L. (1991). Family nursing research, theory, and practice. *Image: Journal of Nursing Scholarship*, *23*: 19–22.

Goslin, E. (1978). Hospitalization as a life crisis for the preschool child: A critical review. *Journal of Community Health*, *3*:321–346.

Graves, C., & Hayes, V. E. (1996). Do nurses and parents of children with chronic conditions agree on parental needs? *Journal of Pediatric Nursing*, *11*(5):288–299.

Hanson, S. M. H., et al. (1992). Education for family health care professionals: Nursing as a paradigm. *Family Relations*, *41*:49–53.

Harticker, L. (Ed.). (1998). Core principles of family-centered health care. Advances in family centered health care. *Institute for Family-Centered Care*, *4*(1):1–20.

Hauser, S., et al. (1985). The contribution of family environment to perceived competence and illness adjustments in diabetic and acutely ill adolescents. *Family Relations*, *34*:99–108.

Hawkins, J. (1997). Academic performance and school success: Sources and consequences. In R. Weissberg, et al. (Eds.) *Healthy Children 2010: Enhancing Children's Wellness* (pp. 278–305). Thousand Oaks, CA: Sage.

Hill, R., & Gedaly-Duff, V. (1998). Nurses' interactions with families and children during pain management. *Communicating Nursing Research*, *31*(6):176.

Hines, P. (1999). The family life cycle of African American families living in poverty. In B. Carter and M. McGoldrick (Eds.) *The Expanded Family Life Cycle: Individual, Family, and Social Perspectives*, ed 3, (pp. 327–345). Boston: Allyn & Bacon.

Howard, B. (1991). Discipline in early childhood. *Pediatric Clinics of North America*, *38*(6):1351–1369.

Hoyert, D. L., et al. (1999). Final Data for 1997. National vital statistics report, 47(19). Hyattsville, Maryland: National Center for Health Statistics. Http:// www.cdc.gov/nchswww/data/nvs47_19.pdf

Igoe, J. (1993). School-linked family health centers in health care reform. *Pediatric Nursing*, *19*:67–68.

Igoe, J. B., & Giordano, B. P. (1992). *Expanding School Health Services to Serve Families in the 21st Century*. Washington, DC: American Nurses Publishing.

Jackson, P. (1996). The primary care provider and children with chronic conditions. In P. L. Jackson and J. A. Vessey (Eds.) *Primary Care of the Child with a Chronic Condition*, (pp. 3–15). Philadelphia: Mosby.

Jendrek, M. P. (1993). Grandparents who parent their grandchildren: Effects on lifestyle. *Journal of Marriage and the Family*, *55*:609–621.

Johnson, T. W., & Colucci, P. (1999). Lesbians, gay men, and the family life cycle. In B. Carter & M. McGoldrick (Eds.) *The Expanded Family Life Cycle: Individual, Family, and Social Perspectives*, ed 3, (pp. 349–361). Boston: Allyn & Bacon.

Kalafat, J. (1997). Prevention of suicide. In R. Weissberg, et al. (Eds.) *Healthy Children 2010: Enhancing Children's Wellness*, (pp. 175–213). Thousand Oaks, CA: Sage.

Kann, L., et al. (1998). Youth risk behavior surveillance: United States, 1997. Chronic Disease Prevention and Health Promotion, Rockville, Maryland. Http://www.cdc.nccdphp/dash/ MMWRFile/ ss4703.htm.

Kass, B.L., et al. (1996). Racial and ethnic differences in health 1996. MEPS chartbook no. 2. http://www.meps.ahcpr. gov/papers/chartbk2/chrtbk2a.htm

Kelley, S.J., et al. (1997). To grandmother's house we go . . . and stay: Children raised in intergenerational families. *Journal of Gerontological Nursing, 23*(9):12–20.

Kirby, S.N., et al. (1999). Supply and demand of minority teachers in Texas: Problems and prospects. *Educational Evaluation and Policy Analysis, 21*(1):47–66.

Kivett, V. R. (1991).The grandparent-grandchild connection. In S. P. Pfeifer & M. B. Sussman (Eds.) *Families: Intergenerational and Generational Connections*, (pp. 267–290). New York: Haworth Press.

Klein, D. M., & White, J. M. (1996). The symbolic interaction framework. In *Family Theories: An Introduction*, (pp. 87–118). Thousand Oaks, CA: Sage.

Kleinman, A. (1988).*The meaning of symptoms and disorders. In The Illness Narratives*, (pp. 3–30). New York: Basic Books.

Kleinman, A., et al. (1978). Culture, illness, and care. Clinical lessons from anthropologic and cross-cultural research. *Annals of Internal Medicine, 88*:251–258.

Kohlberg, L. (1984). *The Psychology of Moral Development.* San Francisco: Harper & Row.

Kramer, R., (1989). Remembering Lara. In P. Benner, & J. Wrubel. *The Primacy of Caring*, (pp. 298–307). Menlo Park, CA: Addison-Wesley.

Lash, M., & Wertlieb, D. (1993). A model for family-centered service coordination for children who are disabled by traumatic injuries. *The ACCH Advocate, 1*:19–27, 39–41.

Loveland-Cherry, C. J. (1996). Family health promotion and health protection. In P.J. Bomar (Ed.) *Nurses and Family Health Promotion: Concepts, Assessment, and Interventions*, ed 2, (pp. 22–35). Philadelphia: W.B. Saunders.

Maslow, A. H. (1970). *Motivation and Personality*, ed 2. New York: Harper & Row.

McGoldrick, M., & Carter, B. (1999). Remarried families. In B. Carter and M. McGoldrick (Eds.) *The Expanded Family Life Cycle: Individual, Family, and Social Perspectives*, ed 3, (pp. 417–435). Boston: Allyn & Bacon.

McGoldrick, M., & Walsh, F. (1999). Death and the family life cycle. In B. Carter and M. McGoldrick (Eds.) *The Expanded Family Life Cycle: Individual, Family, and Social Perspectives*, ed 3, (pp. 185–201). Boston: Allyn & Bacon.

McQuillan, R., & Finlay, I. (1996). Facilitating the care of terminally ill children. *Journal of Pain and Symptom Management, 12*(5):320–324.

Mead, G. H. (1934). *Mind, Self, and Society*. Chicago: University of Chicago Press.

Melnyk, B. M. (1998). The COPE program: A strategy to improve outcomes of critically ill young children and their parents. *Pediatric Nursing, 24*(6):521–527, 539–540.

Meister, S. B. (1991). Family well-being. In A. L. Whall & J. Fawcett (Eds.), *Family Theory Development in Nursing: State of the Science and Art*, (pp. 209–231). Philadelphia: F.A. Davis.

Mikhail, B. I. (1994). Hispanic mothers' beliefs and practices regarding selected children's health problems. *Western Journal of Nursing Research, 16*(6):623–638.

Miles, M., et al. (1989).The pediatric intensive care unit environment as a source of stress for parents. *Maternal-Child Nursing Journal, 18*:199–206.

Minkler, M., & Roe, K. M. (1993). *Grandmothers As Caregivers: Raising Children of the Crack Cocaine Epidemic.* Newbury Park, CA: Sage.

Morrison, L. (1997). Stress and Siblings. *Pediatric Nursing, 9*(4):26–27.

Murray, J. S. (1999). Siblings of children with cancer: A review of the literature. *Journal of Pediatric Oncology Nursing, 16*(1):25–34.

Murray, M., et al. (1997). Violence prevention for the 21st century. In R. Weissberg, et al. (Eds.) *Healthy Children 2010: Enhancing Children's Wellness*, (pp. 105–128). Thousand Oaks, CA: Sage.

National Institute of Nursing Research (NINR).(1993). Health promotion for older children and adolescents: A report of the NINR priority expert panel on health promotion. Bethesda, MD: US Department of Health and Human Services, USPHS, NIH.

Newacheck, P. W., et al. (1998). An epidemiologic profile of children with special health care needs. *Pediatrics, 102*(1):117–121.

Paget, M. (1982). Your son is cured now; you may take him home. *Culture, Medicine, and Psychiatry, 6*:237–259.

Patterson, J. M., & Garwick, A. W. (1994). Levels of meaning in family stress theory. *Family Process, 33*:287–304.

Pesznecker, B. L., et al. (1989). The mutual-participation relationship: Key to facilitating self-care practices in clients and families. *Public Health Nursing, 6*:197–203.

Pierce, P. (1998). He wants to be America's family doctor. *Parade Magazine*, Sep *13*:14, 16.

Piaget, J., & Inhelder, B. (1969). *Psychology of the Child.* New York: Basic Books.

Pillitteri, A. (1992). *Maternal and Child Health Nursing.* Philadelphia: J. B. Lippincott.

Pridham, D. F. (1993). Anticipatory guidance of parents of new infants: Potential contribution of the internal working model construct. *Image Journal of Nursing Scholarship, 25*:49–55.

Pruchno, R. (1999). Raising grandchildren: The experiences of black and white grandmothers. *Gerontologist, 39*(2):209–221.

Purnell, M., & Bagby, B. H. (1993). Grandparents' rights: Implications for family specialists. *Family Relations, 42*:173–178.

Rankin, S. H. (1989). Family transitions. In C. L. Gilliss, et al. (Eds.) *Toward a Science of Family Nursing*, (pp. 173–186). Menlo Park, CA: Addison-Wesley.

Robinson, C. A. (1985). Double bind: A dilemma for parents of chronically ill children. *Pediatric Nursing, 11*: 112–115.

Rolland, J. (1999). Chronic illness and the family life cycle. In B. Carter and M. McGoldrick (Eds.) *The Expanded Family Life Cycle: Individual, Family, and Social Perspectives*, ed 3, (pp. 492–511). Boston: Allyn & Bacon.

Sameroff, A. J., & Feil, L. A. (1985). Parental concepts of development. In I. E. Sigel (Ed.) *Parental Belief Systems*, (pp. 83–105). Hillsdale, NJ: Larence Erlbaum.

Schultz, P. R., & Meleis, A. I. (1988). Nursing epistemology: Traditions, insights, questions. *Image: Journal of Nursing Scholarship, 20*:218–220.

Schumacher, K. L. & Meleis, A. I. (1994). Transitions: A central concept in nursing. *Image, 26*(2):119–127.

Selekman, J., & Snyder, M. (1996). Learning Disabilities and/or Attention Deficit Hyperactivity Disorder. In P. L. Jackson and J. A. Vessey (Eds.) *Primary Care of the Child with a Chronic Condition*, ed 2, (pp. 553–579). Philadelphia: Mosby.

Sells, W., & Blum, R. (1996). Morbidity and mortality among U.S. Adolescents: An overview of data and trends. *American Journal of Public Health, 86*(4):513–519.

Shapiro, B. (1993). Management of painful episodes in sickle cell disease. In N. Schechter, et al. (Eds.) *Pain in Infants, Children, and Adolescents*, (pp. 385–410).Philadelphia: Williams & Wilkins.

Shelton, K., & Gedaly-Duff, V. (1999). Validity testing of two instruments for primary care of families: a work in progress. *Communicating Nursing Research Conference Proceedings, 32*(7):214.

Sirkia, K., et al. (1998). Pain medication during terminal care of children with cancer. *Journal of Pain & Symptom Management, 15*(4):220–226.

Solari-Twadell, A., et al. (1995). The pinwheel model of bereavement. *Image: Journal of Nursing Scholarship, 27*(4):323–326.

Spitz, R. (1945). Hospitalism. *Psychoanalytic Study of the Child, 1*:53–74.

Spruhan, J. B. (1996). Beyond traditional nursing care: Cultural awareness and successful home healthcare nursing. *Home Healthcare Nurse, 14*(6):445–449.

Story, M. & Harnack, L. (1999). Nutrition issues for mothers, children, youth, and families. In H.R. Wallace, et al. *Health and Welfare for Families in the 21st Century*, (pp. 419–440). Boston: Jones & Bartlett.

Thomas, R. M. (1992). In *Comparing Theories of Child Development*, ed 3. Belmont, CA: Wadsworth.

Thompson, R. (1986). Where we stand: Twenty years of research on pediatric hospitalization and health care. *Children's Health Care, 14*:200–210.

Tiedeman, M. E. (1997). Anxiety responses of parents during and after the hospitalization of their 5- to 11-year-old children. *Journal of Pediatric Nursing: Nursing Care of Children and Families, 12*(2):110–119.

Tilden, V. P. (1998). Dying in America: Ethics and end-of-life care. *Communicating Nursing Research, 31*(6): 39–56.

Tuchfarber, B., et al. (1997). Prevention and control of injuries. In R. Weissberg, et al. (Eds.) *Healthy Children 2010: Enhancing Children's Wellness*, (pp. 250–277). Thousand Oaks, CA: Sage.

Tyler, D. (1990). Pain in infants and children. In J. J. Bonica (Ed.) *The Management of Pain*, vol *1*, (pp. 538–551). Philadelphia: Lea & Febiger.

U.S. Department of Health and Human Services. Agency for Health Care Policy and Research (AHCPR). (1994). U.S. guideline for management of cancer pain (AHCPR Pub. No.94–0592). Rockville, MD: Agency for Health Care Policy and Research, Public Health Service, U.S. Department of Health and Human Services.

U.S. Department of Health and Human Services. National Center for Health Statistics. (1993). Highlights. Health, United States, 1992. In Health, United States, 1992 and Healthy People 2000 Review (DHHS Pub. No. PHS 93–1232), pp. 3–7, 52–60, 68. Hyattsville, MD: Public Health Service.

Waechter, E. (1971). Children's awareness of fatal illness. *American Journal of Nursing, 71*:1168–1172.

Wald, L. D. (1904). The treatment of families in which there is sickness. *American Journal of Nursing, 4*:427–431, 515–519, 602–606.

Wallace, H. M., et al. (Eds.). (1999). *Health and welfare for families in the 21st century*. Boston: Jones & Bartlett.

Weissberg, R., & Kuster, C. (1997). Introduction and overview: Let's make "health children 2010" a national priority! In R. Weissberg, et al. (Eds.) *Healthy Children 2010: Enhancing Children's Wellness*, (pp. 1–16). Thousand Oaks, CA: Sage.

Woodwell, D. A. (1999). National Ambulatory Medical Care Survey: 1997 Summary. Advance data from vital and health statistics, no. 305. Hyattsville, Maryland: National Center for Health Statistics.

Focus On

FAMILY-FOCUSED MEDICAL-SURGICAL NURSING

This chapter provides insight into the experiences of families in medical-surgical settings. When adults are ill and need hospitalization, they are generally admitted to a medical or surgical unit in a hospital. Regardless of the reason for the patient's hospital admission, the experience is a stressful one for patients and their families; both need nursing care.

This chapter describes issues for nurses to consider as they plan care for families in medical-surgical settings. You will find a summary of the stressors that families face during hospitalization and a discussion of the use of the therapeutic quadrangle to analyze family needs during an illness episode. Students will be particularly interested in the section that deals with caring for families before illness, during acute and chronic illness, and during the terminal phase of illness.

The discussion of the application of theoretical models to family medical-surgical nursing addresses typical student concerns about the connection between theory and practice. In addition, broad categories of family nursing interventions that may be used during any phase of illness are described, including family support, promotion of family integrity, and family mobilization. The case study that is presented realistically portrays the agony and the growth often experienced by families dealing with AIDS. The chapter closes with a discussion of the implications of developments in family nursing on medical-surgical education, research, and health care policy.

Chapter 12

FAMILY-FOCUSED MEDICAL-SURGICAL NURSING

Nancy Trygar Artinian

OUTLINE

OBJECTIVES

On completion of this chapter, the reader will be able to:

- Discuss various approaches to assessing the impact of illness or injury on families.
- Use the structural-functional model, family systems model, and family stress model to design and implement care for families in medical-surgical settings.
- Identify family needs and related interventions before illness and during the acute, chronic, and terminal phases of care.
- Analyze factors to consider when determining hospital visitation policies.
- Discuss family participation in "do not resuscitate" (DNR) decisions.
- Describe how nurses can help families prepare advance directives.
- List advantages and disadvantages to having families present to watch nurses and physicians carry out resuscitative efforts.
- Identify stages in relationships between the family and health care team as defined by Thorne and Robinson.
- Identify factors that may influence family readiness for hospital discharge.
- Determine the potential impact of family nursing knowledge on medical-surgical nursing theory, practice, education, research, and health care policy.

Once considered to be the domain of only community health, mental health, or maternal-child nursing, family nursing is now recognized as a key factor by most nurses in medical-surgical settings. Unfortunately, there is a broad range of skill relative to the care of families in acute care settings—some nurses do not see the value of including the family in care. Other nurses are able to provide creative, expert, and innovative care to families in the midst of continual demands for highly complex and technologic care to patients (Chesla, 1996). Providing care to the entire family unit as well as caring for patients in the context of their families is crucial regardless of the setting for nursing care delivery.

The purpose of this chapter is to describe issues for nurses to consider as they plan care for families in medical-surgical settings. Included is a review of the stressors that families often face during hospitalization and a discussion of the use of the therapeutic quadrangle to analyze family needs during an episode of illness. This chapter examines caring for families before illness, during acute and chronic illness, and during the terminal illness experience and reviews broad categories of family nursing interventions to use during any of the phases of illness. The discussion of the application of theoretical models to family medical-surgical nursing highlights the connection between theory and practice. The case study that is presented realistically portrays the agony and growth often experienced by families dealing with AIDS. The chapter closes with a discussion of the implications of developments in family nursing on medical-surgical education, research, and health care policy.

Several factors contributed to the increasing concern for families in medical-surgical settings. First, there is a growing body of evidence that families influence patient recovery, quality of life, and treatment adherence (Frederickson, 1989; Holder, 1997; Hoskins et al, 1996; King et al, 1993; King, 1996; Kulik & Mahler, 1989; Trief et al, 1998; Wang & Fenske, 1996; Yates, 1989). Hanson and colleagues (1995) found that families that maintain positive family functioning during the chronic diabetes of a family member have lower levels of family life stress, which positively influences patient adherence to diabetes self-management tasks and leads to subsequent metabolic control. Second, there is a growing consumer demand for unfragmented, holistic, humane, and sensitively delivered health care. Finally, the prospective payment system for health care results in early hospital discharge of patients to the care of their families. In such cases, family-focused care throughout the patient's hospitalization helps prepare the family to give care after discharge.

FAMILY STRESSORS DURING HOSPITALIZATION

Families experience many stressors during hospitalization (Johnson et al, 1995). Not only are hospital environments foreign, but nurses and doctors are strangers who speak another language. To add to the stress, families are separated from their ill member soon after entering the hospital doors and are asked to go to a small, sometimes crowded, waiting room. There, they wait endlessly for someone to give them information as they deal with emotions such as fear, anger, and guilt. Some families are better prepared to deal with these stressors than others. Leske and Jiricka (1998) found that, among 51 family members of patients who had motor vehicle accidents or gunshot wounds, increases in prior stressors, strains, and transitions were negatively related to family adaptation outcomes and that family hardiness, resources, coping, and problem-solving communication were positively related to family adaptation outcomes. Depending on past experiences and family resources, some family members may be more vulnerable to stressors associated with an intensive care unit (ICU) hospitalization than others.

Illness or injury requiring hospitalization of a loved one has been termed a nonnormative stressor event for families; that is, it is unexpected and unpredictable. Experiencing such an event may help some families to grow but cause conflicts in others. In the case of illness or injury, home routines are disrupted and some family members may need to assume responsibilities they have never had before. In addition, parents may struggle with how much to tell their children, or children may fear they are going to lose a parent.

Figley and McCubbin (1983) have described the characteristics of nonnormative events that can be used to assess the impact of illness or injury on families. The degree to which these characteristics exist determines the degree of family stress. These characteristics are:

- The amount of time the family has had to prepare for the event, in this case, illness or injury
- The family's previous experience with the illness or injury
- The availability of resources to assist the family in managing the illness or injury
- The prevalence of the illness or injury event
- The extent of loss associated with the illness or injury (e.g., loss of life, loss of body part, loss of roles, loss of income)
- The amount of family disruption or number of family changes caused by the event

THE THERAPEUTIC QUADRANGLE

Medical-surgical nurses need to assess the impact of hospitalization on families and deliver care accordingly. Rolland (1988) describes the therapeutic quadrangle as an aid to analyzing family care needs. The therapeutic quadrangle contains four parts: the illness, the family, the health care team, and the patient. Caring for families in medical-surgical settings requires analyzing all these components and designing and implementing tailor-made plans for family care accordingly.

Illness

Illness is the first element of the therapeutic quadrangle. There is a great deal of variability associated with illness, and this variability is characterized by differences in the onset, course, outcome, and degree of incapacitation of the illness (Rolland, 1988). The onset of illness may be sudden or gradual. Strokes and myocardial infarctions have sudden onsets: arthritis and emphysema have gradual onsets. The type of onset may explain the amount of family readjustment needed. The course of the disease may be progressive, constant, or relapsing. Cancers, rheumatoid arthritis, and emphysema are progressive; a spinal cord injury is constant; and multiple sclerosis and asthma are relapsing. Relapsing illnesses require a different kind of family adaptability from that needed in an illness with a progressive or constant course (Rolland, 1988); in addition, the extent to which an illness is likely to cause death also affects the family. Metastatic cancer and AIDS are progressive and usually fatal, whereas hypertension and arthritis are not likely to end in death if treated properly. Illness outcome influences the degree to which the family experiences anticipatory grief (Rolland, 1988). Thus, the expectation of future loss can alter family perceptions and problem-solving abilities. "The tendency to see the family member as practically 'in the coffin' can set in motion maladaptive responses that divest the ill member of important responsibilities" (Rolland, 1988, p. 25). The degree of illness incapacitation also determines the specific adjustments required of a family. Incapacitation can result from impairment of cognition (e.g., Alzheimer's disease), sensation (e.g., blindness), movement (e.g., stroke with paralysis), or energy production (e.g., cardiovascular and pulmonary diseases). Illness incapacitation can also result from social stigma (e.g., AIDS).

The complexity, frequency, and efficiency of treatment; the amount of home care and hospital-based care required; and the frequency and intensity of symptoms vary widely across illnesses and have important implications for family adaptation (Rolland, 1988). The phases of an illness, which are designated as crisis, chronic, and terminal, also affect family adjustment to the illness.

Family

The family is the second element in the therapeutic quadrangle. Family flexibility, cohesion, structure, cultural background, past experience with illness, resources, problem-solving ability, coping skills, and perceptions are just a few of the qualities that influence the family's relationships with the other elements in the therapeutic quadrangle.

There are a number of family tasks to consider in relation to illness. Moos (1984) described these illness-related tasks as (1) learning to deal with pain, incapacitation, or other illness-related symptoms of their ill member; (2) learning caregiving procedures; and (3) establishing workable relationships with the health care team.

Health Care Team

The third element in the therapeutic quadrangle is the health care team. Health team members vary in the priority they assign to family care, in their sensitivity to family needs, and in their knowledge and ability to assess and intervene with families. Hupcey (1998) found strategies used by nurses to develop relationships with families include demonstrating commitment (e.g., responding to the family member as a person spending time with the family, anticipating family needs), persevering (e.g., getting to know a lot about the family, spending time with more difficult families), and being involved (e.g., being an advocate for the family, bending or breaking rules). Strategies that inhibit relationships with families include depersonalizing the family, maintaining an efficient attitude, and displaying lack of trust in the family (Hupcey, 1998).

Patient

The final element in the therapeutic quadrangle is the patient. The identity of the sick person (e.g., mother, father, grandmother, spouse, sister) and the way the patient handles illness affect family adjustment. The point in the individual's life span at which the illness occurs also influences the family's adjustment. Often illness in the prime of life is unexpected, whereas illness in old age may be anticipated. In general, the more emotionally significant the sick family member, the more disruptive the illness will be. For example, if the ill person is the one everyone in the family depended on or turned to when they needed advice or other types of help, it is more likely that the loss of their contributions to the family will be acutely missed.

APPLICATION OF THEORETICAL MODELS

Chapter 2 describes several theoretical frameworks for nursing of families. Some family theoretical models are more helpful to medical-surgical nurses than others. In this setting, the short hospital stays involved, the sometimes overwhelming needs of patients, and the many other demands on their time influence nurses' abilities to plan and deliver care to families. For the family, the first priority is to help them cope with the immediacy of the hospitalization. Therefore, models that are concise and easy to use and do not depend on long-term relationships with families probably are most useful to acute care nurses. The goal is to help nurses assess and provide care for families within a short period of time. Three models from the family social science genre of theories are particularly useful in this.

Structural-Functional Model

The structural-functional perspective provides a useful framework for assessing families in a medical-surgical setting. The illness of a family member alters the family structure and may have an impact on family role relations. For example, illness may prevent one family member from carrying out his or her usual roles, so that it becomes necessary for another member to take on more responsibilities to compensate. If a single mother is ill, she cannot carry out her various roles, and a grandparent or sibling may have to assume her child care responsibilities. Illness may incapacitate the family if the power structure is patriarchal and it is the husband-father who is ill. Communication may cease if the wife-mother is the person in the family through whom all communication passes and she is ill.

Using the structural-functional framework, assessment focuses on the impact of the illness on family structure and on the family's ability to carry out its roles and functions. This model highlights functions that are important to assess during crisis, such as family coping, affective functioning, economic functioning, and health care functioning. Interventions become necessary when a change in the family structure alters the family's ability to function. Interventions include reinforcing, modifying, or changing the family organization or structure to strengthen, modify, or change its functioning (Berkey & Hanson, 1991). For example, a nurse may use the structural-functional model to plan care for a family whose 18-year-old daughter has paraplegia as a result of a motor vehicle accident. Assessment revealed the family is unable to carry out the coping function, that is, they were unable to manage the stress associated with their perception that their daughter's life was over. An intervention may include assisting the family to explore an alternate value structure related to family or individual productivity and achievement. Other appropriate interventions may include:

- Assisting the family to modify its organization so that role responsibilities can be distributed
- Respecting and encouraging adaptive coping skills used by the family
- Counseling family members on additional effective coping skills
- Telling the family it is safe and acceptable to use typical expressions of affection
- Providing family visitation
- Encouraging family members to recognize their own health needs
- Assisting the family in using existing support structures

Family Systems Model

Another model that can be easily applied in medical-surgical settings is the family systems model, as discussed in Chapter 2 relative to the family social science genre of theories. This model focuses on the interaction of various members of the system rather than simply describing functions of the members (Friedman, 1998). The family system perspective encourages medical-surgical nurses to expand their view of the patient to include family members.

Using a family systems perspective, nurses can explore the effects of the illness or injury on the entire family system; that is, they can place emphasis on wholeness rather than reduction into parts. Assessment includes:

- How does the illness event affect all the members of the family?
- How are members of the family system relating to one another?
- How is the family system relating to the health care team and hospital environment?
- What are the inputs into the family system? What else is the family dealing with? Who makes the decisions about care for family members?
- What is the educational level of family members? What information does the family need or want? What significant family members need to be involved in decision making?
- Is the family system internally processing inputs? Is the family coping?
- What are the family system outputs? Are family responses appropriate?
- How open is the family system? Is the family receptive to help or advice from the health care team?
- How does family behavior affect the patient?
- How does patient behavior affect the family?

Interventions may be designed to assist individual system functioning, family subsystem functioning, or the functioning of the whole family. Interventions may also facilitate family processing capabilities (e.g., family problem solving or family decision making) or enhance the interchanges among members or among systems, with the goal of restoring family stability. For instance, infusing energy into the family by giving information about possible treatment options may facilitate family process by helping them solve a problem that previously caused many disagreements. Other interventions to consider to strengthen family system functioning include:

- Encouraging nurse-family interactions through establishing trust and using communication skills and checking for discrepancies between nurse and family expectations
- Establishing a mechanism for providing the family with information about the patient on a regular basis
- Fostering the family's ability to get information
- Listening to the family's feelings, concerns, and questions
- Orienting the family to the hospital environment
- Answering the family's questions or assisting them to get answers
- Discussing strategies for normalizing family life with ill family members
- Providing mechanisms for the patient and family members to interact with one another (e.g., pictures, videos, audiotapes, open visiting)

- Monitoring family relationships and facilitating open communication among family members
- Collaborating with the family in problem solving
- Providing knowledge to help the family make decisions

Family Stress Theory

The family stress theories that Hanson describes in Chapter 2 fit medical-surgical situations because of the stress on the family that is due to the medical or surgical problem and to the hospitalization. A medical-surgical nurse assessing the impact of illness or injury on the family, first examines the stressor event. A number of questions should be considered: Did the family have time to prepare for the event, or was it unexpected? What family hardships and demands are associated with the event? Has the family previously experienced similar stressful events (Artinian, 1994)?

Assessment also includes a review of the physical, psychological, spiritual, and social resources available to the family. Identification of the meaning that the illness or injury has for the family is also important—for example, whether the family views the situation as a threat or a challenge, whether they blame themselves or place blame outside themselves. Assessment of the level of crisis the family is experiencing, and how much the crisis has disrupted or incapacitated the family, is essential. The nurse may need to enhance family resources or help the family to modify their subjective perceptions of the event.

Interventions to consider include:

- Helping the family to cope with imposed hardships, such as economic burdens imposed by the illness, or demands related to managing illness-related treatments
- Introducing the family to other families undergoing similar experiences
- Discussing existing social support resources (e.g., support groups) available to the family
- Assisting the family to capitalize on its strengths
- Assisting the family to resolve feelings of guilt
- Helping the family visualize successfully handling all the hardships associated with the illness or injury
- If possible, encouraging the family to focus on the positive aspects of the situation or cognitively reappraise the situation as positive

In sum, personal philosophy, hospital unit philosophy, the nature of the nurse's clinical practice, and patient and family needs will influence the nurse's use of models to guide practice in a medical-surgical setting.

VARIOUS PHASES OF ILLNESS

Before Illness: Health Promotion

Medical-surgical nurses may care for families before illness and during periods of acute illness, chronic illness, and terminal illness. Caring for families before illness has two aims. The first is to help all family members develop healthy lifestyles. Studies have shown that families play a key role in determining the health-promoting behaviors of their members (Crooks et al, 1987; Kristeller et al, 1996) and that family support is important in changing both health attitudes and behaviors (Bovbjerg et al., 1995). Nurses have a crucial role in facilitating health promotion within the family (Bomar, 1996). Before illness develops, nurses caring for patients at high risk for familial diseases such as heart disease, stroke, or cancer can suggest to the whole family ways to lower the risk of developing these diseases. Not only can this be done in the same amount of time that it takes to teach the patient alone, but the family benefits as a whole and, at the same time, can help the patient make necessary changes in lifestyle.

The consequences of genetic research add another dimension to family care before illness. The Human Genome Project is one of the most ambitious areas of research in the twentieth century. The goal of this research is to locate, map, and sequence the entire human genome, which consists of almost 100,000 genes (Dwyer, 1998). Even though completion of this project is not anticipated until the year 2005, researchers already anticipate how knowledge of human genetics will alleviate illness and disease. Family nurses in medical-surgical settings will need to grapple with ethical issues associated with human genetics and discuss ways to counsel and advise families about accessing their genetic information and how to act once they know they are at higher risk for illness (Driscoll, 1998).

A second aim during this period is to prevent a stress-filled hospitalization from negatively affecting the family's health (Artinian, 1989; Holicky, 1996; Turk & Kerns, 1985). Well family members are at risk of numerous physical, mental, emotional, social, and financial problems of their own (Bengston et al, 1996; Holicky, 1996). Hathaway and colleagues (1987) conducted a study to determine how the health-related activities and health of significant others are altered by patients' hospitalizations. The sample (n = 50) included wives, daughters, mothers, fathers, husbands, in-laws, cousins, and a nephew. The investigators found that significant others altered their health practices and experienced a worsening of health because of a family member's hospitalization. The health practices most severely affected were exercise, sleep, nutrition, and relaxation. Of the respondents, 40 percent believed they were less healthy than before the patient's hospitalization, 40 percent currently were experiencing a health problem, and 20 percent believed the problem had either started or gotten worse since the hospitalization of the patient. Blood pressure problems were reported most frequently, followed by severe headaches, severe weight problems, arthritis, stomach problems, and other miscellaneous conditions. When asked what could be done to help patients' families cope with hospitalization, significant others suggested caring attitudes by the staff, counseling, religious activities, overnight sleeping arrangements, long-term parking, waiting room amenities, a nursery, and resources for diversional activities. Asking families what would be helpful to them is an important part of nursing assessment.

Despite short hospital stays, there are several ways that nurses can systematically structure care to promote family health. During hospitalization of a family member, nurses can facilitate family health promotion by including families in admission assessments; involving families in plans of care; determining the effects of patient hospitalization on the family; developing caring, open relationships with families; and intervening to address family needs.

Acute Illness

The acute phase refers to the immediate aftermath of illness, for example, the period immediately following a heart attack (Steinglass, 1992). Families with members who are acutely or critically ill are often seen in ICUs, cardiac care units, or emergency rooms under conditions in which they are greatly stressed because a member of their family is experiencing a life-threatening illness or injury.

Rolland (1988) described five tasks that families must accomplish during the crisis phase of illness: (1) creating a meaning for the illness event that preserves a sense of mastery over their lives, (2) grieving for the loss of the family identity before illness, (3) moving toward a position of accepting permanent change while maintaining a sense of continuity between the past and the future, (4) pulling together to undergo short-term crisis reorganization, and (5) developing family flexibility about future goals.

Admission to a critical care unit signals to the family that the patient is seriously ill and that death or major disability is a possibility. Communication among family members may become distorted because the fear, anger, and guilt that members experience may be too intense for them to handle. In some families, conflicts may be blocked or submerged during the initial period of a critical illness, but as time goes on and the family resources become depleted, conflict between members may become more obvious (McClowry, 1992, p. 561).

Many nurses have investigated the needs of families in facing acute or life-threatening illness (Blackmore, 1996; Johnson et al, 1998; Leske, 1986; Lindsay et al, 1997; Lorenz, 1995; McLennan et al, 1996; Molter, 1979; Quinn et al, 1996; Wagner, 1996). The following needs were frequently found to be important:

- To have questions answered honestly
- To know the facts about what is wrong with the patient
- To be informed about the patient's progress, outcome, and chance for recovery
- To be called at home about changes in the patient's condition
- To receive understandable explanations
- To receive information once a day; to have hope; to believe hospital personnel care about the patient; to have reassurance that the patient is receiving the best possible care
- To see the patient frequently

Leske (1992) summarized these as needs for assurance, proximity, information, comfort, and support. In general, families' needs in a critical care unit or during the acute illness period are similar, regardless of their age, gender, relationship to the patient, and patient diagnosis (Leske, 1991). A nurse supports the family by showing compassion, concern, and sensitivity to all family needs (Leske, 1992; Wesson, 1997).

Leske's five family need categories can be used to direct nursing interventions, which should begin on initial contact with family members (Titler et al, 1995). Providing assurance entails establishing a calm and relaxed atmosphere that will support a trusting and empathetic relationship (Leske, 1992). Enhancement of proximity means allowing family members to be near the patient by exercising flexible family visitation policies.

The need for information about the patient has

been shown to be the number one identified need of families of critically ill patients, regardless of diagnosis or length of stay (Jastremski & Harvey, 1998). There are several ways to provide family information: educational orientation programs, classes that provide social support and information about illness management and recovery, informational packets, or unit tours. Learning the balance between too little and too much information and how to deliver it is an important skill for acute care nurses to learn (Goodell & Hanson, 1999). Additionally, the nature of the information to be conveyed to the family should be considered when deciding the best way to provide the information. Malacrida and colleagues (1998) investigated reasons for family dissatisfaction among 390 families of patients who died in an ICU. Although the majority of the respondents (82.6 percent) expressed no criticism of the patient's hospital stay, 17 percent felt the information received concerning diagnosis was insufficient or unclear, and 30 percent expressed dissatisfaction regarding the information received on the cause of death (particularly among family who were informed of the death by telephone and not in person). A face-to-face meeting may best convey information about patient progress or prognosis and perhaps information about self-management activities or visiting hours can be best addressed in a classroom setting or through the use of a booklet.

Recently investigators have tested the effectiveness of interventions to meet information needs. Researchers have found communication by the same health provider is important when meeting ICU family information needs (Johnson et al, 1998). Medland and Ferrans (1998) tested a structured communications program for family members to determine whether the program would increase family members' satisfaction with care, meet their needs for information better, and decrease disruption for the ICU nursing staff caused by incoming calls from family members. The intervention consisted of three components: 1) a discussion with a nurse approximately 24 hours after admission of the patient, 2) an informational pamphlet given at the time of the discussion, and 3) a daily telephone call from the nurse who was caring for the patient that day. The number of incoming calls from family members was significantly lower in the experimental group than in the control group. In the experimental group, satisfaction with care increased significantly from before to after the test, as did the members' perception of how well their information needs were being met.

Lynn-McHale and colleagues (1997) used a pretest-posttest quasi-experimental design to examine the usefulness of a preoperative tour of the ICU on patient and family member anxiety levels before and after cardiac surgery. The majority of patients in this study perceived a benefit or a future benefit from an ICU tour, even though the tour did not significantly reduce anxiety of the patients or family members. Leske (1996) used a four-group quasi-experimental posttest design to examine the effect of intraoperative progress reports on 200 family members' anxiety. Group one received standard perioperative care, which did not include intraoperative progress reports. Group two received in-person progress reports from perioperative nurses. Group three received an "attention" protocol (i.e., a checklist explaining hospital routines and waiting room procedures). Group four received progress reports delivered by telephone. The in-person intraoperative progress report group reported lower state anxiety scores and had significantly lower mean arterial pressures and heart rates than the other three groups.

Increasing numbers of nurses are evaluating technological methods to provide information to families. Technologies that are being explored to enhance communication with families and thus meet their information needs include the Internet, pagers, e-mail, and telephone help lines (Brennan et al, 1995; Carlsson et al, 1996; Olson, 1997; Topp et al, 1998).

Comfort measures may include waiting rooms conducive to rest and relaxation, the availability of private rooms for conferences between the health team and family, placement of telephone and bathroom facilities near the waiting room, and helping families to take care of their needs, such as adequate rest, nutrition, and personal hygiene. Making the waiting room more humane involves addressing environmental factors, such as noise, lighting, temperature, views, privacy, and distraction therapy (Jastremski & Harvey, 1998). The Guidelines/Practice Parameters Committee of the American College of Critical Care Medicine, Society of Critical Care Medicine, (1995) recommends that a visitors' lounge be provided near each ICU and that there should be on average one to two seats per critical care bed. Public telephones with privacy enclosures, television and music, public toilet facilities, and a drinking fountain are also recommended. Warm colors, carpeting, indirect soft lighting, windows, and a variety of seating (including upright, lounge, and reclining chairs) are desirable. The Guidelines/Practice Parameters Committee also suggests that educational materials and lists of hospital and community-based resources be displayed.

Cultural affiliation may moderate the expression of family needs. Waters (1999) compared African-American, Hispanic, and white family members' perceptions of the professional support they expect from critical care nurses during a family member's critical illness. In a sample of 90 family members, 30 from each cultural group, she found significant differences between the groups and suggested critical care nurses develop interventions that respect the cultural uniqueness of family members. Interestingly, most of the white family members were wives of critically ill husbands with cardiac-related problems. African-American family members represented a variety of relatives and responsibility for managing the physiological crisis was a collaborative effort, suggesting critical care nurses be flexible and willing to communicate and interact with a variety of family members. In comparison to white family members, both African-American and Hispanic family members had significantly higher expectations for the critical care nurse to visit the waiting room at least once a shift to check out their concerns. In contrast to white and Hispanic family members, African-American family members had significantly lower expectations for critical care nurses to reassure them that their family member is stable enough that they could leave the waiting room or hospital for a while. Consistent with other findings in the literature, there was similarity across cultural groups. All wanted to be called at home about major changes, to have their questions answered honestly, or to be assured that their family member is receiving the best care. In sum, equitable care, dignity, and respect are universal values, but delivery of culturally effective family-centered care requires an appreciation and understanding of cultural diversity.

Nurse-family relationships in critical care are extremely important, especially if a nurse-patient relationship is compromised by the patient's physiological state. Hupcey (1998) explored strategies used by nurses and families to either develop or inhibit the development of the nurse-family relationship. Strategies used by nurses to develop relationships included: demonstrating commitment to the patient and the patient's family; persevering (spending time with the family, getting to know them); and being involved (being an advocate for the family). Strategies used by families to develop relationships included: (1) determining whether the nurse is a good nurse—families felt better when they believed the nurse was kind and competent; (2) making overtures—trying to please the nursing staff and be good visitors; and (3) displaying trust (opening up with the nurse, asking for advice, accepting the nurse's explanations). Depersonalizing the patient and family, maintaining an efficient attitude, and displaying a lack of trust in the family were actions by nurses that inhibited nurse-family relationships. Preventing the nurse from knowing about the patient and family, becoming overinvolved or underinvolved in caring for the patient, and displaying lack of trust in the nurse were family behaviors that inhibited the development of therapeutic relationships with critical care nurses. Nurse-family relationships benefit the patient; identifying behaviors that affect nurse-family interactions will assist nurses in reevaluating their practice and enhance understanding of the behaviors of family members.

Goodell and Hanson (1999) used Bowen's family system theory to further highlight the intricacies of nurse-family relationships. Highly differentiated nurses, that is, nurses who can remain emotionally separate from, yet connected to family members, can be less reactive and able to cope more effectively with the stress of working in critical care environments. Nurses who sense strong emotional reactions in themselves to certain family members may be drawn into the family system in a reactive and less than therapeutic manner. Goodell and Hanson (1999) suggest that nurses who find themselves frequently drawn into families' emotional systems need to examine their own levels of differentiation and methods of coping with anxiety in relationships. In doing so, nurse-family relationships may be more satisfying to both family members and critical care nurses.

Family Concerns During Hospitalization

Three specific concerns for families during hospitalization for acute illness are family visitation policies, DNR decisions, and policies surrounding cardiopulmonary resuscitation. Each of these concerns is discussed below.

Visitation Policies

During the period of acute illness, families usually encounter restrictive hospital visiting policies. They may not be able to visit their loved one in the hospital when it is convenient for them or when their work schedule permits, and frequently, they must rearrange their plans and routines to fit the policies set by the hospital. Investigators have found that visiting policies in ICUs restricted the number and length of visits and the number and ages of visitors, as well as limiting visitors to members of the immediate family (Younger et al, 1984).

Originally, hospital visiting periods were limited so that the patient could rest and recover. Recent studies challenge the premise that visiting in the ICU should be restricted because of adverse effects on patients. Research findings suggest that family-patient interactions do not alter hemodynamic stability any differently than nurse-patient interactions (Fuller & Foster, 1982). Moreover, one recent study found that "restricting visits to short time periods and terminating visits prematurely contribute to adverse hemodynamic responses in critically ill patients" (Titler & Walsh, 1992, p. 625). Lazure and Baun (1995) investigated whether patient control of family visiting would minimize psychophysiologic effects of coronary care unit visiting. Results showed that, over time, perceived control of visits and rests between visits were greater and heart rate and diastolic blood pressure were lower for subjects who used a visitor control device. Thus, a combination of patient and family factors influences the nature of family visits in ICU.

Research has uncovered several factors that should be considered when planning visiting periods with families (Clark, 1995; Gurley, 1995). Simpson (1991) found that age, patients' personality characteristics, and patients' perceptions of the illness influenced patients' visiting preferences. For instance, older patients preferred longer visits, and extroverted patients preferred more frequent visits. Surprisingly, the more severely ill patients perceived themselves to be, the more visitors they preferred.

The diversity of patient responses to visiting policies suggests that policies should be tailored to patient and family preferences. Hamner (1990) suggested that visiting preferences should be included in patient-family assessments. One way to do this is to ascertain the answers to questions such as: How would you like visiting times to be handled while you are here? Who would you like to be allowed/disallowed to visit? When do you want to see visitors? How often? For how long? The answers to these questions help to tailor visiting policies to meet patient-family needs. Recent evidence suggests that critical care nurses are tailoring visiting to the needs of the patient and family. Simon and colleagues (1997) found that nurses did not restrict visitation, regardless of whether restrictive policies were in place. They found most nurses based their visitation decisions on the needs of the patient and the nurse.

Decisions About Life-Saving or Life-Extending Measures

Families may have to face decisions regarding the use of life-saving or life-extending measures during the acute illness period. Frequently, illness occurs without preparation, and sometimes families must deal with illnesses or injuries in which there is no hope for recovery. In the acute illness period, patients and families are in a crisis situation with little time to discuss the options regarding life-saving measures. Often there is little, if any, discussion about resuscitation preferences while the patient is competent to make a decision, so that health care professionals and families must make end-of-life decisions without the guidance of the patient. Bedell and associates (1986) found that 86 percent of decisions regarding resuscitation measures involved the family, while only 22 percent of the patients were included in the decision making.

Several issues should be kept in mind with regard to DNR orders. First, physicians may discuss many variations of DNR orders with families. Sometimes it is appropriate, for example, to withhold chest compressions and intubation but still administer antiarrhythmic and vasopressor drugs. At other times no life-saving measures may be administered. Nurses can help families by clarifying the various options presented to them and offering opportunities for discussion. Needless to say, decisions about DNR status are difficult to make.

The appropriate timing of discussion of DNR orders is also difficult to determine. It is hard for the physician to know when it is best to discuss the DNR status of the patient with the family. Because nurses develop special insights as a result of the time they spend at the bedside getting to know the patient and family, they can help physicians schedule these important discussions.

Bedell and colleagues (1986) found that four factors assisted families to make decisions about DNR status. First, an explanation of brain death criteria by the physician eased the family's ability to make a decision, as did the second factor, physician and nurse support for the family. Third, families wanted assurance that comfort measures would continue. Fourth, families found any previous discussion they had had with the patient about life decisions was helpful in the decision-making process.

Jacob (1998) found that family members of patients in the ICU are willing and able to take responsibility for decisions about the use of life-sustaining treatment for their loved ones. The long-term acceptance of the experience and the decisions made depend greatly on the interactions between the family members, who makes the decisions, and nurses and physicians in the clinical setting.

Nurses can help families prepare for the possibility of a DNR decision through community education about living wills and durable power of attorney for health care. Such education will enable family members to discuss end-of-life decisions before a crisis event occurs and in less stressful circumstances. Ideally the patient makes decisions about end-of-life care with the family prior to admission to the hospital.

In December 1991, the Patient Self-Determination Act (PSDA) went into effect. The PSDA requires that all health care facilities receiving Medicare or Medicaid funds provide written information to adult patients about their rights to make treatment decisions and execute advance directives (Marsden, 1992). Advance directives may be in the form of a living will or in the form of durable power of attorney. A living will is a written statement that tells a person's family, friends, and doctor(s) what medical treatment he or she would want in the future should he or she become unable to express his or her wishes. An advance directive is a written statement that allows individuals to select in advance someone to speak for them when they can no longer state their wishes. An advance directive applies only to those who are unable to make their own decisions because they are incapacitated, or who, in the opinion of two physicians, are otherwise unable to make decisions for themselves (American Nurses Association, 1992; White, 1997). Different states have different laws about advance directives. Patients and families need to be informed about advance directives, to know that the directive is intended to help others make decisions for the patient, and to know that it can be as simple or as complex as they feel necessary. Nurses can help patients and families prepare advance directives by showing sample forms and providing the support and reassurance the family needs as these important decisions are being made.

A critical care nurse is most likely to be called on to counsel families in the context of some emergency. Families in medical crises are facing hard and painful choices and look to the nurse for advice and counseling (White, 1997). White cautions that there are three risks to giving affirmative advice about advance directives to patients' families: (1) a nurse should not say anything that will undermine a physician's treatment orders—the physician retains legal authority for orders that are given; 2) if a nurse enters overtly into the discussion of what the intent of the patient's advance directive is, she or he risks being perceived by family members who disagree as not being unreservedly committed to the patient's best interests; and 3) an advance directive is a legal document—it is seldom a good idea for a layperson to advise others about how to interpret the language, import, or effect of a legal document.

Should Families Witness CPR Efforts?

During the acute illness period, the patient may suffer a sudden arrest of heartbeat and respiration, requiring cardiopulmonary resuscitation (CPR). When a patient has an arrest, the CPR team is called to the bedside. Physicians, nurses, and other health team members crowd around the patient to administer chest compressions, manually ventilate the patient, perform defibrillation, give drugs, or carry out other life-restoring activities. Until the patient's heart rhythm and respiration are restored, this is a tension-filled situation.

There is no general answer to the question of whether families should witness resuscitation efforts (Rosenczweig, 1998; van der Woning, 1997). Investigators are examining attitudes of hospital staff towards permitting relatives to be present during a resuscitation (Chalk, 1995).

Martin (1991) suggests that there are advantages to having families present to watch nurses and physicians carry out resuscitative efforts. The advantages for families include recognizing that the patient is dying, knowing that everything possible is being done, being able to touch the patient while he or she is still warm and to say whatever they need to say while there is still a chance the patient can hear, recognizing the futility of further resuscitation efforts, and accepting the reality of death. Family presence may eliminate the terrible fear of being left alone (Eichhorn et al, 1995).

On the other hand, there may be disadvantages to having families observe CPR (Osuagwu, 1991; Redheffer, 1989). The experience is traumatic and frightening to watch; families may interfere with protocols and procedures; there is not enough space at the patient's bedside for the CPR team as well as the family; and staff is not available to provide family information and support during the resuscitation.

If hospital and unit policies permit families to witness resuscitation efforts, decisions about family visitation should be made on a case-by-case basis. Martin (1991) provides guidelines for nurses deciding when families are to be permitted in the patient's room during CPR. Martin's guidelines include the following directions:

- Discuss the option with the family and give them a description of what will be going on in the room.
- Check the code status with the doctor and the nurse in charge.
- Assess the room from the point of view of the family.
- Accompany the family member into the room to ensure that the family member gets an accurate explanation and has an appropriate perception of what is being done.
- Do not permit family members to enter the code area while intravenous lines are being placed or while the patient is being intubated.
- Let family members in once the code is under way.
- If a family member cannot handle the visit, escort him or her from the room.

Hopefully nurses will be sensitive to family needs during this stress-filled time and will consider the benefits and risks of witnessing CPR. Some families will not be able to cope with the experience, whereas others will not want to be involved. It is important to assess the family to determine whether their presence might be appropriate (Eichhorn et al, 1995).

Chronic Illness

Chronic illness imposes another set of concerns for families. Chronic illness is "the irreversible presence, accumulation, or latency of disease states or impairments that involve the total human environment for supportive care and self-care, maintenance of function, and prevention of further disability" (Lubkin, 1986, p. 6). Many factors influence the effect of chronic illness on families: the type of illness, the stage of illness, the structure of the family, the role of the patient, the life-cycle stage of the patient, and the life-cycle stage of the family (Biegel et al, 1991; Young, 1995).

The entire family system is affected when chronic illness strikes. "Normal patterns of interaction are disrupted, and there are often reassignments in tasks and roles assumed by particular family members" (Biegel et al., 1991, p. 20). The family must reorganize itself around the chronic illness or disability (Steinglass, 1992). Families may make changes related to work schedules, household tasks, or provision of family income or in interpersonal areas, such as solidarity and belonging, sexuality, and love (Leventhal et al, 1985).

Families and patients face both social and psychological challenges during the course of chronic illness (Biegel et al, 1991, pp. 20–21; Hanson, 1988). These include:

- Preventing medical crises and managing them once they occur
- Controlling symptoms
- Carrying out prescribed regimens
- Preventing or living with the sense of isolation caused by lessened contact with others
- Adjusting to changes in the course of the disease
- Normalizing interactions with others and finding the necessary money to pay for treatments or to survive, despite partial or complete loss of employment
- Confronting attendant psychosocial, marital, and familial problems

Families in the chronic phase may have to deal with a member's illness for a long time—an illness that may be constant, progressive, or episodic in nature. A key family task is to maintain normal life in the "abnormal" presence of this chronic illness and the resulting heightened uncertainty (Rolland, 1988).

As they manage their family member's illness on a day-to-day basis, families become expert caregivers. Exacerbation of a chronic illness, when it leads to hospitalization, brings expert family caregivers in contact with the health care team. Thorne and Robinson (1988), who analyzed relationships between the family and the health care team from the perspective of the family members, found that these relationships moved through three stages. These stages reflected shifts in family trust of health care professionals.

Family members who had not had much experience with chronic illness described the first stage, naive trusting. These family members trust that health care professionals have the same perspective about caring for their ill member that they did. Families believed that their involvement on a day-to-day basis as the primary health care providers would be acknowledged and respected and that professionals would be cooperative and collaborative. Family members naively trusted that health care professionals would act in their ill member's best interests. Over time, however, family members learned that their long experience was often disregarded, as was their involvement and expertise in illness management.

The second stage, the disenchantment phase, was characterized by dissatisfaction with care, frustration, and fear. Families found that it was difficult to be effectively involved in care because they had difficulty obtaining information. As trust diminished, family relationships with health care professionals became adversarial, and families saw their ill member as vulnerable and needing protection.

During the last stage, the guarded alliance phase, families renegotiated trust with health care professionals. They actively sought information and understood the differences in their perspective and that of health care professionals. Families were able to state clearly their own expectations and perceptions, an ability which led to more satisfying care. Families and health care professionals developed a partnership in care. Nevertheless, families still experienced the frustration of waiting, fear that they would not know the right questions to ask, and anger at the recognition that their own expertise was devalued.

Leahey and Wright (1987) have described interventions for families experiencing chronic illness that focus on the family's cognitive, affective, and behavioral levels of functioning. Cognitive interventions include giving information about the chronic illness and its treatment, giving advice about potential family responses to the illness (e.g., need for respite, possible strain on family relationships), giving information about community resources, and helping with family decision making. Others highlight the importance of families receiving education and support to help them cope with chronic illness (Boise et al, 1996). Douglas and Spellacy (1996) found that social support for the family was a significant predictor of positive family functioning among family members of patients with traumatic brain injury.

Cultural factors have significant impact on the clinical encounter between the health care professional and the family. A good continuing relationship is essential for successful management of chronic disease. Misunderstandings predicated on implicit cultural assumptions are a potential hazard (Gropper, 1998).

Affective interventions are designed to modify intense emotions, such as guilt or anger, which may block a family's problem-solving efforts (Leahey & Wright, 1987). They include validating family members' emotional responses and helping them understand that those responses are normal; discussing with families ways to reduce their isolation; referring families to an appropriate support group; helping families open channels of communication; and helping families identify and mobilize their strengths and resources. Johnson and Roberts (1996) report that the family's adaptation to a head injury has a significant impact on the patient's rehabilitation. A family's response of denial or lack of hope in the future has been identified as a major obstacle to successful patient adaptation; thus, hope-facilitating strategies need to be devised. The hopeless family may be unable to make the necessary changes at home or learn the important aspects of the patient's care.

Interventions targeted at behavioral functioning are designed to help family members interact more effectively (Leahey & Wright, 1987). This goal can be accomplished by assigning specific behavioral tasks to some or all family members (Leahey & Wright). For example, families may need help to coordinate responsibilities for particular caregiving activities (Gilliss et al, 1989). They may also need caregiving training to feel comfortable with the tasks at hand.

Other nursing interventions may be directed toward helping health care personnel work with families who are coping with chronic illness. Findings from Thorne and Robinson (1988) suggest strategies to improve relationships between the family and the health care team. Nurses need first to recognize the stage of their relationship (naive trust, disenchantment, or guarded alliance) with these families. Activities to promote cooperative caring must be negotiated between the nurse and the family, and being sensitive to what caregivers have experienced before hospitalization and recognizing their experience is essential to this process. Helping families access the information they need is also important; in fact it is a prerequisite to developing a shared understanding that will help in the development of goals on which there is mutual agreement.

Caring for families with chronic illness presents many challenges for medical-surgical nurses. The problems and concerns that families experience differ from those in the acute illness stage. Nurses need to keep these differences in mind as they plan care.

Terminal Illness

Sometimes nurses in medical-surgical settings encounter families who are coping with the terminal phase of an illness. Knowledge about the process of dying can help nurses work effectively with families during this very difficult time. The more the nurse knows about the family, the better, since how families deal with death is affected by the family's cultural background, stage in the life cycle, values and beliefs, the nature of the illness, whether the loss is sudden or expected, the role played by the dying person in the family, and the emotional functioning of the family before the illness (Rosen, 1990; Leonard et al, 1995).

Phases of Adaptation

Families move through phases of adaptation in response to the news that a family member has a fatal illness (Rosen, 1990), and various emotional responses may emerge during these phases, including disorganization, anxiety, emotional lability, or turning inward. The first phase is the preparatory phase. This phase begins when symptoms first appear and it continues through the initial diagnosis. During the preparatory phase, families experience fear and denial and may refuse to accept the prospect of death. Some family members decide to withhold all information from those who they consider vulnerable, such as children or elderly parents (Rosen, 1990). During the period of initial symptoms, diagnosis, and treatment plan, the family may be highly disorganized and display emotional lability.

Once the family accepts the prospect of loss and begins to live with the reality of the fatal illness and the caretaking tasks of the illness, they move into the middle phase. Families live the day-to-day challenge of dealing with physical symptoms, treatment, and care (Rosen, 1990). The family becomes less disorganized; indeed, it reorganizes to assume new roles. On the other hand, the tedium of daily care may tax the physical and financial resources of the family. Further, if hospitalizations are lengthy or frequent, the logistics of visitation may create discord among family members (Rosen, 1990); some members of the family may feel others are visiting too little or too much—and unresolved family issues from the past may emerge.

The final stage, acceptance, comes when the family accepts the imminent death and concludes the process of saying farewell. Family emotions that surfaced during the first phase but subsided during the middle phase may resurface. Family members may draw together in anticipation of their loved one's death (Rosen, 1990).

Nurses can help families with a dying relative by informing them that it is natural to pass through phases of adaptation and that they can expect to address complex issues in each phase of a fatal illness. Helping families accept their feelings and directing them to appropriate resources, such as hospice, family support groups, social workers, and family conferences, may be useful.

Caring for families when a member is dying is not easy. It is challenging for nurses to facilitate families to cope (Leonard et al, 1995). Rarely do nurses feel comfortable and confident discussing death with patients or families. Two issues are especially difficult for nurses: conveying news of sudden death and offering families the option of organ donation.

Conveying News of Sudden Death

Family grief reactions may be manifested as guilt, self-reproach, anxiety, loneliness, fatigue, shock, numbness, sleep and appetite disturbances, crying, overactivity, or confusion (Swanson, 1993). Informing the family of the death of a loved one is a challenging task. A health care professional's initial contact with the family about a death or about dying has a significant impact on the family's grief reaction. "Bad news, conveyed in an inappropriate, incomplete, or uncaring manner may have long-lasting psychological effects on the family" (Swanson, p. 352).

Respecting the family's cultural background and use of rituals, customs, or styles to deal with death is important. Also important are allowing enough time for questions, allowing the family the opportunity to view the body, describing the events at the time of death, and conveying sensitivity and caring (Leash, 1996; Swanson, 1993). Features of successful interventions have been efforts to provide services tailored to promoting family contact with the dying patient, consultation to facilitate care planning, and communication with families (Danis, 1998). Buchanan and colleagues (1996) demonstrated the importance of specialized follow-up care for surviving family members and loved ones during the year after death. Sudden, traumatic death leaves the survivors in shocked disbelief and intense emotional pain. Appropriate support and intervention can make a significant contribution to the family's eventual recovery by assisting in the normal grieving process and thus avoiding prolonged pathologic grieving (Buchanan et al, 1996).

Offering the Option of Organ Donation

Discussing organ donation with a family whose loved one has suddenly died is difficult. "Often the deceased is a young, previously healthy person who died suddenly in a tragic accident" (Hoffman & Malecki, 1990, p. 24).

Once approached, consent to donation by potential donor families is disappointingly low (Siminoff, 1997). In a study of 124 nurses, Malecki and Hoffman (1987) found that those who felt uncomfortable about requesting donation got more negative responses from potential donor families than nurses who were sad but comfortable and confident.

If organ donation is viewed as a consoling act, rather than an imposition on a grieving family, offering the option of organ donation becomes easier. Organ donation benefits the family of the donor as well as the organ recipient. Hoffman and Malecki (1990) have noted that donation of organs can help families cope with their loss. Perceiving that organ donation can help someone else live, that functioning organs are not wasted, that something positive can come out of death, or that a family member can live on in someone else through donation can help families cope with their loss.

Common courtesy and sensitivity to the family's grief are important (Siminoff, 1997). The following have been found to facilitate offering of the option of organ donation:

- Using a private area
- Clearly communicating about the loved one's death
- Allowing family time to absorb the news regarding their loved one's death before asking about donation
- Assuring the family that the decision is theirs to make
- Informing the family of the possible benefits of donation
- Providing information that will assuage the family's fears regarding donation (Siminoff, 1997)

Many families worry that donation is disfiguring or delays the funeral—neither is true (Siminoff, 1997). Finally, families may be confused about the costs of donation and need to be informed that the organ procurement agencies pay for all costs pertaining to the maintenance or removal of the donor organs once the family has agreed to donation (Siminoff, 1997).

INTERVENTIONS IN A MEDICAL-SURGICAL SETTING

Medical-surgical nurses must intervene with families during all phases of an illness. "Nursing interventions for families are nursing treatments that assist families and their members to promote, attain, or maintain optimal health and functioning or to experience a peaceful death" (Craft & Willadsen, 1992, p. 520). Craft and Willadsen have identified nine categories of family nursing interventions: family support, family process maintenance, promotion of family integrity, family involvement, family mobilization, caregiver support, family therapy, sibling support, and parent education. Leske (1996) highlights that individuals over the age of 65 occupy a substantial number of beds in medical-surgical settings; interventions to meet the needs of aged family members require age-specific considerations.

Support

Families in medical-surgical settings are experiencing life changes and stressors and are frequently in need of support. Nurses can support the family in several ways.

- Use effective, open, and honest communication, that is, listening to family concerns, feelings, and questions, and answering all questions or assisting the family to get answers.
- Help the family acquire information.
- Respect and support family coping mechanisms.
- Foster realistic hope.
- Assist families to make decisions through providing information about options.
- Provide opportunities to visit.
- Arrange family conferences to allow ventilation of family feelings.
- Permit the family to make some decisions about patient care.
- Clarify information.

Henneman and colleagues (1992) note that flexible visiting hours and information booklets are two practical and specific methods to support families. Leske and Heidrich (1996) point out that family support groups provide the opportunity for participants to share common experiences, build mutual support, express common concerns, foster a sense of hope, reduce anxiety, and obtain information common to the group's needs. Leske and Heidrich note however that some aged family members may feel that sharing feelings, personal issues, and private family matters is unacceptable; thus a support group may not be a beneficial intervention for an aged family member. Support groups may be more acceptable if the content focuses on information and tasks rather than sharing feelings and concerns (Leske & Heidrich, 1996, p. 99).

Process Maintenance

The illness and hospitalization of a family member upsets family routines and activities. Identifying how the acute illness episode has altered family roles and consequently disrupted typical family processes is a necessary part of maintaining family process. Offering flexible opportunities for visiting will help to meet the needs of family members and patients and can also promote maintenance of typical family processes. Family members may want to discuss with the nurse other strategies for normalizing family life.

Promotion of Integrity

Stressful hospitalizations may adversely affect the emotional bonding that family members have with one another. Nurses can promote family cohesion and unity through allowing for family visitation and facilitating open communication among family members. Scheduling a family conference to encourage all family members to voice their concerns about care management with one another and with the health care team is a way to facilitate open communication. Telling family members that it is safe and acceptable to use typical expressions of affection may also be appreciated. For example, a wife may appreciate knowing she won't disrupt the technological equipment at her husband's bedside or disrupt equipment attached to his body if she kisses his cheek or holds his hand. Providing opportunities for private family visits can make the visits more satisfying.

Involvement

Giving physical care to their loved one during hospitalization may comfort family members, especially if the family member has routinely provided physical care for the patient at home. Before encouraging family members to become involved in patient care, however, it is important to identify their preferences, the patient's preferences, and family members' capabilities. Family members can be involved with care in a number of ways, such as helping during meal times, assisting with brushing teeth or other comfort measures, and assisting with patient positioning or range of motion.

Mobilization

Family caregivers may be experts in caring for the patient because of their many years of experience with a chronic illness. Nurses can acknowledge this family expertise and use the family's strengths through family mobilization techniques. For example, discussing how family strengths and resources can be used to enhance the health of the patient and establishing realistic goals with the patient and family are two ways to mobilize families. Collaborating with family members in planning and implementing patient therapies and lifestyle changes is another. Families may want to share information about the patient's favorite position when lying in bed, preferences in music, bedtime habits, or preferred comfort measures. Determining family cultural practices and incorporating these into plans for care is yet another way to mobilize the strengths of the family.

PREPARING FOR PATIENT DISCHARGE

Although hospitalization is stressful for families, leaving the hospital is also stressful. As a result of the prospective payment system and other efforts to control health care costs, patients nowadays are discharged quickly from the hospital (Brooten et al, 1988; Feigin et al, 1998). As a result, patients and families must manage most of the patient's recovery at home. Early discharge requires careful attention to discharge planning to help patients and families anticipate problems after discharge.

Numerous investigators have described the preparation of patients for discharge (Duryee, 1992; Garding et al, 1988; Steele & Ruzicki, 1987). Feigin and colleagues (1998) described the use of one-session group meetings to help families reduce anxieties over discharge and increase their capabilities to organize and cope with discharge. Phelan and colleagues (1996) described an education-intensive unit incorporating a living-in family member or friend acting as a care partner who assumes responsibility for administering all medications as a way of reducing medication error rates after discharge. Other clinicians (Franco et al, 1996) described using active family participation in hospital care delivery as a way to prepare family for the transition to home.

In a study involving patients who experienced a coronary artery bypass graft (CABG), Artinian (1993) found that spouses identified four factors as helpful in readying them for their partner's hospital discharge: (1) availability of social support, (2) use of coping strategies, (3) personal resources, and (4) knowledge of what to expect. Consideration of these four factors suggests ways to prepare other types of families for discharge. For instance, available social support can include persons who are available to give necessary information about recovery at home before discharge. Such information should include the trajectory of an uncomplicated recovery, how to distinguish between normal and unusual symptoms during recovery, signs and symptoms of complications, and activities family members can do to make the patient comfortable. Giving a phone number of someone the family can call if they have concerns is also helpful. Supplying bandages, canes, medicines, or other materials to families before they go home may be of assistance, because families do not want to have to run to the store and leave the patient alone. Post-discharge contact also may support family management of recovery at home. Various strategies for doing this have been described, including follow-up contact by telephone (Beckie, 1989; Garding et al, 1988; Gortner et al, 1988; Nicklin, 1986).

Families need coping skills to manage recovery at home. These skills include problem-solving ability, ability to seek help if needed, ability to manage worry and anxiety, and ability to acquire needed information. Nurses need to assess family coping strategies to devise interventions that will fit the individual family's needs.

Four categories of personal resources can help family members feel ready to take a patient home from the hospital. These categories, health and energy, time, self-confidence, and positive beliefs (Artinian, 1993), need to be assessed by the nurse. For example, if the family member taking the patient home has numerous chronic health problems leaving them with feelings of fatigue, discharge activities and recovery at home may seem overwhelming to them. Assessing family members' perceptions of their own health may indicate whether the family needs additional help to manage care at home. Families who lack time to prepare for discharge because of multiple responsibilities may need encouragement to arrange for help or to plan ahead. Assessing family confidence about recovery and managing caregiving activities at home may be beneficial. Or, if a family member does not have positive beliefs about the patient's recovery and does not believe the patient is physically ready to go home, they also will not feel ready. Because optimistic beliefs can help families feel ready for discharge, it is useful to point out to families the positive signs of recovery.

The goal of preparing families for discharge is to help them know what to expect and how to assist in the patient's recovery. Inadequate preparation for discharge can contribute to hospital readmission (Buls, 1995; Martens & Mellor, 1997; Dennis et al, 1996). Making the necessary arrangement for home care visits may complement discharge preparation. Buls (1995) compared 30 clients after CABG surgery and their spouses, who had received home visits from the nurse, with 30 clients after CABG surgery who did not receive home visits. Families who received the home visits had significantly lower anxiety levels; the authors concluded home visits were a useful method to consider to prevent costly rehospitalizations.

IMPLICATIONS FOR EDUCATION, RESEARCH, AND HEALTH CARE POLICY

The body of knowledge about medical-surgical family nursing is growing, and there are many opportunities for nurses to apply this knowledge to practice. It is no longer appropriate to study medical-surgical nursing only from the perspective of individual patient care. Faculty need to clearly define family health care practice in medical-surgical settings (Hanson & Heims, 1992) and incorporate family care into medical-surgical nursing courses and appropriate practice settings. Family assessment frameworks that lead to specific strategies for intervention also need attention in medical-surgical nursing curriculums (Hanson et al, 1992). Relegating the bulk of family content to specialty courses, such as community health nursing or childbearing family nursing, misleads students about the practice of family nursing. Nursing staff on medical-surgical units also need to be educated about family nursing, especially because many staff members were educated at a period when family nursing was not considered important in medical-surgical settings.

Identification of family practice problems (e.g., difficulties associated with delivering care to families) and investigating the validity, relevance, cost, and benefits of potential solutions to those problems will help to promote research-based practice (Lindquist et al, 1990). Designing, implementing, and testing family nursing interventions will foster the growth of medical-surgical family nursing knowledge. However, research findings about families only become valuable to families after they pass through the research utilization process. The goal of research utilization is to improve nursing care, which results in optimal family outcomes. Through research utilization, knowledge about families that is obtained from research is transferred into clinical practice. Nurses who seek to improve family care through research utilization engage in critically analyzing research literature about families, select from the literature interventions that are appropriate for their practice setting, implement the interventions, and then evaluate the family outcomes.

Health care policies clearly influence nursing practice. Family nursing practice in medical-surgical settings can be enhanced through hospital and unit-based philosophy statements that include the family. Policies about family visitation, family participation in care, family presence during CPR, families staying overnight in patient rooms, and families bringing in favorite foods should be evaluated in light of a family care philosophy.

SUMMARY

There is a growing demand for family-focused care within medical-surgical settings. Hospital environments are foreign to family members, a situation that adds to the stress of illness and injury for patients and families. When planning interventions, nurses caring for families need to consider the nature of the illness, family characteristics, the health care team's philosophy about family care, and the characteristics of the patient. Family theoretical models, including the structural-functional model, family systems model, and family stress model, can provide a basis for family assessment and intervention.

RESEARCH BRIEF

Purpose

The purpose of this research is to compare perceptions of ideal levels of support from critical care nurses to levels of perceived receipt of support among African-American family members of critically ill adults.

Methods

The Professional Support Questionnaire for Critical Care Nurses Working with Family Members (PSQ) was administered by mail or telephone to a convenience sample of 36 African-American family members. The PSQ consists of three domains of support, that is, information, comfort, and assurance. Paired *t*-test analyses were used to determine if there were significant differences (differences that did not occur by chance) between levels of perceived ideal and perceived received support from critical care nurses caring for their family member.

Results

Although there was not an absence of professional nursing support, the degree and frequency to which African-American family members wanted nurses to support them were not comparable to the support that nurses provided them.

Implications

This study highlights the importance of assessing family expectations, wants, and needs before providing interventions. This study is an important one because it used a sample of African-American family members: individuals who are not often included in studies about family members in acute care settings. Most studies have targeted easy-to-reach populations, rather than describing family phenomena or testing the effectiveness of family interventions in diverse ethnic and minority groups.

Source: Waters, C. M. (1998). Actual and ideal professional support for African American family members. *Western Journal of Nursing Research, 20*(6):745–764.

Medical-surgical nurses may care for families before illness and during periods of acute illness, chronic illness, or terminal illness. Before illness, nurses should direct interventions at health promotion. During the acute illness phase, nursing interventions should focus on providing assurance, enhancing the proximity of patient and family, managing information, facilitating comfort, and reinforcing support. Families in the chronic phase have been dealing with illness for a long time; thus acknowledging their experiences with illness management is important. Common family concerns in chronic illness, such as guilt, fear, uncertainty, anger, and lack of knowledge about the illness, care requirements, or resources, may require interventions. During the terminal phase, interventions are directed toward helping families move through the phases of adaptation in response to the fatal illness of a family member. In any illness stage, family support, family process maintenance, promotion of family integrity, family involvement, or family mobilization may be helpful.

Efforts to control health care costs have resulted in a pattern of early patient discharge from the hospital. Research suggests that the availability of social support, use of coping strategies, availability of personal resources, and knowing what to expect once at home positively influence a family's perception of readiness for discharge. Nurses should assess these family characteristics to determine family needs at discharge.

Nurses in medical-surgical settings should use the growing body of knowledge about medical-surgical family nursing in practice. They also must advocate for changes in hospital policies and procedure to reflect such knowledge, and update this knowledge through future research. Only when medical-surgical nurses include families in plans for care can they hope to provide unfragmented, holistic, humane, and sensitively delivered health care.

Case Study

THE DEPPS

Alex Depp, a 26-year-old single teacher, received a diagnosis of AIDS a year ago. He has been HIV-positive for 4 years. His only known risk factor for AIDS is promiscuous homosexual activity when he was younger. Alex's immediate family consists of his mother Viola and his sister Jane. Both Viola and Jane were deeply saddened when they learned Alex had AIDS. They believed he would die before he could accomplish what he wanted to do with his life. Soon after Alex's diagnosis, Jane noticed frequent mood swings in her mother and they began to have constant arguments over small things.

Alex regularly experiences night sweats, fatigue, and weakness, and he has ongoing weight loss, diarrhea, and malaise. Yesterday he was admitted to the hospital for a diagnostic bronchoscopy to determine the cause of his persistent nonproductive cough, dyspnea, tachypnea, fever, chills, and chest pain. He had had one episode of *Pneumocystis carinii* pneumonia (PCP) in the past and was at that time diagnosed with AIDS. For the last year, Alex has feared that the next opportunistic infection would bring about his death.

Before his diagnosis, Alex was a healthy, active man. He became debilitated and has been unable to work because of extreme fatigue. He is dependent on his mother and sister for help with activities of daily living. Viola left her job as a cashier in a grocery store, in part to care for Alex and in part because she found it difficult to deal with her coworkers' concerns that she was handling food. Jane is a student. She is angered by the fact that her friends distanced themselves from her after she told them about her brother's illness. Her anger is compounded by guilt and fear: guilt because she once rejected her homosexual brother and fear because she is concerned that she may get AIDS from spending so much time caring for Alex.

Alex underwent bronchoscopy without complications. The bronchial biopsy confirmed PCP. To treat the causative organism, Alex was placed on intravenous pentamidine isoethionate (Pentam), an antiprotozoal drug used to fight PCP infections. After a brief stay in the ICU, Alex was transferred to one of the hospital's medical units. Because his arterial oxygen levels continued to be low, he was given oxygen supplementation. Other care included liquid nutritional supplements, positioning in semi–Fowler's to high Fowler's position, frequent nose and mouth care to prevent candidiasis, and his activities were clustered, so that there would be periods of time to designate as rest periods.

Throughout his hospital stay, Alex's mother and sister felt that no one listened to them. They wanted to talk to the doctor and nurse every day about Alex's condition, but this never seemed possible. At times, the family felt the staff was afraid of Alex because they rarely came into the room and they stood at the door of the room to talk to them. Sometimes they waited 20 minutes for Alex's light to be answered. Alex's mother was bothered by the fact that bedclothes and linens were moist from Alex's fever and sweats. She wondered why the staff didn't change his gown and sheets more often.

Alex was discharged from the hospital 3 weeks after his admission. Six months later he contracted PCP again. He was readmitted to the hospital, where he died 3 days later of respiratory failure. Viola, Jane, and their minister were at his bedside when he died. Nurses noted that the family appeared to accept the reality of Alex's death and mobilized themselves to participate in Alex's funeral and other tasks that would assure their ultimate adjustment.

Discussion The Depp family illustrates many features common to families coping with the phases of illness, and in particular with AIDS. Viola, Jane, and Alex, that is, the Depp family system, were all affected by AIDS. The frequent arguments that occurred between Jane and her mother after they learned of the AIDS diagnosis may have served as a distraction from the harsh reality of Alex's eventual death. It may have been the family's way to avoid addressing their imminent loss. This behavior is common during the preparatory phase of a family's adaptation to a fatal illness.

After the family initially adapted to the prospect of loss, they began to live with the reality of the chronic nature of AIDS. During this "settling-in," or middle phase, Jane and her mother adjusted to illness-related stressors and their caregiving roles. They focused on preventing opportunistic infections and spent time managing Alex's symptoms of fever, night sweats, malaise, and weight loss. Jane and Alex's mother also took over some of the other family functions that had once been assumed by Alex.

Families adjusting to the chronicity of illness endure many stressors. In families facing AIDS, decisions regarding who to tell about the diagnosis can create great stress (Serovich et al, 1992) and families may disagree about the level of disclosure that feels safe to them. Alex's mother, for example, learned that it was not safe to disclose the news of her son's illness to her coworkers. As a consequence, the boundaries of the Depp family system changed. Many families of patients with AIDS desire privacy because of the possibility of stigma and discrimination.

Like Jane Depp, almost everyone who has a family member with AIDS or HIV infection will experience the fear of becoming infected, even when they know rationally that there is no basis for the fear (Macklin, 1988). Partners may hesitate to share a bed, relatives may hesitate to share a meal, grandmothers may hesitate to baby-sit, and family members in general may not want to become involved (Macklin, 1988). In other words, a diagnosis of AIDS affects internal family system processes.

Like Alex, persons with AIDS may have fears that affect the whole family and stress family relationships. They may be hesitant to be tested for fear of learning the results and reluctant to express physical affection, such as hugs or kisses, for fear of infecting loved ones; they may fear abandonment, picking up an infection that the immune system cannot handle, or that treatment for infection will not be effective; they may fear painful treatments, death, or the process of dying (Macklin, 1988).

Jane Depp experienced guilt, which is another stressor that families of persons with AIDS may experience. Jane's guilt was the result of her having once rejected her now very ill brother because he was gay. Guilt may also result from abandoning a partner because of fear of infection. Frequently, well partners experience guilt because they have been spared (Macklin, 1988).

It is not uncommon for families of patients with AIDS to experience anger. The anger may be at fate for the illness, at the disease itself, at the partner for behaviors that led to the infection, or, as in Jane Depp's case, at friends for being judgmental and unsupportive (Macklin, 1988). In addition, families may grieve about the loss of a healthy and active family member, the loss of dreams for the future, the loss of family normalcy, the loss of the pre-AIDS relationship, the loss of personal freedom as the person with AIDS becomes more homebound, and the impending loss of the loved one who has AIDS (Macklin, 1988; Brown & Powell-Cope, 1991).

Uncertainty pervades the lives of families of persons with AIDS. As in Alex's case, the uncertainty may be related to not knowing which opportunistic infection will herald death. Because of Alex's immunodeficiency, infectious agents that rarely cause disease in persons with normal immune systems could unexpectedly cause death in Alex. There may also be uncertainty about when death will occur or uncertainty about staying in a relationship (Brown & Powell-Cope, 1991). Persons with AIDS may be uncertain that they want to put their families through the difficulties associated with their illness, and they may consider dissolving relationships. Family members may not be able to cope with the stigma and the opportunistic illnesses, and they may consider withdrawing from relationships.

According to the family stress model, a stressful event is accompanied by many hardships. For instance, families frequently suffer economic hardship as a result of an AIDS diagnosis. In the Depp family, Alex and his mother gave up full-time jobs. Families may find themselves poverty-stricken because of the loss of earning power, the loss of health insurance, the high cost of treatment, lack of financial assistance, and missed financial opportunities (Brown & Powell-Cope, 1991; Macklin, 1988). Some family members must take sick leave, vacation days, or personal days to care for the person with AIDS. Other family hardships may be associated with taking on additional family responsibilities, such as caregiving responsibilities.

During Alex's hospitalization, Jane and her mother experienced the acute illness phase of AIDS. They displayed behaviors characteristic of the Thorne and Robinson (1988) disenchantment stage in the relationship between the family and the health care team. They were dissatisfied with care and frustrated by the difficulty of obtaining information. Nursing interventions classified as family support (e.g., effective communication, answering questions), family involvement (e.g., changing some of the bed linens), and family mobilization (e.g., permitting the Depps to describe how they cared for Alex at home) might have helped.

The Depps' guess that hospital staff was afraid of Alex because they talked to them from the door of the room was probably correct. During a hospital stay, families and persons with AIDS may meet health care personnel who are fearful of contracting AIDS from patients. Some staff believe that they have the right to refuse to care for persons with AIDS. Others believe that caring for persons with AIDS would be upsetting to their own significant others (Scherer et al, 1992).

Nurses caring for Alex and similar patients need help to cope with their fears about caring for persons with AIDS. Discussion groups can afford nurses the opportunity to voice their feelings and foster the development of positive attitudes, and staff members who are more comfortable in caring for AIDS patients and their families can serve as role models or preceptors for nurses who object to caring for patients like Alex (Scherer et al, 1992).

The Depp family appeared to cope effectively with the terminal phase of illness. Viola and Jane coped by clinging together in anticipation of Alex's death, and nurses helped by permitting their minister to stay with them at the bedside.

This case study illustrates one family's experiences with the various phases of illness, each of which presents different challenges to families. Medical-surgical nurses must be prepared to help families face the challenges and concerns of all these stages. Clinicians can facilitate family involvement by addressing the informational and emotional needs that are salient to both persons with AIDS and their families (Pomeroy et al, 1996; Smith & Rapkin, 1996)

Overview of AIDS Increasing numbers of families are coping with AIDS today. The number of adult and adolescent AIDS cases reported in the United States as of December 1992 was approximately 250,000 (Davis, 1993), and AIDS continues to spread. Persons and families with AIDS are double victims: first, of debilitating disease and, second, of social stigmatization (Davis, 1993).

The clinical symptoms of AIDS are the end result of infection by the human immunodeficiency virus (HIV), which infects the body's cells and then disrupts the immune system. HIV can lie dormant in the body for a long time, and clinical manifestations of AIDS may not appear for 5 years or longer after infection (Rice, 1992). According to the Centers for Disease Control and Prevention (CDC), the diagnosis of AIDS is made when patients meet the following criteria:

- Laboratory evidence of HIV
- Laboratory evidence of unexplained immunodeficiencies
- Documentation of an indicator or opportunistic disease, such as Kaposi's sarcoma, *Mycobacterium tuberculosis,* or *Pneumocystis carinii* pneumonia (Rice, 1992).

"Medical treatment of AIDS is aimed at the early detection and treatment of opportunistic infections and malignancies, the management of symptoms, and prevention of complications" (Jones, 1993, p. 381). Nursing diagnoses for AIDS may include:

- Infection, risk for
- Gas Exchange, impaired

- Tissue Integrity, impaired
- Nutrition, altered, less than body requirements
- Diarrhea
- Pain
- Anxiety
- Thought Processes, altered
- Knowledge Deficit (patient and family)
- Self-esteem Disturbance
- Fluid Volume Deficit, risk for
- Social Isolation (patient and family)
- Fluid Volume Deficit, actual
- Powerlessness
- Coping, Individual, ineffective
- Family Coping, ineffective
- Family Processes, altered

Study Questions

1. Which of the following factors have led to the growth of family nursing in medical-surgical settings?
   a. Consumer demands for unfragmented and holistic care
   b. Early hospital discharge
   c. Empirical evidence that families influence patient recovery
   d. All of the above
2. All of the following characteristics are likely to increase the degree of family stress associated with hospitalization *except:*
   a. Sudden illness onset with no time to prepare.
   b. Repeated family experience with the illness.
   c. Few sources of guidance for the family.
   d. Significant disruption of family functioning as a result of the hospitalization.
3. Nurses caring for families in medical-surgical settings need to consider the following factors of the "therapeutic quadrangle":
   a. Illness, family, doctor, patient
   b. Illness, doctor, nurse, patient
   c. Illness, family, health care team, patient
   d. Family, health care team, social work services, chaplain services
4. Helping families maintain healthy lifestyles is a major aim for nurses during the:
   a. Pre-illness phase.
   b. Acute illness phase.
   c. Chronic illness phase.
   d. Terminal illness phase.
5. Establishing a calm and relaxed atmosphere that will support a trusting and empathetic relationship describes which of the following family nursing interventions?
   a. Proximity enhancement
   b. Information management
   c. Assurance provision
   d. Comfort facilitation
6. Minimization of family disruption effects describes which category of family nursing interventions?
   a. Family support
   b. Family process management
   c. Promotion of family integrity
   d. Family involvement
7. Which of the following family behaviors is rarely displayed during the chronic phase of illness?
   a. Accepting the imminence of death
   b. Carrying out prescribed treatment regimens
   c. Finding the necessary money and resources to facilitate care
   d. Preventing the social isolation caused by lessened contact with others
8. Relationships between the family and the health care team move through stages. The stage characterized by family renegotiation of trust with health care professionals is called the stage of:
   a. Naive trust.
   b. Disenchantment.
   c. Guarded alliance.
   d. None of the above
9. What factors should be considered when determining hospital visiting policies?
   a. Patient preferences
   b. Family preferences
   c. Nursing care needs
   d. All of the above
10. Which of the following is not an advantage to having families present when nurses and physicians carry out resuscitative efforts?
    a. Assurance that the patient is dying
    b. Less nursing staff time is needed for giving explanations, since the family has witnessed activities firsthand.

c. It helps the family accept the reality of death.
d. It provides the family with an opportunity to say what they need to say while there is still a chance the patient can hear.

11. Families of patients with AIDS may experience:
   a. Social stigmatization
   b. Guilt
   c. Economic hardship
   d. All of the above

References

American Nurses Association. (1992). Nurses to educate for end-of-life decisions. *American Nurse, 24*:9.

Artinian, N. T. (1989). Family member perceptions of a cardiac surgery event. *Focus on Critical Care, 16*:301–308.

Artinian, N. T. (1993). Spouses' perceptions of readiness for discharge after cardiac surgery. *Applied Nursing Research, 6*, 80–88.

Artinian, N. T. (1994). Selecting a model to guide family assessment. *Dimensions of Critical Care Nursing, 14*(1),4–16.

Beckie, T (1989). A supportive-educative telephone program: Impact of knowledge and anxiety after coronary artery bypass graft surgery. *Heart & Lung, 18*,46–55.

Bedell, S., Pelle, D., Maher, P. & Cleary, P. (1986). Do-not-resuscitate orders for critically ill patients in the hospital. *Journal of the American Medical Association, 256*, 233–237.

Bengtson, A., Karlsson, T., Wahrborg, P., Hjalmarson, A., & Herlitz, J. (1996). Cardiovascular and psychosomatic symptoms among relatives of patients waiting for possible coronary revascularization. *Heart & Lung, 25*(6), 438–443.

Berkey, K. M., & Hanson, S. M. H. (1991). *Pocket guide to family assessment and intervention*. St. Louis: Mosby Year Book.

Biegel, D. E., Sales, E., & Schulz, R. (1991). *Family caregiving in chronic illness*. Newburv Park, CA: Sage Publications.

Blackmore, E. (1996). A study to investigate needs of relatives of patients on a cardiothoracic ICU, following routine cardiac surgery. *Nursing in Critical Care, 1*(6), 268–277.

Boise, L., et al. (1996). Facing chronic illness: The family support model and its benefits. *Patient Education and Counseling, 27*(1):75–84.

Bomar, P. J. (1996). Family health promotion. In S. M. H. Hanson, & S. T. Boyd. *Family Health Care Nursing: Theory, Practice, and Research* (pp. 174–199). Philadelphia: F. A. Davis.

Bovbjerg, V. E., et al. (1995). Spouse support and long-term compliance to lipid-lowering diets. *American Journal of Epidemiology, 141*(5):451–460.

Brennan, P. F., et al. (1995). The effects of a special computer network on caregivers of persons with Alzheimer's disease. *Nursing Research, 44*(3):166–172.

Brooten, C., et al. (1988). Early discharge and specialist transitional care. *Image: Journal of Nursing Scholarship, 20*:64–68.

Brown, M. A., & Powell-Cope, G. M. (1991). AIDS family caregiving: Transitions through uncertainty. *Nursing Research, 40*:338–345.

Buchanan, H. L., et al. (1996). Trauma bereavement program: A review of development and implementation. *Critical Care Nursing Quarterly, 19*(1):35–44.

Buls, P. (1995). The effects of home visits on anxiety levels of the client with a coronary artery bypass graft and of the family. *Home Healthcare Nurse, 13*(1):22–29.

Carlsson, M. E., et al. (1996). Telephone help line for cancer counseling and cancer information. *Cancer Practice, 4*(6):319–323.

Chalk, A. (1995). Should relatives be present in the resuscitation room? *Accident and Emergency Nursing, 3*(2):58–61.

Chesla, C. A. (1996). Reconciling technologic and family care in critical-care nursing. *Image: Journal of Nursing Scholarship, 28*(3):199–204.

Clark, S. P. (1995). Increasing the quality of family visits to the ICU. *Dimensions of Critical Care Nursing, 14*(4):200–212.

Craft, M. J., & Willadsen, J. A. (1992). Interventions related to family. *Nursing Clinics of North America, 27*:517–540.

Crooks, C. E., et al. (1987). The family's role in health promotion. *Health Values, 11*:7–12.

Danis, M. (1998). Improving end-of-life care in the intensive care unit: What's to be learned from outcomes research? *New Horizons, 6*(1):110–118.

Davis, M. C. (1993). Understanding AIDS. *Caring Magazine, 12*:5–13.

Dennis, L. I., et al. (1996). The relationship between hospital readmissions of Medicare beneficiaries with chronic illnesses and home care nursing interventions. *Home Healthcare Nurse, 14*(4):303–309.

Douglas, J. M., & Spellacy, F. J. (1996). Investigators of long-term family functioning following severe traumatic brain injury in adults. *Brain Injury, 10*(11):819–839.

Driscoll, K. M. (1998). The application of genetic knowledge: Ethical and policy implications. *AACN Clinical Issues, 9*(4):588–599.

Duryee, R. (1992). The efficacy of inpatient education after myocardial infarction. *Heart & Lung, 21*:217–226.

Dwyer, M. (1998). Genetic research and ethical challenges: Implications for nursing practice. *AACN Clinical Issues, 9*(4):600–605.

Eichhorn, D. J., et al. (1995). Family presence during resuscitation: It is time to open the door. *Capsules & Comments in Critical Care Nursing, 3*(1):8–13.

Feigin, R., et al. (1998). The use of single-group sessions in discharge planning. *Social Work in Health Care, 26*(3):19–38.

Figley, C. R., & McCubbin, H. I. (Eds.). (1983) *Stress and the Family*: Vol. 2. Coping with Catastrophe. New York: Brunner/Mazel.

Franco, T., et al. (1996). Developing patient and family education programs for a transplant center. *Patient Education & Counseling, 27*(1):113–120.

Frederickson, K. (1989). Anxiety transmission in the patient with myocardial infarction. *Heart & Lung, 18*:617–622.

Friedman, M. M. (1998). *Family Nursing: Theory and Practice*, ed 4. Stamford, CT: Appleton & Lange.

Fuller, B.F., & Foster, G. M. (1982). The effects of family/friend visits vs. staff interaction on stress/arousal of surgical intensive care patients. *Heart & Lung, 11*, 457–463.

Garding, B. S., et al. (1988). Effectiveness of a program of information and support for myocardial infarction patients recovering at home. *Heart and Lung, 17*:355–362.

Gilliss, C. L., et al. (1989). The family and chronic illness. In C. L. Gilliss, et al. (Eds.). *Toward a Science of Family Nursing* (pp. 287–299). Menlo Park, CA: Addison-Wesley.

Goodell, T. T., & Hanson, S. M. H. (1999). Nurse-family interactions in adult critical care: A Bowen family systems perspective. *Journal of Family Nursing, 5*(1):72–91.

Gortner, S. R., et al. (1988). Improving recovery following cardiac surgery: A randomized clinical trial. *Journal of Advanced Nursing, 13*:649–661.

Gropper, R. C. (1998). Cultural basics and chronic illness. *Advances in Renal Replacement Therapy, 5*(2):128–133.

Guidelines/Practice Parameters Committee of the American College of Critical Care Medicine, Society of Critical Care Medicine. (1995). Guidelines for intensive care unit design. *Critical Care Medicine, 23*(3):582–588.

Gurley, M. J. (1995). Determining ICU visiting hours. *MEDSURG Nursing, 4*(1):40–43.

Hamner, J. B. (1990). Visiting policies in the ICU: A time for change. *Critical Care Nurse, 10*:48–53.

Hanson, S. M. H., & Heims, M. L. (1992). Family nursing curricula in U.S. schools of nursing. *Journal of Nursing Education, 31*:303–308.

Hanson, S., et al. (1992). Education for family health care professionals: Nursing as a paradigm. *Family Relations, 41*:49–53.

Hanson, S. M. H. (1988). Family nursing and chronic illness. In L. M. Wright & M. Leahey, *Families and Chronic Illness* (pp. 2–32). Springhouse, PA: Springhouse.

Hathaway, D., et al. (1987). Health promotion and disease prevention for the hospitalized patient's family. *Nursing Administration Quarterly, 11*(3):1–7.

Henneman, E. A., et al. (1992). An evaluation of interventions for meeting the information needs of families of critically ill patients. *American Journal of Critical Care, 1*(3):85–93.

Hoffman, M., & Malecki, M. (1990). Organ procurement and preservation. In K. M. Sigardson-Poor & L. M. Haggerty, *Nursing Care of the Transplant Recipient* (pp. 13–34). Philadelphia: W. B. Saunders.

Holicky, R. (1996). Caring for the caregivers: The hidden victims of illness and disability. *Rehabilitation Nursing, 21*(5):247–252.

Hoskins, C. N., et al. (1996). Patterns of adjustment among women with breast cancer and their partners. *Scholarly Inquiry for Nursing Practice, 10*(2):99–123.

Hupcey, J. E. (1998). Establishing the nurse-family relationship in the intensive care unit. *Western Journal of Nursing Research, 20*(2):180–194.

Jacob, D. A. (1998). Family members' experiences with decision making for incompetent patients in the ICU: A qualitative study. *American Journal of Critical Care*, 7(1):30–36.

Jastremski, C. A., & Harvey, M. (1998). Making changes to improve the intensive care unit experience for patients and their families. *New Horizons, 6*(1):99–109.

Johnson, D., et al. (1998). Measuring the ability to meet family needs in an intensive care unit. *Critical Care Medicine, 26*(2), 266–271.

Johnson, L. H., & Roberts, S. L. (1996). Hope facilitating strategies for the family of the head injury patient. *Journal of Neuroscience Nursing, 28*(4):259–266.

Johnson, S., et al. (1995). Perceived changes in adult family members' roles and responsibilities during critical illness. *Image-The Journal of Nursing Scholarship, 27*(3):238–243.

Jones, A. (1993). Hematology/immunology. In J. Hartshorn, M. Lamborn, & M. L. Noll. *Introduction to Critical Care Nursing* (pp. 348–385). Philadelphia: W. B. Saunders.

King, K. B., et al. (1993). Social support and long term recovery from coronary artery surgery: Effects on patients and spouses. *Health Psychology, 12*:56–63.

King, R. B. (1996). Quality of life after stroke. *Stroke, 27*(9):1467–1472.

Kristeller, J. L., et al. (1996). Attitudes toward risk behavior of relatives of cancer patients. *Preventive Medicine, 25*(2):162–169.

Kulik, J.A., & Mahler, H. 1. (1989). Social support and recovery from surgery. *Health Psychology, 8*:221–238.

Lazure, L. L. A., & Baun, M. M. (1995). Increasing patient control of family visiting in the coronary care unit. *American Journal of Critical Care, 4*(2):157–164.

Leahey, M., & Wright, L. M. (1987). Families and chronic illness: Assumptions, assessment, and intervention. In L. M. Wright & M. Leahey, *Families and Chronic Illness* (pp. 55–76). Springhouse, PA: Springhouse.

Leash, R. M. (1996). Death notification: Practical guidelines for health care professionals. *Critical Care Nursing Quarterly, 19*(1):21–34.

Leonard, K. M., et al. (1995). Prolonged cancer death: A family affair. *Cancer Nursing 18*(3):222–227.

Leske, J. S. (1986). Needs of relatives of critically ill patients: A follow up. *Heart and Lung, 15*:189–193.

Leske, J. S. (1991). Internal psychometric properties of the Critical Care Family Needs Inventory. *Heart and Lung, 20*:236–344.

Leske, J. S. (1992). Needs of adult family members after critical illness. *Critical Care Nursing Clinics of North America, 4*:587–596.

Leske, J. S. (1996). Intraoperative progress reports decrease family members anxiety. *AORN Journal, 64*(3):424–425, 428–436.

Leske, J. S., & Heidrich, S. M. (1996). Interventions for aged family members. *Critical Care Nursing Clinics of North America, 8*(1):91–102.

Leske, J. S., & Jiricka, M. K. (1998). Impact of family demands and family strengths and capabilities on family well-being and adaptation after critical injury. *American Journal of Critical Care*, 7(5):383–392.

Leventhal, H., et al. (1985). Reactions of families to illness: Theoretical models and perspectives. In D. C. Tlurk & R. D. Kerns (Eds.), *Health, Illness and Families: A Life-Span Perspective* (pp. 108–145). New York: John Wiley & Sons.

Lindquist, R., et al. (1990). Research utilization: Practice considerations for applying research to nursing to practice. *Focus on Critical Care, 17*:342–347.

Lindsay, P., et al. (1997). Educational and support needs of patients and their families awaiting cardiac surgery. *Heart and Lung, 26*(6):458–465.

Lorenz, B. T. (1995). Needs of family members of critically ill adults. *MEDSURG Nursing, 4*(6):445–451.

Lubkin, I. M. (1986). *Chronic Illness: Impact and Intervention.* Boston: Jones & Bartlett.

Lynn-McHale, D., et al. (1997). Preoperative ICU tours: Are they helpful? *American Journal of Critical Care, 6*(2):106–115.

Macklin, E. D. (1988). AIDS: Implications for families. *Family Relations, 37*:14–149.

Malacrida, R., et al. (1998). Reasons for dissatisfaction: A survey of relatives of intensive care patients who died. *Critical Care Medicine, 26*(7):1187–1193.

Malecki, M., & Hoffman, M. (1987). Getting to yes: How nurses' attitudes affect their success in obtaining consent for organ and tissue donations. *Dialysis and Transplantation, 16*:276–218.

Marsden, C. (1992). Making patient self-determination a reality in critical care. *American Journal of Critical Care, 1*:122–124.

Martens, K. H., & Mellor, S. D. (1997). A study of the relationship between home care services and hospital readmission of patients with congestive heart failure. *Home Healthcare Nurse, 15*(2):123–129.

Martin, J. (1991). Rethinking traditional thoughts. *Journal of Emergency Nursing, 17*(2):67–68.

McClowry, S. G. (1992). Family functioning during a critical illness: A systems theory perspective. *Critical Care Nursing Clinics of North America, 4*:559–564.

McLennan, M., et al. (1996). Rehabilitation learning needs: Patient and family perceptions. *Patient Education & Counseling, 27*(2):191–199.

Medland, J. J., & Ferrans, C. E. (1998). Effectiveness of a structured communication program for family members of patients in an ICU. *American Journal of Critical Care*, 7(1):24–29.

Molter, N. C. (1979). Needs of relatives of critically ill patients. *Heart and Lung, 8*:332–339.

Moos, R. H. (Ed.). (1984). *Coping with Physical Illness, 2*: New Perspectives. New York: Plenum Press.

Nicklin, W. M. (1986). Post discharge concerns of cardiac patients as presented via a telephone callback system. *Heart & Lung, 15*:268–212.

Olson, D. (1997). Paging the family: Using technology to enhance communication. *Critical Care Nurse, 17*(1):39–41.

Osuagwu, C. C. (1991). ED codes: Keep the family out. *Journal of Emergency Nursing, 17*:363–364.

Phelan, G., et al. (1996). Self-administration of medication by patients and family members during hospitalization. *Patient Education & Counseling, 27*(1):103–112.

Pomeroy, E. C., et al. (1996). A psychoeducational group intervention for family members of persons with HIV/AIDS. *Family Process, 35*(3):299–312.

Quinn, S., et al. (1996). The needs of relatives visiting adult critical care units as perceived by relatives and nurses. Part I. *Intensive & Critical Care Nursing, 12*(3):168–172.

Redheffer, G. M. (1989). A trauma nurse's opinion. *Nursing, 19*(3):45.

Rice, R. (1992). The patient with AIDS. In R. Rice (Ed.), *Home Health Nursing Practice* (pp. 203–217). St. Louis: Mosby-Year Book.

Rolland, J. S. (1988). A conceptual model of chronic and life-threatening illness and its impact on families. In C. S. Chilman, et al. (Eds.) *Chronic Illness and Disability. Families in Trouble Series*, Vol. 2 (pp. 17–68). Newbury Park, CA: Sage.

Rosen, E. J. (1990). *Families Facing Death*. New York: Lexington Books.
Rosenczweig, C. (1998). Should relatives witness resuscitation? Ethical issues and practical considerations. *CMAJ, 158*(5):617–620.
Scherer, Y. K., et al. (1992). AIDS: What are critical care nurses' concerns? *Critical Care Nurse, 12*(7):23–29.
Serovich, J. M., et al. (1992). Boundaries and AIDS testing: Privacy and the family system. *Family Relations, 41*:104–109.
Siminoff, L. A. (1997). Withdrawal of treatment and organ donation. *Critical Care Nursing Clinics of North America, 9*(1):85–95.
Simon, S. K., et al. (1997). Current practices regarding visitation policies in critical care units. *American Journal of Critical Care, 6*(3):210–217.
Simpson, T. (1991). Critical care patients' perceptions of visits. *Heart and Lung, 20*:681–688.
Smith, M. Y., & Rapkin, B. D. (1996). Social support and barriers to family involvement in caregiving for persons with AIDS: Implications for patient education. *Patient Education & Counseling, 27*(1):85–94.
Steele, J. M., & Ruzicki, D. (1987). An evaluation of the effectiveness of cardiac teaching during hospitalization. *Heart & Lung, 16*:306–311.
Steinglass, P. (1992). Family systems theory and medical illness. In R. J. Sawa (Ed.), *Family Health Care* (pp.18–29). Newbury Park, CA: Sage.
Swanson, R. W (1993). Psychological issues in CPR. *Annals of Emergency.Medicine, 22*(2; part 2):350–353.
Thorne, S. E., & Robinson, C. A. (1988). Health care relationships: The chronic illness perspective. *Research in Nursing and Health, 11*:293–300.
Titler, M. G., & Walsh, S. M. (1992). Visiting critically ill adults: Strategies for practice. *Critical Care Nursing Clinics of North America, 4*:623–632.
Titler, M. G., et al. (1995). Developing family focused care. *Critical Care Nursing Clinics of North America, 7*(2):375–386.
Topp, R., et al. (1998). Can providing paging devices relieve waiting room anxiety? *AORN Journal, 67*(4):852–854, 857–861.
Trief, P. M., et al. (1998). Family environment, glycemic control, and the psychosocial adaptation of adults with diabetes. *Diabetes Care, 21*(2):241–245.
Turk, D. C., & Kerns, R. D (Eds.). (1985). *Health, Illness, and Families: A Life-Span Perspective*. New York: John Wiley & Sons.
van der Woning, M. (1997). Should relatives be invited to witness a resuscitation attempt? A review of the literature. *Accident & Emergency Nursing, 5*(4):215–218.
Wagner, C. D. (1996). Family needs of chronic hemodialysis patients: A comparison of perceptions of nurses and families. *ANNA Journal, 23*(1):19–26.
Wang, C. Y., & Fenske, M. M. (1996). Self-care of adults with non-insulin-dependent diabetes mellitus: Influence of family and friends. *Diabetes Educator, 22*(5):465–470.
Waters, C. M. (1998). Actual and ideal professional support for African American family members. *Western Journal of Nursing Research, 20*(6):745–764.
Waters, C. M. (1999). Professional nursing support for culturally diverse family members of critically ill adults. *Research in Nursing & Health, 22*:107–117.
Wesson, J. S. (1997). Meeting the informational, psychosocial and emotional needs of each ICU patient and family. *Intensive & Critical Care Nursing, 13*(2):111–118.
White, P. D. (1997). The role of the critical care nurse in counseling families about advance directives. *Critical Care Nursing Clinics of North America, 9*(1):53–61.
Yates, B. C.(1989). Stress and social support during recovery from a cardiac illness event. *Oklahoma Nurse, 34*(5):7.
Younger, S. J., et al. (1984). ICU visiting policies. *Critical Care Medicine, 12*:606–608.

Bibliography

Doherty, W. J., & Baird, M. A. (Eds.). (1981). *Family-Centered Medical Care: A Clinical Casebook*. New York: Guilford Press.
Doherty, W. J., & Campbell, T. L. (1988). *Families and Health*. Newbury Park, CA: Sage.
Feetham, S. L., et al. (Eds.). (1993). *The Nursing of Families: Theory/research/education/practice*. Newbury Park, CA: Sage.
Furukawa, M. M. (1996). Meeting the needs of the dying patient's family. *Critical Care Nurse, 16*(1): 51–57.
Hanson, C. L., et al. (1995). Empirical validation for a family-centered model of care. *Diabetes Care, 18*(10):1347–1356.
Hickey, M. L. (Ed.). (1992). Family issues in critical care. *Critical Care Nursing Clinics of North America, 4*:549–649.
Leahey, M., & Wright, L. M. (1987). *Families and Life-Threatening Illness*. Springhouse, PA: Springhouse.
Leske, J. S. (Ed.). (1991). Family interventions. *AACN Clinical Issues in Critical Care Nursing, 2*:181–354.
Sawa, R. J. (Ed.). (1992). *Family Health Care*. Newbury Park, CA: Sage.
Titer, M., et al. (1991). Impact of adult critical care hos-

pitalization: Perceptions of patients, spouses, children, and nurses. *Heart & Lung*, *20*:174–182.

Wright, L. M., & Leahey, M. (1987). *Families & Chronic Illness*. Springhouse, PA: Springhouse.

Young, J. B. (1995). Black families with a chronically disabled family member: A framework for study. *ABNF Journal*, *6*(3):68–73.

Focus On

FAMILY MENTAL HEALTH NURSING

The experience of most nursing students in psychiatric mental health settings involves *individuals* with either acute or chronic conditions. In contrast, this chapter examines the intricacies of *family* mental health nursing.

A historical overview of trends in family mental health nursing is followed by an outline of common theoretical perspectives. The topics covered include Bowen's theory, structural, contextual, and communication theory, the multiple systems view, and nursing conceptual models, so that students are provided with an excellent background on the theoretical bases of family mental health nursing practice.

The chapter continues with a discussion of the importance of health promotion and identifies strategies that, regardless of the practice setting, will assist the nurse in creating a healthy environment for families. The case examples are realistic and address family mental health treatment on both inpatient and outpatient units.

The discussion of chronic mental illness is timely and demonstrates a sensitivity to the cultural issues that pervade our care of families and individuals with mental health problems. The use of case studies helps the student to understand chronic mental health problems and the multiple roles of the family mental health nurse. The chapter concludes with a consideration of the implications of the family approach to mental health nursing for practice, education, research, and health policy.

Chapter 13

FAMILY MENTAL HEALTH NURSING

Helene J. Moriarty • Margaret P. Shepard

OUTLINE

OBJECTIVES

On completion of this chapter, the reader will be able to:

- Describe family mental health nursing.
- Explain how conceptualizations of the family and family interventions have evolved over the past 200 years in psychiatric and mental health nursing.
- Identify and describe five common theoretical perspectives used in family mental health nursing.
- Identify the goals for family mental health nursing interventions in health promotion, acute illness, and chronic illness.
- Describe the implications of the family approach to mental health nursing for theory development, practice, education, research, and health policy.

Psychiatric and mental health nursing is a specialized area of nursing practice that is based on the science of theories of human behavior and on the art of the therapeutic use of self (American Nurses Association [ANA], 1994). The practice is directed to both preventive and corrective efforts for mental disorders and their sequelae. We are concerned with promotion of optimum mental health for society, communities, families, and individuals. Family nursing is an integral component of psychiatric and mental health nursing, though not all nurses in this field practice family nursing. Family mental health nursing recognizes the interaction between families and the mental health of family members. It addresses the psychiatric and mental health care needs of the individual client in the context of the family, while also addressing the needs of the family as a whole.

In the changing health care environment, the shift towards shortened hospital stays and increased outpatient care, along with more manageable medication protocols, have all influenced clients' treatment needs and the system of care delivery in psychiatric and mental health treatment (Baker, 1993). Increasingly, short-term psychiatric hospital admissions are designed for intensive management of acute symptoms, and early discharge places the client with continuing symptoms back in the care of the family and the community. Although there are many benefits in caring for mentally ill clients outside the hospital, it also increases the burdens on the families of mentally ill persons. Extended care for an ill family member strains family resources and often leaves the family ill-equipped to manage the stigma, guilt, and loss that may be experienced (Baker, 1989, 1993). Family caregiving brings an extraordinary number of stressors, placing relatives in what may be a situation of risk. Stressors experienced by the family include difficulties in coping with disturbed behavior, the uncertainty and unpredictability of symptoms, and loneliness and isolation as a result of the stigma of having a mentally ill family member (Baker, 1993; Sveinbjarnardottir & Dierckx de Casterle, 1997). In some families, the burden of providing informal care is likely to contribute to higher levels of affective and anxiety disorders (Cochrane et al., 1997). It is essential for caregivers to receive support to manage these stressors, as well as information about symptom management and community resources, to effectively manage the mentally ill family member at home. Mental health nurses practicing family-centered care are in a position to meet the needs of the client within the context of the family and to meet the needs of the family as a whole.

Contemporary psychiatric mental health nursing practice includes the domains of prevention, intervention, and rehabilitation (ANA, 1994). Thus, nurses practicing mental health and psychiatric care may be found in many settings, providing many levels of care. The American Nurses Association (ANA) has delineated two practice levels of psychiatric and mental health nursing: the psychiatric mental health registered nurse and the advanced practice registered nurse. Both are prepared to use the nursing process and theoretical frameworks to address a broad range of physical and psychosocial problems presented by clients and their families. And both collaborate with a variety of other professions working with and on behalf of the client. The clinical examples in this chapter illustrate the different roles of the nurse in psychiatric and mental health nursing.

HISTORICAL OVERVIEW

Psychiatric and mental health nurses have a long history of working with the family. However, concepts of families and family interventions have changed over the last 200 years with advances in knowledge and changes in health care delivery.

During the Colonial period in American history, there was no organized system of care for people with mental illness. Responsibility for the care of mentally ill persons lay primarily with the family. In the absence of a family, mentally disturbed people were supported and maintained through the charity of neighbors and the community (Burgess, 1997). It was not until the advent of the "asylum," or the public mental hospital, in the nineteenth century that any systematic care was provided for mentally ill persons. In this period, the insane were taken away from the stimulation of the home environment and placed in institutions that had orderly and structured routines. However, because there were few professional tools available to understand and treat mental illness and the debilitating effects of institutionalization had not yet been recognized, patients often stayed in the hospital indefinitely.

Twentieth-century psychiatric treatment was greatly influenced by the Freudian psychoanalytic movement (Bowen, 1976). Before Freud, psychiatric illness was believed to be caused by some unidentified brain pathology. Freud's research led to a theory that proposed that psychiatric symptoms were a function of the mind rather than a brain disease. In addition, Freud introduced the concept of transference, which led to one of the cornerstones of psychiatric treatment, the therapeutic relationship. During this period, however, psychiatric treatment was still provided primarily in institutions, within the framework of the medical model. The role of the nurse was to provide custodial care and companionship for patients. Family participation in treatment was discouraged (Peplau, 1993). This mode of treatment persisted until the National Mental Health Act of 1946, which represented the first national commitment to solving the problem of mental illness through funding for research, services, and training. As part of this commitment, the relationship between psychiatric patients and nurses began to be studied, in an effort to identify how the nurse-patient relationship could be therapeutic for patients. The result was the emergence of the clinical specialty of psychiatric nursing (Peplau, 1993).

In the middle of the twentieth century, biomedical research led to the development of phenothiazines, the medications that help to control the major symptoms of psychosis. Effective use of these antipsychotic medications made it possible for clients who had formerly been "out of touch with reality" to enter into significant therapeutic relationships with psychiatric staff. Thus, this was an exciting time for mental health nurses, who began to implement therapeutic relationships with their patients. This period also marked the beginning of a trend toward less restrictive treatment and discharge of chronically ill patients to the community and the family. Simultaneously, researchers started to examine the reciprocal relationship between the mentally ill client and the family (Rose, 1996). There was increased recognition that caring for mentally ill persons placed a burden on families and that families may play a major role in maintaining the symptoms of mental illness in an individual member.

Efforts to provide community-based services for mentally ill persons resulted in the Community Mental Health Centers Act of 1963, which marked a significant shift away from institutional services to community-based services for mentally ill persons (Burgess, 1997). The act authorized funding for continuous and comprehensive services in community mental health centers and led to what has been called the "deinstitutionalization movement." Large numbers of chronically ill individuals were released from hospitals, and the focus of care shifted toward the community, a change that led to expanded roles for psychiatric nurses as individual, group, and family therapists (Peplau, 1993).

Initially, family therapists tended to blame families for the client's illness, based on the view that the client's symptoms were a manifestation of family pathology. In particular, the mother was often blamed for improperly nurturing her young children, and a disturbed mother-child relationship was thought to be the cause of the psychiatric disturbance in the child. Too often, families felt blamed by nurses and other mental health professionals, through overt or covert implications that they had been responsible for causing or maintaining the individual's symptoms. Other factors related to symptoms received little attention. Experiences such as these only exacerbated family burdens of guilt and shame. Further, there is little empirical evidence supporting the efficacy of treatment strategies that regard the patient as the victim and other family members as villains (Walsh, 1987).

The deinstitutionalization movement was expected to bring sweeping solutions to the problems of the seriously mentally ill. Yet many communities were not able to provide the comprehensive services required to treat this population. As a result, many patients experienced the "revolving door phenomenon": early discharge to the community without adequate treatment programs and supportive services resulted in frequent readmissions to the hospital. In the absence of adequate services, many families had to assume even more responsibility for caring for their mentally ill family member. Frustrated with inadequate services and the tendency of mental health professionals to blame families for individuals' illnesses, families formed consumer advocacy groups such as the National Alliance for the Mentally Ill (NAMI) (Jones, 1999). Groups such as these became very active in lobbying Congress and the public for increased research on mental illness and its treatment. And indeed, research in the last two decades has produced major breakthroughs in genetics, immunology, and knowledge of brain function and has increased scientists' and mental health practitioners' understanding of biologic factors related to mental illness. For example, specific structural and functional changes in the brain have been found to be linked with schizophrenia, and DNA markers for the genetic predisposition to certain affective disorders have been identified (McBride, 1990). Although a familial vulnerability to schizophrenia has been demonstrated, scientists still have not identified specific genetic linkages in this complex disorder (NIMH, 1999).

Growing recognition of the biopsychosocial correlates of mental illness, shorter hospital stays, and the necessity for families to take primary responsibility for their member's care have led nurses and other mental health professionals to enter into a relationship with families as "partners in care." Professionals now acknowledge the benefits of basing family interventions on respect for the needs of family members and the family's collaborative role in improving patient functioning. Mental health professionals are thus combining information about brain function with a consideration of the psychological, social, cultural, and familial factors that also influence human behavior (McBride, 1990). This integrated approach (McKeon, 1990) has propelled nurses and other mental health professionals to identify and study the most effective strategies for mental health promotion in the family (O'Brien, 1998), the most effective ways to share information about a family member's schizophrenia with the family (Main et al, 1993), and the most effective ways to support families in caring for a schizophrenic family member in the community (Brooker & Butterworth, 1991; Zastowny et al, 1992).

COMMON THEORETICAL PERSPECTIVES

Psychiatric mental health nurses typically use therapeutic principles from a number of family systems theories to guide their assessments and interventions with families. Psychiatric mental health advanced practice nurses, many of whom are family therapists, are more apt to base their practice on one *specific* theoretical framework; however, some advanced practice nurses use multiple frameworks. Five major theoretical frameworks are commonly employed in family mental health nursing: Bowen's family systems theory, structural family theory, contextual family theory, communication theory, and the multiple systems view. There is some conceptual overlap among theories. The five theories are summarized in the following sections. Three of these theories (i. e., Bowen's, structural, and communication) are described in detail in Chapter 2.

Bowen's Family Systems Theory

One theory commonly used in family mental health nursing is Bowen's family systems theory (Bowen, 1976; Brown, 1991; Gillis, 1973; Kerr & Bowen, 1988). This theory views the nuclear family as part of the multigenerational extended family and theorizes that patterns of relating tend to repeat themselves over generations. The theory does not "pathologize" families but, rather, encourages individuals to see their families in positive ways. Family members are guided to acknowledge that parents and relatives "did the best with what they had" (Brown, 1991).

The central assumption in this theory is that chronic anxiety is the underlying basis for dysfunction. The theory consists of eight interlocking concepts that address anxiety and emotional processes: (1) differentiation of self, (2) triangles, (3) the family projection process, (4) the nuclear family emotional system, (5) the multigenerational transmission process, (6) sibling position, (7) emotional cutoff, and (8) societal regression. Understanding families requires understanding these concepts and the relationships among the concepts.

The central concept is *differentiation of self;* it has two aspects. First, it refers to the capacity to be a separate yet related human being, and second, it refers to the ability to separate thought from reactive feeling. Differentiation exists on a continuum; the level of differentiation influences the ability to manage anxiety. Those at the higher end of the continuum are able to have intimate relationships, while still maintaining a sense of self. They also exhibit more thinking than reactive feeling. Because they are less reactive, they are better able to manage anxiety and to cope with stress. Those at the lower end of the continuum have more fused relationships; they are extremely close to others but are unable to maintain a basic sense of self. They also show less thinking and more reactive feeling. Because they are more reactive, they are more anxious in times of stress and less able to cope with stress.

A *triangle* describes a relational pattern among persons, objects, or issues. It is an emotional configuration of three members; the members may be three persons or two persons and a group, an issue, or an object. When tension mounts between two persons, one or the other moves toward the third member of the triangle to relieve the anxiety between the twosome. Triangles operate in all families but become problematic over time when they are rigid and entrenched.

The *family projection process* is the process by which parental anxiety is transmitted to children via triangles. The *nuclear family emotional system* describes how anxiety is managed: (1) through marital conflict or distance; (2) through dysfunction of a spouse; or (3) through projection onto a child or children. *The multigenerational transmission process* is the family projection process in action over several generations. *Sibling position* refers to the place and role a child assumes in the family. There is a tendency for siblings in certain positions to take on certain roles and behaviors. For example, the oldest child tends to be a responsible caretaker in the family. *Emotional cutoff* is the process of physically or emotionally separating from the family of origin as a way to handle the anxiety of fusion. *Societal regression* refers to the idea that a high level of anxiety in a society (e.g., from war or economic problems) can lead to reacting emotionally rather than in a thinking way (e.g., through riots).

Using Bowen's family systems approach, the therapist may meet with only one family member, with some members, or with all members. No matter who is present, however, the work is seen as family therapy because the therapist takes a multigenerational view of the family. The therapist and family develop a three- to four-generation genogram to examine family processes. The therapist uses this genogram to assess patterns of relationships, patterns of behavior, significant nodal events (life events), level of differentiation, level of anxiety, and triangles.

The goal of therapy is to increase the level of differentiation in the family and thus decrease anxiety within individuals and in the family. Therapy starts by helping family members learn about the family system: to see patterns of relationships and triangles over generations. It also helps individuals take responsibility for changing their position in generational patterns of relating. Family members are encouraged to develop one-to-one relationships with different family members to get to know the family system, know the triangles, and "detriangulate self." For example, a husband and wife may be encouraged to talk directly to one another about their marital problems rather than using their typical triangle (e.g., the wife complains about the husband to her mother and the husband uses work to escape from the marital tension). Family members are also assisted to take an "I position"; that is, each member is encouraged to speak for himself or herself rather than speaking for the entire family with statements such as "We feel" or "We think." In addition, therapy helps members to think instead of reacting in an impulsive, reflexive way.

Structural Family Theory

A second family systems theory is structural family theory, developed by Minuchin (1974) and his colleagues (Minuchin & Fishman, 1981; Minuchin et al, 1978). This theory emphasizes the relationship between the presenting problem and the structure of the family. Nurses and other health professionals have applied this theory to families facing problems as diverse as diabetes, asthma, eating disorders, juvenile delinquency, family violence, drug abuse, and divorce.

The family structure consists of the "invisible set of functional demands that organize the ways in which family members interact" (Minuchin, 1974, p. 51). Structure encompasses three major areas: (1) power, (2) subsystems, and (3) boundaries. The family's structure may be dysfunctional in any of these areas.

Power refers to the influence that each family member has on family processes. The theory views a hierarchy of power as necessary for effective family functioning. Subsystems are sets of family relationships, each with specific functions. For example, in the spousal subsystem, one function of spouses is to support each other in a relationship that fosters individual growth. The parental subsystem performs the tasks of nurturing and socializing children. In the sibling subsystem, siblings learn about peer relationships, power, and alliances. The last area, *boundaries,* includes the rules that differentiate the tasks of different subsystems. For families to function effectively, there must be clear boundaries between subsystems, with some connectedness between them. Families with boundary problems may be disengaged or enmeshed. In disengaged families with rigid boundaries, there is little communication and support among family members; only a high level of stress will evoke support from other members. In enmeshed families with diffuse boundaries, the intense togetherness hinders individuation of members; in these families, stress of one member elicits strong reactions from other members.

The goal of structural family therapy is to solve problems by altering the underlying structure of the family. The initial assessment includes these overlapping phases: (1) joining with the family to temporarily become part of the family system; (2) obtaining a description of the problem; (3) exploring the family structure by observing transactions around the problem; and (4) assessing boundary flexibility, sensitivity to members' actions, family developmental stage, family life context (sources of support and stress), and the way in which the identified patient's symptoms are related to dysfunctional family structure.

The structural therapist focuses primarily on the individual and family in the present. This approach, however, does not negate history but acknowledges transactional patterns from the past. Nevertheless, its primary focus is on present interactions. As Minuchin (1974) noted, "Structural family therapy is a therapy of action. The tool is to modify the present, not to explore and interpret the past" (p. 14).

The therapist takes an active role in the therapy and tries to create change by transforming those aspects of the family structure that are related to the problem. Restructuring techniques results in a shift of power, subsystems, and boundaries. These techniques include: (1) actualizing transactional patterns; (2) marking boundaries; (3) assigning tasks; (4) relabeling communication; (5) modifying mood and affect; (6) escalating stress; and (7) supporting, educating, and guiding (Minuchin, 1974).

Contextual Family Theory

Another major family theory is contextual family theory, which was developed by Boszormenyi-Nagy and his colleagues (Boszormenyi-Nagy & Spark, 1973; Boszormenyi-Nagy & Krasner, 1986; Cotroneo, 1982, 1986; Cotroneo & Moriarty, 1992). This is a multigenerational family theory that links concern for individuation with concern for rootedness and for significant others in one's relationship network. The relationship network includes: (1) one's legacy—the facts, events, and circumstances of the family and culture into which one is born; (2) the quality of current relationships with nuclear and extended family, peers, friends, colleagues, and the world; and (3) relational connections to the next generation (Cotroneo, Hibbs, & Moriarty, 1992). The theory has been applied to families with a wide variety of problems, such as disturbed parent-child relationships, divorce, family violence, incest, and chronic mental illness.

In contextual family theory, trust and loyalty are key multigenerational dynamics that shape a person's relationships, commitments, and expectations through the interactive process of giving and receiving care. A fundamental assumption of this theory is that living in a family requires a balance of giving and receiving care (Cotroneo et al, 1992).

In relationships based on trust, family members are able to live as separate persons, while at the same time they are connected and available to others as resources. The contextual therapist focuses on behaviors that enhance trust and those that diminish it. The therapist assists family members to identify sources of trust and mistrust in their past and present relationships and to rebalance mistrust with resources that can be used constructively. This process of building trust requires family members to consider the merit of positions taken by other family members even when these positions oppose each other (this is termed "multidirected partiality"). The contextual therapist guides families in this process (Cotroneo et al, 1992).

Loyalty, the other key dynamic in this theory, signifies commitments, obligations, and attachments that bind family members to each other over time. Loyalty forms the basis for family members' obligations to care for one another. In addition, whether or not one received the care one deserved and how one received care shape one's relationships with others outside the family. For example, expectations for care that were not met in the family of origin may be assigned to partners and children, tending to overburden these relationships and often distorting their reality. An assessment of at least three generations is needed to understand how loyalty expresses itself among members of a family (Cotroneo, Moriarty, & Smith, 1992).

The contextual family therapist guides family members in:

- Examining the balance of give and take and individuals' sense of fairness or unfairness in past and present relationships
- Inquiring into the "other side"of family members, for example, exploring one's parents' side
- Guiding family members to rebalance unfairness and helping adults make a claim on their family of origin for consideration (Cotroneo et al, 1992)

Communication Theory

Communication theorists such as Bateson (Bateson et al, 1956), Haley (1963, 1976), Jackson (1965a, 1965b), Watzlawick (Watzlawick et al, 1967; Watzlawick et al, 1974) and Weakland (1976) propose that verbal and nonverbal communication among family members influences behaviors within the family. Watzlawick and colleagues (1967) presented four axioms of communication that can serve as guides for assessing communication within families:

1. All behavior, whether nonverbal or verbal, is communication and conveys a message.
2. All communication defines a relationship.
3. Persons communicate both verbally and nonverbally; the former presents more content, whereas the latter informs more about the relationship.
4. All communications are either symmetrical (equality exists and either person is free to take the lead) or complementary (one leads and the other follows).

According to this theory, dysfunctional communications, such as disconfirmation, disqualification, and incongruent messages (double-bind), are related to problematic family behaviors. Disconfirmation refers to the invalidation of a family member's perception of himself or herself or invalidation of his or her experience. Disqualification includes unclear communications such as contraindications, changes of subject, and incomplete sentences. Incongruent messages consist of verbal and nonverbal messages that conflict that are given at the same time. Strategic family therapy tries to change dysfunctional communications to clear, direct communications to change family behaviors (Haber et al, 1987).

Strategic family therapists, often working with a consultation team of mental health professionals, begin by observing sequences of problematic behaviors and then identifying behaviors that maintain the problems. For example, the therapist asks the family to define a goal for treatment, stated in measurable behavioral terms. The therapist then assigns tasks to families, tries to break dysfunctional communication loops, and uses paradox. Paradoxical instruction "prescribes the symptom" or encourages the family to do more of what it has been doing (i.e., continue the status quo) rather than change. The instruction is based on the assumption that the family will instinctively resist what is suggested by the therapist and, therefore, will do the opposite and begin to change (Haber et al, 1987; Hare-Mustin, 1976; Stanton, 1981).

Multiple Systems View

A multiple systems view incorporates the consideration of many levels in work with families—familial, biological, psychological, cultural, environmental, and spiritual—and explores the interactions of these different levels. Treatment modalities may be offered at these different levels of systems. Use of a specific treatment modality does not necessarily imply an intervention directed toward the cause of the problem. Rather, treatment modalities may address issues and concerns that are present in individuals and families regardless of the possible causes of the problem.

The choice of which systems to work with and the relative importance of each system depends on the problem. Current research indicates that severe mental illnesses, such as schizophrenia and affective disorders, have a biologic basis that interacts with other factors to influence the course of the illness (Harvard Mental Health Letter, February 1997, December 1997; Moltz, 1993; Walsh & Anderson, 1987). This suggests the use of pharmacologic interventions complemented by psychosocial and environmental supports for patients with these illnesses. There are other individual and family problems, however, where the biologic component is less obvious or may not be present—for example, in adjustment disorders, intrafamilial abuse, incest, juvenile delinquency, problems after divorce, problems after bereavement, parent-child relationship problems, and marital problems. In these cases, working with the family and possibly other psychosocial and biologic systems is warranted.

Nursing Conceptual Models

In addition to the five theories previously summarized, some family mental health nurses have used nursing conceptual models to guide their assessment, conceptualization, and goal setting with families (Berkey & Hanson, 1991; Clements & Roberts, 1983; Fawcett & Whall, 1991; Herrick & Goodkoontz, 1989). Neuman and colleagues (Clements & Roberts, 1983) have all discussed how their models address the family and can be applied to nursing practice with families. (Descriptions of specific nursing models are provided in Chapter 2.) Some family nurse theorists have noted that there is a lack of congruence between the conceptualizations of family in the nursing models and in the family systems theories. In response to this problem, Whall (1991) reformulated some family systems theories to make them more congruent with the nursing conceptual models.

Herrick and Goodkoontz's report (1989) exemplifies how a nursing model is helpful for family nursing in mental health settings. They described how Neuman's systems model guided their assessment of individual, family, and environmental stressors in a family referred to an outpatient clinic for assistance with an emotionally disturbed teenager. The assessment identified multiple stressors present in different family members, in family dynamics, and in the family's environment. Based on this assessment, family therapy was chosen as the appropriate intervention.

HEALTH PROMOTION

In family mental health nursing, health promotion falls in the domain of primary mental health care. This care is defined as "continuous and comprehensive services necessary for the promotion of optimal mental health, prevention of mental illness, management and/or referral of mental and physical health problems, diagnosis and treatment of mental disorders, and their sequelae, and rehabilitation" (Burgess, 1997, pp. 19–20). To help prevent mental illness, psychiatric nurses consult with health agencies and schools, provide mental health education, develop and evaluate community programs, and offer family therapy. The family may be considered the unit of care, or the family may be seen as influencing lifestyle choices that may prevent illness for individual members of the family (Danielson, Hamel-Bissell, & Winstead-Fry, 1993).

Promotion of mental health is a nursing phenomenon that is not restricted by specialty or place of health care delivery. Whether the nurse seeks to reduce the stresses experienced by the family caring for the child with a chronic condition or the stresses experienced by the aging caregiver of a terminally ill spouse, the goal is to preserve mental health.

Risk Factors for Mental Health

Many stressors in life have been identified as risk factors contributing to the vulnerability of individuals and family as a whole. The two most consistently identified risk factors are low socioeconomic status and female gender (Institute of Medicine, 1989; Lavigne et al, 1998; US Department of Health and Human Services Office of Public Health and Science, 1998). Poverty is the most tenacious threat to mental health of individuals, families, and communities; it has consistently been associated with higher rates of both individual dysfunction (Raine et al, 1996) and family dysfunction (Costello et al, 1997; Lavigne et al, 1998). Moreover, poverty is complex and encompasses additional factors, such as low income, unemployment, lack of education, and poor housing.

The higher rates of mental illness among women is also extremely complex and may be related to role overload (Lavigne et al, 1998). Women are more likely to juggle work, family, and domestic demands; and women are more likely to be single parents and to live in poverty. Both poverty and female sex may be amenable to family-level nursing preventive measures, such as identifying health and economic resources for families and assisting partners to negotiate domestic responsibilities equitably.

Risk factors may also vary according to sociocultural contexts. For example, in a comparative study of psychiatric disorders among Native American and white youth in Appalachia, Costello and colleagues (1997) identified higher family risk factors (including poverty, violence, and substance abuse) but a lower incidence of mental illness in the Native American children. White children in this study were more likely than native children to seek and use mental health services to deal with problems related to poverty and family deviance. The authors concluded that the relative influence of risk factors varied by the cultural context. The influence of culture on symptom expression and health-seeking behavior cannot be underestimated (Canino & Spurlock, 1997). The relative influence of risk factors, such as poverty, may vary in association with other factors, such as bereavement and physical disability, in diverse cultural contexts (Patel et al, 1998).

Interventions for Promotion

Health promotion, by definition, means early intervention targeted at specifically identified risk factors. Successful mental health promotion must be acceptable to the communities and families for whom they are intended. To that end, collaboration among community members, mental health care providers, and consumers is essential. School-based clinics that bridge the gaps between isolated individuals and families and needed mental health care services are examples of effective community-based health promotion programs (Armbruster et al, 1997). Promotion of family cohesion and resilience have been found to diminish the influence of risk factors among low income school-age children (Reynolds, 1998; Thienemann et al, 1998). The family is likely to serve protective functions in relation to risk factors, although further research is necessary to identify other family variables that may mediate against the pervasive influence of major risks for common mental illnesses.

Example: Divorce

Another life stressor that may place families at risk is divorce and the custody disputes that sometimes arise. Child custody disputes signal parental conflicts that have negative implications for all parties, especially children (Hetherington, 1981; Wallerstein & Kelley, 1980). In situations of intense parental conflict, children are at high risk for emotional and behavioral disturbances such as depression, low self-esteem, school problems, and antisocial behavior (Emery, 1982; Hetherington et al, 1978; Hetherington, 1981). The contextual approach to custody decisions, which is derived from contextual family systems theory, can be used to minimize or prevent mental health problems in families by helping families negotiate a custody and visitation agreement (Cotroneo, Hibbs, & Moriarty, 1992; Cotroneo, Moriarty, & Smith, 1992). This approach is based on the view that the best interests of children cannot be separated from the welfare of their parents. Examining the interests of children in an intergenerational context reflects the full reality of their relationship network and family loyalties.

In this approach, family meetings are held that include both parents and all siblings; they may also include grandparents, aunts, uncles, and other significant persons. Each family member is asked to identify his or her own needs and commitments regarding parenting. The therapist helps the family examine the full relational context of the parents as well as the children, particularly the kind of parenting that the parents themselves received. The therapist also helps family members explore family loyalty issues and unfinished family business that may undermine trust. Cotroneo and colleagues speculate that parents who struggled with loyalty conflicts in their families of origin may use marriage and parenting of their children to re-enact that struggle. Thus parents' perception of what is at stake in a custody dispute may be distorted, and their capacity for giving and sharing may be impaired (Cotroneo, Hibbs, & Moriarty, 1992).

Topical guidelines for structuring these meetings are outlined in Box 13–1. These meetings redirect the focus from blame to trust-building, so that parents can see themselves less as adversaries and more as collaborators in the care of their children. Parents learn to differentiate between issues that belong to the marriage and issues of parenting, and they also address issues from their families of origin. In this context of trust, parents are encouraged to negotiate an arrangement that they can live with and that protects the child's access to both parents (Cotroneo, Hibbs, & Moriarty, 1992).

Cotroneo and colleagues (1992) have illustrated the use of the approach with a small sample of families and through a case study. The findings suggest that the approach can help families create alternatives to continued disputation. The authors suggest using the approach as soon as a parent files for custody or visitation to minimize damage to the child.

Example: Family Violence

The problem of family violence is another area for family health promotion. It is a sad fact that relatedness increases the likelihood of physical or sexual abuse.

Box 13–1

GUIDELINES FOR FAMILY MEETINGS ABOUT CHILD CUSTODY DISPUTES

I. Current family situation
  a. Response of family members to separation or divorce
  b. Effects on family members
    1. What has been done to help the children deal with the situation?
    2. Contact made with significant legal, religious, psychological, social, and health care resources

II. Family genogram information
  a. Ways in which parents define and validate themselves in relation to significant others, particularly their own families of origin
    1. Patterns of expectations and commitments across three generations
    2. Gender-related issues
    3. Intergenerational history of losses, relational injuries, and injustices

III. An exploration of parenting of children (past, present, and future) and the developmental burdens and demands that are placed on children
  a. Acknowledgment of children for their contributions to the family that may have been taken for granted
  b. Exploration of the worries that children may be experiencing and how they get help when it is needed
  c. Acknowledgment of the parents for the losses, relational injuries, and injustices experienced in their families of origin
  d. Exploration of ways in which family members can work to correct injustices and exploitation in past and present relationships and repair injuries that have already been sustained
  e. Consideration of the consequences of any imbalances in giving and receiving care and fairness that exist in the family

IV. Family task (conjoint session)
  a. Describe the family situation as you see it. What are the conflicts for you?
  b. In thinking about what to do, what are you considering and why?
  c. If you could have things your way (according to your preferences), what would you do now?
  d. If you were to put your plan into action, what would happen? Do you think your plan would be successful? Why? Why not?
  e. What would be the consequences of your plan for you, your spouse or partner, and each individual child?

Source: Uses and Implications of the Contextual Approach to Child Custody Decisions by M. Cotroneo, B. J. Hibbs, and H. Moriarty, 1992, *Journal of Child and Adolescent Psychiatric and Mental Health Nursing, 5*(3):17. Copyright 1992 by Nursecom, Inc. Reprinted with permission.

One out of every five American families experiences family violence. One out of four American women report that they have been physically abused by a husband or boyfriend at some time in their lives (Lieberman Research, 1996). The rate of child abuse reports in the United States grew 4 percent, from 45 per 1,000 children in 1992 to 47 per 1,000 children in 1997. Since 1988, the nationwide increase is 41 percent (Daro & Wang, 1997). As Dobash and Dobash (1979) stated, "Despite fears to the contrary, it is not a stranger but a so-called loved one who is most likely to assault, rape, or murder us."

Family violence may be viewed as a severe stressor that is a symptom of family dysfunction and that leads to adverse sequelae for individual family members and the family as a whole. The term encompasses child abuse and neglect, spouse abuse, sibling abuse, teenage violence towards parents, and elder abuse. Child abuse and spouse abuse often exist together in a family.

Four forms of abuse are described in the literature—physical, emotional, neglectful, and sexual. Physical abuse is a nonaccidental injury inflicted by someone whose intent is to cause physical harm. Emotional abuse is a means of controlling through fear and degradation. It may include threats of harm, extreme and constant criticism, physical and social isolation, and false accusations. Neglect is a deliberate failure to provide for the basic human needs, e.g., food, shelter, hygiene, safety, and health care. Sexual abuse is assaultive and nonassaultive sexual exploitation; it refers to any form of sexual interaction. Incest is sexual abuse among family members; it occurs most commonly between a parent and child within a family, but it may also involve siblings. Sexual activity between a parent and a child or between an adult and a child always constitutes abuse. It does not matter whether it involves physical force or whether the child is perceived by the adult as freely engaging in sexual activity. Because of a child's age, the child cannot give informed consent. Therefore, this sexual activity always involves exploitation of the child by the adult.

Prevention of child abuse is critical, given the potential for intergenerational patterns of abuse. Children who are abused and neglected in their families of origin are at higher risk for tolerating and using violence in their adult relationships (Finkelhor, 1988). Oliver (1993) reviewed 61 studies for rates of intergenerational transmission of child abuse and concluded that one-third of child victims go on to become neglectful or abusive parents.

Research indicates that there are three sets of factors that place families at risk for child abuse and neglect: parental characteristics, child characteristics, and family ecosystem characteristics. Parental factors include: (1) the parent was abused or neglected by his or her parents, (2) the parent believes in physical punishment, (3) the parent has unrealistic expectations of the child, (4) the parent is under great stress, e.g., unemployment, (5) the parent is a loner with few friends, (6) the parent sees the child as willful and purposely "bad," and (7) the parent is a substance abuser. Child characteristics include: (1) the child is different as a result of illness, prematurity, or disability; and (2) the child is difficult (e.g., fussy, hyperactive, demanding). Familial factors include: (1) the family is under great stress (e.g., poor, single-parent family, unemployed, or with other health problems), (2) the family is socially isolated, (3) the family is a patriarchal (male-dominated) household, and (4) the family has a history of abuse in the nuclear or extended family (Strong & DeVault, 1992). Identification of these risk factors is critical for family assessment and early intervention with families at risk or with families with abuse.

Nurses in all clinical areas must be knowledgeable of the symptoms of abuse and neglect, the risk factors for abuse, and the reporting system for their states. In the United States, the Child Abuse and Prevention and Treatment Act (1974) was amended in 1996 to mandate that specific persons, including nurses, physicians, and health care professionals, report any suspicion of child abuse (AMA, 1996).

Primary prevention of abuse involves strengthening individuals and families to enable them to better cope with multiple life stressors. For example, nurses can conduct community classes to teach parents about normal developmental challenges, such as toilet training, ways to discipline without physical punishment, and methods of conflict resolution. Secondary prevention involves identification of families at risk for violence and those who are beginning to use violence, followed by early intervention to prevent or stop the violence.

Advanced practice family mental health nurses and other mental health professionals may provide treatment to victims, perpetrators, and families. The aim is to protect the victim, stop the violence, and prevent further violence by changing family processes. Most treatment approaches over the last 10 years have focused on the victim as the primary context for treatment. However, family system approaches that consider the whole family as the unit of assessment and treatment have evolved in the United States and Europe (Cirillo & DiBlasio, 1992; Colgan-McCarthy & O'Reilly-Byrne, 1988; Cotroneo, 1986; Cotroneo & Moriarty, 1992; Gelinas, 1986).

Families who are not experiencing severe stressors such as poverty, divorce, or violence may choose to work on issues such as stress reduction and strengthening relationships among family members. There is no such thing as a perfect family. All families have issues and concerns even if they are not experiencing severe distress. A basic goal for mental health promotion is to assist healthy, functioning families to maintain and enhance the health of both the family and family members. Health promotion for these families may take place in community educational programs or through counseling. A nurse working with the family can use a variety of approaches to enhance the family's communication and relationships. Other examples of nursing interventions that promote family health are discussed in Chapter 9.

FAMILY MENTAL HEALTH NURSING IN ACUTE ILLNESS

Some clients and families experience acute symptoms, such as suicidal ideation associated with major depression. It is estimated that 300,000 people attempt suicide each year (Centers for Disease Control and Prevention, 1999). Clients and families may also present with an acute exacerbation of a chronic illness; for example, a client with chronic schizophrenia may experience a resurgence of psychotic symptoms. Acute distress may also be associated with a severe stressor that triggers psychiatric symptoms, such as a panic attack (American Psychiatric Association [APA], 1994). Acute symptoms require early diagnosis and treatment and prompt referral for additional consultation as necessary.

When the nurse is caring for the family as client, acute individual distress is often associated with a familial crisis. For example, 15-year-old Angela attempted suicide by swallowing "a handful" of her grandmother's medication for hypertension. During the assessment, the advanced practice nurse learned that Angela thought she was pregnant. She was afraid to tell her parents because she thought it would hurt and disappoint them. When the nurse cares for the client within the context of the family, the relationship between the individual's symptoms and the family response to the symptoms is considered. In either case, the meaning the family attaches to the symptom can influence the family's decision to seek care (Danielson et al, 1993).

Acute psychiatric and mental health disturbances often compel families to seek immediate care. They may seek care from the general family practitioner or go directly to an emergency department or community mental health center. In many cases the initial screening is done by a nurse who has not been prepared as a psychiatric mental health nurse. The nurse assesses the presenting problem and then makes appropriate referrals. In the case of Angela, the nurse would first determine if Angela had ingested a potentially lethal dose of medication, which would require immediate medical intervention. If Angela needed to be stabilized in an intensive care unit, she and her family might be seen by the psychiatric consultation liaison nurse. The role of this nurse in a medical treatment setting is to help the client and the family begin to understand the implications of the crisis that has occurred and the options for family treatment.

Once Angela's physiological safety had been established, she might be referred to a psychiatric mental health advanced practice nurse for a comprehensive assessment. Using a multiple systems perspective, the nurse would assess: (1) Angela's physiological condition, (2) her mental status, including any persistent suicidal ideation, (3) the availability of family resources and support to keep the client safe, (4) the meaning the crisis had for the family, and (5) the need for psychiatric hospitalization.

In acute situations, the nurse collaborates with the family and other mental health professionals in planning for the client's care. Initial treatment may focus on assisting the client and family to open lines of communication. After resolution of the crisis, the family may be referred for family therapy to help them develop more effective coping strategies.

Care of the client experiencing acute distress may involve a brief admission to an inpatient psychiatric unit. Traditionally, hospitalization reinforces an individualistic view of care, in which one member is seen in the sick role and the other members of the family are seen as peripheral to the illness. Merely adding family therapy to the treatment program does not make the inpatient experience a family experience. Family-focused care can be more fully integrated into inpatient treatment programs through use of the following time-honored strategies identified by Bowers and McNally (1983):

- Plan intake conferences at the time of admission. An intake conference with the family makes it possible to assess the family as a unit and the needs of each of its members. It also serves to inform the family that care will be family-centered and indicates how they may be involved in treatment.
- Structure intensive family therapy into the treatment program. Family therapy may help the family view the presenting problem as a family problem rather than as solely the problem of the hospitalized client.
- Make family conferences a regularly scheduled activity. In inpatient settings, interdisciplinary treatment teams typically meet frequently to evaluate the client's progress toward the goals of treatment, but families are not usually included in these meetings. Family conferences involve the family in setting treatment goals and evaluating progress for the individual and family.
- Plan therapeutic leaves of absence for the individual so that family members may work together outside the hospital setting on family treatment goals.
- Use psychiatric mental health advanced practice nurses to supervise family treatment. These specialists, who have education and experience in working with families, can both conduct family sessions and supervise others involved in family meetings and conferences.

A family-centered approach alters the traditional concept of milieu therapy (Bowers & McNally, 1983). Traditionally, the family members were seen as "intruders" or visitors to the inpatient milieu and not as a part of the treatment process. Integrating the family into the milieu may involve restructuring traditional components of the milieu; for example, families need to be included in community meetings, medication groups, and discharge groups. New components may also need to be added to milieu treatment—for example, family intake conferences, multifamily therapeutic groups, and joint meetings of client, family, and staff.

Case Study: Family Treatment on an Inpatient Unit

The following case example depicts family-focused inpatient treatment. The therapeutic goals and treatment strategies reflect a multiple systems view in addressing many levels of systems. Interventions at the family level are derived from Bowen's (1978) multigenerational family systems theory.

Jeremy G., an 18-year-old high school senior, was experiencing severe mood swings along with escalating angry, defiant behavior, school failure, and suicidal ideation. At times, Jeremy felt "on top of the world." During these periods, he felt he could accomplish almost anything. At other times, Jeremy reported "subzero" self-esteem. An intensive outpatient evaluation indicated that Jeremy was a gifted student and an artistic young man. His longstanding pattern of mood swings supported a diagnosis of a bipolar mood disorder called cyclothymia (APA, 1994).

The family evaluation revealed that his parents had a long history of marital problems. The parents maintained emotional distance from one another, and Jeremy was distant from his father. Jeremy felt that he had tried, for many years, to get along with his father but that his father was "cold and impossible to please." Mr. G. reported having a very distant relationship with his own father. Jeremy and his mother had an unusually close, fused relationship. Jeremy's two sisters, aged 13 and 15 years, were relatively free of the triangular emotional system that occurred between Jeremy and his parents.

Jeremy and his family agreed to a 2-week hospitalization for Jeremy. He was referred for a neurological evaluation and magnetic resonance imaging (MRI) to rule out any biologic causes for his mood swings, and he began a trial of antidepressant medication for management of cyclothymia. The family agreed to participate in family therapy sessions. The therapeutic goal was to decrease emotional reactivity among family members and increase the family's level of differentiation.

In therapy, family members were encouraged to take an "I position" and to become more thoughtful in their responses to one another, rather than emotionally reactive. In addition, Jeremy was encouraged to participate in age-appropriate peer relationships. This helped Jeremy remove himself from the three-person triangular emotional system and begin to improve his self-esteem. Treatment staff helped Jeremy identify his strengths and encouraged him to pursue his dream of going to art school. In addition to attending family sessions and treatment conferences, Jeremy's parents attended a medication group to learn about the medication prescribed for Jeremy. They also attended a parenting group that focused on learning from and sharing with other parents about childrearing issues. In separate sessions, the parents began to focus on their own marital issues. The Gs had managed their problems by submerging them and projecting their marital anxiety onto Jeremy. When the couple began to address their problems in therapy, less anxiety was projected onto Jeremy.

Mr. G.'s parents also attended several family therapy sessions. Mr. G. was encouraged to be less reactive with his own father and to work on developing a one-to-one relationship with him. As he did so, Mr. G. became more open to developing a relationship with his son. As Jeremy began to assume an "I position" in his family, he was able to express his desire for a rewarding relationship with his father. This goal was incorporated into the plans for therapeutic leaves of absence. Jeremy and his father went on several outings together to work on their relationship. Following the 2-week hospitalization, Jeremy was discharged and the family began monthly family therapy sessions to build on the successes in the hospital.

Special Considerations: When a Child Is Hospitalized

When a child with acute psychiatric symptoms requires hospitalization, the staff need to keep in mind how radical and strange hospitalization may seem to the family, which is used to having responsibility for the child. Many hospitals have rules that shut out families from the process of goal setting and treatment for the child (Goren, 1992). Goren stresses the need for inpatient staff to work in partnership with families because family participation is essential for effective problem solving. She presents the following guidelines for engaging families in inpatient treatment of a child:

- Recognize the family's competencies. Given that "all families have competencies" (p. 45), staff should point out parents' strengths and emphasize the importance of using these strengths in the child's treatment.
- Replace therapeutic relationships with therapeutic systems. That is, rather than relying heavily on the traditional one-to-one therapeutic relationship, rely on the therapeutic system of child, family, and staff.
- Involve the child, family, and staff as partners in treatment planning conferences and in developing the treatment contract.
- Work through the family rather than in its place. Given that the family is the natural caregiver for the child, staff should assist the family to intervene with the child.
- Consider family-support alternatives to out-of-family placement. Rather than removing the child from the family, try to build up the family's strengths and bring in supports from the extended family and community.
- Decrease the barriers between the hospital and the community and minimize the hospital's interference with parenting. Encourage parents to take part in activities such as meals, classes, and bedtime preparation.

When these guidelines are followed, treatment becomes a process between the staff system and the family system, with the involvement of community services as well. As Goren said, "The child belongs, in the sense of what is ordinary and usual, to the family and community. The responsibility of the staff is to intervene in ways that support the child's belongingness and that increase the likelihood of rapid return to normal life" (1992, p. 46).

Outpatient Care

For some acute problems, outpatient treatment may be appropriate if there is no danger to family members or others. The following case study illustrates outpatient family treatment when a mother reported feeling overwhelmed by raising her children and questioned her ability to continue. Treatment was based on structural family theory.

Case Study: Family Treatment in an Outpatient Setting

Caroline M., the mother, was a 30-year-old, single woman, who was referred to the community mental health center by a female friend. Caroline lived in a three-bedroom row home with her five children: Paul, age 12; Tametrice, age 10; Sam, age 8; Nina, age 6; and Vera, age 4. Caroline had held various jobs over the last 10 years as kitchen helper, typist, and factory worker. She had been unemployed for several months, since she quit her job because of her boss's verbal abusiveness. Presently, the family was subsisting on welfare. Caroline came to the clinic because she was very "edgy and nervous." She reported difficulty in expressing her anger toward family and friends and felt physically explosive. She was raising five children with little outside support and felt overwhelmed by this. She cared deeply about her children but questioned her ability to raise them. She had had two previous contacts at the clinic for the same reasons but reported withdrawing from therapy because she "did not like" the therapists. During the present contact, she began work with two nurse co-therapists. Nine sessions were conducted: six sessions with the entire family, two sessions with Caroline, and one session with the children.

During the sessions, the therapists joined with the family to attempt to better understand the family system and assess the family structure. The mother and Paul made up the parental subsystem. As the oldest son, Paul was a "parentified child," who was assuming many parental functions in the family; when Caroline felt overwhelmed by her parental functions, she delegated these to Paul. He attempted to meet his mother's expectations of him to receive her love and approval, but she did not acknowledge his contributions. Figure 13–1 depicts some aspects of the family's structure and the therapeutic goals for transforming these aspects. Box 13–2 outlines therapeutic goals for strengthening the parental subsystem, strengthening the sibling subsystem, and supporting the mother's personal needs.

FAMILY MENTAL HEALTH NURSING IN CHRONIC ILLNESS

Chronic mental illness is characterized by diagnosis, duration, and disability (Bachrach, 1991). Health care providers are now also using the term "severe and persistent illness" to denote chronic mental illness. For example, schizophrenia, chemical dependence, and eating disorders are considered severe and persistent mental illnesses. A mental illness that persists for 2 years or more is considered chronic. A lingering disability such as one that precludes the ability to return to work full-time also characterizes a disorder as chronic. Prevalence rates for chronic mental illness in the United States range from 1.9 million to 2.4 million (CDC, 1999a). Further, it has been estimated that about one-third of the homeless population is chronically mentally ill (Burgess, 1997). Given the prevalence of chronic mental illness, nurses and other health care professionals in many settings are likely to encounter mental illness and its related problems. For example, medical management of a client with diabetes may be complicated by severe and persistent schizophrenia. A woman's pregnancy may be complicated by a 10-year history of bulimia. Treatment of a client's alcohol abuse may need to include consideration for the client's depression.

Because of the encompassing nature of the label "chronic mental illness," it is difficult to generalize about treatment needs for this population. One client may lack family support and require supportive services for housing, management of medications, and a daily routine. Another client may receive family and community support, but the family may require assistance in managing the burdens associated with caring for a chronically ill family member. Wraparound services may be required for a family caring for a child with complex needs (Handron, Dosser, McCammon, & Powell, 1998). The goal of wraparound services is to create an individualized package for intensive care in the home, school, and community settings. It encompasses a strength-based, family-driven orientation that focuses on the unique needs of each child and family. In addition to improving behavioral outcomes for children engaged in wraparound serv-

Present Map

M and PC (executive subsystem)
....
Children (sibling subsystem)

Therapeutic Goal

M

PC ⋮ Other siblings

KEY

M = Mother
PC = Parentified child
... = Diffuse boundary
--- = Clear boundary

FIGURE 13-1
The map under therapeutic goal represents a clear boundary between mother and children, with Paul, the parentified child, returning to the sibling subsystem, but maintaining a position of leadership among his siblings.

Box 13–2

THERAPEUTIC GOALS FOR THE M. FAMILY BASED ON STRUCTURAL FAMILY THEORY

I. Strengthening the parental subsystem
   a. Acknowledge Caroline's stressors as a single parent.
   b. Teach Caroline about age-appropriate expectations for the children.
   c. Teach her new ways to enforce limits (e.g., through rewards or through withholding privileges).
   d. Assign tasks both inside and outside the therapy session that reinforce the parental subsystem (e.g., designation of assigned days for dishwashing).
   e. Help Caroline identify her double-bind messages and her inconsistent expectations for the children.
   f. Facilitate mobilization of supports (e.g., family, friends, church, community groups).

II. Strenghtening the sibling subsystem
   a. Emphasize individual differences to mark boundaries between the children and between mother and children.
   b. Role play or assign tasks to teach siblings ways to resolve conflicts without calling for mother.
   c. Decrease the children's competition for mother's attention by encouraging mother to designate one "special time" for each child to spend with her alone.
   d. Modify Paul's position as parentified child
      i. Support Paul in his efforts to increase his autonomy outside the family.
      ii. Acknowledge Paul's contributions to the family.
   e. Encourage activities involving only the sibling subsystem by assigning tasks requiring cooperation among siblings (e.g., Paul could teach his siblings about history or all siblings could make a present for their mother).

III. Supporting Caroline's personal needs
   a. Explore Caroline's needs for intimacy and social contact (e.g., through her relationships and social activities). Have some individual sessions with Caroline to discuss sexual issues or other issues she wishes to address without the children present.
   b. Explore the impact of Caroline's present conflict with her partner on her ability to cope with her children.
   c. Discuss possible job opportunities and completion of her general equivalency diploma.

ices, the intensive program has been found to be a cost-effective means of maintaining children in the context of their own family, school, and community.

Cultural Perspectives on Chronicity

The family's cultural beliefs influence their perceptions and management of the client's chronic mental illness. Indeed, cultural psychiatrists (Lefley, 1990; Lefley, 1998a) have suggested that the concept of chronicity in mental illness is an artifact of cultural belief systems and expectations regarding the nature of illness. In Westernized cultures, such as the mainstream culture in the United States, chronicity may be a by-product of the treatment community's belief that serious mental illness is inherently chronic. Also, the bureaucratic treatment system tends to reinforce dependence and the "sick role" behavior associated with chronicity. Further, it has been suggested that the incidence of mental illness is greater in cultures that produce high levels of stress and offer low levels of social support. The incidence of chronicity may also be higher in cultures that provide few work opportunities for chronic patients and few supports to caregivers of chronically mentally ill persons.

In some non–Western cultures, mental illness is perceived as external to the patient and is thought to be caused by supernatural forces or possession (Skultans, 1991). In such cultures, patients and families may experience less blame and stigmatization for the illness. Also, the family and community are likely to be more supportive, and family support is perceived as an integral component of treatment. It is also interesting that in these non–Western cultures, where mental illness is believed to be brief and temporary, the incidence of chronicity is lower (Lin & Kleinman, 1988). The differing rates of chronic mental illnesses in Western and non–Western cultures tend to support the view of cultural psychiatrists that chronicity in mental illness is a cultural artifact.

Within this westernized multicultural society, differences in culturally determined values and belief systems abound. These differences may influence family relationships with professional, legal, and consumer communities. A family's cultural system may influence their perception of the family burden related to caring for a member with severe and persistent mental illness (Hines-Martin, 1998; Lefley, 1998b; Nahulu et al, 1996). Knowledge of culturally determined family beliefs about mental illness and perceptions of care will enhance family-provider relationships and effect treatment outcomes (Solomon, 1998; Vandiver & Keopraseuth, 1998). For example, in their work with Native American families, Johnson and Johnson (1998) found that respectful approaches to family education contributed greatly to diagnostic accuracy, treatment, and rehabilitation efficacy. When the nurse conveyed respect and interest in family cultural beliefs, it enhanced joining with the family and engagement in the treatment program.

Chronic mental illnesses that demonstrate great cultural variations include the eating disorders—anorexia and bulimia. Both disorders are found almost exclusively among women in Westernized cultures (Harvard Mental Health Letter, November 1997). Family systems theories (Minuchin et al., 1978) suggest that certain types of family organization are closely related to the development and maintenance of symptoms of eating disorders. The following case example demonstrates a family mental health nursing approach to assessing eating disorders on an inpatient unit.

Case Study: Assessment on an Inpatient Unit

Carmella was a 19-year-old woman admitted to an inpatient psychiatric unit for bulimia. She was a freshman at an Ivy League university in the United States and had always been a hard-working student who strove for excellence in her academic work. Her physical appearance was striking; many patients on the unit referred to her as the "beautiful" patient who "could be a model." The other patients could not understand why Carmella was in the hospital because she looked so "perfect." On the unit, Carmella tried to be a peacekeeper; she avoided any expression of dissatisfaction or conflict with others and tried to please everyone—patients and staff. Carmella came from a very close and religious Italian family in which three generations lived together. In this family, there was a great emphasis on togetherness; expressions of disagreement and conflict were discouraged. On the third night of her hospitalization, Carmella's mother visited her. Carmella's primary nurse wanted to assess Carmella's responses after the visit, based on her awareness that family factors are often related to eating disorders. Five minutes after the visit, Carmella entered the kitchen, removed two gallons of ice cream from the refrigerator, and began binge eating. The nurse followed Carmella into the kitchen and asked her what she was feeling as she began binge eating. Carmella said she had felt "ready to explode" with anger at her mother during the visit but could not express it. This represented a breakthrough in Carmella's treatment because it was the *first time* Carmella made a connection between her feelings and her binge-eating behaviors. The primary nurse, psychiatrist, and patient continued to explore this connection in treatment. A major goal was to help Carmella to develop new ways to express her anger, conflict, and disappointment in others. Family therapy, group therapy, and milieu therapy were used to address this goal.

Family Support: Psychoeducational Models

Family involvement in the care of clients with chronic mental illness results in better outcomes for the client. For example, family support of the patient has been shown to improve medication compliance (Mulaik,

1992) and to raise levels of satisfaction with family relations and housing (Dixon et al, 1998) in schizophrenic clients with severe and persistent mental illness. Enhanced family interaction has been related to a better quality of life (Sullivan et al, 1992) and higher individual functioning (Thienemann et al, 1998) in families with a schizophrenic member. However, the burden of caring for a mentally ill family member is often overwhelming (Friedmann et al, 1997; Rose, 1996). Without adequate support, caregivers may become exhausted and relinquish their responsibilities. One of the most promising interventions to emerge since the deinstitutionalization movement is psychoeducation (McFarlane, 1997). Psychoeducational programs target the family as a unit; the benefits may be experienced by both the chronically mentally ill member and the family caregivers.

The content of psychoeducational interventions varies with the treatment philosophy as well as the needs of the specific client and family. For example, one psychoeducational model called behavioral family management (Falloon et al, 1984) involves training families in family communication and problem solving. Another approach called supportive family management (Zastowny et al, 1992) provides clients and families with detailed information about the illness, treatment plan, and services. Supportive family management may also include information on the availability of community services, advice on daily living, and management of client symptoms and family issues. A study (Zastowny et al, 1992) comparing these two psychoeducational interventions found similar clinical improvements with both approaches. Both interventions prevented frequent relapses and rehospitalization, decreased psychiatric symptoms, allowed a reduction in drug dosage, and improved the quality of life for patients and their families. The following case example illustrates the use of the supportive family management approach for a client with chronic schizophrenia.

Case Study: Supportive Family Management Model

Walter J., age 38, was first diagnosed with schizophrenia when he was 19 years old. He had not been able to work gainfully since his initial diagnosis, and he remained at home with his mother Agnes J., age 68, and her sister Grace W., age 63. Walter's father died when Walter was 7 years old. Thus, Walter's mother had been his only caregiver for most of his life. Walter had had more than 20 hospitalizations over the course of his illness. Hospitalization was usually precipitated by Walter's refusal to take his medications regularly. During his brief hospitalizations, Walter was stabilized on his medication and then discharged back to the care of his mother. The only follow-up care that Walter received was monthly meetings with his psychiatrist for medication management. Walter rarely kept those appointments because, in his delusional thinking, he was convinced that his medications had caused him to have cancer. Walter's mother was afraid to push him too hard to take the medications because she feared it would cause his symptoms to worsen and Walter would become violent, as he had several times in the past.

During his most recent hospitalization, Walter was referred to the psychoeducational treatment planning team to begin supportive family management. Once Walter was stabilized on his medication, supportive family management focused on the following:

- Education for Walter and the family about Walter's medications
- Instruction for Walter and the family on the signs and symptoms of acute exacerbations of schizophrenia
- Instruction for Walter and the family on behavior modification strategies to reinforce Walter's successful attendance in outpatient treatment and to reinforce compliance with medications
- Information for Walter and the family about the availability of public services to transport Walter to and from his outpatient appointments
- Information for Mrs. J. about the local chapter of the National Alliance for the Mentally Ill (NAMI), a family support group designed to help families understand and cope with the serious mental illness of a member
- Hotline phone numbers and local resources to help Mrs. J. if Walter became violent

A psychiatric mental health advanced practice nurse visited the family's home weekly to determine how the family was managing, to offer advice and information as needed, and to provide Mrs. J. with support. Weekly visits continued for the first 3 months after discharge from the hospital. Eventually the visits were tapered to an as-needed basis. Walter was able to stay out

RESEARCH BRIEF

Family caregivers of persons with chronic illnesses are at high risk for emotional problems and psychiatric disorders. In the study summarized here, the researchers tested the effectiveness of an intervention designed to decrease depression in family caregivers of persons with dementia.

There is convincing evidence of higher rates of distress and depression among caregivers of persons with dementia. The goals of this study were: (1) to evaluate the efficacy of a community-based psychoeducational nursing intervention designed to teach home caregivers to manage behavioral problems of persons with Alzheimer's disease and related dementias (ADRD) using the progressively lowered stress threshold (PLST) model and (2) to compare the intervention with routine information and referrals for case management, community-based services, and support groups. The PLST is based on the assumption that modifying environmental demands will reduce stress and promote functional adaptive behavior. The PLST model addressed three dimensions of the caregiver's situation: (1) patient symptoms, (2) level of patient behavior, and (3) staging of the disease.

Study participants were randomly assigned to either the experimental PLST training group (n = 132) or to the comparison group (n = 108), which received routine information and referral. All caregivers were asked to complete the Profile of Mood States (POMS) and the Geriatric Depression Rating Scale (GDRS), both reliable measures of affective states in the elderly. Data were collected at baseline and at 3, 6, and 12 months. There were no significant differences between the two groups in age, gender, ethnicity, amount of caregiving, relationship to care recipient (i.e., spouse, adult child, or other), or caregiver diagnosis.

Multiple regression techniques were used to test the following hypothesis: Caregivers who receive home care management training based on the Progressively Lowered Stress Threshold will report less depression than those who receive routine information, case management, and support group referral as a basis for providing home care for the ADRD patient" (Buckwalter et al, 1999, p. 84). The data from the GDRS clearly lent support to the hypothesis at each study time; however, the data from the POMS supported the hypothesis at 6 months. Although the differences in depression scores remained in the hypothesized direction, the difference was no longer significant.

Although modest, the positive impact of the PLST intervention on caregiver depression is significant, given the prevalence of depression in this group. Opportunities for family mental health nursing intervention include: 1) screening high-risk caregivers; 2) encouraging the use of mental health services; 3) providing referrals for support groups and services, such as respite care; and 4) developing independent and collaborative interventions, such as the psychoeducational intervention tested in this study.

Source: Buckwalter, K. C., et al. (1999). A nursing intervention to decrease depression in family caregivers of persons with dementia. *Archives of Psychiatric Nursing, 13*:80–88.

of the hospital for 16 months following the implementation of supportive family management. This was a dramatic change for the J. family, given Walter's history of frequent admissions to the hospital.

Although psychoeducational programs do not offer a cure for serious and persistent mental illness, they do assist clients to remain relatively free of the debilitating symptoms associated with the illness and they also provide support for family caregivers to allow them to continue in that role. Minimally, family intervention programs for the chronically mentally ill should include: (1) reduction of the stressful impact of the illness on the family; (2) information about the illness, patient abilities, and prognosis; (3) methods of stress reduction and problem solving; and (4) linkages to supplementary services to support the efforts of family members to maintain their patient in the community (Walsh & Anderson, 1987).

IMPLICATIONS FOR THEORY, PRACTICE, EDUCATION, RESEARCH, AND HEALTH POLICY

It is exciting that the body of knowledge about family mental health nursing is expanding. As shown in the case examples in this chapter, nurses may apply this knowledge in many different settings—in inpatient psychiatric and nonpsychiatric settings, in outpatient psychiatric and nonpsychiatric settings, in other community settings, and in the home. The expanding knowledge also has clear and compelling implications for theory development, research, education, and health policy.

Concepts of families are changing. Some family systems theories appear to emphasize the relationship between family interactions and illness in a unidirectional flow from family to illness. However, clinicians and researchers are now recognizing the reciprocal influences between the family and illness within a sociocultural context: illness in a family member influences the family and the family may influence the course of an illness. The challenge for mental health professionals is to integrate this view into research and care of individuals and families. Traditional theories may need to be expanded or modified to consider these reciprocal influences. It is not helpful to point a finger and blame individuals or families for illness. It is more helpful to engage the individual and family in a partnership for the benefit of both. It is also useful to draw on the patient's and family's resources in a collaborative process of goal setting and treatment. Those theories that are more resource-based need further development and testing. No matter what the debate about the causes of problems, it is clear that both individuals and families suffer with them, and both deserve our empathy and care.

In the current context of health care reform, increased emphasis must be placed on theory and research in the promotion of mental health in families, prevention of mental illness in families, and treatment of acute and chronic mental illness within families. Research on families is necessary to provide empirical support for funding family-based services. Most health care services in the United States are not organized around the family but around a health problem in the individual. Furthermore, reimbursement for health care is based on the individual; most third-party payers do not see the family as a client and do not accept family-level diagnoses. They provide coverage only for individual diagnoses included in the Diagnostic and Statistical Manual of Mental Disorders (DSM–IV) (APA, 1994), the diagnostic classification system for psychiatric illnesses.

Nursing education needs to incorporate a stronger family systems mental health focus in the curriculum, not only in mental health nursing, but also in every clinical area, because all nurses encounter families that are confronting mental health issues. Undergraduate students need to learn how to assess the mental health of individuals and the family and how to intervene therapeutically with families in hospital, home, and clinic. Graduate students in psychiatric and mental health nursing need an in-depth understanding of family theories and clinical experience with family therapy in varied settings. As advanced practice nurses, they will be called on to perform comprehensive assessments and to intervene with families within shorter periods than in the past.

Education of the public is also critical; people need to become more aware of the role families play in their own health and in the health of their members. This is particularly important with the greater emphasis on preventive care.

As stated in *Nursing: Social Policy Statement,* "the family is the necessary unit of service" (ANA, 1980, p. 5). The challenge now is for mental health nurses to embrace this idea and make it a reality in their thinking, practice, and research.

Study Questions

1. Which of the following recent trends have influenced both the client's treatment needs and the system of care delivery in family mental health nursing?
   a. Freudian psychoanalytic movement, deinstitutionalization
   b. Downward turn in the economic market, consumer advocacy

c. Health care reform, shortened length of hospital stay, more manageable medication protocols
d. Freudian psychoanalytic movement, the medical model

2. Family mental health nurses who are using structural family theory to guide their practice would assess which of the following areas in families?
a. Differentiation of self, anxiety, and triangulation
b. Power, subsystems, and boundaries
c. Multigenerational trust, multigenerational loyalty, and other multigenerational family processes
d. Disconfirmation, disqualification, and double-bind messages

3. Family mental health nurses who are using Bowen's family theory to guide their practice would assess which of the following areas in families?
a. Differentiation of self, anxiety, and triangulation
b. Power, subsystems, and boundaries
c. Multigenerational trust, multigenerational loyalty, and other multigenerational family processes
d. Disconfirmation, disqualification, and double-bind messages

4. Family mental health nurses who are using contextual family theory to guide their practice would assess which of the following areas in families?
a. Differentiation of self, anxiety, and triangulation
b. Power, subsystems, and boundaries
c. Multigenerational trust, multigenerational loyalty, and other multigenerational family processes
d. Disconfirmation, disqualification, and double-bind messages

5. Family mental health nurses who are using communication theory to guide their practice would assess which of the following areas in families?
a. Differentiation of self, anxiety, and triangulation
b. Power, subsystems, and boundaries
c. Multigenerational trust, multigenerational loyalty, and other multigenerational family processes
d. Disconfirmation, disqualification, and double-bind messages

6. Family mental health nurses who are using a multiple systems view to guide their practice would assess which of the following areas in families?
a. Family interactional patterns
b. Biologic factors
c. Psychological factors
d. Cultural, environmental, and spiritual factors
e. All of the above

7. Nancy is an advanced practice nurse practicing family nursing in a community mental health center. She is developing a health promotion program for the community. Health promotion seeks to:
a. Increase positive coping abilities and counteract harmful conditions that may produce disability
b. Provide early diagnosis and treatment and prompt referral as necessary
c. Assist the client and the family to resume the highest level of productivity in all aspects of daily living
d. Assist the client and the family to cope with residual disability that warrants continued assistance

8. After a potentially lethal suicide attempt by drinking rat poison, 33-year-old Maria was admitted to the intensive care unit for stabilization of her physical condition. The nurses sought a consultation from the mental health consultation liaison nurse. The role of the consultation liaison nurse in a medical treatment setting is to:
a. Refer the client for inpatient psychiatric treatment
b. Help the client and the family begin to understand the crisis that has just occurred and options for family treatment
c. Provide intensive psychotherapy
d. Focus on assisting the client and the family to open lines of direct communication

9. John has experienced the debilitating effects of schizophrenia for the past 10 years. After his most recent discharge from the hospital, he was admitted to a psychoeducational program. A psychoeducational program might include all of the following elements *except:*
a. Information about the availability of specific community services
b. Helping the family to understand how they caused John's illness
c. Detailed information about the illness, treatment plans, and medications
d. Home visits by a mental health nurse specialist

10. Melissa is a 19-year-old woman who has recently received a diagnosis of bipolar disorder. She was admitted to an inpatient treatment setting that emphasizes family-focused treatment. Family-focused treatment is likely to include:
a. Use of therapeutic leaves of absence to provide a break from the demands of treatment

b. Custodial care and companionship from the nurses
c. Regular scheduled conferences that include the family in setting treatment goals
d. The use of psychopharmocologic interventions only

References

American Medical Association (AMA). (1994). *Diagnostic and treatment guidelines on domestic violence.* Chicago: AMA.

American Medical Association (AMA). (1996). *Facts about family violence.* Chicago: AMA.

American Nurses Association (ANA). Council on Psychiatric and Mental Health Nursing (1994). Statement on Psychiatric Mental Health Clinical Practice and Standards of Psychiatric Mental Health Clinical Nursing Practice. Washington, DC: ANA.

American Nurses Association. (1980). Nursing: Social policy statement. Kansas City, MO: ANA.

American Psychiatric Association (APA). (1994). *Diagnostic and statistical manual of mental disorders,* ed 4. Washington, DC: APA.

Armbruster, P., et al. (1997). Bridging the gap between need and service utilization: a school based mental health program. *Community Mental Health Journal,* 33:199–211.

Baker, A. F. (1989). Living with a chronic schizophrenic can place great stress on individual family members and the family unit: How families cope. *Journal of Psychosocial Nursing,* 27:31–36.

Baker, A. F. (1993). Schizophrenia and the family. In C. S. Fawcett (Ed.) *Family Psychiatric Nursing* (pp. 342–355). St. Louis: Mosby Year Book.

Bateson, G., et al. (1956). Toward a theory of schizophrenia, *Behavioral Science,* 1(19):251–275.

Berkey, K. M., & Hanson, S. M. (1991). *Pocket Guide to Family Assessment and Intervention.* Philadelphia: Mosby Year Book.

Boszormenyi-Nagy, I., & Krasner, B. (1986). *Between Give and Take: A Clinical Guide to Contextual Theory.* New York: Brunner/Mazel.

Boszormenyi-Nagy, I., & Spark, G. (1973). *Invisible Loyalties.* New York: Harper & Row.

Bowen, M. (1976). Theory in the practice of psychotherapy. In P. J. Guerin (Ed.) *Family Therapy: Theory and Practice* (pp. 42–90). New York: Gardner Press.

Bowen, J. (1978). *Family Therapy in Clinical Practice.* New York: Jason Aronson.

Bowers, J., & McNally, K. (1983). Family-focused care in the psychiatric inpatient setting. *Image: The Journal of Nursing Scholarship, 15*:26–31.

Brooker, C. & Butterworth, C. (1991). Working with families caring for a relative with schizophrenia: The evolving role of the community psychiatric nurse. *International Journal of Nursing Studies, 28*:189–200.

Brown, F. H. (Ed.). (1991). *Reweaving the Family Tapestry.* New York: W.W. Norton.

Buckwalter, K. C., et al. (1999). A nursing intervention to decrease depression in family caregivers of persons with dementia. *Archives of Psychiatric Nursing, 13*:80–88.

Burgess, A. W. (1997). Psychiatric Nursing. In A. W. Burgess (Ed.), *Psychiatric Nursing: Promoting Mental Health* (pp. 11–34) Stamford, CT: Appleton & Lange.

Canino, I. A. & Spurlock, J. (1997). Mental health issues of culturally diverse and underserved children. *Journal of the Association for Academic Minority Physicians, 8*:63–66.

Centers for Disease Control and Prevention (1999a). Fastats A-Z, Mental Health. [on-line]. Available: http://www.cdc.gov/nchswww/fastats/mental.htm.

Centers for Disease Control and Prevention (1999b). Fastats A-Z, Suicide. [on-line]. Available: http://www.cdc.gov/nchswww/fastats/suicide.htm

Chafez, L., & Barns, L. (1989). Issues in psychiatric caregiving. *Archives of Psychiatric Nursing, 3*(2):61–68.

Child Abuse Prevention Treatment Act (1974). United States Federal Legislation. Publication No. 93–247. Washington, DC: U.S. Government.

Cirillo, S., & DiBlasio, P. (1992). *Families that Abuse: Diagnosis and Therapy* (J. Neugroschel, Trans.) New York: Norton.

Clements, I. W., & Roberts, F. B. (Eds.). (1983). *Family Health: A Theoretical Approach to Nursing Care.* New York: Wiley & Sons.

Cochrane, J. J., et al. (1997). The mental health of informal caregivers in Ontario: an epidemiological study. *American Journal of Public Health, 87*:2002–2007.

Colgan-McCarthy, I., & O'Reilly-Byrne, N. (1988). Mistaken love: Conversations on the problem of incest in an Irish context. *Family Process, 27*:181–199.

Costello, E. J., et al. (1997). Psychiatric disorders among American Indian and white youth in Appalachia: the Great Smoky Mountains Study. *American Journal of Public Health, 87*:827–832.

Cotroneo, M. (1982). The role of forgiveness in family

therapy. In A. Gurman (Ed.), *Questions and Answers in Family Therapy*: Vol. 2. (pp. 241–244). New York: Bruner/Mazel.

Cotroneo, M. (1986). Families and abuse: A contextual approach. In M. Karpel (Ed.), *Family Resources* (pp. 413–437). New York: Guilford Press.

Cotroneo, M., Hibbs, B. J., & Moriarty, H. (1992). Uses and implications of the contextual approach to child custody decisions. *Journal of Child and Adolescent Psychiatric and Mental Health Nursing, 5*(3):13–26.

Cotroneo, M., & Moriarty, H. (1992). Intergenerational family processes in the treatment of incest. In A. Burgess (Ed.), *Child Trauma: Issues and Research* (pp. 293–305). New York: Garland.

Cotroneo, M., Moriarty, H., & Smith, E. (1992). Managing family loyalty conflicts in child custody disputes. *Journal of Family Psychotherapy, 3*(2):19–38.

Danielson, C. B., et al. (1993). *Families, Health, and Illness: Perspectives on Coping and Intervention.* St. Louis: Mosby Year Book.

Daro, D., & Wang, C. (1997). Current trends in child abuse reporting and fatalities: Annual fifty state survey. Chicago, Ill: NCPCA.

Dixon, L., et al. (1998). The participation of families of homeless persons with severe mental illness in an outreach intervention. *Community Mental Health Journal, 34*:251–259.

Dobash, R. E., & Dobash, R. (1979). Violence against wives: A case against the patriarchy. New York: Free Press. Cited in B. Strong and C. DeVault (1992). *The Marriage and Family Experience*, ed 5, (p. 468). New York: West.

Emery, R. (1982). Interparental conflict and the children of discord and divorce. *Psychological Bulletin, 92*:310–330.

Falloon, I. R. H., et al. (1984). *Family Care of Schizophrenia.* New York: Guilford Press.

Fawcett, J., & Whall, A. (1991). Family Theory Development In *Nursing: State Of The Science And The Art.* Philadelphia: F. A. Davis.

Finkelhor, D. (1988). *Stopping Family Violence.* Newbury Park, CA: Sage.

Friedmann, M. S., et al. (1997). Family functioning and mental illness: a comparison of psychiatric and nonclinical families. *Family Process, 36*:357–367.

Gelinas, D. (1986). Unexpected resources in treating incest families. In M. Karpel (Ed.), *Family Resources* (pp. 327–358). New York: Guilford.

Gillis, J. M. (1973). *Family therapy in clinical practice: An abstract.* Unpublished manuscript. University of Pennsylvania School of Nursing, Philadelphia.

Goren, S. (1992). Practicing in partnership with families in the inpatient setting. *Journal of Child and Adolescent Psychiatric and Mental Health Nursing, 5*(3):43–46.

Haber, J., et al. (1987). *Comprehensive Psychiatric Nursing*, ed 3. New York: McGraw-Hill.

Haley, J. (1963). *Strategies of Psychotherapy.* New York: Grune & Stratton.

Haley, J. (1976). *Problem-solving Therapy.* San Francisco: Jossey-Bass.

Handron, D. S., et al. (1998). "Wraparound": The wave of the future: theoretical and professional practice implications for children and families with complex needs. *Journal of Family Nursing, 4*:65–86.

Hare-Mustin, R. (1976). Paradoxical tasks in family therapy: Who can resist? *Psychotherapy: Theory, research and practice, 13*:128–130.

Harvard Mental Health Letter (February 1997). Brain imaging and psychiatry. Part I. *13*(8):1–4.

Harvard Mental Health Letter (November 1997). Eating disorders. Part II. *14*(5):1–4.

Harvard Mental Health Letter (December 1997). Mood disorders: An overview. Part I. *14*(6):1–4.

Herrick, C. A., & Goodkoontz, L. (1989). Neuman's systems model for nursing practice as a conceptual framework. *Journal of Child and Adolescent Psychiatric Nursing, 2*(2):61–67.

Hetherington, E. (1981). Children and divorce. In R. Henderson (Ed.), *Parent-child Interaction: Theory, Research, and Practice* (pp. 35–58). New York: Academic Press.

Hetherington, E., et al. (1978). The aftermath of divorce. In J. Stevens & M. Mathews (Eds.), *Mother/child, Father/child Relationships* (pp. 149–176). Washington, DC: National Association for Education of Young Children.

Hines-Martin, V. P. (1998). Environmental context of caring for severely mentally ill adults: an African American experience. *Issues in Mental Health Nursing, 19*:433–451.

Institute of Medicine. (1989). Research on children and adolescents with mental, behavioral and developmental disorders. Report of a study by a committee of the Institute of Medicine (Division of Mental Health and Behavioral Medicine), National Academy of Sciences. Washington, DC: National Academy Press.

Jackson, D. D. (1965a). Family rules: Marital quid pro quo. *Archives of General Psychiatry, 12*:589–594.

Jackson, D. D. (1965b). The study of the family. *Family Process, 4*:1–20.

Johnson, C. A. & Johnson, D. L. (1998). Working with Native American Families. *New Directions for Mental Health Services, 77*:89–6.

Jones, S. L. (1999). NAMI: a convention worth noting. National Alliance for the Mentally Ill. *Archives of Psychiatric Nursing, 13*:1–2.

Kerr, M. E., & Bowen, M. (1988). *Family Evaluation.* New York: W. W. Norton.

Lavigne, J. V., et al. (1998) Psychiatric disorders with onset in the preschool years: II. Correlates and predictors of stable case status. *Journal of the American Academy of Child and Adolescent Psychiatry, 37*:1255–1261.

Lefley, H. (1990). Culture and chronic mental illness. *Hospital and Community Psychiatry, 41*:277–286.

Lefley, H. P. (1998a). The family experience in cultural context: implications for further research and practice. *New Directions for Mental Health Services, 77*:97–106.

Lefley, H. P. (1998b). Family culture and mental illness: constructing new realities. *Psychiatry, 61*:335–355.

Lieberman Research Institute Inc. (July–October, 1996). Tracking survey conducted for the Advertising Council and the Family Violence Prevention Fund.

Lin, K. M., & Kleinman, A. M. (1988). Psychopathology and clinical course of schizophrenia: A cross-cultural perspective. *Schizophrenia Bulletin, 14*:555–567.

Main, M. C., et al. (1993). Information sharing concerning schizophrenia in a family member: Adult siblings' perspectives. *Archives of Psychiatric Nursing,* 7(3):147–153.

McBride, A. B. (1990). Psychiatric nursing in the 1990s. *Archives of Psychiatric Nursing, 4*:21–28.

McFarlane, W. R. (1997). Fact: Integrating family psychoeducation and assertive community treatment. *Administration and Policy in Mental Health, 25*:191–198.

McKeon, K. L. (1990). Introduction: A future perspective on psychiatric mental health nursing. *Archives of Psychiatric Nursing, 4*:19–20.

Minuchin, S. (1974). *Families and Family Therapy*. Cambridge, MA: Harvard University Press.

Minuchin, S., & Fishman, H. C. (1981). *Family Therapy Techniques*. Cambridge, MA: Harvard University Press.

Minuchin, S., et al. (1978). *Psychosomatic families: Anorexia nervosa in context*. Cambridge, MA: Harvard University Press.

Moltz, D. A. (1993). Biopolar disorder and the family: An integrative model. *Family Process, 32*:409–423.

Mulaik, J. S. (1992). Noncompliance with medication regimens in severely and persistently mentally ill schizophrenic patients. *Issues in Mental Health Nursing, 13*:219–237.

Nahulu, L. B., et al. (1996). Psychosocial risk and protective influences in Hawaiian adolescent psychopathology. *Cultural Diversity and Mental Health, 2*:107–114.

National Institute of Mental Health (1999). Schizophrenia Research at the National Institute of Mental Health. [on-line]. Available: http://www.nimh.nih.gov/publicat/schizresfact.htm

O'Brien, S. M. (1998). health promotion and schizophrenia. Year 2000 and beyond. *Holistic Nursing Practice, 12*:38–43.

Oliver, J.E. (1993). Intergenerational transmission of child abuse: Rates, research, and clinical implications. *American Journal of Psychiatry, 150*(9):1315–1324.

Patel, V., et al. (1998). Outcome of common mental disorders in Harare, Zimbabwe. *British Journal of Psychiatry, 172*:53–57.

Peplau, H. E. (1993). Foreword. In C. S. Fawcett (Ed.), *Family Psychiatric Nursing* (pp. vii–ix). St. Louis: Mosby Year Book.

Raine, A., et al. (1996). High rates of violence, crime, academic problems, and behavioral problems in males with both early neuromotor deficits and unstable family environments. *Archives of General Psychiatry, 53*: 544–549.

Reynolds, A. J. (1998). Resilience among black urban youth. Prevalence, intervention effects, and mechanisms of influence. *American Journal of Orthopsychiatry, 68*:84–100.

Rose, L. E. (1996). Families of psychiatric patients: a critical review and future research directions. *Archives of Psychiatric Nursing, 10*:67–76.

Shepard, M.P., & Moriarty, H.J. (1996). Family mental health nursing. In S.M. H. Hanson & S. T. Boyd (Eds.), *Family Health Care Nursing*. (Chapter 13, pp. 303–326). Philadelphia: F.A. Davis.

Skultans, V. (1991). Women and affliction in Maharashtra: A hydraulic model of health and illness. *Culture, Medicine and Psychiatry, 15*:321–359.

Solomon, P. (1998). The cultural context of interventions for family members with a seriously mentally ill relative. *New Directions for Mental Health Services,* 77:5–16.

Stanton, M. D. (1981). Strategic approaches to family therapy. In A. Gurman & D. Kniskern (Eds.), *Handbook of Family Therapy*. New York: Brunner/Mazel.

Strong, B., & DeVault, C. (1992). *The Marriage and Family Experience*. New York: West.

Sullivan, G., et al. (1992). Clinical factors associated with better quality of life in a seriously mentally ill population. *Hospital and Community Psychiatry, 43*:794–798.

Sveinbjarnardottir, E., & Dierckx de Casterle, B. (1997). Mental illness in the family: An emotional experience. *Issues in Mental Health Nursing, 18*:45–56.

Thiemann, M., et al. (1998). Defense style and family environment. *Child & Human Development, 28*:89–198.

US Department of Health and Human Services Office of Public Health and Science (1998). Healthy People 2010 Objectives: Draft for Public Comment. Washington, DC: US Government Printing Office.

Vandiver, V. L. & Keopraseuth, K. O. (1998). Family wisdom and clinical support: culturally relevant practice strategies for working with indochinese families who care for a relative with mental illness. *New Directions for Mental Health Services,* 77:75–88.

Walsh, F. (1987). New perspectives on schizophrenia and the family. In F. Walsh & C. M. Anderson (Eds.), *Handbook of Family Therapy* (pp. 3–18). New York: Haworth Press.

Walsh, F., & Anderson, C. M. (1987). Chronic disorders

and families: An overview. In F. Walsh & C. M. Anderson (Eds.), *Chronic Disorders and the Family* (pp. 3–18). New York: Haworth Press.

Wallerstein, J., & Kelly, J. (1980). *Surviving the Breakup*. New York: Basic Books.

Watzlawick, P., et al. (1967). *The Pragmatics of Human Communication*. New York: Norton.

Watzlawick, P., et al. (1974). *Change: Principles of Problem Formation and Problem Resolution*. New York: W. W. Norton.

Weakland, J. H. (1976). Communication theory and clinical change. In P. J. Guerin, Jr. (Ed.), *Family Theory: Theory and Practice*. New York: Gardner Press.

Whall, A. L. (1991). Family system theory: Relati nship to nursing conceptual models. In A. L. Whall & J. Fawcett (Eds.), *Family Theory Development in Nursing: State of the Science and Art* (pp. 317–341). Philadelphia: F. A. Davis.

Zastowny, T. R., et al. (1992). Family management of schizophrenia: A comparison of behavioral and supportive family treatment. *Psychiatric Quarterly*, *63*:159–186.

Focus On

GERONTOLOGICAL FAMILY NURSING

In our society, nearly every family is concerned with the well being of at least one elderly member. Because current health care delivery is oriented primarily toward meeting the needs of the individual, not the family unit, many families "go it alone" and seek professional help only during emergencies or periods of acute illness. The family is where members learn about health and illness and also where most care is given and received throughout life. Consequently, the family has great potential as an ally in maintaining and restoring the health of its members.

The purpose of this chapter is to provide an overview of the practice of intergenerational family caring. Although this practice has long been the established norm, it is not without negative consequences. Thoughtful, well-planned nursing interventions that recognize and use family strengths can promote the health of the members and prevent or alleviate many of the negative outcomes of illness. Using a holistic, theory-based approach to working with families, nurses are uniquely able to exert a positive influence in the lives of older persons and their loved ones by assisting them both physically and psychologically. The challenges, decisions, and transitions faced by many families as they move through later life are also examined in this chapter, as are the many facets of the nurse's role in working with the family to provide care and services to their older members.

Chapter 14

GERONTOLOGICAL FAMILY NURSING

Beverly S. Richards • Mary Luanne Lilly

OUTLINE

OBJECTIVES

On completion of this chapter, the reader will be able to:

- Describe the nature, scope, and goals of gerontological family nursing, including goals and implications for practice.
- Discuss demographic and social trends that are influencing the dynamics and structure of the contemporary older family.
- Describe the normative changes and nonnormative events that challenge today's older families in relation to family functioning and caregiving.
- Demonstrate the use of the family life cycle model and the resiliency model of family stress, adjustment, and adaptation as a basis for assessing the family and for formulating intervention within a family systems framework.
- Provide guidelines and direction for the nurse to develop and maintain a therapeutic alliance with the family.
- Present implications for future research and social policy.

GERONTOLOGICAL FAMILY NURSING PRACTICE

Changing demographic and social trends make it imperative to respond to the complex, growing health care needs of our aging citizens and their families. Families vary greatly in their ethnicity, histories, structures, coping styles, values, resources, living circumstances, and needs. Likewise, older adults as individuals vary in their past life experiences as well as in their current physical, financial, and other living circumstances. The goal of family gerontological nursing is to work in partnership with the family to maintain optimal functioning, restore health, and prevent or reduce the effects of illness in the older members. To accomplish this, the nurse must help families provide care to their older loved ones that promotes the optimal health and functioning of all members, regardless of age. The nurse must use skillful, thoughtful communication to assist family members to define and clarify problems, solve problems, set limits, and clarify boundaries and family roles. Sometimes when the demands of family caring exceed the family's resources and compromise their well-being, the nurse is called on to help the family choose other forms of care. To be successful, the nurse must focus assessment, planning, management, intervention, and evaluation of care on the family as a unit. An extensive background in the biological sciences and the physical aspects of health and illness is important in working with older families because it allows the nurse to monitor physical symptoms and teach family members to carry out medical regimens and nursing care procedures.

Because the types and levels of care needed by older persons vary widely, gerontological family nurses practice in a variety of settings. For example, home health agencies such as visiting nurse services have special programs that provide various levels of care in the elderly person's home. Some general hospitals in urban areas provide follow-up care of older patients after hospitalization for acute illness. Gerontological family nurses also practice in long-term care facilities, mental health centers, inpatient psychiatric units, specialized clinics such as Alzheimer's centers or geriatric institutes, interdisciplinary group practices with primary care physicians, and nurse-managed clinics in the community.

By its very nature, gerontological family nursing challenges the nurse to assume a variety of roles that includes advocate, health care broker, liaison, health teacher, family counselor, consultant, and case manager. Because many conditions and illnesses in the elderly are chronic, the nurse's relationship with a family may extend over time. During periods of greatest need, the nurse may even be viewed as a part of the family.

DEMOGRAPHIC AND SOCIAL TRENDS

The older population—persons 65 years or older—numbered 34.1 million in 1997. They represented 12.7 percent of the U.S. population, about one in every eight Americans. The number of older Americans increased by 2.8 million, or 9.1 percent, since 1990, compared to an increase of 7.0 percent for the under-65 population. The older population itself is getting older. In 1997, the 65- to 74-year-old age group (18.5 million) was eight times larger than in 1900, but the 75- to 84-year-old group (11.7 million) was 16 times larger and the over 85 years group (3.9 million) was 31 times larger (AARP, 1998).

Advances in biomedical science have reduced early deaths from acute diseases and prolonged life for those with chronic conditions like cancer and heart disease. Unfortunately, living longer also brings increased possibilities for debilitating illnesses and conditions, such as Alzheimer's disease, diabetes, arthritis, and stroke. A national survey revealed that four out of five persons 65 years of age have at least one chronic condition, and the incidence of multiple conditions increases with age (Porterfield & St. Pierre, 1992). Because age is commonly accompanied by one or more chronic health problems, an older person can be deprived of independence by limitations in the ability to function and carry out self-care activities. Help may be needed with at least one of the following daily activities: bathing, dressing, transfers, toileting, indoor mobility, and taking medications. Assistance may also be required with household tasks, meal preparation, shopping, transportation, and management of finances.

Many individuals who live to age 85 or older experience a period of dependence and need for care before reaching the end of life (Brody, 1985). These persons are called "frail" or "fragile" elders. More women than men are in need of help, because older women are more likely to be widowed and to live alone, they have less income than elderly men, and they have more chronic health problems, such as arthritis, osteoporosis, and diabetes (AARP, 1998; AARP, 1991).

In spite of these facts, only 5 percent of the population 65 years of age and older live in long-term care facilities. The majority of elderly persons who live in nursing homes are older, female, single, childless, and have multiple health problems. Over 40 percent of nursing home residents have some form of dementia (AHCPR, 1997). It can thus be safely concluded that many older persons with chronic conditions are able to remain in the community with the care and assistance of family and friends.

Over the past few decades, an immense body of research has focused on the nature of family relationships, including the informal caregiving network within the aging family. (See Given & Given, 1991, for a comprehensive review.) Approximately two-thirds (67 percent) of older noninstitutionalized persons (81 percent of older men and 56 percent of older women) live in a family setting. The remaining 32 percent live alone. They represent nearly 42 percent of older women and 16 percent of older men. Also, 8 of 10 noninstitutionalized older persons have at least one living child (AARP, 1991). Two-thirds live within 30 minutes of a child. The majority (66 percent) had at least weekly visits with children and even more (76 percent) had weekly phone conversations. Studies have firmly established that aging is a family affair and elderly members continue as integral parts of their family networks until death (AHCPR, 1997; Aldous 1987; Shanas, 1979; Tennstedt et al, 1993). Reciprocal patterns of intergenerational support and care extend throughout the life cycle of the family, although they tend to shift as the older generation experiences more financial and health problems (Brody, 1985; Kain, 1990; Townsend & Poulshock, 1986).

CAREGIVING IN OLDER FAMILIES

What Is the Extent of Family Caregiving?

The family, not the formal health care system, provides 80 to 90 percent of care to their elderly members, including medical and nursing care, personal services such as transportation, and help with household tasks and shopping (Brody, 1985; Hanley et al, 1991). The family responds to emergencies, provides acute care and assistance, and initiates and maintains links with the formal care system as necessary. Also, the more frail an elderly member becomes, the more responsibility for care the family assumes (Biegel & Blum, 1990; Hanley et al, 1991). Despite this evidence, there is a lingering myth among many nurses that family members, especially adult children, do not provide care for elderly family members when they need it but instead rely on formal services such as nursing homes. In truth, adult children are providing more assistance and more difficult care to their elderly parents than in the "good old days" (Brody, 1985; O'Neill & Sorenson, 1991). Further, the prospective payment system has shortened hospital stays, sending people home "quicker and sicker" and creating more pressure on the family to provide care for which they may be unprepared. Unfortunately, help in the form of community-based support services is sparse, poorly funded, uncoordinated, or absent altogether. This is especially true for families in rural areas (Henderson, 1992; Lee, 1993).

Who Provides the Care?

The support and care given by all family members are usually lumped together under the term "family caregiving." Closer examination reveals, however, that one individual assumes primary responsibility of caregiver, and it usually is given by one member at a time (Tennstedt et al, 1993). When the elderly person is married, the spouse is first in line. Adult children are usually less involved in the care of a married parent, relying instead on the other parent to provide the majority of care. This may work satisfactorily unless the caregiving parent's health is also declining. Unfortunately, many elderly couples do not receive the assistance they need because they hide the seriousness of the difficulties from the rest of the family until a crisis occurs.

When there is no spouse available, the children, usually a daughter or daughter-in-law, assume the caregiving role. If there are no children, another family member, such as a sibling, niece, or nephew, may step in to help provide care. These more distant relatives generally do not provide the intensity of care that spouses or children provide; instead, they serve more as intermediaries to obtain care from formal sources.

Women have always been the traditional caregivers and they continue to provide nearly three-fourths (72 percent) of the family care given to older members. This figure remains constant, even though more women than ever are in the work force (the percentage of working women rose from 38 percent in 1960 to 55 percent in 1987) (Select Committee on Aging, 1987; United Hospital Fund, 1997).

Daughters outnumber sons as caregivers by four to one (Brody, 1990). Also, women provide more hours of care and they are more likely to give assistance with personal hygiene, household tasks, and meal preparation. Men, on the other hand, more typically help with financial management, transportation, and home repairs (Dwyer & Coward, 1991; Stone et al, 1987). Although women provide the bulk of care, the contributions of men should not be overlooked. They frequently provide support and affection to the primary caregiver. Also, many elderly husbands assume the role of primary caregiver if their wives become ill or disabled, meeting both their personal care needs and taking over household tasks.

At What Price is Family Caregiving?

Research findings over the past several decades have consistently pointed to the key role that family relationships play in helping older members maintain their independence and health (Field et al, 1993: Fletcher & Winslow, 1991; Shanas, 1979; Stone et al, 1987), and indeed, the term "family caregiving" has become so common that its meaning is taken for granted. Providing informal assistance to family members is a normative and usual activity throughout life. When does it cross the bounds of what is expected and ordinary and become extraordinary care? Biegel and colleagues (1991) point out that " . . . caring for a family member who has a chronic illness involves a significant expenditure of time and energy over potentially long periods of time, involves tasks that may be unpleasant and uncomfortable, is likely to be nonsymmetrical, and is often a role that had not been anticipated" (p.17). Depending on the type and stage of the illness, the tasks and responsibilities can vary greatly over time.

While family caregiving of elderly members will no doubt continue, researchers have raised questions about the capacity of family caregivers to provide the bulk of long-term care to the elderly (Baille et al, 1988; Brody, 1981, 1985; Brody et al, 1992). Brody (1985) notes that ". . . parent care has become a normative but stressful experience for individuals and families and its nature, scope, and consequences are not yet fully understood" (p.19).

Some of the negative consequences of caring for older loved ones, especially those with dementing illnesses such as Alzheimer's disease have been well documented over time. Those caregivers have been found to be at greater risk for physical and emotional illness, especially depression; greater social isolation and lack of social support; and an increase in financial burdens (Cattanach & Tebes, 1991; Cohen & Eisdorfer, 1988; Cohen et al, 1990; Gallagher et al, 1990; Neundorfer, 1991a, 1991b; United Hospital Fund, 1997).

Research findings also suggest that long-term family care during chronic illness may increase the potential for abuse and neglect among family members (Paveza et al, 1992; Pillemer & Finkelhor, 1988, 1989; Semple, 1992; Williams-Burgess & Kimball, 1990). This includes mistreatment of an elderly ill member and mistreatment of other family members by the ill person. Risk may increase when the elderly person has a dementing illness such as Alzheimer's disease, with reports of 57 to 65 percent of those persons becoming aggressive toward family members at some time (Hamel et al, 1990; Ryden, 1988).

Other Pressures Facing Families

Conflicts between caregiving and other responsibilities can produce tremendous role strain and overload. These conflicts can strain the adult child's relationship with the elderly parent (Sherrell & Newton, 1996). Research findings suggest that the competing demands contribute to the most pervasive consequence of caregiving: emotional stress (George & Gwyther, 1986). Two important sources of caregiver stress are competing familial obligations and conflict with work (Stone et al, 1987). One large study found that many women either quit their jobs or cut their hours to care for their elderly relative (Brody, 1985).

Societal trends influence the structure of contemporary families and thus affect their caregiving capacity. The increasing divorce rate has brought about more single-parent families, most of them headed by working women. Also, the steadily decreasing birth rate since World War II means that as the need for caregivers increases there will be fewer family caregivers available. Many couples are postponing childbearing, which means that in the future they will be providing care to their elderly parents while they are still responsible for dependent children.

The demands on family caregivers are intensified as hospital stays are shorter and care shifts into the community. At the same time, more elders are going to need more long-term care, which is rarely covered by insurance. These trends have created a dilemma for many older families. Faced with the need for expensive long-term care, many elderly couples are forced to "spend down" their assets to qualify for Medical coverage. This may leave the healthier spouse with seriously reduced resources.

The fierce pride that many older people take in their independence and lifelong self-sufficiency means that they try to avoid accepting government assistance at any cost. To protect hard-earned assets, these older persons may attempt to get by, denying their need for formal care until a medical crisis occurs. This can place added stress on the entire family because they may be unaware of the seriousness of an elderly member's health problems until the crisis occurs. This situation can also place unanticipated demands on family members for immediate care and assistance for which they are unprepared.

THEORETICAL PERSPECTIVES

Background

Families are like individuals in that each has a life cycle with predictable developmental stages and changes (see Chapter 2). The changes that families experience over time are like those in a kaleidoscope. The turn of events, whether an accumulation of small changes or the advent of a major stressor, results in the creation of a new pattern from the existing components of family life. While some changes are subtle, others are more dramatic, but the changing patterns unfold progressively and unidirectionally.

Until the occurrence of a stressor event or crisis that demands change, families maintain fairly stable patterns of interaction over time. Events that demand change take two forms: normative and nonnormative. Normative changes or transitions are those expected, somewhat predictable maturational life events, such as marriage, birth of the first child, retirement, and death of a spouse in old age. Although these are expected changes, a period of floundering or crisis may occur until adjustment is achieved. Nonnormative crises, on the other hand, are not predicted or expected and may occur with little warning. Examples include the diagnosis of a serious chronic illness, the accidental death of a family member, a job transfer, the unexpected unemployment of a primary breadwinner, or adult children having to move back home with parents. The suddenness of the event does not allow the family to plan or rehearse options, and there can be considerable family disequillibrium, confusion, and distress until new patterns in roles and responsibilities are established.

Many years ago, Neugarten (1968) pointed out a still-useful insight. He observed that biological and social clocks create a framework for change in both individuals and families alike. As the family grows older, the health status of members may change as a result of natural aging or illness. At the same time, living arrangements, financial concerns, and alliances ebb and flow in response to marriages, deaths, divorces, remarriages, relocations, retirements, and illnesses. Parent-child relationships change as caregiving responsibilities shift. Changes may also result from social and environmental pressures that occur outside the family, such as bad economic times, an increase in crime, or natural disasters.

The ways in which families work together to meet these demands and changes, maintain equilibrium, and meet the needs of members have been studied extensively from the perspective of family systems theory (see Chapter 2). Two system-based models provide a framework for understanding and working effectively with aging families. The first is the family life cycle model, which provides a view of how families change over time (Aldous, 1978; Carter & McGoldrick, 1980; Duvall & Miller, 1985). It points out places in family development where changes in status and roles are likely to occur and it can be useful in predicting many facets of family behavior and vulnerability. The second model is the resiliency model of family stress, adjustment, and adaptation (McCubbin & McCubbin, 1993). This approach to the family is concerned with how families negotiate change and adapt to stressful life events over time, particularly to stressors such as illness. The approach is especially useful because it incorporates the characteristics of the individual members, the family system, and the community, all of which interact to shape the course of family behavior and adaptation. It also stresses the importance of family resilience and the natural healing qualities of family life.

Life Cycle of Older Families

The family's life cycle includes the various stages of development of the family system over time. These stages are convenient divisions that help to study a process that, in real life, flows from one stage to another without a pause or break. The family's life cycle is like a chain, with each stage (link in the chain) beginning in a previous one and coming to fruition in a future one (Duvall & Miller, 1985).

Stages divide the lifetime of a family into distinctive periods that are marked by changes in status and roles. Stages are initiated by critical events that can originate either inside or outside the family system. Internal events in the older family include becoming a couple again after launching the last child, becoming grandparents, experiencing the onset of physical or cognitive incapacity in a spouse or elderly parent, or the death of the spouse. Events originating outside the family may occur in connection with education or work life and include retirement or starting a second career.

As with the development of individuals, each stage requires the completion of certain tasks to move on to the next stage. Duvall and Miller (1985, p. 318) identify eight family developmental tasks of the aging couple:

1. Making satisfying living arrangements as aging progresses
2. Adjusting to retirement income
3. Establishing comfortable routines
4. Safeguarding physical and mental health
5. Maintaining love, sex, and marital relations
6. Remaining in touch with other family members
7. Keeping active and involved
8. Finding meaning in life

As families move from one stage into the next, changes in earlier interaction patterns create changes within the family system. Schumacher and Meleis (1994) identified transitions as a concept central to nursing. Client-nurse contact may occur as a result of individual or family response to situational, developmental, or health status transitions. In an earlier work, Brubaker (1983) identified four common events that initiate significant transitions in the careers of aging families. Each requires family members, either willingly or unwillingly, to participate in negotiating the change. These are

- The empty nest, or launching of children into independence
- Retirement of one or both spouses from employment
- An incapacitating illness that compromises independence or requires institutionalization
- Disruption of the family through death
- Need for relocation or change in living arrangements because of declining health or functional abilities

Assessment of the Life Cycle

The family development model provides a framework from which to assess both existing and potential strengths and vulnerabilities in the family. The results of the assessment can be built into the plan of care using anticipatory guidance, education, and support. In the life cycle of the family, roles, responsibilities, individual developmental tasks, career demands, and resources are rarely synchronized. Therefore, understanding the timing and intersection of internal and external events is crucial in determining family vulnerability. It is especially important to examine critical role transitions within the family—recent, current, or anticipated—because some have greater potential than others for causing stress and vulnerability.

Transitions within older families occur when roles and responsibilities start to shift across the generations. Middle-aged children often find their aging parents coming to them for emotional support, advice, and other forms of help. This may occur at a time when their own children are leaving home, the family's financial resources are stretched to pay for college tuition, and the mother is returning full time to the work force. For the older generation, the changes brought by retirement, possible loss of income, and physical decline may bring fear and trepidation. Reaching out to their children for help is often a disturbing and even humiliating experience. As much as they need the help, they may have great difficulty in asking for it.

As elderly members begin to develop signs of physical or cognitive decline that threaten their independence and capacity for self-care, several things are likely to happen. There may also be a shift in the traditional hierarchical structure as parental authority and influence decline, which brings shifts in roles, responsibilities, and boundaries. Adult children are confronted with the filial crisis, a concept introduced by Blenkner (1965) in an attempt to explain the experience of adult children when parent care becomes necessary. The children are forced to face the fact that their belief that their parents will "be there" forever is a fantasy. Instead of continuing to be the recipient of parental nurturance, they must become the nurturing ones—both to their parents and to the younger generation. Middle-aged children's sense of loss and distress may be intensified because they must admit to their own mortality as their aging parents must acknowledge their decline, need for help, and loss of independence (King et al, 1990).

As the parents' need for care and assistance increases, the adult children, particularly adult daughters, may find themselves caught in the middle between the needs of the older and the younger generation. This group has been described as the sandwich generation (Brody, 1981). These family members are a vulnerable group because as the need to provide care for others increases, the caregivers often neglect their own needs (Bunting 1989).

RESILIENCY MODEL OF STRESS, ADJUSTMENT, AND ADAPTATION

The resiliency model of family stress, adjustment, and adaptation developed by McCubbin and McCubbin (1993) (see Chapter 2) provides a framework for understanding a family's response, adjustment, and finally, adaptation to stress over time. These authors have worked extensively with families responding to a loved one's chronic illness or condition. Their framework is useful for understanding the demands and challenges that older families experience and allows for assessment and intervention at many points to promote adaptation. The resiliency model evolved from Hill's (1958) earlier formulation of family vulnerability to crisis events and the subsequent development of the double ABCX family stress and adaptation model developed by McCubbin and Patterson (1983). The model is oriented toward adaptation, which is its central concept. Adaptation is the outcome of family efforts to bring a new level of balance, harmony, coherence, and functioning to a family crisis situation over time.

The model includes a number of interacting components that influence successful or unsuccessful family adjustment. These are illustrated in Figure 14–1. The stressor (A) and its severity interact with the family's vulnerability (V). Vulnerability is influenced by the pileup, or number and timing, of other family stresses, transitions, and strains that occur along with the main stressor. Family vulnerability interacts with the family typology (T), that is, the patterns of family interaction that have been established over time. These components then interact with the family's resistance resources (B) and, in turn, interact with the family appraisal (C) of the stressor. Their appraisal interacts with the family's problem-solving and coping strategies (PSC) (McCubbin & McCubbin, 1993). All of these components work together to influence the family's adjustment.

The Stressor and Its Severity

"A stressor is a demand placed on the family that produces, or has the potential of producing, changes in the family system" (McCubbin & McCubbin, 1993, p. 28). The event or demand can influence many aspects of family life including health, roles and responsibilities, and boundaries. Severity is determined by the degree to which the stressor threatens the stability of the family. In many older families, the stressor event is the onset, or recognition through diagnosis, of the deterioration in health of an older member.

Family Vulnerability: Pileup and Life-Cycle Changes

Vulnerability is the degree of fragility in the interpersonal and organizational state of the family. It is influenced by the number of normative changes in the family's life cycle and by the accumulation or pileup of demands from inside or outside the family. The model outlines six categories of stresses and strains that contribute to a pileup of demands as a family attempts to adapt to a stressor such as illness.

1. The illness and related hardships over time
2. Normative transitions in individual family members and the family as a whole
3. Prior family strains accumulated over time
4. Situational demands and contextual difficulties
5. The consequences of family efforts to cope

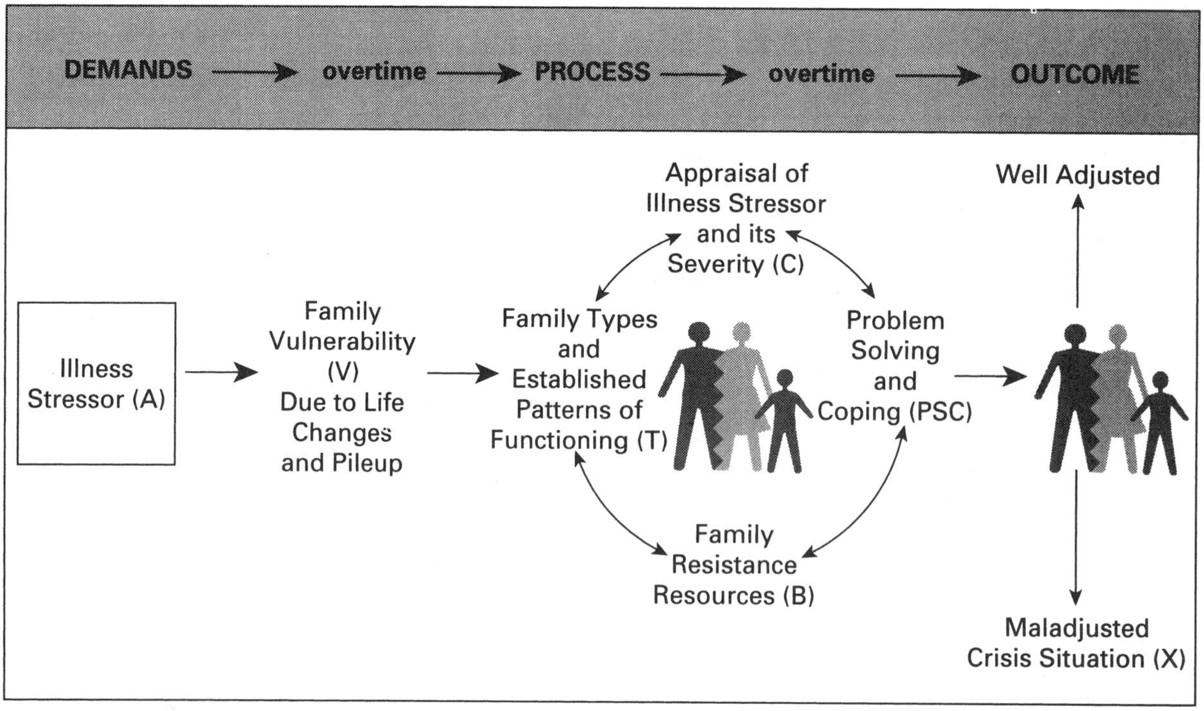

FIGURE 14-1
Adjustment phase of the resiliency model of family stress, adjustment, and adaptation. (From Danielson, C.B., Hamel-Bissell, B., and Winston-Frey, P.: *Families, Health, and Illness: Perspectives on Coping and Interventions.* C.V. Mosby, St. Louis, 1993, p. 67, with permission.)

6. Intrafamilial and social ambiguity that provides inadequate guidelines on how families should act or cope effectively (McCubbin & McCubbin, 1993, p. 37)

Specific demands might include economic stress due to poor health, heavy health care expenses, need to relocate, death of a member, or adult children leaving or returning home.

Family Types: Family-Established Patterns of Functioning

The family type is characterized by fairly stable, observable patterns of functioning. Two family attributes that are important in helping families manage chronic illness are a moderate degree of cohesion and flexibility. These facilitate a spirit of cooperation, open communication, and negotiation as change becomes necessary.

Family Resistance Resources: Capabilities and Strengths

Resistance resources are capabilities and strengths that enable the family to manage the stressor and prevent major upheaval in their functioning. The following critical family resources have been identified by McCubbin and McCubbin (1993): economic stability, cohesiveness, flexibility, hardiness, shared spiritual beliefs, open communication, traditions, celebrations, routines, and organization.

Resources outside the family are also important to adaptation. These include the family's social support network of friends and neighbors, as well as community-based agencies such as day-care centers, respite programs, and self-help groups. Social support serves to protect and insulate the family from the effects of stress and promotes recovery from crisis. The elders, especially the very old elders, or those without available family, may have a limited social support network because of poor health, restricted mobility, limited finances, deaths of friends, and lack of transportation.

Family Appraisal of the Stressor

Appraisal includes the family's perceptions and definition of the stressor and its accompanying hardships, as well as the family's perceptions of their available resources and the actions needed to meet the demands and regain family balance. If family members perceive the situation as hopeless or beyond their ability to manage, they may not be able to recognize and use available resources or seek additional resources. Therefore, they will be at high risk for maladapation. On the other hand, if they can accept the situation and see it as a challenge they can deal with, they are more likely to engage in constructive efforts to manage the situation.

Family Problem Solving and Coping

The model includes a consideration of the problem-solving skills and coping strategies the family uses to manage the demands created by the stressor. Steps in the problem-solving process include: (1) organizing the stressor into manageable components, (2) identifying alternative management strategies, and (3) taking steps to resolve the problem. Coping includes family patterns and a wide range of efforts to maintain and strengthen the family, obtain family and community resources, and attend to the well-being and developmental needs of family members.

Family Response: Stress and Distress

When a stressor occurs that necessitates family management or change, it causes tension in the family. If this tension is not resolved or at least brought within manageable limits, it becomes stress. Stress occurs when there is a perceived imbalance between the demands on the family and its resources and capabilities. If balance is not restored, family distress may occur and the stress can even threaten the stability and integrity of the family system.

Together, the family life cycle model and the resiliency model of family stress, adjustment, and adaptation provide a comprehensive framework for assessing the aging family's strengths and areas of vulnerability in times of stress and change. This is a crucial aspect of assisting families to adapt positively to their changing lives.

PRACTICE CONSIDERATIONS

Relational and Emotional Considerations

The role of the gerontological family nurse includes teaching, giving advice, providing encouragement and support, and advocating for the family within the health care delivery system. The first step is to establish a therapeutic alliance with the elderly members and the rest of their family. To do this successfully, it is necessary to view the family as a system, not as individual victims who need to be rescued. It is important to recognize that adult children often experience powerful feelings of abandonment, anger, and guilt when their parents' health fails. These emotions may alternate with denial of the seriousness of the health problems. Older spouses may also experience these feelings, especially when the healthier spouse has always been dependent on the person who is declining; frequently, it is the nurse in the home, hospital, or clinic who first notices the frustration and tension in family caregivers. The family's negative or angry feelings may be temporarily displaced onto the nurse or other professional caregivers and mistakenly interpreted as hostility or treatment resistance. In reality, these feelings are a natural response to a tragic, sad, irreversible situation (King et al, 1990). It is often helpful at this point to explain to the family that these are normal reactions and help them explore their perceptions of the situation and its meaning for them. In situations that involve long-term caregiving, it may be useful to refer family members to support groups or to teach them stress management techniques (Dellasega, 1990).

Cultural Considerations

Families may differ culturally, ethnically, and racially from the personal identity of the gerontological family nurse. Culture refers to "a group's way of life: the values, beliefs, traditions, symbols, language, and social organization that become meaningful to group members" (Aranda & Knight, 1997, p. 342). Ethnicity refers to "groups whose members share a common social and cultural heritage passed on to each successive generation" (Giger & Davidhizar, 1995, p. 63). An essential characteristic of ethnicity is a shared sense of identity or peoplehood (Aranda & Knight; Giger & Davidhizar). Race refers to "biological grouping within the human species, distinguished or classified according to genetically transmitted differences" (Encyclopaedia Britannica, 1995). Research on the influence of culture, ethnicity, and race on the process and outcomes of family caregiving is in the early stages. It is likely that these variables influence multiple aspects of caregiving. However, other variables, such as socioeconomic status, educational level, and historical experience, may have equal or greater influence on the process and outcomes of family care (Aranda & Knight, 1997; Connell & Gibson, 1997). Therefore, it is important for the gerontological family nurse to assess for, but not assume the influence of, these variables on individuals and family caregivers.

In addition to working with families, nurses belong to families. Working intensively with families who are under stress has the potential to evoke powerful feelings in the nurse. Awareness of the beliefs, values, and practices of the nurse's own family, along with its accompanying emotional challenges, can help the nurse understand the client family's responses to the decisions and changes they are facing. Sometimes health professionals stereotype or show bias toward families that do not share their personal values and views of effective family functioning (Danielson et al, 1993). Stereotype or bias may be present in spite of efforts to include diversity content in the educational process, particularly if such content is applied indiscriminantly to individuals identified as belonging to a particular cultural or ethnic group. To avoid bias, it is crucial that the nurse be open and sensitive to the family's beliefs, values, and practices in relation to health and family functioning. In addition, it is important to recognize the great diversity within the various groups (e.g., Hispanic Americans may be of Cuban, Puerto Rican, or Mexican origin) as well as between groups (e.g., Hispanic, Caucasian, African, or Asian American). It is imperative to recognize the similarities inherent in the shared experience of the human condition. Families must never be stereotyped: each family is unique and families vary widely even within identified ethnic and racial groups.

Goals and Intervention Strategies

Health Promotion and Disease Prevention

One of the challenges of gerontological family nursing is incorporating both health promotion and disease prevention strategies along with participating in the monitoring and management of acute and chronic illness. The twentieth century has seen an impressive increase in life expectancy for elders because of advances in health care (e.g., improved control of hypertension) and alterations in health behaviors (e.g., smoking cessation, dietary modification). Elders in the twenty-first century will have even greater opportunities to benefit from research-based information on maintaining health and avoiding illness and disability (Rubenstein, 1996–97). The gerontological family nurse is in a key position to inform and influence the health-related interactions and behaviors of elders and family members.

Currently, the leading causes of death among the elderly include cardiovascular disease, cancer, stroke, respiratory disease, falls and other accidents, diabetes, renal disease, and hepatic disease. Major chronic conditions include arthritis, dental disease, high blood pressure, cardiac disease, vision problems, osteoporosis, hearing problems, depressive disorders, diseases of the vascular system and activities of daily living (ADL) and instrumental activities of daily living (IADL) dependencies (American Association for World Health, 1999; Rubenstein, 1996–97).

Most causes of mortality and morbidity are amenable to primary or secondary preventive interventions. Primary interventions aim to prevent the onset of illness; secondary interventions aim to detect disease before the appearance of symptoms (Rubenstein, 1996–97). Examples of primary interventions include influenza immunizations, regular dental exams, regular physical activity, avoidance of tobacco and excessive alcohol use, avoidance of excessive sun exposure, elimination of environmental hazards, maintenance of a nutritionally adequate diet and maintenance of prosthetic devices (e.g., hearing aids, glasses, dentures). Examples of secondary interventions include screening and early intervention for cancer, elevated blood pressure, cholesterol, and blood sugar. Secondary preventive interventions also include screening, treatment, and referral for depression, dementia, and functional loss in elderly individuals (American Association for World Health, 1999; Rubenstein, 1996–97).

Research indicates that primary and secondary preventive practices can greatly improve the health status of elderly individuals and add to the quality of life for elders and involved family members. Recommendations, interventions, referrals, and follow-up should be research-based, systematic, and proceed from a thorough history and physical, hopefully with the participation of elders, family, and the interdisciplinary treatment team. To increase elder participation in and compliance with health promotion and illness prevention strategies, it is imperative that gerontological family nurses be up to date and proactive in providing information, education, intervention, and referral to elders and their families.

Acute and Chronic Illness

The initial contact with the older person frequently occurs when help is sought for an acute or worsening health problem. Following the medical evaluation, the family nurse should set up a conference that includes the patient and all other family members who may be involved in providing care and assistance. The physician and other members of the health care team, such as the social worker, visiting nurse, and physical therapist, are to be included as needed. The first step is to establish a working partnership with the family so that they are comfortable in expressing their feelings, ideas, and concerns. The goal is to provide support and information, and also to help them set realistic goals by clarifying what needs to be done, establishing a plan of action, and determining the best way to carry it out.

Start by obtaining a picture of the family using the concepts from the family life cycle model and resiliency model of family stress, adjustment, and adaptation described earlier. First explore their perceptions of the current stressor: the elderly member's illness or condition. Do they understand the diagnosis? What do they believe that it will mean in terms of changes or demands on the family? How are they defining the situation in relation to themselves, to a spouse, or to a parent? What resources are available to them personally, within the family, and in the community? How do they perceive those resources? What other stressful events and transitions are occurring, for example, health problems, job stress, or other family disruptions? How have they coped with other stressful events or periods in the past? Did they pull together (cohesion) and make adjustments (flexibility) or did they freeze and pull apart?

Next, the family's priorities, both as individuals and as a group, should be brought into the open and discussed. Priorities include both what they hope to accomplish in their elderly member's care as well as their individual personal goals. Financial concerns, time constraints, and generational responsibilities should be discussed openly. The elderly member's wishes, priorities, and expectations must be included for a plan to be successful.

The next step is to help the family establish caregiving goals that are realistic and acceptable (Kashner et al, 1990). Some elderly members' desire to remain in their own home may be so strong that rather than leave, they would accept mediocre care or no care at all. They may also have an unspoken expectation that the adult children will "pitch in" and help. This may create increasing tension and stress in the family because the adult children, while wanting their loved one to have the best care possible, may be unaware of this expectation or be unable to deliver the assistance needed because of other demands.

It may also be helpful to inquire whether any family members have ever promised the elderly member that "I will never put you in a nursing home. I will always take care of you, no matter what happens." Many family members, especially wives and daughters, make this well-meaning but unrealistic commitment either under duress, as a result of guilt or denial, or as a form of reassurance to an aging relative. It can, however, have a profoundly negative effect on the family when they face difficult caregiving decisions. Through open, guided discussion, the nurse can help them see the situation realistically so that they can face appropriate alternatives when necessary.

After all family members have had an opportunity to express their priorities and goals for caregiving, role clarification needs to occur. At this point, the nurse should help the family evaluate how they plan to work together to meet not only the needs of the elderly member, but also those of the other members; the effects of the illness require inevitable role and structural changes in the family. The day-to-day care expectations should be made explicit, including the responsibilities of individual members and the plan for emergencies and other contingencies, such as illness or vacations.

Whatever their role in caregiving, all family members should be taught about the illness or condition, including the actual caregiving activities and the resources required. Then both the designated caregiver and those less directly involved in day-to-day care will know the actual requirements for care and the resources necessary. This can prevent conflict and misunderstanding between family members at a later time.

The nurse must ensure that decisions are made with the full participation of the elderly person whenever possible, even if the person has an early dementing disorder. It is also necessary to help the family coordinate their caregiving activities over time. The nurse can lay the groundwork for formal assistance by connecting the family with appropriate community resources, such as adult day care, respite care, in-home health services, support groups, and family workshops or classes.

It is highly desirable, whenever possible, to visit the elderly person at home with family caregivers present. This is a useful strategy because visiting on family's "turf" tends to strengthen the nurse's therapeutic alliance with the family; at the same time, it is possible to see their usual patterns of interaction and evaluate the home in terms of safety and available resources.

Legal counsel is an important aspect of caregiving that is often overlooked until a crisis occurs. Not only do families need to know about the benefits of their elderly members, including health care insurance, Medicare, pensions, and social security, but they also need to know about advance directives, living wills, health care representatives, and estate planning. With elders who have progressive dementing disorders, it is particularly important to plan for the time when the person is no longer competent to handle legal or financial matters. Many families are hesitant to discuss these matters and need encouragement and assistance to do so. Yet, such planning assures that the elderly person's wishes are known and honored and may prevent later family guesswork, hassles, and conflicts.

The older members' spiritual needs must not be overlooked (Reed, 1991). Religious affiliation and spiritual beliefs have an important place in many older persons' lives. Also, the church, parish, synagogue, or temple is often a great source of formal and informal support to its elderly members.

SOCIAL POLICY CONSIDERATIONS

Given current social and demographic trends, it is certain that the future will bring increasing demands for family caregiving of elderly members. At a time when biomedical breakthroughs are succeeding in slowing or halting chronic conditions, managed care is shifting more care into the community and placing even greater responsibility for care on family members. The difficulty of caring for an elderly family member is compounded by economic pressures and additional demands at work and at home. While elderly husbands and wives care for one another as long as possible, this responsibility is often assumed by an adult daughter or daughter-in-law when one parent dies or either of them becomes disabled (Stone et al, 1987). The strain experienced by these adult daughter caregivers has been well documented (Brody, 1990).

As the population continues to age, more adult daughters will be widowed or divorced. This is because women outlive men and also tend to have a lower remarriage rate than men after divorce or death of their husbands. Recently, caregiving daughters without husbands have been shown to be at higher risk for mental health problems than those with husbands. They are also less well off economically than their married sisters (Brody et al, 1992). The Family Leave Act will not solve the dilemma of caregivers who cannot afford to take leaves without pay. For such families a tax credit similar to the Child and Dependent Care Tax Credit should be explored (Stone et al, 1987).

The vulnerability of the growing group of caregivers must be addressed. Failure to do so will result in increased mental and physical health problems for overburdened family members, and ultimately, increased costs to society. The informal family caring system is a national resource that must be protected and supported, not overwhelmed. No institution can replace the support and care given by family members; rather, elderly persons' needs for care are best served by a combination of formal and informal services. This requires the development of affordable support services in the community that supplement family caregiving, such as respite care, homemaker services, adult day care centers, and neighborhood wellness clinics. The challenge is to provide appropriate, accessible forms of tangible assistance with caregiving and not simply view family members as unpaid workers who need to be "cheered on" in their caregiving work (Brody, 1985; United Hospital Fund, 1997).

IMPLICATIONS FOR FUTURE RESEARCH

The challenges facing the aging family are complex. To meet the needs of our noninstitutionalized elderly, we need answers to many questions. For example, what functions do formal and informal care systems perform best? What balance of formal and informal services is needed to meet the care needs of the elderly? How can caregivers balance competing family and work demands, and what interventions are effective in reducing caregiver distress (Knight et al, 1993)? Only recently has it been recognized that abuse and violence are serious problems in older caregiving families. What are the factors that contribute to the aggression and violence, and under what conditions do they occur?

Studies of interventions for elders with various illnesses and chronic conditions need to be conducted with family caregivers in the home, to test the effectiveness of approaches to specific care situations. Finally, further research is needed to determine the best ways to reach older families of various ethnic and racial backgrounds and develop care options that they will accept.

SUMMARY

Family members are concerned and involved in the care of their elderly. The current health services system, where care is directed toward the individual, falls short in the provision of and payment for services designed to assist families providing care and assistance to their elderly members. Nevertheless, the gerontological family nurse is likely to encounter families in situational, developmental, and health-related crises and transitions, and in need of assistance. The nurse's ability to recognize the family as a potential ally will guide the depth and breadth of her or his assessment, evaluation, and intervention strategies. Likewise, recognition of the potential negative consequences of family participation in elder care will prompt the nurse to provide anticipatory counseling, guidance, and referrals for family members involved in emotionally and physically taxing situations. It is important to approach elderly individuals and their families using a holistic, theory-based approach if the gerontological family nurse is to exert a positive influence on their health and well-being.

Our society is aging rapidly. While this demographic shift is influencing every institution in our society, none are more affected than the family and health care. With increasing longevity, there is an increase in chronic, incapacitating conditions. At the same time, as efforts to contain health care costs intensify, more and more responsibility for care and assistance is being shifted into the community. The family is the single most important resource to elderly persons, but the burdens of responsibility for caregiving are compounded by increasing demands at work and home. Some family researchers have raised questions about the family's capacity to continue to assume increasing responsibility for informal care. Gerontological family nurses are in an excellent position to understand the challenges facing older families, the dynamics of family caregiving, and the stress it produces; they can work with the families to lighten their load. To do so, however, the nurse must build an effective partnership with the family to maximize their capabilities, minimize their vulnerabilities, and serve as a bridge to the formal care system.

RESEARCH BRIEF

Sample and Setting

The sample consisted of 245 community-based dementia caregivers in 4 states: Iowa, Minnesota, Indiana, and Arizona.

Methodology

This was a 4-year, longitudinal, quasi-experimental design, aimed at testing a theory-based, psychoeducational intervention.

Findings

Caregivers in the treatment group experienced improved outcomes in mood, distress over care recipient's problem behaviors, decreased burden related to caregiving, and increased satisfaction and mastery related to caregiving compared with controls.

Implications

Nurses can have a positive impact on caregiving outcomes using a theory-based, psychoeducational intervention in the community setting.

Source: Buckwalter, et al. (2000). Family caregiver home training based on the progressively lowered stress threshold model. Sigma Theta Tau Monograph on Aging.

Case Study

THE JOHNSONS

Mary Johnson lives in the family home, where she and her husband James raised their three children. Mary is a 72-year-old woman and has been living alone since the death of James, 10 years earlier. Thanks to a small pension from James' retirement, along with Mary's social security pension, Mary has been able to live comfortably but not extravagantly through careful management of her resources. Mary has led an active life, walking daily, babysitting for grandchildren, teaching in Sunday school, participating in the church Ladies' Club, and volunteering at the neighborhood Senior Center. Mary has a close relationship with her three daughters and their families and enjoys regular, if not daily, contact. In the past few years, Mary's daughters have expressed concerns about the changing character of the neighborhood. Many of Mary's friends and neighbors have either died or moved away.

Recently Mary was taken to the hospital emergency room after a fall at church. Mary became dizzy and then "blacked out"; she sustained a broken wrist and evulsion wound to her right shin. Mary's condition was stabilized and she was transferred to a transitional care unit for rehabilitation. Mary made good progress in her recovery; discharge is anticipated within the week.

Mary is adamant about returning to the family home when discharged. She recognizes that she will need continued assistance and is concerned about burdening her daughters and their families with her care. Discharge planning is complicated by the following factors: (a) Mary will need some assistance with activities of daily living (ADLs) and instrumental activities of daily living (IADLs) for at least 6 weeks, (b) special wound care is necessary because of Mary's diabetes and impaired circulation, (c) Mary's bedroom and bath are on the second floor—there is a half bath on the first floor, and (d) although Mary's daughters live within a 10-minute drive, they work full time and have teenage children involved in numerous school and extracurricular activities. A family conference is scheduled by Mary's primary nurse to plan for her care after discharge.

Discussion This case illustrates how a nonnormative change in a parent's health status can create disequilibrium in a previously smoothly functioning family system. Mary, her daughters, and the gerontological family nurse must negotiate the complicating factors to allow Mary to return to the family home. The negotiation process will entail determination of family members' appraisal of the situation and an assessment of resources available to manage the situation. Information gathering about the family's typical problem-solving skills and coping strategies is a critical component of the gerontological nurse's database. Immediate and long term planning will be necessary to ensure that Mary's health status remains stable and her living situation satisfactory to all involved.

The gerontological family nurse helps the family identify, coordinate, and use all their available resources to facilitate continuing family functioning and adaptation.

The short term plan developed during the family conference included: (a) daily visits by a home health aid to assist with activities of daily living, (b) Mary's daughters are to assist with instrumental activities of daily living (IADLs) in the evening and on weekends, (c) biweekly visits by a home health nurse to assess wound healing and diabetes management, (d) the Ladies' Club is to provide a daily lunch and visit, and (e) the grandchildren and spouses are to call after school and help with yard work and household chores.

Although this plan was satisfactory in meeting Mary's short-term convalescence needs, Mary and her daughters agreed that Mary's oldest daughter and high school-aged son would move in with Mary. This decision was influenced by the following considerations: (a) Mary suffered from residual disability from her wrist fracture, (b) she needed careful dietary and medication management to prevent complications from the diabetes, and (c) Mary could no longer rely on the immediate response of close and trusted neighbors.

To implement this new plan, Mary's daughters arranged for a shower to be added to the downstairs bathroom. The family room was converted to a bedroom for Mary. Mary's oldest daughter and her son occupied the bedrooms on the second floor. This arrangement allows for the privacy of all household members and accommodates Mary's wish to stay in the family home.

Fortunately, this family seemed to have little difficulty working through the short-term and long-term demands resulting from Mary's accident. However, the nurse must realize that this is the beginning, not the end of the Johnsons' story. Mary's accident served as a wake-up call for her daughters, reminding them of Mary's age and the possibility of gradual or abrupt changes in her health status and level of independence. Redefining and renegotiating both family roles and responsibilities and patterns of communication while maintaining multi-generational responsibilities will be a challenge for all family members. Mary's oldest daughter, her son, and Mary will have to adjust to their new living arrangement. Mary's daughters plan to share the additional filial responsibilities, the increased dependence of Mary, and their own family transitions. The grandchildren will also be affected by the changes. This family has resources to help them adjust and make changes: strong family bonds, adequate financial resources, and flexibility. The gerontological family nurse needs the knowledge and skills necessary to assist them with these adjustments and to facilitate their adaptation over time.

Study Questions

1. Which of the following statements are true?
   a. Adult children should be discouraged from talking to their elderly parents about their benefits and finances.
   b. Older families, like older people, seem more alike than different.
   c. Families provide the bulk of health care to older people.
   d. Sons and daughters share the care of elderly parents equally.
2. List and describe three common, normative events that can trigger significant transitions in older families.
3. Social support outside the family is important in helping older individuals remain independent and functioning in the community. Name four factors or conditions that may hinder or limit the availability of social support.
4. A major goal of gerontological family nursing is:
   a. To help the family system restore and maintain the functioning and health of its older members.
   b. To assist the family in making health care placement decisions for its older members.
   c. To set appropriate caregiving goals for the family.
   d. To help the family avoid the need for institutionalization of elderly members.
5. List and discuss three potential stressors that are commonly experienced by the "sandwich generation." How might these affect their coping and adaptation to a decline in health of aging parents?
6. Which of the following are true statements?
   a. Most older persons tend to rely heavily on the formal health care system to meet their needs.
   b. The formal health care system is set up to meet the needs of the family.
   c. Older people tend to rely on family assistance and "make do" until a crisis occurs.
   d. Families caring for an elderly member with a dementing illness are at greater risk for poor health and elder mistreatment.
7. Which of the following statements are true?
   a. Chapters and articles which describe the unique characteristics of various cultural and ethnic groups provide universally accurate information about individuals and families.
   b. Variability within cultural groups may be as great as variability between cultural groups.
   c. The inclusion of diversity content in the nursing curriculum eliminates the problems of stereotyping and bias in nursing assessments.

References

American Association of Retired Persons (AARP), Administration on Aging (AOA). (1998). Profile of older Americans: 1998. http://www.aoa.dhhs.gov/aoa/stats/profile/#older

AARP. (1991). A profile of older Americans. Washington, DC: AARP and AOA.

Agency for Health Care Policy and Research (AHCPR). (1997). AHCPR Research on Long-term Care. Rockville, MD: AHCPR.

Aldous, J. (1978). *Family Careers. Developmental Change in Families.* New York: John Wiley & Sons.

Aldous, J. (1987). New views on the family life of the elderly and the near-elderly. *Journal of Marriage and the Family, 49*:277–234.

American Association for World Health. (1999). *Healthy aging, healthy living: Start now!* Washington, DC: Author.

Aranda, M., & Knight, B. (1997). The influence of ethnicity and culture on the caregiver stress and coping process: A sociocultural review and analysis. *Gerontologist, 37*:355–364.

Baille, V., et al. (1988). Stress, social support, and psychological distress of family caregivers of the elderly. *Nursing Research, 37*:217–222.

Biegel, D. E., & Blum, A. (1990). *Aging and Caregiving: Theory, Research, and Policy*. Newbury Park, CA: Sage.

Biegel, D., et al. (1991). *Family caregiving in chronic illness.* Newbury Park, CA: Sage.

Blenkner, M. (1965). Social work and family relationships in later life with some thoughts on filial maturity. In E. Shanas & G. J. Streib (Eds.) *Social Structure and the Family: Generational Relations*. Englewood Cliffs, NJ: Prentice-Hall.

Brody, E. M. (1981).Women in the middle and family help to older people. *Gerontologist, 25*:19–29.

Brody, E. M. (1985). Parent care as a normative family stress. *Gerontologist, 25*:19–29.

Brody, E. M. (1990). *Women in the Middle: Their Parent Care Years*. New York: Springer.

Brody, E. M., et al. (1992). Differential effects of daughters' marital status on their parent care experiences. *Gerontologist, 32*:58–67.

Brubaker, T. H. (Ed.) (1983). *Family Relationships in Later Life*. Newbury Park, CA: Sage.

Buckwalter, K.C.; Gerdner, L.A.; Hall, G.R; Kelly, A.; Kohont, F.; Richards, B.S.; and Sime, M. (2000) in Gerontological Nursing Issues for the 21st Century. Indianapolis, IN: Center Nursing Press: a Division of Sigma Theta Tau International.

Bunting, S. (1989). Stress on caregivers of the elderly. *Advances in Nursing Science, 11*:63–73.

Carter, G. A., & McGoldrick, M. (1980). *The Family Lifecycle: A Framework for Family Therapy*. New York: Family Press.

Cattanach, L., & Tebes, J. K. (1991). The nature of elder impairment and its impact on family caregivers' health and psychosocial functioning. *Gerontologist, 31*:246–255.

Cohen, D., & Eisdorfer, C. (1988). Depression in a family member caring for a relative with Alzheimer's disease. *Journal of tbe American Geriatric Society, 36*:885–889.

Cohen, D., et al. (1990). Caring for relatives with Alzheimer's disease: The mental health risks to spouses, adults, children and other family caregivers. *Behavior, Health, and Aging, 1*:171–182.

Connell, C., & Gibson, G. (1997). Racial, ethnic and cultural differences in dementia caregiving: Review and analysis. *Gerontologist, 37*:355–364.

Danielson, C. B., et al. (Eds.). (1993). *Families, Health, and Illness: Perspectives on Coping and Interventions*. St. Louis, MO: C. V. Mosby.

Dellasega, C. (1990). Coping with caregiving: Stress management for caregivers of the elderly. *Journal of Psychosocial Nursing, 28*:15–22.

Duvall, E.M., & Miller, B.C. (1985). *Marriage and Family Development*, ed 6. New York: Harper & Row.

Dwyer, J. W., & Coward, R. T. (1991). A multivariate comparison of the involvement of adult sons versus daughters in the care of impaired parents. *Journal of Gerontology, 46*:S259–269.

The New Encylclopaedia Brittanica. (1995, vol 9, p. 876). Chicago: Encyclopaedia Brittanica.

Field, D., et al. (1993). The influence of health on family contacts and family feelings in advanced old age: A longitudinal study journal of gerontology. *Psychosocial Sciences, 48*:8–28.

Fletcher, K.R., & Winslow, S.A. (1991). Informal caregivers: A composite and review of needs and community resources. *Family Community Health, 14*(2):59–67.

Gallagher, D., et al. (1990). Depression and other negative affects in family caregivers. In E. Light & D. Lebwitz (Eds.) *Alzheimer's Disease Treatment and Family Stress: Directions for Research*, (pp. 218–244). New York: Hemisphere.

George, L. K., & Gwyther, L. P. (1986). Caregiver well-being: A multidimensional examination of family caregivers of demented adults. *Gerontologist, 26*:259–259.

Giger, J., & Davidhizar, R. (1995). *Transcultural Nursing.* St. Louis: Mosby.

Given, B. A., & Given, C. W. (1991). Family caregivers for the elderly. In J. J. Fitzpatrick, et al. (Eds.). *Annual Review of Nursing Research*, Vol. 9, (pp. 77–101). New York: Springer.

Hamel, M., et al. (1990). Predictors and consequences of aggressive behavior by community-based dementia patients. *Gerontologist, 30*:206–211.

Hanley, R., et al. (1991). Will paid home care erode informal support? *Journal of Health Politics, Policy, and Law, 16*:507–521.

Henderson, M.C. (1992). Families in transition: Caring for the rural elderly. *Family Community Health, 14*(4): 61–70.

Hill, R. (1958). Generic features of families under stress. *Social Casework, 49*:139–150.

Kain, J. (1990). *The Myth of Family Decline*. New York: W.W. Norton.

Kashner, T M., et al. (1990). Family size and caregiving of aged patients with hip fractures. In D. E. Biegel & A. Blum (Eds.). *Aging and Caregiving: Theory, Research, and Policy* (pp. 184–203). Newbury Park, CA: Sage.

King, D.A., et al. (1990). Families of cognitively impaired elders: Helping adult children confront the official crisis. *Clinical Gerontologist, 10*:3–15.

Knight, B. G., et al. (1993). A meta-analytic review of interventions for caregiver distress: Recommendations for future research. *Gerontologist, 33*:240–248.

Lee, H. J. (1993). Health perceptions of middle, "new

middle," and older rural adults. *Family Community Health, 16*:19–27.

McCubbin, H. I., & McCubbin, M.A. (1993). Families coping with illness: The resiliency model of family stress, adjustment, and adaptation. In C. B. Danielson, et al. (Eds.), *Families, Health and Illness: Perspectives on Coping and Intervention* (pp. 21–63). St. Louis: C.V. Mosby.

McCubbin, H. I., & Patterson, J. M. (1983). Family Transitions: Adaptation to Stress. In McCubbin & C. R. Figley (Eds.), *Stress and the Family*, Vol 1, Coping with Normative Transitions (pp. 5–25). New York: Brunner/Mazel.

Neugarten, B. L. (1968). Adult personality: toward a psychology of the life cycle. In B. L. Neugarten (Ed.), *Middle Age and Aging* (pp. 137–147). Chicago: University of Chicago Press.

Neundorfer, M. M. (199la). Coping and health outcomes in spouse caregivers of persons with dementia. *Nursing Research, 40*:261–265.

Neundorfer, M. M. (1991b). Family caregivers of the frail elderly: Impact of caregiving on their health and implications for interventions. *Family Community Health, 14*:48–58.

O'Neill, C., & Sorenson, E. S. (1991). Home care of the elderly: A family perspective. *Advances in Nursing Science, 13*(4):28–37.

Paveza, G. J., et al. (1992). Severe family violence and Alzheimer's disease: Prevalence and risk factors. *Gerontologist, 32*:493–497.

Pillemer, K., & Finkelhor, D. (1988). The prevalence of elder abuse: A random sample survey. *Gerontologist, 28*:51–57.

Pillemer, K., & Finkelhor, D. (1989). Causes of elder abuse: Caregiver stress versus problem relatives. *American Journal of Orthopsychiatry, 59*:179–187.

Porterfield, J. D., & St. Pierre, R. (1992). *Healthful aging*. Guitford, CT: Dushkin Publishing Group.

Reed, P. G. (1991). Self transcendence and mental health in the oldest-old adult. *Nursing Research, 2*(1): 43–163.

Rubenstein, L. (1996–97). Update on preventative medicine for older people. *Generations*, (Winter):47–53.

Ryden, M. (1988). Aggressive behavior in persons with dementia living in the community. *Alzbeimer's Disease and Associated Disorders International Journal, 2*(4):342–355.

Schumacher, K., & Meleis, A. (1994). Transitions: A central concept in nursing. *Image: Journal of Nursing Scholarship, 26*:119–127.

Select Committee on Aging, U.S. House of Representatives. (1987). Exploding the myths: Caregiving in America. Committee Publication No. 99-61 I. Washington, DC: U.S. Government Printing Office.

Semple, S. H. (1992). Conflict in Alzheimer's caregiving families: Its dimensions and consequences. *Gerontologist, 32*: 648–655.

Shanas, E. (1979). The family as a social support system in old age. *Gerontologist, 19*:3–9.

Sherrell, K., & Newton, N. (1996). Parent care as a developmental task. Families in Society: *The Journal of Contemporary Human Services,* ___:174–181.

Stone, R., et al. (1987). Caregivers of the frail elderly: A national profile. *Gerontologist, 27*:616–626.

Tennstedt, S., et al. (1993). Is family care on the decline? A longitudinal investigation of the substitution of formal long-term care services for informal care. *The Millbank Quarterly, 71*:601–624.

Townsend, A. L., & Poulshock, S. W. (1986). Intergenerational perspectives on impaired elders' support networks. *Journal of Gerontology, 41*:101–109.

United Hospital Fund. (1997). Initiatives: Facts about family caregiving. http://www.uhfnyc.org/initiat/fhcpfaq.htm

Williams-Burgess, C., & Kimball, M.J. (1990).The neglected elder: A family systems approach. *Journal of Psychosocial Nursing, 30*(10):21–25.

Additional Bibliography

Archbold, P. G. (1983).The impact of parent-caring on women. *Family Relations, 32*:39–45.

Cohen, D., & Eisdorfer, C. (1986). *The Loss of Self: A Family Resource for the Care of Alzheimer's and Related Disorders*. New York: W.W. Norton.

Dillehey, R. C., & Sandys, M. R. (1990). Caregivers for Alzheimer's patients: What we are learning from research. *International Journal of Aging and Human Development, 30*:263–285.

Given, C. W., et al. (1988). Sources of stress among families caring for relatives with Alzheimer's disease. *Nursing Clinics of North America, 23*: 69–83.

Hogstel, M. O. (1990). *Geropsychiatric Nursing*. St. Louis: C.V. Mosby.

Pratt, C. C., et al. (1985). Burden and coping strategies of caregivers to Alzheimer's patients. *Family Relations, 34*:27–33.

Pruchno, R. A., & Potashnik, S. L. (1989). Caregiving spouses: Physical and mental health in perspective. *Journal of the American Geriatric Society, 37*:697–705.

Focus On

FAMILIES AND PUBLIC HEALTH NURSING IN THE COMMUNITY

The purpose of this chapter is to provide students with an opportunity to explore the commonalities and linkages between family nursing and public health nursing in the community. The complementary principles of each of these practice areas are carefully described. Historical roots of the connections between family and community are explained, and their continued importance to practice is emphasized as changes in health care delivery increase the need for both community-based and population-focused health care.

The authors discuss models that provide a perspective for viewing the family as the client within the community setting. Through the use of examples, students are helped to understand these models and their usefulness to practice. The importance of prevention-focused frameworks of community public health and community interventions is explored in a similar fashion. The core functions of public health, as defined by the Institute of Medicine (1988), will be discussed in the framework of nursing and family.

Students are reminded that public health nurses working for public health agencies or private home health agencies and family nurses in clinics and acute care settings must use their knowledge of both families and communities to provide nursing care. To practice at a single level excludes a large and inportant area of nursing practice. Family nursing practice is in a unique position to bridge the gap between individuals and communities and has the potential to make significant contributions in assuring a healthy population.

Chapter 15

FAMILIES AND PUBLIC HEALTH NURSING IN THE COMMUNITY

Debra Gay Anderson • Cecelia Capuzzi • Diane C. Hatton

OUTLINE

OBJECTIVES

On completion of this chapter, the reader will be able to:

- Describe the practice of community public health nursing.
- Understand the historical antecedents of family and community public health nursing.
- Understand the interface between the practices of family and community public health nursing.

- Describe selected theoretical models that guide the practice of community public health family nursing.
- Describe selected concepts from community public health nursing and their application to family health.
- Apply the concept of "levels of prevention" to family and community public health.
- Identify community public health nursing interventions that promote health and that provide care for acute and chronic illnesses in families.
- Discuss the implications of community public health nursing for family nursing theory, practice, research, education, and social policy.

Community public health nurses have a long history of working with families, and they recognize that the health of individuals is intertwined with the health of families and the community. Families have a major impact on the health of individuals—that impact can be positive or negative. For example, families are assumed to provide social support, which is both health-promoting and health-restoring for their members. However, this support may instead be negative or absent, in which case family members' health is compromised (Anderson, 1996). There is recognition in the existing literature that the home is more dangerous for American women than are the city streets (Novella, 1992). Similarly, the health of families is important to every community's well-being. In fact, the health of communities is measured by the collective health of its individuals and families (e.g., the rate of low-birth-weight infants born to single mothers in a community; number of children without health insurance in a region). Violence, poverty, employment rates, and homelessness are indicators of the community's and family's health. Lastly, the character of the community and its ability to deal with health issues influences the well-being of all that live there. This chapter describes how the principles and practice of family nursing and community health nursing are integrated to yield what might be called family-centered community public health nursing.

WHAT IS COMMUNITY PUBLIC HEALTH NURSING?

Community as client is inherent in community health nursing practice. The community client may be a location in space and time, such as a neighborhood, a city, or a state. The community may be an aggregate of people with similar characteristics, such as all people infected with HIV, diagnosed with juvenile onset diabetes, or defined as homeless. The community client may describe groups who have a specific function (Shuster & Goeppinger, 1996), such as a nurse's organization that provides education on gun safety or a group of parents who work to decrease teen suicide. The use of the term "community" in this chapter reflects all of these populations. The practice of community public health nursing encompasses both caring for the community as a whole and caring for individuals and families within the community. According to the Association of Community Health Nursing Educators (ACHNE, 1995) the definition of community health nursing is:

> The synthesis of nursing theory and public health theory applied to promoting and preserving the health of populations. The focus of community health nursing is the community as a whole, with nursing care of individuals, families, and groups being provided within the context of promoting and preserving the health of community (p. 2).

For the purpose of this chapter, the public health nurse definition from the Public Health Nursing Section of the American Public Health Association (1996) is most useful:

> Public health nursing is the practice of promoting and protecting the health of populations using knowledge from the nursing, social, and public health sciences.

This definition of community public health nursing suggests that the target of care is the community: the community is the client receiving care. Individuals, families, and groups are subunits of the community. Nurses working in community settings direct care toward individuals, families, and groups, and the community serves as the context within which care is given.

Although family nursing should be evident in every

clinical setting, it is particularly applicable in community public health nursing, in which nurses seek to empower families to achieve and maintain wellness through health promotion and primary prevention (Duffy et al, 1998).

Traditional Community Health Nursing Roles

Working with individuals, families, and groups in the context of the community involves one set of nursing roles and interventions, while working directly with the community as a client involves others. Clark (1996) categorizes these nursing roles as: (1) client-oriented, (2) delivery-oriented, and (3) group-oriented. Client-oriented roles are directed toward providing services to clients, and include the roles of caregiver, educator, counselor, referral source, role model, advocate, primary care provider, and case manager. Delivery-oriented roles are directed toward facilitating the operation of the health care delivery system and indirectly enhancing the care of clients. These roles include those of coordinator, collaborator, liaison, and discharge planner. Lastly, group-oriented roles are directed toward promoting the health of the population of a community, and include the roles of case finder, leader, change agent, community care agent, and researcher. Client-oriented and delivery-oriented roles are used most frequently when providing care to individuals, families, and groups in community settings, while group-oriented roles are used when care is directed toward the community.

Not all community health nurses perform all of these roles. Often the setting and employing agency determine which roles are used. In addition, the core functions of public health have changed and strengthened many community health roles. These ideas will be further explained later in this chapter.

Historical Roots

Initially, the focus of care in the community was on individual patients; the family was a source of care for sick household members. Usually care was provided in the patients' homes and the nurses were called "visiting" nurses. Visiting nurses were described as early as the pre–Christian era in India, Egypt, Greece, and Rome (Gardner, 1928). Visiting nursing is documented from the eleventh to sixteenth centuries in Europe, with both secular and religious orders providing care (Rue, 1944).

In the mid-1800s, the importance of health promotion and disease prevention began to be recognized. Community health nurses, or visiting nurses, expanded their roles to include health education as well as sick care, and to function effectively, they directed their care not only to individuals, but also to families (Gardner, 1928; Rue, 1944). Recognizing that nurses were more effective when care involved all family members, Lillian Wald established a home-visiting service in the homes of the sick poor more than 100 years ago (Kuss et al, 1997). Wald developed guidelines for nursing of families in the home (Rue, 1944; Wald, 1986). Furthermore, Wald went beyond caring for families during an illness to being a forceful advocate of economic and social reform to effect social change that would improve the overall health of families and communities (Kuss et al, 1997).

In the early 1900s, subspecialties in community health nursing developed. Some nurses cared for mothers and infants, others cared for those with communicable diseases, and still others worked with mentally ill people. Also, community health nurses began seeing individuals in other settings besides the home, including clinics, tenements, day nurseries, schools, and industries (Spradley, 1996). In each instance, the importance of families was recognized. Despite these early trends, community health nurses did not fully direct their practice to the family as a unit of care until the 1950s. The family as a unit of care remained the orienting perspective for community health nurses until the 1970s (Spradley, 1996).

Community Public Health Nursing Today

Over the past 30 years, community public health nursing has undergone a major shift, in part because of societal developments beginning in the late 1960s. First, nurses began to recognize that the entire community needs health services, not just the sick poor. Second, other nursing specialists, such as home health nurses, began practicing outside the hospital setting, and some of these stated that the family was their focus of practice. Third, changes in the health care delivery system began to blur the distinctions between private, public, and nonprofit services. All of these developments led community public health nurses to re-examine their scope of practice (Spradley, 1996).

As a result, some community health nurses have redirected their care toward the *community as client,* with the family as an important subunit; others have continued to emphasize the family as the central unit of service. Despite the differing viewpoints of community health nurses, knowledge about families remains an important component of community public health nurses today.

In 1998, the World Health Organization's (WHO) European Region identified 21 health targets for the next century (Fawcett-Henesy, 1998). Comprehensive primary health care is the method to be used in achieving the goals. Of particular importance is the focus on families, work places, the local community, and other settings that include multiple generations living together. The importance of targeting families in the community to improve health is a challenge for health care providers worldwide.

THEORETICAL PERSPECTIVES

Many theoretical perspectives on the family are available to guide community health nursing practice. Not surprisingly, nursing models for families reflect two prevalent schools of thought in community public health nursing today. Some consider the family as the unit of care and the community as context; others focus on the community as client and view the family as a subunit (see Chapter 1).

Nursing Models

Most early nursing models focused on individuals as recipients of care. Both family nurses and community health nurses criticized these models because they did not represent the perspective of their practice. In addition, community health nurses criticized these early models for directing care primarily toward the restoration of health rather than toward maintaining wellness. The models either did not mention the community, or they considered it part of the environment.

Two current models that do address family and community as client will be discussed in detail: Zerwekh's (1991) family caregiving model for public health nursing and the public health nursing within the core public health functions model (Public Health Nursing Directors of Washington, 1993). Both provide guidance in the provision of nursing care for families and the communities in which they are a vital part.

Family Caregiving Model

Zerwekh's (1991) family caregiving model for public health nursing continues to be a useful framework for providing care to families in the community (Ackerman, 1994). Expert community health nurses created this model on the basis of descriptions of home-visiting activities that made a difference in the outcomes for maternal-child clients. From these descriptions, 16 competencies were identified and a model of their relationships was developed (Figure 15–1). The focus of this model is the family and developing the ability of members to take charge of their lives and make their own choices. Nurses' actions are aimed at encouraging family self-help through believing in the family's ability to make choices and aiding them to believe in themselves. Appropriate actions include listening to the family's needs, expanding the family's vision of choices, and feeding back reality so that the family can see patterns in their lives and the consequences of their decisions.

The first three competencies establish the foundation for family caregiving: (1) locating the family, (2) building trust, and (3) building strength. After this foundation is laid, eight encouraging self-help competencies are employed when working with families:

1. Being available
2. Mobilizing resources

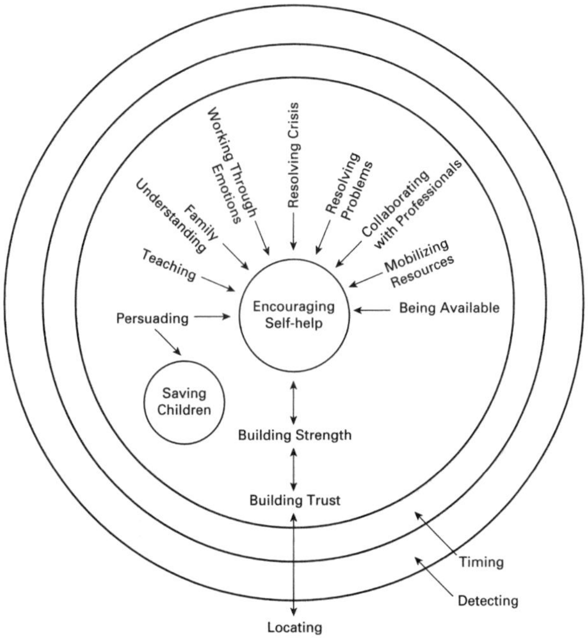

FIGURE 15-1
Zerwekh's family caregiving model for public health nursing. (From Zerwekh, J.V.: A family caregiving model. *Nursing Outlook* 1991, 39:214, with permission.)

3. Collaborating with other professionals
4. Resolving problems
5. Resolving crises
6. Working through emotions
7. Fostering family understanding
8. Teaching
9. Persuading

Three of these competencies help to foster community: being available, mobilizing resources, and collaborating with other professionals. Thus, the model acknowledges that the community is the context for family care.

If family self-help cannot be achieved and the nurse finds a family member is still at risk, two additional forceful competencies are employed: (1) persuading, which includes the use of reasoning, confronting, and threatening action (for example, calling child protective services); and (2) saving the children. In these at-risk situations, the nurse's responsibility for children (or individuals at risk) becomes primary.

Two competencies are used simultaneously with the other competencies and are ongoing during the care of the family. These are called encompassing competencies. The first of these, timing, relates to the speed of introducing an intervention and has three dimensions: (1) detecting the right time to initiate the action, (2) persisting in implementing the intervention, and (3) futuring, whereby the nurse considers the present action based on a view of the future (e.g., the child's development). The second encompassing competency, detecting, uses comprehensive assessment to identify potential and actual health problems.

Zerwekh's (1991) model is an important step in providing an original model of family nursing care in the community setting. It has been affirmed as being important to effective public health nursing (Ackerman, 1994). Public health nurses in Ackerman's study identified additional competencies. These additional competencies need further testing for validation for use in community public health nursing.

Core Public Health Function Model

A recent model of community public health nursing (Public Health Nursing Directors of Washington, 1993) is based on the core functions of public health (IOM, 1988) The purpose of the core public health function model (Figure 15–2) is to provide a model for public health professionals within today's rapidly

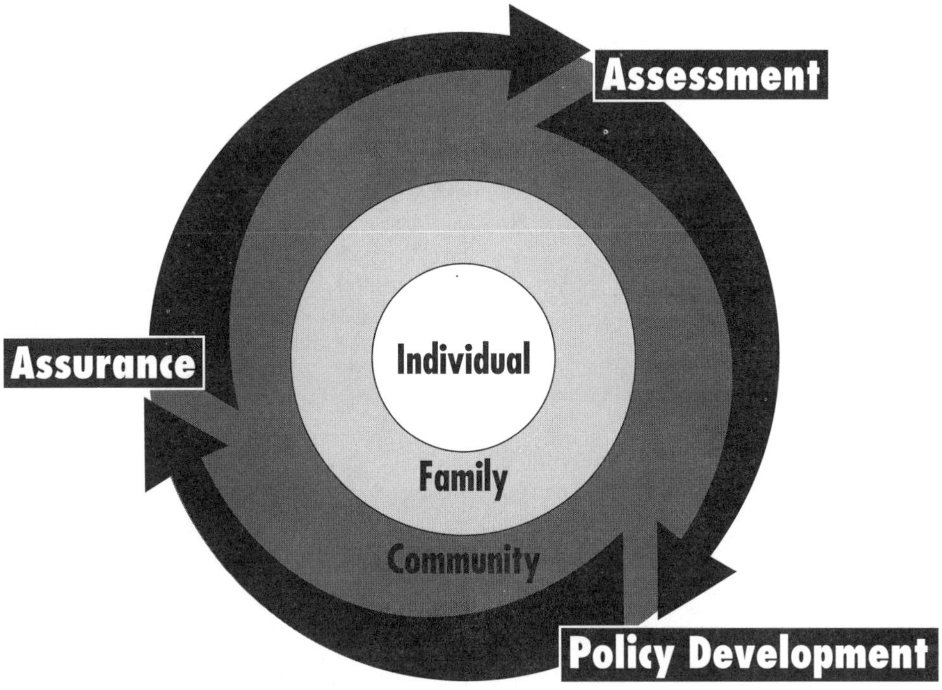

FIGURE 15-2
Public Health Nursing within the Core Public Health Functions Model.

changing health care environment. The core functions of assessment, policy development, and assurance address three core areas of service: the community, the family, and the individual. This model was developed in response to the 1988 Institute of Medicine (IOM) report, *The Future of Public Health*. The IOM identified assessment, policy development, and assurance as the three primary functions of public health (IOM, 1988). The IOM report provided the setting for dialogue in Washington State that resulted in the definitions of the core functions for Washington State (WSDOH, 1993) and provided the background for the development of the nursing model.

The core public health function model addresses each of these areas. Public health nurses, administrators, and educators from Washington State collaborated to develop the public health nurse's role within the core public health function model. Each core function is described and the role of the public health nurse for each is discussed. Individual, family, and community levels will be included because each level affects family.

Assessment

The trust that public health nurses have earned from their clients, agencies, and private providers enable ready access to populations that are otherwise difficult to access and engage in health care. In addition, they have knowledge of current and emerging health issues through their daily contact with high-risk and vulnerable populations. This trust and knowledge provides the foundation for the activities listed in Box 15–1.

Box 15–1 ASSESSMENT

Community

1. Analyze data on and needs of specific populations or geographic areas.
2. Identify and interact with key community leaders, both formally and informally.
3. Identify target populations that may be at risk. These populations may include high-density, low-income areas; preschools; primary and secondary schools; and elderly people.
4. Participate in data collection on a target population.
5. Conduct surveys or observe targeted populations, such as preschools, jails, and detention centers, to gain a better understanding of needs.

Family

1. Evaluate a specific individual family's strengths and areas of concern. This involves a comprehensive assessment of the physical, social, and mental health needs of the family.
2. Evaluate the family's living environment, looking specifically at support, relationships, and other factors that might have a significant impact on family health outcomes.
3. Assess the larger environment in which the family lives (the block or specific community) for safety, access, and other related issues.

Individual

1. Identify individuals within the family who are in need of services.
2. Evaluate the functional capacity of the total individual through the use of specific assessment measures, including physical, social and mental health screening tools.
3. Develop a nursing diagnosis for the individual that describes a problem or potential problem, cause, and contributing factors.
4. Develop a nursing care plan for the individual.

Source: Public Health Nursing Directors of Washington (1993).

Policy Development

Public health nurses are uniquely qualified to develop policy at the individual, family, and community level. The information obtained at the assessment level is used to make decisions at the organizational and community level. Public health nurses synthesize and analyze data collected from individuals, families, and communities in making policy decisions. Activities include those listed in Box 15–2.

Assurance

Assurance activities are the direct individual-focused services that public health nurses have provided over the past several years. This was due, in large part, to programmatic funding and Medicaid reimbursement that focused on the individual rather than population-focused services. Although the current shift in emphasis is toward assessment and policy development, there remain critical assurance activities for the

Box 15–2

POLICY DEVELOPMENT

Community

1. Provide leadership in convening and facilitating community groups to evaluate health concerns and develop a plan to address the concerns.
2. Recommend specific training and programs to meet identified health needs.
3. Raise awareness of key policy makers about health regulations, budget decisions, and other factors that may negatively affect the health of communities.
4. Recommend programs to target populations, such as child care centers, retirement centers, jails, juvenile detention facilities, homeless shelters, work sites, and minority communities.
5. Act as an advocate for the community and individuals who are not willing or able to speak to policy makers about issues or programs of concern.
6. Work with business and industry to develop employee health programs.

Family

1. Recommend new or increased services to families based on identified needs.
2. Recommend programs to meet specific families' needs within a geographic area.
3. Facilitate networking of families with similar needs and issues. Make recommendations to policy makers about specific issues affecting clusters of families.
4. Request additional data and analyze information to identify trends in a group or cluster of families.
5. Identify key families in a community who may be either in opposition to or in support of specific policies or programs and develop appropriate and effective intervention strategies to use with these families.

Individuals

1. Recommend or assist in the development of standards for individual client care.
2. Recommend or adopt risk classification systems to assist with prioritizing individual client care.
3. Participate in establishing criteria for opening, closing, or referring individual cases.
4. Participate in the development of job descriptions to establish roles for various team members who will provide service to individuals.

Source: Public Health Nursing Directors of Washington (1993).

public health nurse. These include those listed in Box 15–3.

BASIC COMMUNITY PUBLIC HEALTH CONCEPTS

Several concepts basic to community health nursing have set the direction for care provided to individuals, families, groups, and communities. Health promotion, disease prevention, primary prevention, secondary prevention, tertiary prevention, epidemiology, risk, and case-finding are defined and examples from the Healthy People 2000 document (U.S. Public Health Service, 1996) are used to demonstrate each concept. Health promotion includes activities that improve or maintain the well-being of people (Albrecht & Swanson, 1993). Teaching families conflict resolution skills is an example of a health promotion activity. Disease prevention includes those activities that protect families from actual or potential dis-

Box 15–3 ASSURANCE

Community

1. Provide service to target populations such as child care centers, preschools, work sites, minority communities, jails, juvenile detention facilities, and homeless shelters. Interventions may include health screening, education, health promotion, and injury prevention programs.
2. Improve quality assurance activities with various health care providers in the community. Examples include education on new immunization policies; educational programs for communicable disease control; assistance in developing effective approaches and support techniques for high-risk populations.
3. Maintain safe levels of communicable disease surveillance and outbreak control.
4. Participate in research or demonstration projects.
5. Provide expert public health consultation in the community.
6. Assure standards of care are met within the community.

Family

1. Provide services to a cluster of families within a geographic setting. Services may be provided in a variety of settings including homes, childcare centers, preschools, and schools. Services may include physical assessment; health education and counseling; and health and developmental screening.
2. Provide care in a nursing clinic to a specific group of families in a geographic location.

Individual

1. Provide nursing services based on standards of nursing practice to individuals across the age continuum. These services may encompass a variety of programs including First Steps, children with special health care needs, child abuse prevention, immunizations, well child care, and HIV/AIDS programs.
2. Assess and support the individual's progress toward meeting outcome goals.
3. Consult with other health care providers and team members regarding the individual's plan of care.
4. Prioritize individuals' needs on an ongoing basis.
5. Participate in quality assurance teams to measure the quality of care provided.

Source: Public Health Nursing Directors of Washington (1993).

eases and disabilities and their consequences (Albrecht & Swanson, 1993). Water fluoridation and accident control programs are examples of preventive activity.

Disease prevention occurs at three different levels: primary, secondary, and tertiary (Leavell & Clark, 1958). Primary prevention focuses on preventing the occurrence of health problems. The four leading causes of death for adolescents and young adults aged 15 to 24 are motor vehicle crashes, other unintended injuries, homicide, and suicide. Schools can be instrumental in decreasing youth violence and injury through education, the expansion of after-school sports, and other activities for young people (U.S. Public Health Service, 1996). In rural New Mexico, tribal leaders and other members of the Jicarilla Apache tribe have engaged in a suicide prevention effort in schools and a public education campaign to make the community aware of the problem. The number of suicide attempts has dropped and no suicides were recorded in 1995 (U.S. Public Health Service, 1996). Secondary prevention activities are designed to identify and treat health problems early. The Milwaukee Women's Center initiated a public awareness campaign designed to decrease violence against women. Milwaukee Transit Company buses display the center's messages about family and intimate partner violence. The numbers of calls to domestic violence hotlines and agencies have increased, including calls from men admitting they need help (U.S. Public Health Service, 1996).

Secondary prevention activities are carried out during the early stage of an acute or chronic illness. Tertiary prevention is aimed at correcting health problems and preventing further deterioration and is used for both acute or chronic health problems. Littleton, Colorado was the site of one of the nation's recent school shootings. Twelve students and one teacher were killed and the two student gunmen committed suicide. Tertiary prevention should focus on rebuilding the community; dealing with the grief and fears of individuals, families, and the entire community; and developing community prevention strategies to help prevent such a violent act from occurring in the future.

Community health nurses use concepts from epidemiology to promote health and prevent disease. Epidemiology is a science that is concerned with health events in human populations (Valanis, 1999). An important epidemiological concept is risk, which refers to the probability that individuals in a community will be affected by a health problem. Community health nurses attempt to identify those individuals, families, and populations at risk for health problems using case-finding methods that include review of health statistics, screening programs, and contact tracing (Freeman & Heinrich, 1981). An example of using risk assessment has been demonstrated at a school-based program in Dayton, Ohio. Adolescents who are identified as at high risk of becoming perpetrators or victims of violence are enrolled in the Positive Adolescent Choices Training (PACT) program. Adolescents in the program have shown reductions in violent confrontations and improvements in managing conflict.

These concepts are useful both when the family is the focus of care and when the community is client. Likewise, while the major focus of community health nursing is on health promotion and disease prevention, these concepts may be applicable during various other phases of the health-to-illness trajectory.

Strategies for Health Promotion and Disease Prevention

Many health promotion and disease prevention strategies are directed at both families and communities. Clark (1996) outlines five categories of health promotion and disease prevention strategies: (1) health appraisal, (2) health education, (3) lifestyle modification, (4) provision of a healthy environment, and (5) development of effective coping skills. In addition, *Promoting Health/Preventing Disease: Objectives for the Nation* (U.S. Department of Health and Human Services, 1980) suggests that (1) planning and providing health services (e.g., family planning clinics), (2) instituting health legislation and regulations, (3) offering economic incentives, and (4) developing health technology (e.g., websites for support groups) are additional measures that may promote health. While community health nurses are not usually involved in technology development, they frequently use all the other measures in the care of the family as client in the community setting and in the care of community as client. These strategies also can be employed in a variety of community settings (e.g., the family's home, schools, and clinics).

The Family as Client

An initial health-promoting and disease-preventing strategy is to conduct a health appraisal of families and their environments to identify strengths and potential risks to health. Appraisal of the family's environment is often a unique function of community health nursing. If the community health nurse is able to make a home visit, that environment can be directly observed. Realistic interventions can then be developed, based on the availability of resources or referrals for resources. Likewise, the community health nurse who works in a school or occupational setting can directly appraise the effects of these environments.

An environmental appraisal includes assessment of physical, psychological, social, and economic environments. Assessment of the physical environment of the home includes examination of safety hazards (e.g., condition of paint, age of housing, fire extinguishers, dangerous playground equipment), facilities for hygiene (e.g., running water, indoor plumbing), items to meet basic needs (e.g., food, heating, cooking facilities, refrigeration), and objects that promote social, emotional, and physical development (e.g., toys, books). A similar assessment can be applied to other settings. The neighborhood also should be assessed for level of violence, safety hazards, availability of transportation, access to needed goods and services, access to recreational facilities, and the presence of environmental pollutants (Clark, 1996).

The community health nurse also appraises the family's psychological, social, and economic environment. In the home, family communication patterns, role relationships, family dynamics, emotional strengths, coping strategies, and childrearing and discipline practices can be assessed directly. Likewise, the effects of the social environment (e.g., religious practices, culture, social class, economic status, and social support system) on health can be assessed. Specific methods of assessing factors in the psychological and social environment are discussed in Chapters 4 through 7 of this book. In settings other than the home, factors that promote the psychological and social growth of individual family members also should be assessed. Textbooks on school health and occupational health nursing frequently contain guides for assessing these aspects of the environment.

Another community health nursing strategy to promote health and prevent disease in families is health teaching and information giving. After completing the health appraisal, the community health nurse reinforces those behaviors that are health-promoting and provides health information and teaching in areas identified as risky. Again, the four determinants of health provide a useful framework for developing a health teaching plan. For example, topics such as child development and childrearing are based on normal human development (human biology).

The community health nurse uses a variety of strategies to modify risky lifestyles identified in the health appraisal. Teaching and health information can be used to discuss immunizations, nutrition, rest, exercise, use of seat belts, and abuse of harmful substances, such as alcohol and drugs. The community health nurse may also refer the family to programs and resources that assist in lifestyle modifications (e.g., smoking cessation classes, exercise programs). Furthermore, the community health nurse might also promote a healthy lifestyle and influence lifestyle changes as a counselor and role model.

Healthy environments also promote health. Health teaching based on appraisal of the physical environment might include information on child safety and prevention of falls. Other teaching might focus on psychological or social environmental problems, such as improving family communications or dealing with peer pressure. In some situations, the community health nurse promotes a healthy environment by providing information to community members outside the family. For example, community health nurses working in schools might need to inform officials about playground hazards or poor food-handling practices.

Helping families develop effective strategies for coping with stress is another health promotion strategy. The chapter on family mental health nursing discusses the effects of stress and provides detailed information on how to assist families in coping with stress. Health education, referral to community agencies, counseling, and role modeling are among the strategies used by community health nurses.

Finally, a major health promotion strategy is ensuring access to health promotion and prevention services, including immunizations, family planning, prenatal care, well child care, nutrition, exercise classes, and dental hygiene. These services may be provided directly by the community health nurse in the home or in clinics, schools, or work settings. In some cases, the community health nurse facilitates access to these services through referrals, case management, discharge planning, advocacy, liaison, coordination, and collaboration.

Community as Client

When nursing care focuses on the community with the goal of promoting health and preventing disease, nurses use strategies and interventions similar to those used with families, but the strategies are refocused toward the community (e.g., health appraisal, health education).

Nurses also use some additional strategies (e.g., program planning and policy development).

One strategy for promoting the health of families when the community is client is to conduct a community assessment (i.e., health appraisal of a community) to identify potential and actual health risks to all individuals and families living in the community. After these potential health risks are identified, the community health nurse intervenes to reduce these risk factors.

A community assessment involves collecting health and social data about the population, the social institutions (e.g., health and social services, economics, education, safety and transportation, recreation, politics and government, and communication), and the environment (physical, psychological, and social). Demographic information about the population provides information regarding possible health problems. For example, a community with a large population less than 5 years of age might benefit from strategies aimed at increasing competence in parenting and increasing compliance with immunization schedules. Information on social institutions is helpful in assessing the adequacy of the community's resources. Such information can indicate whether there are enough pediatricians, whether municipal transportation is available to go to hospitals and clinics, and whether fire and emergency services are staffed for immediate response. Assessment of the environment includes evaluating the types and adequacy of sewage and water treatment and investigating for the presence of disease-bearing insects, such as the ticks that cause Lyme disease.

Methods of gathering data for a community assessment include windshield surveys; interviews with key informants; analysis of secondary data gathered by health departments, such as morbidity and mortality rates; and large population surveys. A windshield survey is the motorized equivalent of simple observation. Through an automobile windshield many dimensions of a community's life and environment are carefully observed (Stanhope & Lancaster, 1996). Often the data are about families in the community: for example, the proportion of single-parent families or the number of day care facilities. A detailed description of community assessment is beyond the scope of this chapter. However, most community health nursing texts provide guidance for implementing a community assessment.

Once data has been collected, it is analyzed to identify the community's health problems; that is, to make "community diagnoses." An example of a community diagnosis is: "The children are at risk for lead poisoning due to the amount of old housing stock in the community." After community diagnoses are made, goals are developed to correct the problems and plans are made to intervene.

Thus, a second strategy for promoting the health of families in communities is program planning to develop the needed health services identified in the community assessment.

Program planning includes:

- Identification of potential solutions to the problem
- Analysis and comparison of alternative solutions
- Selection of one program or solution
- Development of program goals and objectives
- Identification of resources
- Development of the specific activities of the program
- Development of methods to evaluate the program

Usually program planning involves multidisciplinary teams of health and nonhealth professionals. The community and its families also should be involved in the planning and implementation to assure that the program meets their needs. During this process, community health nurses employ the group-oriented roles of community care agent, leader, and change agent.

Awareness of the need to design community health programs with a family-centered approach has grown over the past 20 years. For example, in 1986, Congress passed PL 99-457, the Education for All Handicapped Children Act and mandated that services be provided to the families of children with developmental disabilities as well as to the child (Shelton et al, 1987). Since then, the Association for the Care of Children's Health (ACCH) has developed a definition of family-centered care that many other groups working with families have adapted (Korteland & Cornwell, 1991, p. 57). Box 15–4 lists the elements of family-centered care. Community health nurses can facilitate development of health programs that are supportive to families by using these elements during program planning and implementation.

The work of David Olds and his colleagues (Olds et al, 1997) has shown the effectiveness of family-centered care, and particularly, the effectiveness of community public health nursing home visitation. In their studies, nurses visited low income, unmarried mothers and their children. The families with home visitation had significantly improved health outcomes. The home visitation reduced the number of the mothers' subsequent pregnancies, use of welfare, child abuse and neglect, and

Box 15-4 ELEMENTS OF FAMILY-CENTERED CARE

- Recognition that the family is the constant in the child's life, whereas service systems and personnel within those systems fluctuate.
- Facilitation of parent-professional collaboration at all levels of health care.
- Sharing of unbiased and complete information with parents about their child's care on an ongoing basis in an appropriate and supportive manner.
- Implementation of appropriate policies and programs that are comprehensive and provide emotional and financial support to meet the needs of families.
- Recognition of family strengths and individuality and respect for different methods of coping.
- Understanding and incorporating the developmental and emotional needs of infants, children, and adolescents and their families into health care delivery systems.
- Encouragement and facilitation of parent-to-parent support.
- Assurance that the design of health care delivery systems is flexible, accessible, and responsive to family needs.
- Respect for the racial, cultural, and socioeconomic diversity of families.

Source: Korteland, C., and Cornwell, J.R. Evaluating family-centered programs in neonatal intensive care. *Children's Health Care,* 1991; 20:56–61. Used with permission.)

criminal behaviors for up to 15 years after their first child's birth.

The nursing home visit program (Olds et al, 1998) also reduced serious antisocial behavior and substance use as the high-risk children in the study entered adolescence. As adolescents, they had fewer instances of running away, fewer arrests, less convictions and violations of probation, fewer lifetime sex partners, and less cigarette smoking and alcohol use than comparable adolescents. In sum, not only have these researchers shown how home visits in the community are beneficial for high-risk families, but they have also shown how community public health nurses are essential for the effectiveness of this visitation program.

A final strategy for promoting health and preventing disease in communities is policy development and implementation. Community health nurses frequently interact in local and state policy arenas by alerting policy makers about the health problems in their communities. Nurses can give direct accounts of the effects these health problems have on families in the community. They can write letters, make telephone calls, testify before committees, and take part in other political activities to create awareness of the health problem. Nurses also sit on advisory boards and task forces at all levels: community, city, county, state, and national. In these positions, nurses can directly influence policy to promote health and prevent disease.

Once a health problem is recognized, community health nurses work with others to propose and shape policy solutions. The community health nurse's perspective on a proposed policy's effect on families is important to the development of health proposals. Community health nurses often implement these policies to ensure optimum results for family health.

Acute and Chronic Illness

Nursing care for families in the community who have either an acute or chronic illness involves secondary and tertiary prevention. Secondary prevention strategies include: (1) early detection of health problems in families and communities, (2) referral for further evaluation and treatment, and (3) health teaching about the potential illness and the need for follow-up.

Tertiary prevention focuses on: (1) monitoring the health problem, (2) providing treatment, (3) providing health education, and (4) promoting adjustment to the illness. Community assessment, program planning and implementation, case finding, community education, and health policy development can also be appropriate as secondary and tertiary prevention measures. Strategies using these measures in relation to the care of the family as client can be carried out in a variety of community settings.

Secondary and Tertiary Prevention

One secondary prevention strategy is early detection of acute or chronic illnesses. Screening for detection of illness is a major function of community health nurses and is accomplished through health appraisals, as described previously in this chapter, and by using screening tools and methods. Many screening procedures are available for detecting health problems in family members of all ages and in the family as a whole. These procedures and instruments are discussed in other chapters in this text.

Once community health nurses detect a health problem, they initiate appropriate nursing care and/or make referrals to nurse practitioners or physicians for medical evaluation of the condition and treatment. The community health nurse is responsible for assuring that the patient receives the needed health care.

The referral process includes identifying the need for referral, identifying appropriate health resources, preparing the client for the referral, communicating with the referral agency, and evaluating the outcome of the referral for the client (Clark, 1996). During this time, the community health nurse also provides health education and information about the significance of positive screening results and the need for follow-up and treatment of the condition. Clients vary in their ability to find and use health care resources. Clemen-Stone and colleagues (1991) suggest that there are three levels of nursing intervention in the referral process. Level 1 clients are dependent on the nurse to identify needed health care resources, coordinate referrals, and assist the patient to use the referral services. Level 2 clients are moderately independent. They seek information from the nurse and may need some help in identifying resources and in completing the referral process. Level 3 clients are independent; after they are given information about health resources, they can complete the referral process.

One tertiary prevention strategy is to monitor the individual's physical condition. Follow-up health appraisals provide information that can be compared to the initial health appraisal data to chart progress. For example, the nurse monitors the diabetic client's blood glucose levels to determine whether the treatment is effective. Another tertiary prevention strategy is to provide nursing treatments to correct the illness and prevent further health problems. In these instances, the community health nurse provides direct patient care, such as dressing changes, medication administration, and range of motion. In some communities, home health nurses employed by private agencies provide these treatments; in other communities, community health nurses from public health departments provide this care. Home health nursing is a subspecialty of community health nursing; however, home health nurses in private agencies tend to provide more intensive technological nursing care. School nurses and occupational health nurses also provide direct nursing interventions.

A third tertiary prevention strategy is to provide health teaching to the patient and the family to help them carry out prescribed treatments. The nurse also provides information about the disease and the ways to prevent further problems. A fourth type of tertiary prevention strategy is to assist the patient and family in coping with the illness through counseling or to help mobilize other support resources within the family and the family's extended network or in the community.

Nursing Interventions

Care for families with acute and chronic illnesses at the community level involves using: (1) community assessment to identify significant acute and chronic health problems in the community, (2) planning and providing screening and treatment services, (3) identifying those at risk for particular acute and chronic illnesses, (4) providing community educational programs, and in some instances, (5) developing health policy. These strategies focus on acute and chronic health problems in the community.

IMPLICATIONS

Practice

Although nurses have focused on the family unit in the community for many years, there are still many obstacles to family-centered care. First of all, nurses must have access to families to provide care; thus, care should be provided in settings where families commonly reside. These include homes, the schools where younger family members spend a large portion of their day, the occupational settings where adult members are easily located, and sites where elders congregate.

Also, barriers to care of families in the community

must be removed. Most health agencies, even those that espouse a family focus, really direct care to the individual. Patient records usually contain only data about the individual. Thus family members have separate records; either family assessment data are only in one family member's record or they are duplicated in all records; or more commonly, they are not recorded at all. This fragmentation makes it difficult to view the family as a unit. In the past, there were legal constraints to recording one individual's assessment information in another's record because of confidentiality. Some agencies have not found ways to overcome this legal barrier.

Education

Nursing education should include a strong family orientation and a strong community orientation to enable students to understand the interplay between the health of the community and the health of families. Undergraduate students need to learn community-focused interventions that can promote the health of families. Graduate students specializing in family and community health nursing need to study the theoretical perspectives of community-focused and family-focused interventions. Practices that include family-centered nursing provide students with opportunities to practice theoretical perspectives and are important at both the undergraduate and graduate level of nursing.

Research

Research is needed to identify common family health problems in the community, resources to meet family needs, and effective organization of services to promote family health and coping. Program evaluation is necessary to determine the effectiveness of interventions and to develop a strong base for funding of programs.

Research is also needed to determine which intervention strategies are most effective in promoting family health and preventing family illness. Research on the effects of home visiting on individual health problems should be broadened to include the effect on family problems. Research conducted by Olds and his colleagues (1998) was discussed earlier. Their research has demonstrated the effectiveness of public health nursing interventions, while research by Ackerman (1994) demonstrated the importance of research in testing a model for effective public health nursing.

Policy

Policy-level barriers to providing family-centered care in the community include the current organization of health services and reimbursement for health care. Health services in the community frequently are not family-focused but are arranged according to specific health problems (e.g., sexually transmitted diseases) or by age or life stage (e.g., prenatal care, teenage clinics). This occurs because funding is allocated for specific services. Such arrangements preclude the health provider from focusing on the family as a unit and force; instead, there is a focus on the specific health problem or life stage of the individual.

Reimbursement for health care also promotes an individual focus. Only specific health conditions or treatments are reimbursable, and furthermore, reimbursement covers only the individual presenting the problem; most insurance does not recognize the family as a client or accept family health diagnoses. Last, it frequently happens that not all family members are covered by health insurance and that reimbursement is thus limited to those who are covered. To remove these barriers, there must be health policy changes; and to effect these changes, there must be a strong nursing voice.

SUMMARY

In summary, community public health nurses are concerned with the health of individuals, families, groups and communities. Community public health nurses work in a variety of settings, including public and private health agencies, schools, and occupational sites. They use concepts from the public health discipline, including epidemiology, health promotion, and illness prevention. Community public health nurses employ a large repertoire of roles. These roles vary according to whether the nurse is focusing on the family as the unit of care in the context of the community or focusing on the health of the community, with families being a subunit. Health intervention strategies used by community public health nurses include individual, family, and group health appraisals, community assessment, health education, referral to community resources, monitoring health problems, providing treatments, coordination of care, planning and providing health services, and instituting health legislation and regulations.

Case Study

THE YORKES

This case study describes a typical community health nursing role. The scope of activities and breadth of responsibility described here are common to many community health nurses. As you read through the case, consider the following:

- Use Zerwekh's family caregiving model for public health nursing or the core public health function model in understanding the Yorkes' situation and planning for care.
- How would the care given by Catherine Parker be different if she had an individual rather than a family focus?
- How do the geography of the community and the availability of resources influence the Yorkes' health?
- What types of prevention strategies is Catherine Parker using in caring for the Yorkes?
- Are there other strategies that would be helpful?
- What actions should Catherine Parker take at the community level to improve the Yorkes' health?

Catherine Parker, PHN, is a community health nurse for Monroe County Health District. She has a caseload of 50 families who live in the northwest section of the county. The health department sponsors 15 clinics a week, including clinics for prenatal care, well children, family planning, immunizations, sexually transmitted diseases, and hypertension. In addition, public health nurses (PHNs) work closely with environmental health professionals. Catherine works Tuesday and Thursday mornings in the prenatal care and well-child clinics. She also works with the hospital's discharge coordinator to identify patients who need community services after leaving the hospital. Monroe County Health District's Nursing Department is responsible for providing school health services to the county's three elementary schools, two middle schools, and one high school; Catherine spends one afternoon a week at the high school. Recently, Catherine was asked to be on a task force to develop protocols for working with mothers with a substance abuse problem; this group meets monthly. Also, the State Health Department is planning to implement a child health information tracking system and has directed each county to conduct a feasibility study. Catherine is surveying the young families in her caseload for their views on having their child's health information available to multiple health providers.

Last week, when Catherine was doing discharge planning at the county hospital, she realized that the Yorke family could use additional services and arranged a postpartum home visit. Gina Yorke, age 23, delivered her fourth child a week ago and is now at home. Gina's husband, Rob Yorke, age 24, is an unemployed logger receiving job retraining at the local community college. The other three children are ages 13 months, 2 years, and 3 years. Rob's parents live nearby. The Yorkes recently moved to Monroe and live in a rural part of the county. Gina received late prenatal care at the Monroe Health Clinic. The family lives in a rented, two-bedroom house 15 miles from town. Rob uses the only car for transportation to classes.

The Yorkes are just one of many families who live in the rural part of the county. There is no public transportation. Most families that live in this area rent their homes because it is less expensive than buying. The median family income of the people residing in this area is $12,120 a year. The mean age of the residents in this area is 25 years. Most houses have indoor plumbing with running water; the water comes from the county system. All houses have septic tanks. In the past year, three methamphetamine labs have been discovered in the area; adolescent substance abuse is a problem.

Catherine returns to visit the Yorke family for a 6-week postpartum follow-up. She weighs and measures the new baby and measures the infant's head circumference. The baby is gaining weight adequately and appears to be healthy. Gina Yorke also is feeling well and has had her 6-week checkup with the nurse midwife at the health department.

Gina mentions that the 2-year-old is not feeling well. He feels hot and has a rash on his chest. Catherine takes the child's temperature and it is 101°F. He has a runny nose and congestion in his chest. The rash on his trunk has vesicles; Catherine determines that he has varicella (chickenpox). None of the other children have had chickenpox, nor do they have any symptoms yet.

Catherine teaches Gina to take the child's temperature and discusses skin care and hygiene. She also emphasizes the importance of giving the child fluids and makes suggestions for diet. Catherine tells Gina that the child should be kept isolated from people outside the household until the vesicles are dried. If the child becomes more ill, Gina should call the doctor at the health clinic. Catherine asks Gina if any of her family can help her with the care, and Gina indicates that Rob's mother is available. Catherine returns in a week to find that the family is coping well, although the other children now all have chickenpox.

County health statistics indicate that there is a high incidence of lead poisoning in young children, particularly children in rural areas. It is possible that the source of lead is water pipes, since older homes have plumbing that used to be soldered with lead; also, many of these older homes were painted with lead-based paints. Nearby, there also is a factory that makes lead pipe fittings; this factory has been cited by the Environmental Protection Agency for high levels of toxic waste emission.

While working in the well-child clinic, Catherine Parker screens all children for high levels of lead in their blood. Gina Yorke brings her children to this clinic for preventive care, and when the children are tested, all are found to have lead in their blood. Follow-up care is planned and implemented. This comprehensive and interdisciplinary care is typical of a family receiving health care services from a county health department.

Study Questions

1. Describe the target of care for community public health nursing.
2. Identify nursing's historical roots in caring for families in community settings.
3. Analyze how the practices of family and community public health nursing interface.
4. Define the following: epidemiology, public health nursing, community as client, aggregate of people, health promotion, disease prevention, and primary, secondary, and tertiary prevention.
5. List at least one example of a public health intervention for each level of prevention.

References

Ackerman, P. M. (1994). Competencies for the practice of effective public health nursing: Confirmation of Zerwekh's Family Caregiving Model. Unpublished Doctoral Dissertation, University of Colorado, Denver.

Albrecht, M., & Swanson, J. M. (1993). Health: A Community View. In J. M. Swanson & M. Albrecht (Eds.), *Community Health Nursing: Promoting the Health of Aggregates* (p. 312). Philadelphia: W.B. Saunders.

American Public Health Association, Public Health Nursing Section. (1996). The Definition and Role of Public Health Nursing: A Statement of the Public Health Nursing Section. Washington, D.C.: Author.

Anderson, D. G. (1996). Homeless women's perceptions about their families of origin. *Western Journal of Nursing Research, 18*:29–42.

Association of Community Health Nursing Educators (ACHNE) (1995). *Perspectives on Theory Development in Community Health Nursing.* Louisville, KY: Author.

Clark, M. J. (1996). *Nursing in the Community*, ed 2. Stamford, CT: Appleton & Lange.

Clemen-Stone, et al. (1991). *Comprehensive Family and Community Health Nursing*, ed 3. St. Louis: C.V. Mosby.

Duffy, M. E., et al. (1998). Family Nursing Practice in Public Health: Finland and Utah. *Public Health Nursing, 15*(4):281–287.

Fawcett-Henesy, A. (1998). Speaking Out. *Nursing Times, 94*(23):23.

Freeman, R. B., & Heinrich, J. (1981). *Community Health Nursing Practice*, ed 2. Philadelphia: W.B. Saunders.

Gardner, M. S. (1928). *Public Health Nursing.* New York: MacMillan.

Institute of Medicine (1988). *The Future of Public Health.* Washington, D.C.: National Academy Press.

Korteland, C., & Cornwell, J. R. (1991). Evaluating Family-centered Programs in Neonatal Intensive Care. *Children's Health Care, 20*(1):56–61.

Kuss, T., et al. (1997). A Public Health Nursing Model. *Public Health Nursing, 14*(2):81–91.

Leavell, H. R., & Clark, E. G. (1958). *Preventive Medicine for the Doctor in His Community.* New York: McGraw-Hill.

Novella, A. (U.S. Surgeon General). (1992). In New York State Office for the Prevention of Domestic Violence. New York.

Oberg, C. N., et al. (1994). *America's Children: Triumph or Tragedy.* Washington, DC: American Public Health Association.

Olds, D., et al. (1997). Theoretical Foundations of a Program of Home Visitation for Pregnant Women and Parents of Young Children. *Journal of Community Psychology, 25*(1):9–25.

Olds, D., et al. (1998). Long–term Effects of Nurse Home Visitation on Children's Criminal and Antisocial Behavior. *JAMA, 280*(14):1238–1244.

Public Health Nursing Directors of Washington. (1993). Public Health Nursing within Core Public Health Functions. Olympia, Washington: Washington State Department of Health.

Rue, C. B. (1944). *The Public Health Nurse in the Community.* Philadelphia: W.B. Saunders.

Shelton, R., et al. (1987). Family–centered Care for Children with Special Health Care Needs. Washington, D.C.: Association for the Care of Children's Health.

Shuster, G. F., & Goeppinger, J. (1996). Community as client: Using the nursing process to promote health. In M. Stanhope & J. Lancaster (Eds.), *Community Health Nursing* (pp. 289–314). St. Louis: C.V. Mosby.

Spradley, B. W. (1996). *Community Health Nursing: Concepts and Practice*, ed 2. Boston: Little, Brown.

Stanhope, M., & Lancaster, J. (1996). *Community Health Nursing: Promoting Health of Aggregates, Families, and Individuals*, ed 4. St. Louis: Mosby.

United States Public Health Service. (1996). Healthy People 2000: Progress Review: Violent and Abusive Behavior. Department of Health & Human Services, Public Health Service. Available: http://www.health.gov/healthypeople [1996, November 26].

United States Department of Health and Human Services. (1980). *Promoting Health/Preventing Disease: Objectives for the Nation.* Washington, DC: Author.

Valanis, B. (1999). *Epidemiology in Health Care*, ed 3. Stamford, CT: Appleton & Lange.

Washington State Department of Health (WSDOH). Core Public Health Functions Task Force. (1993). Core Public Health Functions. Olympia, WA: Washington Department of Health.

Wald, A. L. (1986). The Family as the Unit of Care in Nursing: A Historical Review. *Public Health Nursing, 3*(4):240–249.

Zerwekh, J. V. (1991). A Family Caregiving Model for Public Health Nursing. *Nursing Outlook, 39*(5):213–217.

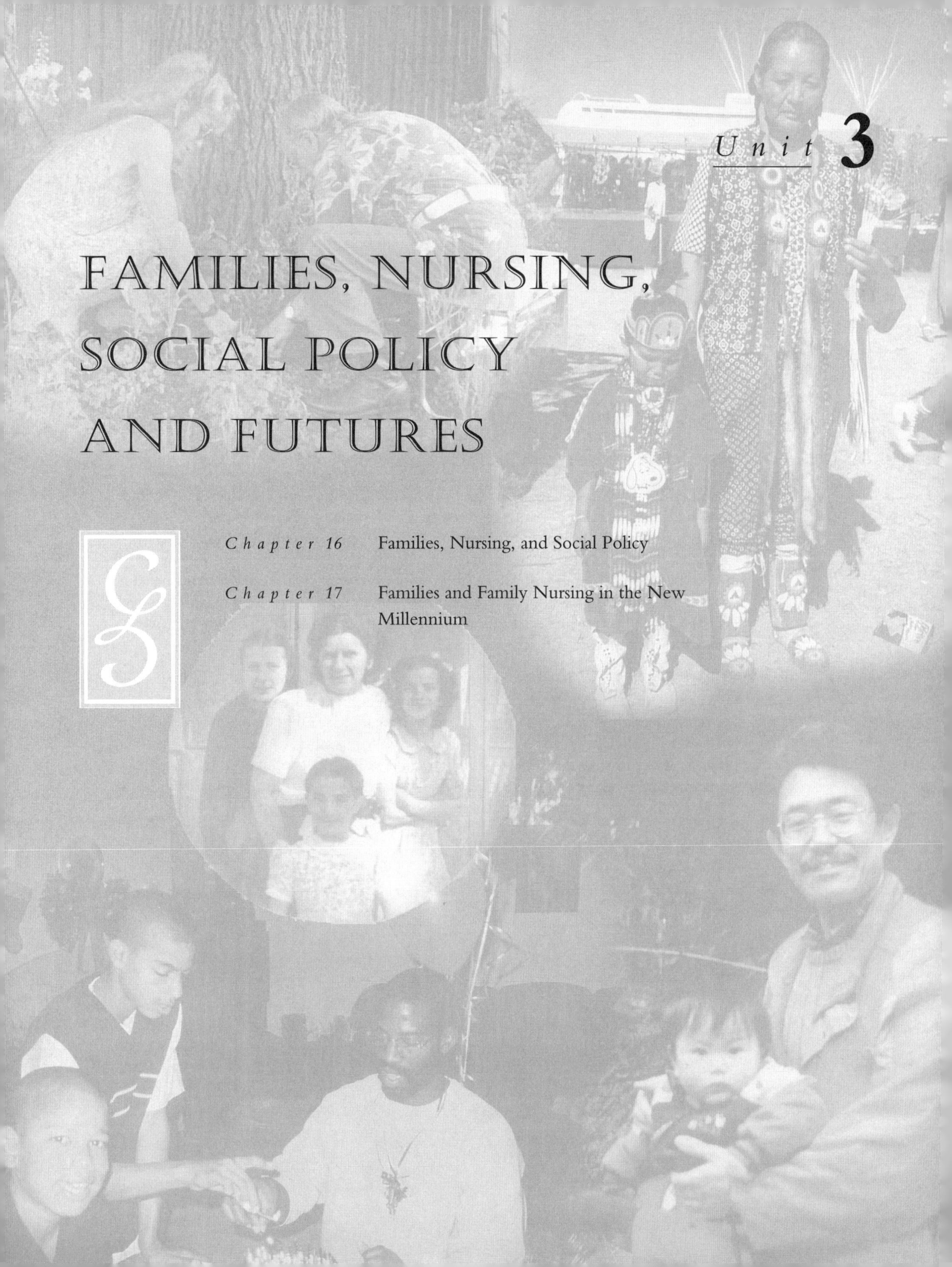

Unit **3**

FAMILIES, NURSING, SOCIAL POLICY AND FUTURES

Focus On

SOCIAL POLICIES THAT AFFECT NURSING OF FAMILIES

Families live within social policies that have evolved in or been legally created by the culture and government surrounding them. These policies have an impact on who can be considered family, how parenting is supported, caregiving for dependents, access to health services, and basic economic welfare. This chapter explores a range of issues that arise because of this social policy context, with indicators of their impact on the provision of nursing care. There is no way in which such a discussion can ever be complete. The nursing student should be alert to evolving social policy and make every effort to consider the impact it will have on families.

This chapter discusses some of the dominant ways in which public social policy affects the family, particularly the health of the family. The material covered includes policies affecting the ability to parent or provide care for family members, gain access to needed health and illness services, and provide for family welfare. The goal of this chapter is to illustrate the variety of lived family experiences influenced by social structure and to review important legal and social policies regarding family in order to facilitate the highest quality of nursing care and health care policy.

Chapter 16

FAMILIES, NURSING, AND SOCIAL POLICY

Kristine M. Gebbie • Eileen Gebbie

OUTLINE

OBJECTIVES

At the completion of this chapter, the reader will be able to:

- Describe how a legal definition of family affects lived experience of families.
- Discuss the impact policy shifts in access, cost, and quality of personal care have on families.
- Discuss at least one example of the role socially structured discrimination plays in family life.
- Identify at least three laws or public policies that affect the range of services available to a family.
- Describe the responsibility of the nurse in response to the these laws or public policies.

THE INTERSECTION OF FAMILY WITH SOCIAL POLICY

As discussed in earlier chapters, the dominant concept of family in American culture has been an idealized *normative* nuclear family, composed of man, woman, and biological children, an image of "how we are" that in fact may never have been (Coontz, 1992). The term "extended family" is commonly used to include not only the nuclear family, but also the circle of biologically and legally related grandparents, aunts, uncles, and cousins. Although we think of "family" as a personal and individual experience, it is also socially, economically, and legally defined. Because of these social structures, we may be bound to individuals for whom we do not care, whom we do not know, or whom we fear. The same structures mean we may have difficulty remaining in touch with others for whom we have strong, positive feelings. For example, the grandparents of a noncustodial divorced parent have no continuing legal relationship to their grandchildren and may be denied access to them because of difficulties between their child (the noncustodial parent) and the custodial parent.

Legal and biological definitions of "father" and "mother" and "child" may or may not coincide with the actual titles or relationships of the adults most important to children. Although all humans have biological ties to at least two individuals and many have biological ties to one or more children, these "family members" may or may not be active participants in each other's lives. There are other times when a person may have no emotional or intellectual experience of others as "family," as a result of isolating quarrels or divergent value judgments, even though the legal and biologic relationships exist.

Rather than be limited by the normative terms, or limit communication by legalistic assumptions, nurses must learn to inquire of a patient in an open manner, "Who do you include in your family?" This will allow individuals to describe their significant others and significant relationships based on personal experience and not on socially conditioned *norms*. After this first discussion, if it is necessary for completing required institutional forms or some other such purpose, questions about specific legal relationships may be asked.

There are no all-right or all-wrong descriptions of family and no universal experience of family and social policy. For example, we are increasingly aware of spousal abuse, partner abuse, child abuse, and elder abuse, in part because of laws requiring health professionals (and others) to make reports of suspected cases of abuse. Are these abuses and ills really new or just newly publicized? And are families really so ineffective now? "While it is clear that many families did not adequately provide services in the past, contrary to myth it is also clear that many contemporary families are currently providing a wide range of services" (Armstrong, 1996, p. 4). This chapter includes examples of situations in which the experience of family appears to come into conflict with the socially acceptable or currently legal definition of family. It is at these points of tension that we can learn a great deal about what is important, both to individuals and the larger social structure. Because "family" is so tied to women and *gender* role concerns, much attention is given to the ongoing criticism of traditional women's roles. And because issues of *sexual orientation* have become the focus of social and legal debate, a number of examples are chosen to illustrate how society has responded to *gay, lesbian, bisexual, and transgender* (GLBT) families.

The reader is encouraged to look beyond the specific examples to the issue of social definition. There may or may not be any genetic or biologic reason for certain definitions or restrictions; situations that on the surface may appear "illegal" or extremely unusual may in fact be extremely functional and positive for those involved. And the legal definitions are grounded in history and community need for stability, particularly economic and political stability, as well as the dominant religious perspective. *It is critical that the nurse encountering an unusual situation be alert to the possibility that judgments based on automatically presumed "normality" can be unhealthy and limiting for the family seeking care and for the nurse.*

DEFINITIONS OF FAMILY

The legal rite of marriage that establishes the classic nuclear family *has* been a constant through many changes and is one of "property rights," based in the sexual relationship seen at the heart of legal marriage (Collins, 1996). Although a couple may have sex without a marriage license, the relationship remains unrecognized unless extended over time as "common law" marriage. Even if backed by a license, an "unconsummated" marriage may be annulled. That is, family made by legal measures can be undone by the lack of sexual ones.

The United Nations declared 1994 the International Year of *the* Family (italics added). One social scientist has criticized the use of "the" in this title as evidence that the pervasiveness of the *nuclear family* "with its gender differentiation is ideologically correct and what should be" (Trost, 1996, p. 2) Today's nurse, given our extremely diverse society, must be prepared to identify such assumptions about family and understand that they may act to exclude some individuals from full participation in community. Whatever one's own preferred family structure, or lived experience of family as positive or negative, effective nursing care requires identifying and *respecting* the meaning of family to each patient and each family encountered.

The traditional definitions of family have assumed that the adult couple at the center are of different *sexes* (Box 16–1). Therefore, the partnerships established by two individuals of the same sex must be established through informal, nonlegal measures, even if they are affirmed by practical, emotional, and sexual activity. Legal privacy rights presumed by most couples may not be claimed by same-sex partners. For example, in 1986, Michael Hardwick was arrested while having oral sex with his male partner in his own bedroom. When Hardwick challenged the arrest made under Georgia anti-sodomy laws, he was found to have no right to engage in oral or anal sex and no right to privacy in his bedroom (Leonard, 1997, p. 460). Hawaii, with a state constitution that expressly forbids sex discrimination, has been the site of the movement to allow GLBT couples fully legal marriages. There has been a consistent blind eye turned to the regular presence in our communities of so-called spinsters and bachelors who just happened to live together their whole lives (Armstrong, 1996, p. 4). Intriguing discussions in state legislatures and elsewhere illustrate that even those who believe that it may be in society's best interests to affirm stable couples of any sexual orientation and sex combination, they may find it extremely difficult to call these couples "families" or grant them the act of affirming "marriage" (Fenn, 1997, p. 3). In March 2000, Vermont became the first state to fully recognize partnerships of same sex couples.

When asked about "family," people have stated that they consider children, spouses, exspouses, former in-laws, children of new spouses, and friends as family members. These people have become family by virtue of providing emotional care or because of shared responsibility combined with domesticity and sex (Trost, 1996, p. 4). "Chosen family" is not a common term in society at large, and perhaps its most extensive use today is within "queer" theory and social science. Whatever nurses or their patients call it, the phenomenon exists. Kath Weston describes her chosen family and their weekly meals, card-playing and TV watching: "In retrospect, the incipient trust and solidarity . . . combined to make Thursdays feel like family occasions" (Weston, 1996, p. 563). Beyond meals, Weston and her chosen family shared a history of material assistance like moving to the same neighborhood, house-sitting, phone calls and attending social events together, which drew this group closer. Weston does not see chosen families as *deviant* from traditional marriage-based relationships but identical to them, apart from legality (Box 16–2). Godparents, in-laws and the extension of family associated with adoption also illustrate the selective aspects of limiting our understanding of family to only "blood relations" or a narrow legal tie.

A moving story illustrative of the role chosen family plays in the health and illness care setting is that of Sharon Kowalski and Karen Thompson, a couple who had been living together for 4 years before the following events began. In 1983, Kowalski was paralyzed and rendered speechless in a car accident. Kowalski's parents became increasingly uncomfortable with their daughter's lesbian relationship with Thompson. When

Box 16–1 TYPES OF FAMILY

- Biological family
- Blended family
- Chosen family
- Extended family
- Foster family
- Nuclear family
- Your family
- Your patient's family

Box 16–2 POSSIBLE MEMBERS OF A FAMILY

Adult members
- Spouse
- Same-sex partner
- Siblings
- Step and foster siblings
- "Best friends"

Previous generation
- Parents
- Stepparents
- Foster parents
- Aunts and uncles

Next generation
- Biological children
- Adopted children
- Stepchildren
- Foster children
- Neighbor children
- Nieces and nephews

Pet members
- Dogs, cats, fish, ferrets, iguanas

Thompson filed a suit for guardianship of her partner, the parents countered; Kowalski was then 27 years old, a college graduate and fully independent. In mid-1985 the Kowalski parents were granted guardianship and placed their daughter in a nursing home without sufficient rehabilitation services, despite Kowalski's progressing state of recovery, which had not been anticipated. Thompson and the couples' friends were denied visitation. Although she did not see Kowalski for 3 years, Thompson continued her legal battle with the help of the American Civil Liberties Union. When Thompson won a suit to have Kowalski tested for competency (which would nullify her parents' claim), Kowalski's first request was to see Thompson. Kowalski was found to have adult-level communication skills and potential for more rehabilitation than the nursing home was providing. Her parents at this point stepped aside and, in 1991, Thompson was given custody of Kowalski, after which her continued recovery (nearly a decade after the accident) allowed her to go home. In this case, the law and tradition (apparently combined with sexism, homophobia, and ableism) were eventually forced to accommodate a demand for recognition that what it meant to be a partner and family can be based on heart, lived experience, and stubborn persistence (Griscom, 1998, pp. 346–351).

The state of Alaska lent some validity to the reality of chosen family when, in 1995, it was found to be illegal for the University of Alaska to cover only opposite sex spouses in health insurance (Moskowitz, 1996, p. 1). To be legal, the university would either have to deny all spouses or cover anyone recognized as dependent on the employee. Many state and local governments and private businesses now allow workers to identify a significant other of either gender as partner for purposes of insurance coverage. Although this expansion challenges definitions of family, the most negative response is not to the general issue but to the inclusion of same-sex partners. One group affected by shifts that allow some recognition of "partnership" without marriage is elders, who may co-habit without marriage to preserve Social Security benefits available only to a widow and canceled if she remarries.

It is not surprising, however, that there is widespread legal discrimination on the basis of sexuality, given that "homosexuality" itself was classified as an illness by the American Psychiatric Association until 1973. GLBT families have only had 25 years of development free of a label of pathology. What is surprising, though, is that the American Association for Marriage and Family Therapy did not include a nondiscrimination clause for sexuality until 1991; their accreditation commission did not follow suit until 1997. Some data suggest that GLBT people seek mental health services two to four times more often than straight folks, and the treatment they received regarding family issues might be related to these stresses. Although GLBT psychology journals, such as the *Journal of Homosexuality,* do exist, it is posited that these are generally only read by lesbian and gay people and those specifically interested in that research, not the treatment community at large. The *assimilationist* representation of GLBT families in the media may give the impression that their dynamics are identical to those of straight families, thus discouraging research into the effects of *heterosexism* and homophobia on the family as a whole (Clark & Serovich, 1997).

The Next Generation

The social impact of legal definitions of family have an impact on the next generation in intriguing ways as well. Courts in many states have affirmed adoption by GLBT couples. However, the standard birth certificate form was created with tradition in mind: there are blanks for "father" and "mother," rather than "parent A" and "parent B" or some other more flexible designation. For all couples, the advent of newer reproductive technologies makes some of these labels even more elusive. Is "mother" the source of the ovum, the possessor of the uterus, or the person who assumes nurturance at birth? Is "father" the source of the sperm, the legal spouse of the mother, or a nurturing and caring single parent who happens to be male? Our dialogue on these issues is in its infancy, pulled along by court decisions, ethical analyses, media exposés, and community exploration.

Likewise, we are relatively early in our experience with open adoption records and state laws allowing adopted children and biological parents to find one another. Our general bias toward information access suggests that this is a good trend, although anecdotes identify problems. These include the problem of explaining to a subsequent family the sudden appearance of an older sibling, or the response of a long-time partner to revelations about a previous sexual liaison.

If the standard definition of "nuclear family" includes parents and children, does it take a child in a home to constitute a family? In 1995, 24 million married couples had no children living in their home. Leslie Lafayette is the founder of the ChildFree Network. The Network links together, for social activities, members who do not have, cannot have, or do not want children. They advocate politically for an end to workplace inequalities, such as expectations that they will perform extra work for co-workers who are out with sick children and see their insurance rates rise because of group coverage for *in-vitro fertilization* (Fost, 1996, p. 1). There is some rising social awareness of the injustice and psychological damage done when a couple without children is treated as if they had neglected some important obligation or are less than complete. Some of them are infertile, with all of the social and psychological burdens that entails. Others are without children deliberately. In either case, respect for the individuals involved argues against leaping to any conclusions about "rightness" or "completeness."

CHILDREN AND PARENTING

The process of somehow getting a child for whom you can be a parent can profoundly challenge *and* perpetuate socially structured notions of parenthood. In Minnesota, Karen Heeney and Julia Beatty, a couple, were denied legal protection for access to artificial reproductive technologies in 1995. "The court also noted that the Minnesota parentage law on artificial insemination applied only to married couples, not single women, and that Minnesota law generally favored the institution of traditional marriage" (Moskowitz, 1996, p. 1) (Box 16–3). Research into the policies supporting and funding fertility clinics illustrates the lengths to which straight couples are allowed to go to achieve both physically and psychologically "normal" births (Cussins, 1998). These experiences are limited to couples who can afford the high costs, which are generally not covered by health insurance plans (although 12 states now ensure some coverage). Economically similar single women and lesbians are referred to sperm banks.

Motherhood, in addition to "fetal personhood," becomes a tricky juggle of semantics because, among the genetic mother, the gestational mother, and the woman who will raise the child, the traditional definitions of parenthood may not be sustainable. Ragoné (1998) found that a surrogate who donates ova, has motherhood attributed to her, but in the case of a gestational surrogate, who "simply" carries the child, motherhood is not. In contrast, men who donate sperm, itself a kind of surrogacy, are never considered parents. In these situations, selective reduction in the case of multiple fertilizations becomes even more complicated. Having

Box 16-3

WHO IS A FIT PARENT?

A Florida court ruled in a custody suit that an 11-year-old girl would be put in the custody of her convicted-murderer father (he killed wife number one), who was over $1,000 behind in child support, instead of her lesbian mother, because the father would be more strict and the daughter would not be forced to live in a lesbian environment (Moskowitz E.H. (1995) In the Courts: Two Mothers. Hastings Center Report [online] Available: FirstSearch/BSSI96029087[7 January 1999]).

asked a woman to be either a genetic or gestational parent to your child for a fee, can you demand she abort excess fetuses or abnormal ones? Furthermore, who or what does this kind of generation serve?

Courts have given some answers. In 1993, the California Supreme Court heard the case of a boy who was carried by a surrogate after implantation of his parents' combined sperm and egg. The justices ruled in favor of the couple, invoking issues of intent, which a dissenting justice felt was "invoking the paradigm of intellectual property law" (Rose 1998, p. 217). For, if "motherhood was ultimately a matter of intention" then this child was akin to property (a notion much more common a century or so ago). It is also interesting that such issues of authorship in the law are expressed in paternalistic terms. Feminists see this as a usurpation of their power as procreators, which in a case of petri dishes and syringes is questionable (or maybe uncategorizable) itself. Beyond gender issues, race became a mitigating factor because the father was white, the genetic mother was Filipina, and the surrogate was African-American. What race would this boy be considered if left to be raised by his surrogate? Or his biological mother? Or his father? Some combination of these three? Another question seems the most significant: Who *is* the parent, in the lived experience of the child? We must be careful not to impose outdated normative limitations on children who owe their lives to new technologies applied to people otherwise limited by their natural capacities (Rose, 1998).

Children can also be viewed as "generated" property to be protected by law. In many cultures, this extends to parental or family decisions on marriage partner, a choice affirmed by exchange of goods, property, or money. The traditional taboo against incest is not as natural or biological as we assume. Children as the property of the family must be protected to remain pure for the selected outsider who eventually will have sexual access. More common in this country are custody debates, which further highlight the owned status of children as both physical and emotional property. Legal intervention may be required, for example, in cases of parental kidnapping. Both parents may have emotional ownership of a child, and associated legal possession is violated by denial of access to the other parent through "theft" (Collins, 1996).

Social theorists Brennan and Noggle (1997) question the tendency to speak about justice *for* families instead of *within* them (Box 16–4). This means seeing parents as the stewards of their children "limited by children's own rights." In terms of public policy, this would change the test of best interests to include the child's own voice in that test. It would also seek to prevent the need to invoke the legal standard of clear and present danger to protect children by supporting intervention while there is still a positive relationship between parent and child. Brennan and Noggle suggest education, financial assistance for single parents, universal child care, drug rehabilitation, and even in-home consultants, such as nutritionists and housekeepers, and presumably child support enforcement. "All these are ways to provide for the nurturing of the child while respecting her right to maintain the personal relationships with her biological parents" (1997, p. 11). This model could lead to such actions as reconsideration of the current nature of adoptions, which are closer to a legal transaction, with children as parental property. Instead, the model would recognize and foster initial emotional attachments that may then lead to adoption, rather than the other way around (Brennan & Noggle, 1997).

Many of today's families also include the role of foster child or foster parent. This form of socially recognized family provides a legal mechanism for short-term placement of children when there are no parents or the parents have been found to be unfit. Foster homes are supposed to fill a temporary role, either until the original parents are once again available or until a new, per-

Box 16–4 CHILDREARING AND ECONOMICS

Family structure affects children's eventual occupational outcome. The lack of two biological parents is associated with lower socioeconomic status. Children living in an alternative home with one male parent are twice as likely to be at the bottom of the career ladder as female-headed alternative homes and homes with two biological parents. (Biblarz, T.J., A.E. Raferty & A. Bucar. (June 1997). Family structure and social mobility. *Social Forces* [online], pp. 1319–1341. Available: FirstSearch/ BSSI97028681 [7 January 1999].)

manent adoptive family is identified. Although foster parents bear the emotional and physical burdens of day-to-day childrearing, they may be paid at least a token amount to do so and do not have the full legal custody of their charges. Legal relatives of the child (grandparents, aunts, cousins) may be asked to assume this role.

Over the course of recent decades, we have experienced an increased concern for the physical and emotional safety of children, arguing for rapid removal of children from potentially dangerous situations, coupled with laws requiring health and education professionals to report suspected child abuse promptly to authorities for investigation. The subsequent decisions about long-term care and rearing of the child have been complex. There is serious concern for the mental health of children moved from one foster care setting to another and of children separated from siblings in the process. The preferential use of biological family members or members of the same ethnic or racial group as foster parents is seen as one antidote to these problems. From time to time, there has been an associated dialogue about the economic responsibility of families to care and whether a related foster parent should be paid as a nonrelative would be paid. Critics of this approach suggest that it is primarily a budget-saving measure rather than a well-considered policy in support of families.

Others have been more focused on questions about re-establishment of the original family group and the negative impact on children of staying in foster care for extended periods. Termination of parental rights and permanent adoption of children can take a very long time, especially when social policies keep child welfare agencies on very short staff and budget. There is some feeling that the prolonged permanent placement process is far more harmful to children than other options. The occasional widely reported death of a child known to child protective agencies but still living with the reportedly abusive parent(s) provides additional emotional fuel to the entire debate, with no tidy resolution in sight.

Social and legal constraints are evident in another area of parenthood: interracial adoption. There is increasing pressure to place children in families of the same race to ensure that the child is given a full opportunity to learn her or his collective past. In the case of Native American children, this has been enacted into law. For example, The Indian Child Welfare Law Center of Minnesota works "with the Indian community to preserve and reunite Indian families by providing culturally appropriate legal services to Indian children, parents, extended family members, and tribes in cases governed by the Indian Child Welfare Act of 1978, and to serve as a community development resource for Indian Child Welfare Act education, advocacy, and public policy" (http://www.glrain.net/icwalc/). These constraints, which make a great deal of sense within the historical context of the United States, are viewed with concern by anxious-to-adopt parents who want to locate an adoptable infant regardless of skin tone. Their search has led to a growth in international adoptions, many of which are interracial. The popular press supports this by devoting much space to discussions of the plight of orphans in various impoverished countries and the "excessive" difficulties American parents experience going through the adoption process in a foreign country. Less time has been devoted to the hidden difficulties encountered on return to the U.S. Children with no English language and having only experienced life in an understaffed institution or during a time of armed conflict may not quickly become the warm and cuddly bundles of joy that the new parents anticipated. And a number of countries have enacted laws limiting these adoptions, out of apparent concern that the children will be denied their heritage.

In one study of African-American mothers, "boundaries distinguishing biological mothers of children from other women who care for children" were found to be in regular flux, giving rise to the term "othermothers," the women who help "bloodmothers" in rearing responsibility. Neighborhood systems of mothers intercaring and interrelating have developed, possibly because the bloodmother was physically unable to care for the child because of illness or employment outside of the home (Hill Collins, 1996, p. 574). One hypothesis is that this represents a group *solidarity* originating in the nature of family under U.S. slavery, in which family units were split through sale without question. These arrangements can be seen as similar to the chosen families discussed earlier.

Women with "disabled" or ill children may find a consistent experience of being labeled "bad mother," implying that mothers are judged by the quality of their products, that is, their children. The women in one study were not bad parents by measures of caring, nurturing, or supporting their offspring. But the situation and "cultural markers" left them feeling second-class, if not as if they were totally failing as parents. Beyond their own questioning why they and their children were made to be different: Is it punishment? Fate? God?, they encountered mixed social messages. One woman has described her response to seeing a poster featuring a sick infant, looking much like her own child, every time she went to get food from her local Women, Infants, and Children prescribed nutrition program. The poster was intended to minimize the incidence of fetal alcohol abuse but seemed to be accusing the woman, even though she had done everything "right" during her pregnancy (food, exercise, temperance). Women have perceived an implicit guarantee of a healthy infant if they commit to these right behaviors, and they feel that society accuses them—that any sick infant is the result of faulty motherhood. When interacting with strangers or acquaintances, these mothers also sensed a need to speak out and prove that they *hadn't* done anything to "deserve" or warrant a sick infant (Landsman, 1998).

Although "alternative" families may be perceived as rare and on the sideline of social acceptability, they do get air time in the news and popular media: Mia Farrow and Woody Allen, Ellen DeGeneres and Anne Heche, television programs such as *Step by Step, Will & Grace,* and *Roseanne.*

Homeless families have not had the same level of attention from the media and academia, although they often arrive at their situation as a direct result of public policy decisions rather than personal choices. In a New York City homeless family, the mother is typically a 20-year-old unmarried woman with one or two children age 6 or younger. She probably did not finish high school, has never worked, and had an abortion by age 16. Her likelihood of having been in foster care is one in five, and if she was, she is over twice as likely as other homeless mothers of having an open case with child welfare agencies. Homeless kids are three times more likely to have been born to a single mother than their nonhomeless counterparts. However, *half of these mothers had two-parent homes themselves,* growing up without public assistance. Ralph da Costa Nunez (1995, p. 1) has found in his work as president of Homes for the Homeless, the composition of homeless families to be "loosely knit, transitory." Education is the ultimate predictor of eventual stability and success, yet education is not (or cannot be) emphasized within homeless communities. The end result is a lack of "critical skills, values, and self-esteem, typically instilled in a traditional family structure [meaning with a home and financial stability]," with people experiencing a persistence of family ideals but lacking structure or experience to fulfill them (1995, p. 1). Public policies about homeless shelters (traditionally serving single men) and available housing ("can't you stay with someone?") leave these young women and their children at risk for any number of problems, physical and emotional (Nunez, 1995).

For those families that do include children and teens today, not only is the structure of their family likely different than their parents but so is their appearance. The "second" baby boom, begun in 1977, consists of 72 million children and teens (28 percent of the total population). As one example of change, by 1990, two million of these youth described themselves to be of a different race than at least one of their parents, making one in every 35 young people mixed-race. To get an idea of what this means, think of a school with classes of 30 to 40 children: *one child in every classroom* is from a family that defies traditional racial or ethnic categorization. This dynamic, as well as a growing desire to avoid stereotyping on racial or ethnic grounds, has led to changes such as the new federal policy adding "mixed race" as an option on census and other government data collection instruments.

Schools

One of our (very few) universal social policies in the United States is the commitment to education for all children. School is an integral part of a child's life, so its structure, location and tone have strong impact. Schools have been a part of the Americanization process for generations of immigrants. Because schools have contact with almost every child, we also turn to them as social gatekeepers, as in the "no shots, no school" laws enacted by states concerned with the control of vaccine-preventable diseases. We expect schools to teach not only basic reading, mathematics, computing, and athletic skills, but also human anatomy and health promotion, sexuality education, and alternatives to violence.

What schools teach (overtly or covertly) about social roles, gender, and family becomes part of later adult life (Box 16–5). Because the broader society is in conflict about sexual orientation, for example, high schools have had difficulty providing appropriate services (or even any explicit services) to GLBT teens as they struggle through adolescence. This lack of good social support during a time of self-discovery may be one of the factors leading to subsequent mental health problems or risk-taking behavior. Stereotyping and social exclusion may further set the stage for problems. Study of internal social structures at four California high schools found an array of cliques (as defined by members and their peers): jocks, cheerleaders, "drama freaks," punks, stoners, losers, "death rockers," brains, preppies, nerds. Each group had its own standards of style, actions, and goals (or lack thereof). Who achieves or fails to achieve privileges from larger disciplinary and social bodies is shaped in large part by these adolescent societies (Wooden, 1996, pp. 532–537). Much analysis of the 1999 violence and death at Columbine High School in Littleton, Colorado, focused on the role preferential treatment of athletes and isolation of others (the black-coated "trenchcoat mafia") played in setting the stage for violence.

After a 1987 group suicide at a New Jersey high school, Donna Gaines (1996, p. 14) spent time with the dead teens' peer group. Outside (or in place of) school, they hung out in an abandoned building, sometimes bored, listening to music, using substances, and having sex. The teens did not lack interest in life, but they did not have any interest in the standard school activities and clubs, preferring their own company. Although after the suicides the town recognized the need for greater outreach and constructive (or at least not destructive) activities, "it was taken for granted that if you refused to be colonized" by such options, you were "looking for trouble." The blame for "failure" was bounced back to those who would be victims, leading some to describe them as "overregulated by adults, yet alienated from them . . . integrated only into the world shared with their peers" (Gaines, p. 22). When young people who did not respond positively to the standard socialization process offered by our schools seek to define their own adult families, it is not clear what they will expect or how they will live.

Overregulation based on social values was clearly one of the biggest problems in the schools run by the Catholic church on American Indian reservations earlier in this century and the previous centuries. Violence, denial of culture, racism, sexism, and absolute separation from blood family defined many of the children's experiences. "All I got out of school was being taught how to pray. I learned quickly that I would be beaten if I failed in my devotions or . . . prayed the wrong way, especially prayed in Indian to Wakan Tanka, the Indian Creator" (Crow Dog & Erodes, 1996, p. 512). Without the religious overtones, the same abrupt separation from family and culture was the norm in schools run by the Bureau of Indian Affairs. Why is this important now? Because the children who lived through these experiences are now adult family

Box 16–5

CONFUSING SOCIAL VALUES

The community response to the behavior of one high-school jock clique, the Spur Posse (widely reported in national media), illustrates social response to behavior. The members of the Posse took turns having sex with women (consensually or through rape) and publicly keeping score. In the aftermath of disclosure, it was more often the involved women who received social condemnation than the sexually aggressive Posse members (Wooden, W. S. (1996). Kicking Back at 'Raging High'. *Mapping the Social Landscape.* Susan J. Ferguson, Ed. Mountain View, CA: Mayfield Publishing).

members with their own responsibilities. Some have become part of movements to reclaim American Indian culture and transmit it to future generations; others continue to experience alienation and associated personal and social pain.

Jonathan Kozol's landmark work, *Savage Inequalities* (1991), captures the two poles of U.S. education: the college prep schools and inner-city wastelands. Swimming pools, computers, foreign languages, and landscaping are compared to the lack of functioning plumbing, ancient textbooks, poor teachers, and little insulation from winter's chill. One set of children has the tools and scores for entrance into the best universities and careers, the other set may see teen pregnancy and truancy as a far better emotional option than the societal disregard evidenced by their education. The impact both will have on the next generation's "parent pool" needs no elaboration. Our collective sense of community has not been extended to eliminate such a disparity of investment, though states have taken steps to set at least minimum expenditure-per-pupil equity across districts.

Given the importance of preparing the next generation for adulthood, this country does have some governmental efforts that should, at least theoretically, help with good parenting. For example, within the Social Security Act, part D of Title IV requires states to provide child support enforcement. In 1984 the Child Support Enforcement Amendments and in 1988 the Family Support Act were passed to encourage the collection of support payments from noncustodial parents. Unfortunately, as of 1992 they had failed to do so (Family Policy, 1997, p. 3). Of the 186 million cases in U.S. Health and Human Services in 1994, only 18 percent had successful collection (Garasky, 1997, p. 2). This results in the poverty in which 35 percent of mother-only families live (Family Policy). Changes associated with 1997 welfare reform have further strengthened this effort. This is a case of government advocating for individual familial responsibility. The push for this policy, however, runs against other concerns, such as protecting a woman's autonomy and safety if she declines to identify the child's father or fears him.

Kentucky's youth services programs provide one example of social policy that is supportive of families. The state has recognized the important role of family in preventing and rehabilitating juvenile offenders and delinquents. "The problem is that they often do not know how to be good parents. By helping parents improve their skills, education and youth service professionals can make a real difference in the lives of at-risk children" (Wolford et al, 1995 p. 1). Parents are included in rehabilitation programs (such as therapy sessions) even if it means videotaping them when the youth are housed too far away for the parents to attend. Within schools (kindergarten through high school) Youth Service Centers funded by the Kentucky Educational Reform Act of 1990 are being established. The services offered are age-appropriate, from pre-school and after-school care, parent education, and health services to job counseling and training and mental health and abuse crisis intervention. All students and families are eligible for the services, which are locally coordinated and facilitated by families, school personnel, and students (Wolford et al, 1995).

HEALTH AND ILLNESS CARE

Assuring access to health and illness care services is one way to improve the health of individuals and families. While many other factors, such as exposure to environmental hazards and genetic heritage, are critical, it is also extremely important that children receive their immunizations and be regularly evaluated for normal growth and development. Likewise, it is important that adults be adequately immunized and be screened for hypertension, diabetes, and cancer at appropriate ages and intervals. Both adults and children need dental care. And if there is an ongoing challenge to health, such as asthma, early detection and comprehensive management will minimize absence from school or work and increase the likelihood of full participation in age-appropriate activities. Finally, a family with healthy members is in a better position to respond to the challenges of daily living.

The absence of a comprehensive commitment to access to universal health insurance coverage for all makes achieving the desired level of interaction with health professionals extremely difficult (Box 16–6). At least one proposal for financing universal health care has been presented to and denied by the Congress every year since 1912 (Chung & Pardeck, 1997, p. 4). In 1999, more than 40 million Americans lacked health insurance, more than the number uninsured at the time of the last major attempt to provide universal coverage, in 1993 and 1994. The majority of those uninsured are those working in low-paying jobs that do not offer an affordable insurance policy as a benefit of employment, or the families of workers who cannot afford to purchase coverage for their dependents. The costs of insurance coverage, or of care purchased directly, con-

Box 16–6

ACCESS TO HEALTH SERVICES

- Children ages 5 to 17 lose 4.5 days of school each year because of acute or chronic illness.
- Only 40.5% of the U.S. population has dental insurance.
- Texas and Arizona have the most uninsured citizens (over 24% of the population); Hawaii has the least (under 9%).

(National Center for Health Statistics, 1999)

tinues to rise, making access ever more difficult. Those who lack insurance are routinely found to seek care later in an episode of illness, when they are sicker, and thus with the need for more, and more expensive, care, which they cannot afford. Lacking a regular source of primary care, the emergency room becomes the caregiver of last, most expensive resort. For example, while it is not surprising that 31.6 percent of all visits to emergency rooms are for injuries and poisonings (they comprise only 9.2 percent of *all* outpatient visits), it should be of concern that 13.3 percent of emergency room visits are for "symptoms, signs, and ill-defined conditions," a category comprising only 6.2 percent of all outpatient visits (NCHS, 1999). The uninsured are also more likely to report not purchasing a recommended prescription for medication after a visit.

The Child Health Insurance Program (CHIP) (Figure 16–1) enacted by Congress in 1997 represents an attempt to protect children by making affordable insurance available to them. The funds (one of the largest sums ever made available for this purpose) may be used by the states either to expand Medicaid through increased eligibility for children in families with income levels higher than those used for regular Medicaid, or to create new programs. Two problems have made progress with CHIP difficult. The process of welfare reform has removed families from Medicaid eligibility, making more children eligible for CHIP than were contemplated when the program began. And there are at least concerns, if not documented evidence, that employers will drop dependent coverage, pushing previously insured children into this publicly supported program. Even with coverage, there are continuous debates about the exact services to be covered, and the level of co-payment or deductible needed. These debates reflect social policies or social conflict, including the debate about whether health and illness services are a consumer commodity to be purchased at individual preference or a social good to be made available equitably to everyone. Medicare, for example, has not provided coverage for prescription drugs, though doing so would probably decrease the need for hospitalization by the elderly. In Congressional debate of medicare, opposition to what might appear to be a natural extension comes from those concerned with the potential economic consequence of making the U.S. government a large purchaser capable of establishing price controls on drugs. Another example is the conflict between full coverage for all reproductive health services and the strong antichoice lobbying of some groups, which has led to limits on funding for abortion in many public programs. An intriguing rebalance has come in that the push by (generally more powerful) men to have the antiimpotence drug Viagra covered by insurance has highlighted the failure of many insurance plans to cover contraception for (generally less powerful) women.

Another attempt to improve access to care for children and adolescents has been the development of comprehensive school health clinics. Schools have long been the site of some health-related services, such as screening for vision or hearing problems, dental caries, or scoliosis. They have also included at least some health education, with the most recent addition being HIV/AIDS education mandated in some or all grades in all states. School nurses have been employed to assure evaluation of health problems that arise in the course of the school day and to oversee medications or other treatments needed by children with disabilities. It has been a natural expansion of traditional school health services to add primary health care through the employment of physicians, nurse practitioners, or physician's assistants. One rationale for placing services in the school has been the difficulties that working parents (either single parents or two working parents) have leaving work to take their children for care during ordinary daytime working hours. The first school-based clinics were for adolescents and included a strong emphasis on access to reproductive health services.

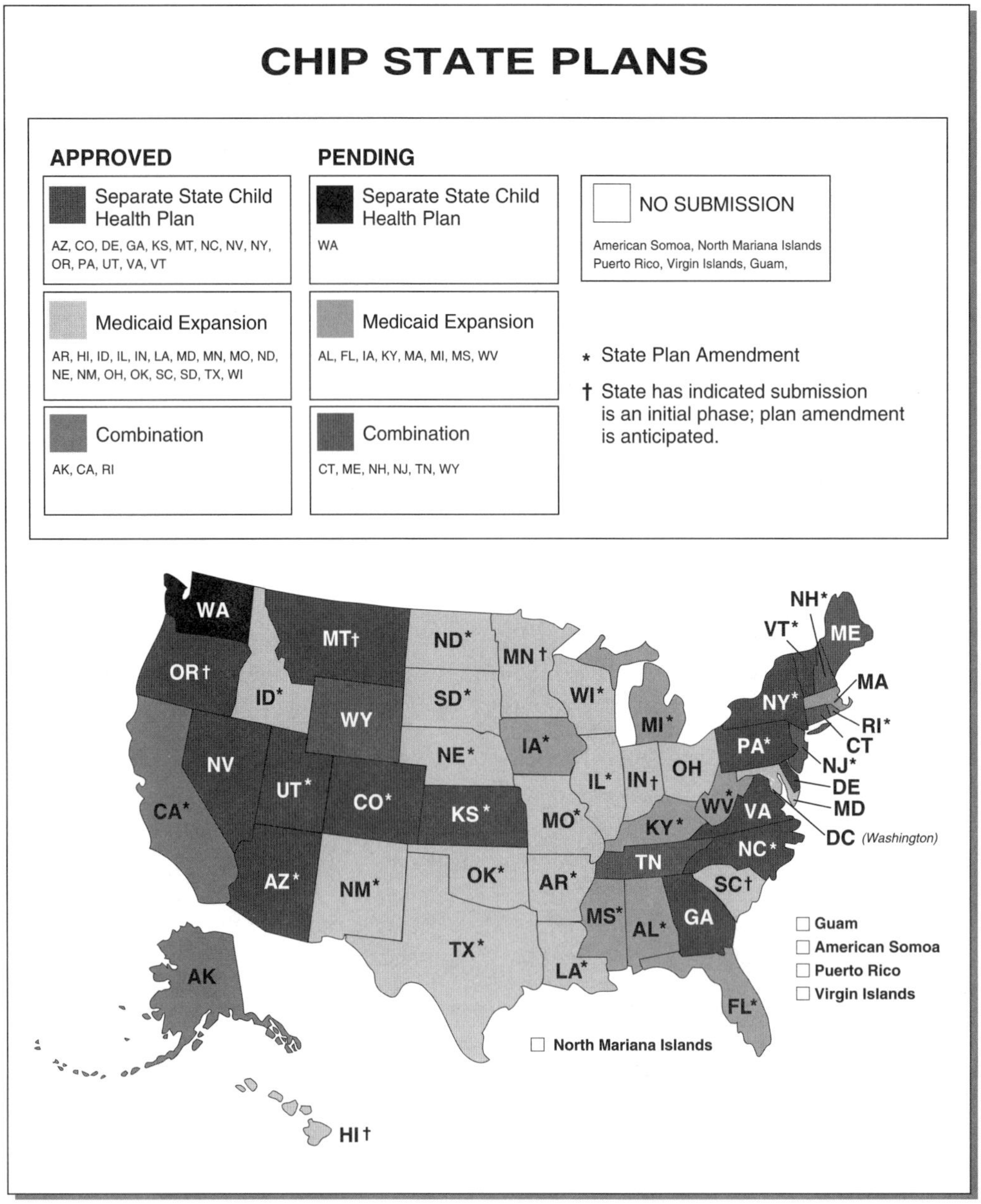

FIGURE 16-1
CHIP state plans

Some school-based programs have considered expansion to cover even the family members of the children.

The health of families has been improved in recent years by more than access to care. National policies regarding desirable levels of immunization and improved quality of the care being rendered are also important. *Healthy People 2010* is the current iteration of national health objectives developed by the Department of Health and Human Services (DHHS) 2000 (http://web. health.gov/healthypeople/). The overall goal for the nation is increased years of healthy life and the elimination of health status disparities across racial, ethnic, sex, gender, or other lines. Developed every 10 years to plan a decade of effort, *Healthy People* has provided a national focus on important areas for investment of resources and has spurred states and localities to develop their own *Healthy People* plans as well. Public dialogue through earlier *Healthy People* efforts revealed the fact that over 50 percent of U.S. children were not fully, age-appropriately immunized. This has led to significant improvements, using a combination of provider education, support for vaccine purchase, registries and recall systems, and community-wide advertising. Other areas of family health that have benefited from the comprehensive, population-focused efforts of this type have been injury prevention, diabetes detection and management, and asthma management.

Nurses have many opportunities to encounter the problems created for families by the lack of health insurance, limited access to primary care, or social policies that are at odds with a family's values. Less visible are those policies about our environment that have a differential impact on families. Environmental health encompasses all those organized activities that endeavor to limit human contact with substances harmful to health by providing some form of barrier or by preventing their general release (Box 16–7). Efforts to assure safe drinking water, clean air, and safe disposal of waste products are all part of environmental health. One of the signal successes of this effort is the dramatic reduction of blood lead levels in children after the removal of lead from gasoline products; additional lead control efforts focus on protection from access to old paint products or paint. As with other areas of health, those at the lowest income levels are those most vulnerable to failures in our policies. This includes poor urban children living in old buildings with lead solder in drinking water pipes and old lead-based paint on the walls, rural poor children living without benefit of a working sewer or septic tank, or the children of migrant laborers living and playing near pesticides and dangerous farm equipment. Community decisions regarding the location of waste disposal sites (both industrial waste sites and domestic waste land fills) means that those of lower income are much more likely to live in proximity to harmful waste products than those more affluent. The environmental justice movement has emerged as a way of bringing attention to these disparities and mobilizing action to protect all of the population.

CAREGIVING FOR OLD AND YOUNG

One of the roles families play within society is that of caregiver for dependent family members. These may include ill, young, or elderly persons or those with long-term disabilities. The level of care needed varies widely, from those who need complete assistance with all activities of daily living, those who can manage personal hygiene and nourishment but need assistance with functional activities, such as shopping or transportation, to those who need regular emotional or social support while maintaining physical independence. As examples of the intersection of social policy and family health, this section will focus on issues of child care and elder care.

Paid child care is the practical outcome of a society that is composed of individuals who both parent and work. Successful, affordable childcare is a persistent concern at all income levels in this country. Some other societies (France, the Scandinavian countries) provide

Box 16–7 ENVIRONMENTAL (IN)JUSTICE

Traditional social science has focused on the intersections of race, class, and gender. However, increased concern about our physical environment has led to a sociology of the environment. Environmental disparities seem to be linked to race, or to not being white. Three out of five African-Americans in the U.S. live near "uncontrolled toxic waste sites." Of the 18 federal research grants available to find new nuclear waste facilities, 15 proposal writers are directing their efforts at sites on American Indian reservations. The public consequences are very real. (Pinderhughes, R. (Summer 1996). The impact of race on environmental quality: an empirical and theoretical discussion. *Sociological Perspectives* [online], pp. 231–248. Available: FirstSearch/BSSI96036145 [22 August 1999]).

universal child care in the neighborhood or at the workplace, believing that parenting is a responsibility shared by the entire community. Overall, 73 to 95 percent of European 3- to 5-year-olds are in public day care (Hertz & Ferguson, 1996, p. 1). In this country, there has been limited support for subsidizing and organizing child care for those at the low end of the income scale, to enable those parents to participate in work training or take entry-level employment. Some businesses provide on-site child care, either as a mechanism to retain or attract skilled workers or because of labor union negotiations. Other options for parents include live-in or day-only caregivers, relatives, home-based day care, center-based day care, backup adults in case of illness, varied hours for parent work schedules, or any combination of these. The transition of women to work outside of the home and their replacement as child caregivers with other child care options (including fathers) can be characterized as a "de-skilling" of the stereotypical mother (Hertz & Ferguson, 1996).

As women of color, especially African-Americans, have joined the middle class, they have gained access to child care options beyond those offered by relatives at no cost. At the same time, those options raise the potential of exposing their children at a young age to experiences of racism within day care programs. Women who place children in day care report feeling less replaced as a parent, in contrast to those who bring someone into the home to provide care (Hertz & Ferguson, 1996, p. 4–5), perhaps because they can see day care as a school, a socially positive step, not replacement parenting, which is subject to criticism.

All of these child care issues are, of course, related to the work schedules given to or developed by parents. While some may be able to organize split shifts or irregular days on and off, others must, by the nature of their work, be away from the home during regular business hours. Those families in which schedules could be juggled to accommodate more parent time in the home, "push the boundaries of maintaining middle class standards . . . [Parents] do pay career costs associated with these choices and they pay economic penalties because they earn less. Yet, they challenge conventional wisdom about what is possible in integrating work and family life: They are not waiting for the State or the workplace to broadly implement 'family friendly' policies." (Hertz & Ferguson, 1996, p. 13)

However, those parents who shift their job time and so lack full "job success" are mainly women, thus "reinforcing the old pattern of women's work ghettos" (Harrington, 1998, p. 4). The most common employer approaches to accommodating parenting are leave (now required by law for larger employers) and options to work part-time. When polled, parents suggest that flexible work hours and child care within the workplace would be better. Furthermore, even in places that allow sick leave and time off for family, employees who felt stigma or disapproval from their peers were reluctant to make use of the policies (Lee & Duxbury, 1998, p. 8). If shifting work schedules becomes the answer, then day care programs may need to adjust *their* hours of operation. This may also increase the participation of fathers in child care. In some studies it was found that, if a mother worked part-time, fathers were more likely to care for the child during mother's work hours than if the mother worked full-time. But fathers' work schedules also had an impact on their availability, and those work schedules are the strongest predictor (over other socioeconomic concerns) of whether they will be child caregivers. Families with more money were also less likely to make use of fathers, although what was more important was how much money the mother made relative to the father's income. Larger amounts of male unemployment in 1990 and 1991 resulted in a noticeable increase in paternal caregiving (Casper & O'Connell, 1998, p. 6).

The Sick Child

The components that produce healthy folks are known, sometimes even facilitated, by the state. But what if the family has a child who is critically ill? The practice of medicine within neonatal intensive care units (NICUs), where paid professionals often make decisions over or without the opinions of parents, calls into question the nature of parenting and, consequently, family. Unless a family is willing to go to court, medical practitioners control care by both overt and subtle means, usually with the best of intentions. NICU doctors, nurses, aids, and the like have been trained to face the multitude of situations that a sick or premature infant presents; most parents are not. Does this necessarily mean medicine knows best? According to Wall and Partridge (1997, p. 69), neonatologists whose armamentarium is now so expansive, "feel culpable when they elect to limit the treatment of marginally viable infants . . . (which) may at times be either inappropriate or inhumane."

Even though most parents do not anticipate or consider the possibility of delivering a sick infant, does this mean they are unable to cope? They are the parents and, as such, "become the natural repositories of what little information there is about their infants' interests and are expected to act as representatives for their infants"

(Heimer & Staffen, 1998, p. 244). Despite this, the research interviews of NICU parents done by Ellenchild and colleagues found an ongoing "underrepresentation" of the parents' position. Parents recalled a "general acceptance of all proffered treatments" but also that "they were not informed sufficiently in the NICU" (Heimer & Staffen, 1998, p. 74–86). Heimer and Staffen posit that parents play only a ceremonial role, in that they get to name the infant "but do not care for it" and are irrelevant in many treatment decisions. They are told of their importance, but the actions of the NICU speak to the preeminence of medical care over parenting (Heimer & Staffen, 1998, pp. 49, 69, 228).

How does this affect the issue of family? Education, which could promote positive parental involvement, is perceived by practitioners studied as impossible and unwelcome. Lack of information has ethical implications: "Without information parents are not in a strong position to be responsible decision makers. They cannot provide informed consent for any treatment of the child—a basic ethical mandate" (Ellenchild, 1996, p. 87). However, informed consent is not required for all or even many procedures (e.g., how much oxygen, how much food, cleaning techniques), although with sick infants their impact can be significant. In Haywood's (1994, p. 432–439) study of physician misassessment of NICU outcomes, the authors make a rather obvious statement that only with complete and cutting edge information can practitioners *and* parents make strategic decisions. A move toward family-centered care and full implementation of the principles on which his text is premised may provide an answer or at least a palliative to prevent some of the clashes described below.

Jehovah's Witnesses who are parents have a difficult time having their religious beliefs dominate over socially approved and medically prescribed procedures, such as blood transfusion. A family (not Witnesses) in New Zealand, having refused a liver transplant for their less than 2-year-old, very sick son, were taken to court for "unreasonableness." This decision was overturned in a higher court, because the mother was acting on behalf of the family and the pain and stress which would make her child's life even worse. Another family, with four children in all, went through a difficult and eventually further debilitating heart procedure with their oldest child. When the same procedure was suggested for their youngest, they refused. An Austrian family refused chemotherapy for a 6-year-old child's abdominal cancer in 1995. Having fled to Spain, the child was returned to Austria by state authorities and forcefully treated (Nicholson, 1997). *Nurses who have not considered the issues of parental rights, parental authority, and family autonomy will not be in a good position to help families in situations such as these.*

At the other end of life, *caregiving* is growing both as an inevitable family responsibility and as a profession. The Administration on Aging predicts that, by 2020, of the 15.2 million persons over age 65 who are living alone, 19.2 percent will need help with daily living. In 1998, three times the number of people than was the case a decade earlier had at least one member of the household caring for a friend or relative. Race is important in this statistic, with Asian-American and African-American homes being more likely to include a caregiver than homes described as Hispanic or white (Braus, 1998).

Caregiving, both lay and professional, is facilitated both by technological advances and need. The tools now exist for home care, as do the chronic diseases that demand them. Home care remains gendered in its nature, continuing to be feminine labor. There persists a perception that it is women's "unique, gender-based obligation to care for others without compensation . . . restrict(ing) women's choices and abilities to work, while at the same time leaving men free to be breadwinners" (Harrington, 1998, p. 4). Even where policies are written to be generally applicable, as in the Family Medical Leave Act, there is a general expectation that women will be the caregivers of first resort, regardless of the burden that places on them.

The fact that these lay caregivers are unpaid benefits greater social structures, especially Medicare and Medicaid. If we did not continue to expect that there will be home caregivers, it would cost us all a great deal more, either in emotional and social cost, earlier death, or increased taxes and fees (Schroeder & Ward, 1998). Women engaged in (lay) home care experienced much higher levels of stress than their other family members, as well as more alienation from those outside of the home because of their relation to the person for whom they cared (Armstrong, 1996, p. 7). These experiences are similar to those reported by many nurses about their workplace roles (Schroeder & Ward, 1998).

At least one observer suggests that "Our family care system is collapsing. When it worked well, it depended on the unpaid labor of women at home . . . our society has no new philosophic consensus for an economic system that would support families as care providers" (Harrington, 1998, p. 1). The Hastings Center, for example, presents a case of the granddaughter of a degenerating 70-year-old woman who asks her grandmother's oncologist for help in encouraging the use of Meals on Wheels and home caregivers. The grandmother lives alone and the granddaughter, her only visitor, is not able to cope with the increasing debility. The doctor declines, as he is listening to the grandmother, who is adamant about her independence and must be respected as a competent adult, a decision consistent with the best of patient autonomy approaches. The granddaughter questions whether her role as lone support is really so unimportant in the decision. (Don't I count?, 1997). It may be that we need a reconsidered ethic of autonomy in circumstances of physical dependency such as this. Family-centered thinking, including in the evaluation the impact of a decision on all participating family members, is at least as appropriate in this case involving adults as it is in the case of care for children.

In 1965, Medicare began funding home-care services for the elderly. In 1997, the cost had gone from $46 million to $20.5 *billion.* Medicaid also contributes, paying one-quarter of those dollars for the poor and some disabled. Less than one-quarter of all home care bills are paid by those using the service and 4 percent are covered by private insurance (Braus 1998: 7). In 1981, Medicaid Home and Community-Based Service Waivers were authorized, providing federal monies to home and community alternatives to nursing homes (Kennedy, 1997, p. 2). By doing so, the federal government is reflecting a valuing of the home, whether for humanitarian or economic reasons. Some states have had active senior groups supporting similar investment of state dollars, based on the assumption that admission to an institution is only occasionally the right choice, even for an older person with serious limitations in activities of daily living.

Even seemingly unrelated policies can have an impact on these commitments, however. The Human Rights Campaign, a GLBT political action organization, believes the U.S. House of Representatives has undermined this strong support for care in the home (and by implication, in the family) by their November 1995 vote to repeal the District of Columbia's domestic partnership law. Supporters of the repeal believed they were standing for the nuclear family, heterosexual marriage, and tradition. However, the law that allowed hospital visits and "equal access to health benefits for two people living together as a family for more than six months" mostly affected old people and those with disabilities who could not live alone and their care providers, not GLBT chosen families (Human Rights Campaign, 1995).

When the family decision is to use paid caregivers, it is important to realize that the family configuration is changed. Paid caregivers enter into homes influenced by their own cultural notions of their role. In the act of intimate care in the home environment, family-like relationships are created, leading to "fictive kin" status between professional caregiver and client. At times these chosen family members can move beyond fictive kin to functional kin status by virtue of the "substantive assistance, whether it be emotional, custodial, physical, or financial" (Karner, 1998, p. 7). *No assumptions should be made in advance about the relationships among identified home patients, their family members and their caregivers, particularly ones who have been involved for some period of time. The financial relationship may or may not be associated with a well-developed emotional and social one.*

WORK AND WELFARE

As indicated at the outset, this chapter can in no way provide a complete discussion of the social policies that affect a family in the U.S. today. As with the earlier sections, this discussion of work and welfare policies is illustrative of the issues and should point the way to questions to include in a family assessment or areas of potential social advocacy.

Social structures beyond the individual almost always include the rest of those who share the person's home. Many European countries, such as Germany, Sweden, and France have "family policies" that support "the well-being of families as an objective or a goal." Although the obvious diversity of U.S. families would make a blanket of identical support difficult, the Consortium of Family Organizations suggested in 1990 that the federal government ought to provide "substitute services only when the family cannot." The substitute services available when needed should include anything that might encourage the stability of parental and marital commitment, while recognizing that it should not discriminate against families with nontraditional make-ups (Family Policy, 1997, p. 1). Although they sound very appealing, these proposals easily become confused with fiscally conservative proposals that would control public spending by pushing responsibility onto "the family," even when the family lacks appropriate resources and would be discriminated against in contrast to those with higher incomes.

Head Start is this country's clearest policy commitment to comprehensive support of childrearing families. This program, begun during the 1960s War on Poverty, is designed to give young children in low-income families the nutrition, health services, and early learning support that makes them ready for learning. A strong bias for family involvement strengthens parents' ability to support their children even after the completion of Head Start participation. This program has never received appropriations sufficient to accommodate all families eligible by reason of income, nor is there any coherent reason why a similar range of services should not be available to all children. The problems experienced by families are made more complicated by this lack of a "coherent national policy"; research has found that the existing family programs are uncoordinated and not useful. The programs that do exist (like Social Security, the former Aid to Families with Dependent Children, and the current Temporary Assistance to Needy Families) "are largely reactive in nature; more importantly, they are not available to all children and families" (Chung & Pardeck, 1997, p. 2). Although the Family and Medical Leave Act was passed in 1993, giving folks time off after the birth of an infant or adoption as well as care of sick family members, time off does not equate to sufficient financial stability to house, clothe, and feed the family, or to coverage for the needed health services.

Poverty in itself is a limiting and at times frightening experience for families. In 1990, 26 percent of the population were children. Children are now the poorest age group of U.S. citizens, with one out of five living in poverty. One quarter of teens have long-term serious health or wellness problems, including pregnancy. Since 1981 the proportion of children needing mental health help has risen 80 percent (Chung & Pardeck, 1997, p. 1). Poverty, which persists in the face of employment and effort, is infuriating and disheartening, and possibly fuels other social problems. As a an example of this, consider Studs Terkel's portrait of C. P. Ellis (1998), which illustrates both the development of serious mental and social problems and the emergence of a solution.

As a white man from North Carolina, Ellis grew up poor, with an alcoholic, depressed father who worked for a textile mill, dying at age 48. At that point, Ellis quit eighth grade to help support his family. After he married, Ellis got a loan to start a service station, which he worked at nonstop until he had a heart attack: "I really began to get bitter. I didn't know who to blame. I tried to find somebody. I began to blame it on black people. I had to hate somebody. Hatin' America is hard because you can't see it to hate it. You gotta have somethin' to look at to hate." (Terkel, 1998, p. 361). Ellis drew on his father's past involvement in the Ku Klux Klan, becoming an exalted cyclops at the height of the civil rights movement. Ellis describes feeling important, like he had a vehicle to change his position in life. City officials began to use the Klan to counter civil rights protests, but not openly, which Ellis later realized was an ugly abuse. When his town received a grant to solve racial problems, the Klan was included. Ellis became co-chair of an education commission with "a militant black woman." "How could I work with her? But after two or three days, it was in our hands. We had to make it a success. This gave me another sense of belongin', a sense of pride . . . Here's a chance for a low-income white man to be somethin . . . My mind was beginnin' to open up . . . I don't want the kids to fight forever." Out of this experience, Ellis went on to put aside his race hatred, to run for the school board, he learned to sleep soundly at night, organized his union, and came to cry when he reflected on the words of Martin Luther King Jr., whose death he had initially celebrated (Terkel, 1998, pp. 365–367).

Women are the largest group receiving public income assistance. White women constitute the majority of those served, but a higher proportion of populations of women of color are enrolled. Women use welfare (what many still refer to by its old name, Aid to Families with Dependent Children, or AFDC) in four ways: in emergencies for the short term, as unemployment insurance, to supplement insufficient income, and in place of work (Schroeder & Ward, 1998). The overwhelmingly negative attitudes about women who remain on welfare for extended periods of time have fueled efforts to change the entire system in ways that would provide support when needed but clearly move people to independence. The Personal Responsibility and Work Opportunity Reconciliation Act, signed by President Clinton in 1996 as an effort to "reform" welfare and its purported abuses, sets lifetime limits on enrollment, with consequences as yet undetermined. The AFDC has been replaced by Temporary Assistance to Needy Families (TANF), with a 5-year lifetime limit. College attendance no longer counts as employment, meaning that those receiving assistance are directed to whatever employment is available at their present skill levels without the option of seeking education for subsequent employment (and tax-paying) at a higher level. It is expected that several hundred thousand disabled children currently receiving funding will lose it, with more stringent requirements of disability for establishing need in the first place. Though many of those no longer eligible for welfare are still able to participate in the Medicaid program, facilitating access to health-related services, it is not clear that states are making this plain to the people. If those previously receiving a combination of assistance and Medicaid are now receiving neither and are working in entry-level jobs with no health insurance benefit, it is likely that this will be reflected in a lowered health status for their children.

The attitudes toward welfare have been complicated by rising *xenophobia,* with legal immigrants also losing substantial social services. This appears to be a process of *blaming the victims,* putting the onus of social standing on the individual instead of the social systems and institutions which perpetuate all the "isms": racism, classism, sexism, heterosexism, and ableism. "Even the use of the word 'personal' in the [Welfare Reform] act's name attests to the conviction that poverty is an individual rather than structural problem and will be solved by individual effort alone" (Schroeder & Ward, 1998).

There are some who argue that governments can hurt families to a vast extent but are very limited in capacity to help (25th anniversary, 1996). With this belief, it is possible to argue that families should not be the focus of public policy at all, either at the federal or the state level. And given the structure of our federal government, states are key actors in what is provided as options to families both in the "market and privately in households, in who does the work in these spheres and how it is done" (Armstrong 1996, p. 2). And nearly every state has developed programs, plans, and rhetoric describing local efforts for improving family situations, while reforming welfare and saving money from the state coffers. For example, Cheryl Sullivan, as director of Indiana's Family and Social Services Administration (FSSA), is "(m)aking the government work for the families and children" she serves. The goal is to invest in independence now for a healthier future in Indiana. In her words, "Government alone cannot solve all the problems that families may have, but neither can it sit idly by. When families fail, everyone pays the cost." This sentiment is embodied by the Partnership for Personal Responsibility (PPR) (part of "welfare reform"), in which participants are restricted to 2 years of assistance, do not receive additional benefits for children born after entry into the program, and teen parents must live with another responsible adult and everyone must sign an agreement to immunize their children, get them to school, and accept any job offered (Sullivan, 1996, p. 1) (Box 16–8).

The FSSA also works with the state Department of Education to develop student educational goals. If a parent PPR member does not participate, their cash benefits are reduced. Noncompliance in the PPR program includes sanctions such as refusal of assistance for 2 to 36 months. A 1991 Indiana gubernatorial initiative, known as Step Ahead, organizes community councils for the creation and management of public service resources. Sixty-four of these 92 councils have begun to resolve transportation issues, which keep parents from successful employment. In 1995, Indiana began a "Most Wanted" campaign to "catch" delinquent noncustodial parents for child support payments. The amount collected that year doubled the 1989 total. Sanctions for failure to pay include loss of driver's or professional licenses (Sullivan, 1996, p. 7). Through county housing authorities, family self-sufficiency programs act as a bridge between welfare and independence (Monnett, 1997, p. 1).

In Hartford, Connecticut, after attending the Million Man March, Executive Director John Wardlaw began the Family Reunification Program. Available for families living in housing authority facilities, the program allows fathers to live with their children and children's mother without risk of losing welfare payments. In turn, the fathers appear jointly on the lease, agree to serve as a role model by abstaining from drug activity, receive job placement, and attend support meetings and life skills classes, while having their rent frozen for 18 months to enable them to break out of welfare (Callahan, 1996). In this case, public health measures have been recognized *and* facilitated by government policy. Many of the most creative and successful of these programs have operated in states with a more dispersed population and a very

Box 16–8

TRANSPORTATION AS KEY TO FAMILY SUCCESS

Minneapolis' McKnight Foundation's Family Loan Program will make loans to families who have been rejected by commercial lenders and have experienced some financial setback that might "hinder a parent's ability to keep a job or stay in school." The no-interest loans (over 80% of which are transportation-related) are in amounts up to $2,200 for 2 years. All of the loan sites are self-renewing after an initial opening grant (Mueller, M. R., & Berde, C. T. (Spring 1996). Minnesota's family loan program. *Public Welfare* [online], pp. 32–41. Available: FirstSearch/BSSI96022731 [7 January 1999].)

healthy economy. States with large cities concentrating poverty in inner city neighborhoods and continuing to experience high rates of unemployment have a much more difficult job of overcoming systemic barriers.

SUMMARY

Families are complex systems that exist within the even more complex system of a society. They are defined by society and the material world, but many seek to change those social definitions when the definitions no longer fit. Nurses are educated to serve individuals within the context of their families or to provide services to families as units. If working with a family does not take into account the ways in which that particular family is being influenced by social policy, it is likely that care will be less than ideal or that desired outcomes will not be achieved. For example, if a 19-year-old unmarried mother of two expresses the desire to work at getting a college degree so that she can fulfill her own career aspirations and improve her children's economic status, a working knowledge of the limits of welfare support, eligibility for tuition assistance, availability of affordable child care, and public transportation all should be taken into account *before* delivering a "you can do it" pep talk. *Yes, encouragement is appropriate, but it must be grounded in reality.*

The above example may seem extremely obvious. What may be less obvious to many are the subtleties of our assumptions about what is ordinary, expected, or right. Choosing carefully the words to use when exploring the configuration of people a new patient may call "family" can be as important as selecting the right position for a stethoscopic examination. A nurse who demonstrates awareness of family as experienced by a patient is going to give better nursing care, because a wider range of information on which a more complete care plan can be based will be forthcoming. A ground rule, both in assessing strengths and problems and in developing interventions, is "*ask first.*" Do not assume that you can determine by observation who is parent, which other is significant, who is central to a child's well-being, or who is willing or able to be accountable for action. And when initial questions indicate that the family configuration you are exploring does not fit any category that is familiar, *admission of ignorance and a request for education is wiser than blind assumption.*

Nurses are also in a position to act as advocates. In their day-to-day work, they see the impact that existing social systems and public policies have on families. Nurses are direct witnesses to limitations on who can participate in decision making at the end and beginning of life, who can take family leave and for how long to provide needed care and support, whether available child care is adequate and appropriate, and in the ways that long established "isms" cause deep pain. Many of those for whom we care are not in a position to actively advocate for changes. The role we can play in giving voice to the concerns and in devising creative alternatives is indispensable.

Each of us has a biological family, the source of our genetic material. Each of us also has a birth certificate naming the individual(s) legally responsible for us. Each of us has been reared by one or more adults, who may have volunteered, inherited the process, or been hired for the job. Each of us has moved through adulthood with or without participating in a shared life that may or may not be definable as a legal marriage. Each of us will make explicit or implicit decisions about the bearing, adopting, rearing, or avoiding of children. And each of us will experience the process of aging and the search for a source of support when frail, support that may or may not come from those considered family. At each step along the way, social policy about eligibility for legal relationship, for economic and social support, and for public recognition will either provide strength for or serve as a deterrent to healthy living. Nurses have multiple opportunities to support positives and to mitigate, at least by evidence of understanding, the negatives experienced today. Doing so not only is of benefit to our patients, but can enrich our individual and personal family life as well.

Study Questions

1. Identify two examples of "family" that are outside and contradict the stereotypical nuclear family.
2. Describe at least one policy shift in access or cost of personal health services that has an impact on the health of families.
3. Describe social discrimination as it affects family experiences.
4. List at least three services available to families because of public policies.
5. Why is it important that a nurse never presume to define "family" for a patient?
6. Discuss areas in which advocacy by nurses could be significant for family social policy.

References

25th anniversary: families in a changing world. *Journal of Comparative Family Studies*, Summer 1996.

Armstrong, P. (Summer 1996). Resurrecting 'the family': interring 'the state'. *Journal of Comparative Family Studies* [online], pp. 224–47. Available: FirstSearch/ BSSI96044131 [7 January 1999].

Biblarz, T.J., Raferty, A.E. & Bucar, A. (June 1997). Family structure and social mobility. *Social Forces* [online], pp. 1319–1341. Available: FirstSearch/ BSSI97028681 [7 January 1999].

Braus, P. (1998). When the helpers need a hand. *American Demographics* [online]. Available: FirstSearch/BSSI 98033092 [7 January 1999].

Brennan, S. & R. Noggle. (Spring 1997). The moral status of children: children's rights, parents' rights, and fam-ily justice. *Social Theory and Practice* [online], pp. 1–26. Available: FirstSearch/BSSI97027892 [7 January 1999].

Bumpass, L.L., et al. (August 1995). The changing character of stepfamilies: implications of cohabitation and non-marital childbearing. *Demography* [online], pp. 425–436. Available: FirstSearch/BSSI95036874 [7 January 1999].

Callahan, A. (November/December 1996). Family reunification: bringing fathers home. *Journal of Housing and Community Development* [online], pp. 25–27. Available: FirstSearch/BSSI96043416 [7 January 1999].

Casper, L.M., & O'Connell, M. (1998). Work, income, the economy, and married fathers as child-care providers. *Demography* [online]. Available: First-Search/BSSI 98022649 [7 January 1999].

Chung, W. S., & Pardeck, J. T. (Summer 1997). Explorations in as proposed national policy for children and families. *Adolescence* [online], pp. 429–436. Available: FirstSearch/ BSSI97032725 [7 January 1999].

Clark, W. M., & Serovich, J. M. (July 1997). Twenty years and still in the dark? Content analysis of articles pertaining to gay, lesbian, and bisexual issues in marriage and family therapy journals. *Journal of Marital and Family Therapy* [online], pp. 239–253. Available: First-Search/BSSI97635455 [7 January 1999].

Collins, R. (1996). Love and Property. Susan J. Ferguson, Ed. *Mapping the Social Landscape*. Mountain View, CA: Mayfield Publishing.

Coontz, S. (1992). *The Way We Never Were: American Families and the Nostalgia Trap*. New York: Basic Books.

Crow Dog, M., & Erodes, R. (1996). Civilize them with a stick. *Mapping the Social Landscape*. S. J. Ferguson, Ed. Mountain View, CA: Mayfield Publising.

Cussins, C. (1998). Producing Reproduction: Techniques of Normalization and Naturalization in Infertility Clinics. *Reproducing Reproduction*. S. Franklin and H. Ragone, Eds. Philadelphia: University of Pennsylvania.

Department of Health and Human Services. 2000. *Healthy People 2010*. http://www.health.gov/healthypeople

Don't I count? (March/April 1997) The Hastings Center Report [online], pp. 23–24. Available: FirstSearch/ BSSI97018864 [7 January 1999].

Ellenchild, W. & Spielman, M.L. (1996) "Ethics in the Neonatal Intensive Care Unit" *Advances in Nursing Science 19*:1 (72–85).

Family Policy. (Spring 1997). *Policy Studies Journal* [online], pp. 69–73. Available: FirstSearch/BSSI97035923 [7 January 1999].

Fenn, R.L. (1997). Just don't call it marriage. *The Gleaner,* North Pacific Union, Seventh-day Adventist Church, Feb 3, 1997, p. 3.

Fost, D. (April 1996). Child-free with an attitude. *American Demographics* [online], pp. 15–16. Available: First-Search/BSSI96013521 [7 January 1999].

Gaines, D. (1996). Teenage Wasteland: Suburbia's Dead-End Kids. *Mapping the Social Landscape*. S. J. Ferguson, Ed. Mountain View, CA: Mayfield Publishing.

Garasky, S. (Spring 1997). User fees and family policy: attempting to recover costs for state-provided child support enforcement services. *Policy Studies Journal* [online], pp. 100–108. Available: FirstSearch/BSSI97035926 [7 January 1999].

Griscom, J. L. (1998). The Case of Sharon Kowalski and Karen Thompson: Ableism, Heterosexism, and Sexism. *Race, Class, and Gender in the United States*, ed 4. P. S. Rothenberg, Ed. New York: St. Martin's Press.

Harrington, M. (July/August 1998). The care equation. *American Prospect* [online]. Available: FirstSearch/ BSSI98021392 [7 January 1999].

Harrison, H. (November 1993). The Principles for Family-Centered Neonatal Care. *Pediatrics*. *92*(5):(643–650).

Haywood, J. et al. (1994). Comparison of Percent & Actual Rates of Survival & Freedom from Handicap in Premature Infants. *American Journal of Obstetrics & Gynecology 171*:2 (432–439).

Heimer, C. A., & Staffen, L. R. (1998). *For the Sake of the Children*. Chicago: University of Chicago.

Hertz, R., & Ferguson, F. I. T. (Summer 1996). Child care choice and constraints in the United States: social class, race and the influence of family views. *Journal of Comparative Family Studies* [online], pp. 249–280. Available: FirstSearch/BSSI96044132 [7 January 1999].

Hill Collins, P. (1996). The Meaning of Motherhood in Black Culture. *Mapping the Social Landscape*. S. J. Ferguson, Ed. (Mountain View, CA: Mayfield Publishing.

Human Rights Campaign. Human Rights Campaign Condemns Congressional Vote to Repeal D.C. Domestic Partners Act. Press Release, 2 November 1995. http://www.hrc.org

Indian Child Welfare Law Center. http://www.glrain.net/icwalc/

Jacques, J.M. (1998). Changing marital and family patterns: as test of the post-modern perspective. *Sociological Perspectives, 41*:281–413.

Karner, T. X. (1998). Professional caring: homecare workers as a fictive kin. *Journal of Aging Studies* [online]. Available: FirstSearch/BSSI98013155 [7 January 1999].

Kennedy, J. (July/September 1997). Personal assistance benefits and federal health care reforms: who is eligible on the basis of ADL assistance criteria? *Journal of Rehabilitation* [online], pp. 40–45. Available: FirstSearch/BSSI97035427 [7 January 1999].

Kozol, J. (1991). *Savage Inequalities.* New York: Crown.

Landsman, G. H. (Autumn 1998). Reconstructing Motherhood in the Age of Perfect Babies: Mothers of Infants and Toddlers with Disabilities. *Signs, 24*:69–99.

Lee, C. M., & L. Duxbury. (1998). Employed parents' support from partners, employers, and friends. *The Journal of Social Psychology* [online]. Available: FirstSearch/BSSI98016268 [7 January 1999].

Leonard, A. S. (1997). Equal Protection and Lesbian and Gay Rights. *A Queer World.* Martin Duberman, Ed. New York: New York University Press.

Mays, V. M., et al.. (1998). African American families in diversity: gay men and lesbians as participants in family networks. *Journal of Comparative Family Studies* [online], pp. 0047–2328. Available: FirstSearch/ BSSI 98027743 [7 January 1999].

Mitchell, S. (1995). The next baby boom. *American Demographics 17*(October):22–27.

Monnett, M. L. (January/February 1997). A successful family self-sufficiency program. *Journal of Housing and Community Development* [online], pp. 6–7. Available: FirstSearch/BSSI97017926 [7 January 1999].

Moskowitz, E. H. (March/April 1995). In the courts: two mothers. The Hastings Center Report [online], p. 42. Available: FirstSearch/BSSI95010874 [7 January 1999].

Moskowitz, E. H. (July/August 1996). In the courts: same-sex couples. The HASTINGS Center Report [online], pp. 47–48. Available: FirstSearch/BSSI96029087 [7 January 1999].

Mueller, M. R., & Berde, C. T. (Spring 1996). Minnesota's family loan program. *Public Welfare* [online], pp. 32–41. Available: FirstSearch/BSSI96022731 [7 January 1999].

Nicholson, R. H. (January/February 1997). In the family's best interests. The Hastings Center Report [online], p. 4. Available: FirstSearch/BSSI97007267 [7 January 1999].

Nunez, R. da Costa. (Fall 1995). Family values among homeless families. *Public Welfare* [online], pp. 24–32.

National Center for Health Statistics (NCHS) 1999. Health US: 1996. Centers for Disease Control & Prevention. Available: FirstSearch/BSSI96004405 [7 January 1999].

Pinderhughes, R. (Summer 1996). The impact of race on environmental quality: an empirical and theoretical discussion. *Sociological Perspectives* [online], pp. 231–248. Available: FirstSearch/BSSI96036145 [22 August 1999].

Ragoné, H. (1998). Incontestable Motivations. *Reproducing Reproduction.* S. Franklin and H. Ragoné, Eds. Philadelphia: University of Pennsylvania.

Robinson, J., et al. (1998). Time and the melting pot. *American Demographics, 20*:6, p. 8.

Rose, Mark. "Mothers and Authors: Johnson Calvert and the New Children of our Imagination." *The Visible Woman.* P.A. Treichler, L. Cartwright, C. Penley, eds. New York: New York University Press, 1998.

Schroeder, C., & Ward, D. (1998). Women, Welfare, and Work: One View of the Debate. *Nursing Outlook, 46*: pp. 226–232.

Sullivan, C. G. (Summer 1996). The partnership for personal responsibility. *Public Welfare* [online], pp. 26–30. Available: FirstSearch/BSSI96037230 [7 January 1999].

Terkel, S. (1998). C. P. Ellis. *Race, Class, and Gender in the United States,* ed 4. P. S. Rothenberg, Ed. New York: St. Martin's Press.

Trost, J. (Summer 1996). Family structure and relationships: the dyadic approach. *Journal of Comparative Family Studies* [online], pp. 395–408. Available: FirstSearch/BSSI96044138 [7 January 1999].

U.S. Commission on Human Rights. (1998). Indian Tribes: A Continuing Quest for Survival. *Race, Class, and Gender in the United States,* ed 4. Paula S. Rothenberg, Ed. New York: St. Martin's Press.

Wall, S. N., & Partridge, J. C. (January 1997). Death in the Intensive Care Nursery: Physician Practice of Withdrawing and Withholding Life Support. *Pediatrics 99*(1): 64–70.

Weston, K. (1996). Families We Choose: Lesbians, Gays, Kinship. *Mapping the Social Landscape.* S. J. Ferguson, Ed. Mountain View, CA: Mayfield Publishing.

Wolford, B. I., et al. (December 1995). Kentucky links at-risk families to education and treatment. *Corrections Today* [online], p. 108. Available: FirstSearch/BSSI 96006863 [7 January 1999].

Wooden, W. S. (1996). Kicking Back at 'Raging High'. *Mapping the Social Landscape.* S. J. Ferguson, Ed. Mountain View, CA: Mayfield Publishing.

Zaichkin, J., Ed. (1996). *Newborn Intensive Care.* Petaluma, CA: NICU Ink Press.

Focus On

FAMILIES AND FAMILY NURSING IN THE NEW MILLENNIUM

This is the final chapter in our journey into family health care nursing. In Unit I, you became acquainted with the origins and development of families and family nursing; learned about the structure, process, and function of families; read about the sociocultural and other influences on family health and functioning; and received an overview of family nursing theory and research. You studied the family nursing process, including how to assess and intervene with families and how to promote family health.

In Unit 2, you read about family health care nursing practice in a variety of settings with a multitude of theoretical and interventional approaches. We know, for example, that family nursing can be practiced with families across the age continuum: childbearing, childrearing, and aging families. Family nursing can be practiced in many settings, including medical-surgical, mental health, and community health environments.

Here in Unit 3, Chapter 16 viewed families, nursing, and health from a social policy point of view. Chapter 17 turns to the future of families and family nursing as society stands at the beginning of the new century and new millennium. The evolving development and implementation of nursing care of families is based on the belief that families are the basic unit of society and that this orientation will continue into the future, despite changing family demographics and value systems, despite the vicissitudes of the health care delivery system and how health care is financed, and despite the pull and tug of nursing between individual and family centered care. This textbook closes with an exploration of the future of American families, families around the world, factors influencing family nursing, and the future of family nursing theory, practice, research, education, and social policy.

Chapter 17

FAMILIES AND FAMILY NURSING IN THE NEW MILLENNIUM

Shirley May Harmon Hanson

OUTLINE

OBJECTIVES

On completion of this chapter, the reader will be able to:

- Describe general patterns of changing families.
- Specify demographic family trends in the U.S.
- Discuss several world demographic trends.
- Summarize other factors influencing family nursing: religion, sexuality, health care technology, and health care reform.
- Be articulate on the future of family nursing theory, practice, research, education, and social policy.

FAMILIES AND FAMILY NURSING IN THE NEW MILLENNIUM

Changing Families

American families changed dramatically during the twentieth century. The nuclear family, consisting of mother, father, and their children together, is no longer the principal family structure; it is now just one of a multitude of well-recognized family forms. Indeed, Spanier (1989) noted that "no normative family structural form exists in contemporary society . . . the dominance of a traditional familial structure has been a fictional notion throughout most of American history" (p.4). Today we recognize that there are a variety of family forms, each of which is tenable and each of which has its own set of characteristics, qualities and values. As family structures have become more diverse, the complexity of preparing health care providers for family care has increased.

General Patterns

Some believe that families as a unit are in jeopardy. Others see the changes as part of an evolutionary process. At times, American families have been romanticized, as the unequaled foundation of positive emotional relationships and security. However, in a classic description of the social history of the American family, Calhoun (1960) provided another view, describing eighteenth-century families as characterized by economic and social domination of women, the selling of wives, the oppression of individual needs, and even infanticide. Coontz (1992) reminded us that families have always been in a state of "flux and often in crisis" (p.2) and noted that idealizing families of previous decades discounts the strengths that families have developed in coping with a changing society. In contrast, Popenoe (1993) asserted that American families are in decline and that action must be taken immediately to strengthen the institution of the family. However, in a recent book on family futures edited by Dreman (1997b), he summarized this age-old dilemma pertaining to the future of families:

> Is there life for the family in the twenty-first century? Who will prevail: the optimists or the pessimists? The pessimists claim that family life in its present form is doomed. This gloomy forecast is attributable to increased demands from the workplace, rampant technological advancement, and the pursuit of personal achievement at the expense of interpersonal needs and values [p. xi] . . . The pessimists among us feel that the traditional family is outmoded and no longer capable of coping with the realities of contemporary living [p. 4].
>
> The optimists claim the opposite, that is, that increasing alienation and emphasis on the occupational sphere necessitates a sense of family, community, and belonging as a haven from work-related stress [p. xi].

Whitehead (1992) and Doherty (1992), who both provided broad overviews of where family life has been and may be going, wrote that the last 50 years of American family life experienced three distinct cultural periods. The first was called *traditional familism* by Whitehead and the *institutional family* by Doherty. This period extended from the mid-1940s to the mid-1960s and was characterized by the dominance of married couples with children, a high birth rate, a low divorce rate and a high degree of marital stability. The period was marked by a robust economy, a rising standard of living, and a growing expanding middle class. Culturally, it was defined by conformity to social norms, the ideology of separate spheres for men and women, and idealization of family life. Younger adults in the post-World War II period tended to have strong identities and small egos. The television emblem of post-war family life was, and still is, *Ozzie and Harriet.* The chief family value for this period was responsibility.

The second period was called the period of *individualism* or the *psychological family.* This period extended from the mid-1960s to the mid-1980s and was characterized by greater demographic diversity, a decline in the birth rate, an accelerating divorce rate, individual and social experimentation, the breakdown of the separate spheres ideology, the creation of a "singles" lifestyle, idealization of career and work life, and the search for meaning in life through self expression. Younger adults in this period could be said to have big egos and weak identities. The emblematic television shows of this period were the *Mary Tyler Moore Show* in the 1970s and *L.A. Law* in the 1980s. Both programs treated work relationships and the workplace as the primary realm of intimacy, nurturing, and fulfillment. Children do not exist in the workplace. The chief family value for this period was satisfaction.

The third period, which we have now entered, may be termed the period of *new familism* or the *plu-*

ralistic family and has resulted largely from the fact that the "Baby Boomers" have reached adulthood and parenthood. This period is characterized by a leveling off of the divorce rates, a leveling off of work force participation among women, and the highest number of births since 1964. Socially, it is less conservative than the first period, but more conservative than the second period. Lifestyles appear to be shifting away from expressive individualism and a fascination with self and toward a greater attachment to family and commitment to others. We are beginning to see couples place happiness and well-being of the family above their individual desires or ambitions. A growing number of men and women are cutting back on work to devote more time to children. Women's career plans are including the time to actively participate in raising young children. These parents of the "Baby Boom" generation have greatly influenced the media culture, and new values and behaviors are being created through televisionm programs such as *Murphy Brown, Thirtysomething,* and *Life Goes On,* and the later programs, *Cosby, Home Improvement,* and *Everybody Loves Raymond.* Flexibility and diversity are the hallmarks of this new period.

If a new family ethos is emerging, it is good news for children. There are many positive aspects to the social and cultural changes of the past 25 years: greater choice for adults, greater freedom and opportunities for women, and greater tolerance for difference and diversity. The period of the "me generation" was not altogether positive for children or families, however. The quality of the family of the future depends on whether family ethics and policies can be established that will help develop and maintain healthy bonds between family members in different living arrangements and between families and their communities.

Future American Demographics

At the beginning of the twenty-first century, profound structural and demographic changes are occurring in family life (Dreman, 1997b, p. 3–4). The traditional two-parent nuclear family is viewed by many as a relic of the past. This is reflected in major changes in divorce, marriage, fertility and longevity rates, increasing rates of employed women, and new family structures, lifestyles, and life cycles. Accelerating rates of stress and violence in the family reflect strain between work and the family, evolving gender conflicts, ambiguity in parental roles of the biologic versus the socializing parent (in the case of stepparents), and parenting roles (as a result of "high-tech" reproduction techniques). At a time of rapid social, industrial, and technological change, family values of community, belonging, and family-related status are often usurped by individualism, autonomy, and the pursuit of career-related prestige.

As noted in Chapter 1, the statistical profile of the American family has changed drastically over the past 20 years. If these trends endure beyond the year 2000, the overall population of the United States will have grown by about 7 percent, or nearly 270 million people. In 2050, America is projected to be 50 percent more populous than it was in 1995. The largest growth is expected to be in the nation's Hispanic and elderly populations, each of which will make up 20 percent of the nation's people. An increase of 6 million persons will occur through immigration alone, with cities and states on the east and west coasts receiving a disproportionate share of these immigrants.

Average household size declined from 2.69 persons in 1985 to 2.48 in 2000. The population is getting older, with the median age above 37. People over age 85 will represent about 13 percent of the population and the "oldest old" or frail elderly persons(over 85 years of age) will increase by about 30 percent. The number of children under age 5 will decline from 18 million to 17 million. In 2000 plus, economic expansion will create 18 million new jobs, and women of all racial and ethnic groups will be the major new entrants into the job market with women making up 47 percent of the workforce. Already it is estimated that nearly 65 percent of preschool children and 80 percent of school-aged children have mothers who work. The occupations growing the fastest include service, professional, technical, sales, and executive and management positions (Children's Defense Fund, 1990; U.S. Public Health Service, 1990).

The decline in the economic status of the American family is another demographic change that gives reason for concern. According to a study by the U.S. Department of Commerce, although in 1992 the official definition of poverty was an income of $14,428 a year for a family of four (U.S. Bureau of Census, 1994a), 18 percent of individuals with full-time jobs earned less than $13,091 in 1992. Thus, trying to support a family on this wage is essentially living in poverty, and poverty is significantly related to health because of the difficulty of obtaining resources to meet health care needs. In addition to low wages being earned by workers, unemployed, uninsured or underinsured, minority, homeless, and undocumented individuals (who are not legally residing in the United States) are all at risk for poor health care. Planning heath care for these groups will continue to be a challenge in the twenty-first century. Family nurses will have the challenge of promoting health in families where health care is a scarce resource. Participating in health care reform that will insure access to care for these populations is a significant role for nurses.

The changing ethnicity in America also creates greater challenges in promoting health in families. As Wisensale (1992) noted, "the United States is evolving into a multiracial, multicultural, and multilingual society . . . in short, we as a nation are changing color" (p. 420). Beyond the year 2000, it is estimated that the proportion of Caucasians in the total population will decrease from 76 to 72 percent. The proportion of Hispanics, African-Americans, American Indian and Alaska Natives, and Asians and Pacific Islanders will increase (U.S. Public Health Service, 1990). Minority families tend to be economically disadvantaged and have less access to health care, which is evident in many health outcomes, such as teenage pregnancy rates, low birth-weight newborns, and a high incidence of alcohol and drug abuse and family violence.

Figure 17–1 shows the racial and ethnic makeup of America in 1995 and projections for the year 2050. In the future, we will see less white and a lot more of everything else. While the population of all races will grow, some will grow faster than others. By 2025, the number of Hispanic Americans will increase dramatically, and their political power is sure to grow proportionately.

Specific Demographic Trends

The following projections and trends for the future of families provide an important lens through which to view the future (U.S. Bureau of the Census, 1991a, 1991b, 1992a, 1992b, 1992c, 1992d, 1994a, 1994b, 1995a, 1995b, 1995c).

- Marriage rates remain high in the United States and are among the highest of all developed nations in the world. But there was a slight decline in the rate of marriage following World War II, largely because of the trend to postpone marriage and the increase in the rates of cohabitation. Nevertheless, marriages continue to dissolve because of abandonment, separation, divorce, or death of a spouse. On the whole, Americans will continue to believe in the institution of marriage.
- Divorce rates during the 1970s and 1980s increased rapidly. More than 60 percent of all marriages are said to end in divorce. In recent years, there has been a slight trend downward that is thought to be a result of the increase in age at first marriage, which lowers the risk of divorce. According to Gelles (1995), divorce will continue to be the typical way the majority of marriages end.
- Children will increasingly live in single-parent households headed by mothers, subsist on earnings below the poverty level, and lack support from fathers.
- Birth rates appear to be generally down after the "Baby Boom" following World War II. Children's overall share of the population has declined since 1970 and will continue to decline in the foreseeable future as fertility rates stay low and "Baby Boomers" age. Delays in first marriage often mean that couples delay having their first child. The birth rate among never-married women is rising and will likely continue; unmarried motherhood currently accounts for almost one-third of all births in the U.S. Fertility rates will likely stay below replacement levels (i.e., 2.0 children per two parents) for the general populations, although there is a significant variation in fertility rates across socioeconomic, racial, and ethnic groups.
- The proportion of married women (with or without children) employed in the workforce has increased rapidly in the past 40 years, with the greatest growth among married women with preschool children. The combined effects of the economy and women's movement will continue the upward trend in maternal employment. Mothers in two-parent households carry increasing economic responsibilities. Working mothers are here to stay.
- The future of families is one of diversity of family forms and structures. There is little evidence that any of the forces will move families back toward the "idyllic nuclear family of the 1950s" (Gelles, 1995). Families and intimate relations will continue to evolve. For example, continued development exists in single-parent families, gay and lesbian relationships, interracial marriages, and multigenerational families (the new extended family). Diversity includes both cohabitation and living as a single adult.
- The future of families will increase and change

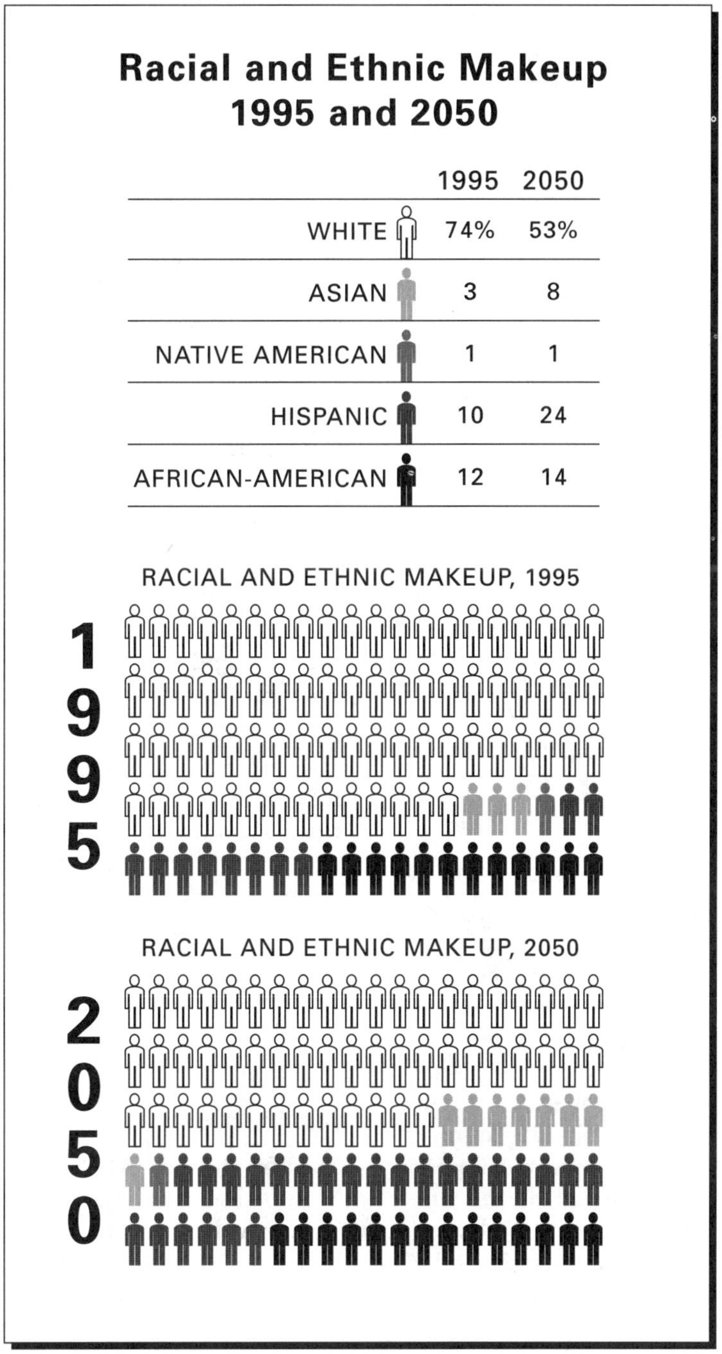
Racial and Ethnic Makeup
1995 and 2050
1995 2050
WHITE 74% 53%
ASIAN 3 8
NATIVE AMERICAN 1 1
HISPANIC 10 24
AFRICAN-AMERICAN 12 14
RACIAL AND ETHNIC MAKEUP, 1995
1995
RACIAL AND ETHNIC MAKEUP, 2050
2050

FIGURE 17-1
Racial and ethnic makeup: 1995 and 2050.

marital roles. Twenty years ago, it was predicted by many that household equality was quickly approaching. However, it appears that working women simply added a second "shift" to their lifestyles. The maintenance of the home and child care are still considered the province and responsibility of women. Although more men are involved in housework and child care, more men have also abandoned their families and failed to provide court-ordered child support after divorce. There is reason to predict that role options in families will continue to become more flexible. There is also reason to believe that families will always have a gender-based division of labor.

- Parents face growing concerns about caring for children through more years of education (and living at home) at the same time that their own longer-living parents survive and need care and attention. Middle-aged adults find themselves in the "sandwich generation," between prolonged dependency of adult children remaining or returning to the home of origin and elderly parents and grandparents living with them on a somewhat permanent basis. It is estimated that 20 percent of the nation's children will be raised by their grandparents (Burton et al, 1995).
- Families will have more complicated family histories and kinship relationships, resulting from divorce, remarriage, and serial relationships. Society will need to come up with a whole new vocabulary to describe the complexity of relationships in modern families.
- The increase in the numbers of elderly accompanied by the decline in the fertility rates and decreased mortality have a direct impact on families. The fastest growing population group are individuals older than 85 years, who are more likely to be frail and dependent and have multiple health needs. The availability of kin to provide family care becomes a major issue for families. Families will be managing care of family members from a distance by means of phone, E-mail, and fax technology (Kaakinen, 1999; Kinsella, 1996). What the future may hold is that the old will be cared for by their children in their 80s or grandchildren in their 60s (Kaakinen, 1999; Dreman, 1997).

Genetic technology will be a part of our future whether we like it or not. Today, we are moving rapidly toward a future when our knowledge of our genetic makeup and its implications for our individual futures will radically transform the world around us. What are the social, legal, political and ethical issues arising for the future from recent advances and discoveries made in genetic research? (Wilcox, 1997).

There are many more future projections and concerns that are outside the purview of this book. However, Gelles (1995) believed that the two major threats and unknowns to families in the future could be predicted. *First,* there is AIDS: "The cloud that hangs over the family and intimate relations is not divorce, cohabitation, working mothers, or alternative lifestyles. Today's cloud is AIDS" (Gelles, p. 508). The disease was barely recognized 10 years ago, and today it has moved far beyond its original impact on gay culture (in the U.S.) to include all parts of the American culture and every nation in the world. The *second* concern is the status of children in this country. The status of children in families has changed and these changes have not all been in their best interest. Although some argue that the key change is the absence of fathers, the major structural change is the poverty that affects children in single-parent homes. There is a significant increase in the percentage of children in the U.S. who live in poverty. The major problems children face do not come from cohabitation, day care, or the fact that their mothers work. Families are not declining because of divorce, working mothers, and lower fertility. The family is declining because this society continues to ignore the needs of a substantial portion of its children. Many children do not get immunizations, are not well fed or clothed, do not get health care, and live in dangerous environments.

World Demographic Trends

Thus far, the focus of demographic changes has been on American families. It is impossible to view U.S. families without looking at two major global trends as well: population and aging. In the book, *Which World? Scenarios for the Twenty-first Century,* Hammond (1998) presented population projections from 1995 totals to the low, medium, and high projections for the year 2050 (Table 17–1). These projections include what Hammond termed "industrialized, transitional, and developing regions." It is clear that global concerns are shared by all. On October 12, 1999, this planet reached

TABLE 17–1
Population Projections, 2050 (in millions)

		2050		
	1995	**Low**	**Medium**	**High**
Industrial Regions				
North America	297	301	384	452
Europe	383	293	346	389
Japan	125	96	110	122
Transitional Regions				
Russia	148	97	114	142
Eastern Europe	152	110	131	156
Developing Regions				
Latin America	471	643	802	991
China	1,220	1,198	1,517	1,765
Southeast Asia	511	664	827	1,010
India[a]	929	1,231	1,533	1,885
Sub-Saharan Africa	586	1,518	1,783	2,089
North Africa and Middle East	348	650	785	930
World Total[b]	**5,687**	**7,662**	**9,367**	**11,156**

[a]The corresponding numbers for South Asia as a whole are 1,225 for 1995 and 1,786, 2,194, and 2,665 (low, medium, and high projections, respectively) for 2050.
[b]The regional numbers do not add up to the world total because a number of countries have been omitted to simplify.
Source: Hammond, A. (1998). *Which World? Scenarios for the 21st Century,* (p. 258). Washington, DC: Island Press.

a population of 6 billion (with the U.S. constituting only 5 percent of the world's population).

The International Conference on Population and Development (ICPD) believes that population concerns are the heart of sustainable development strategies. The United Nations consensus is that population will not level off until it reaches 9 billion in 2050 (247 children are born each minute into the world). (Contact http://www.unfpa.org for more information of the ICPD's plan of action.) Martha Farnsworth Riche (1998), former head of the U.S. Bureau of the Census, developed a report entitled *From Pyramids to Pillars: The New Demographic Reality,* which described the facts of aging, fertility, the new pattern of healthy living, and population change. Check it out through Communications Consortium Media Center under its Global Population Initiative (info@ccmc.org). Figure 17–2 shows the soaring world population trends from 1800 to 2050 and emphasizes that this growth takes place primarily in poor nations.

The final words of the publication are: "When girls are educated and couples have options for planning their families, they exercise these options responsibly everywhere in the world regardless of culture. Only when these options are universal will the old pyramid of aging become the pillar that supports a sustainable world population" (Riche, p. 10).

Figure 17–3 shows the world population by billions with an emphasis on the contributions of China and India. Sixty percent of the world's population increase is being contributed by only 10 countries, with 21 percent contributed by China and India. Net annual additions, averaged from the years 1995–2000, are shown in millions.

The second major world demographic change pertains to the aging of the world population. Figure 17–4 shows a comparison of the global aging patterns over time among the continents. The graying of the world appears to be affecting industrialized countries as a result of their advanced medical technology and standards of living. In North America, the current life expectancy is 77 years; it is 69 in Latin America and the Caribbean, 73 in Europe, 66 in Asia, and 51 in Africa. By 2030 the numbers of Americans over 65 will nearly

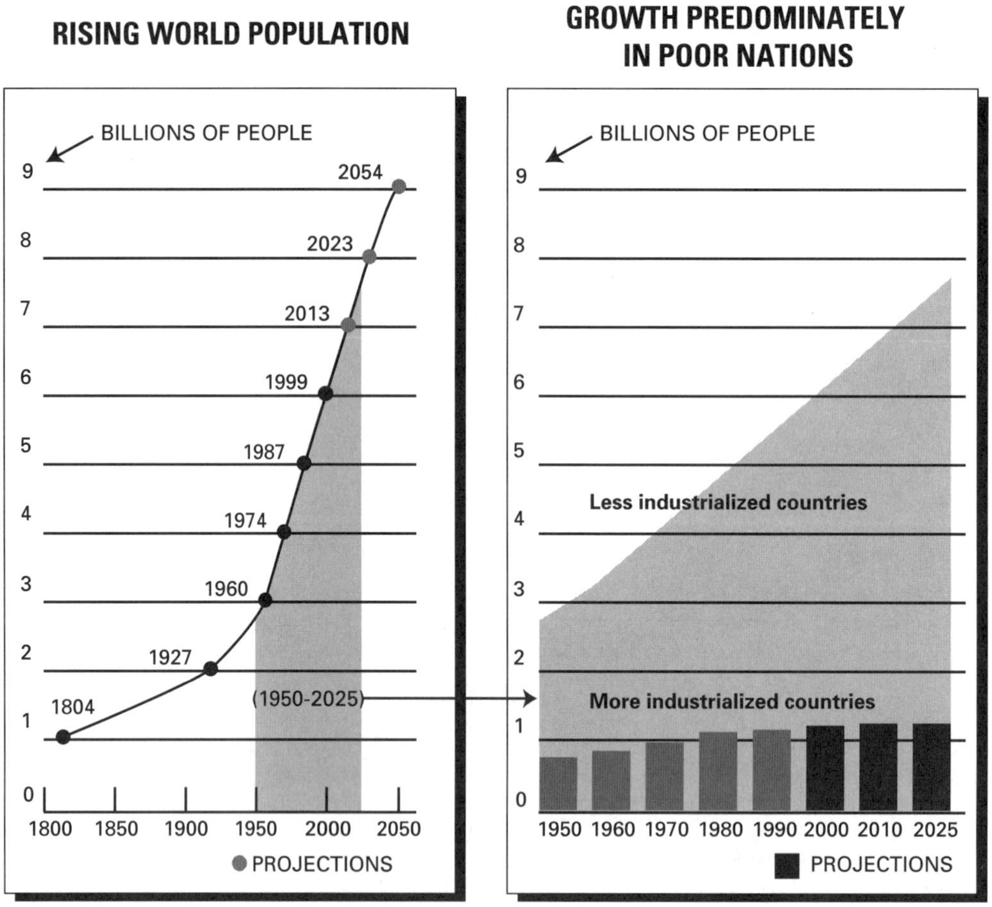

Reference: United Nations Population Division

In 1804 the world's population reached the 1 billion mark. It took 123 years to reach 2 billion while it only took 12 years to go from 5 to 6 billion. Due to a decline in the fertility rate and the aging of the population, the world's population will level off at 10 billion (approx.) by the year 2200.

Because the growth rates of less industrialized countries have been significantly higher than more industrialized countries, in the past 50 years, the net gain in the world's population has taken place in the world's poorest areas.

Note:

More-industrialized countries and areas include: North America, Europe, Japan, Australia, and New Zealand

Less-industrialized countries and areas include: All of Africa, all of Asia except Japan, the Transcaucasian and Central Asian countries of the former Soviet Union, all of Latin America and the Caribbean, and all of Oceania except Australia and New Zealand

FIGURE 17-2
Soaring world population and growth nations.

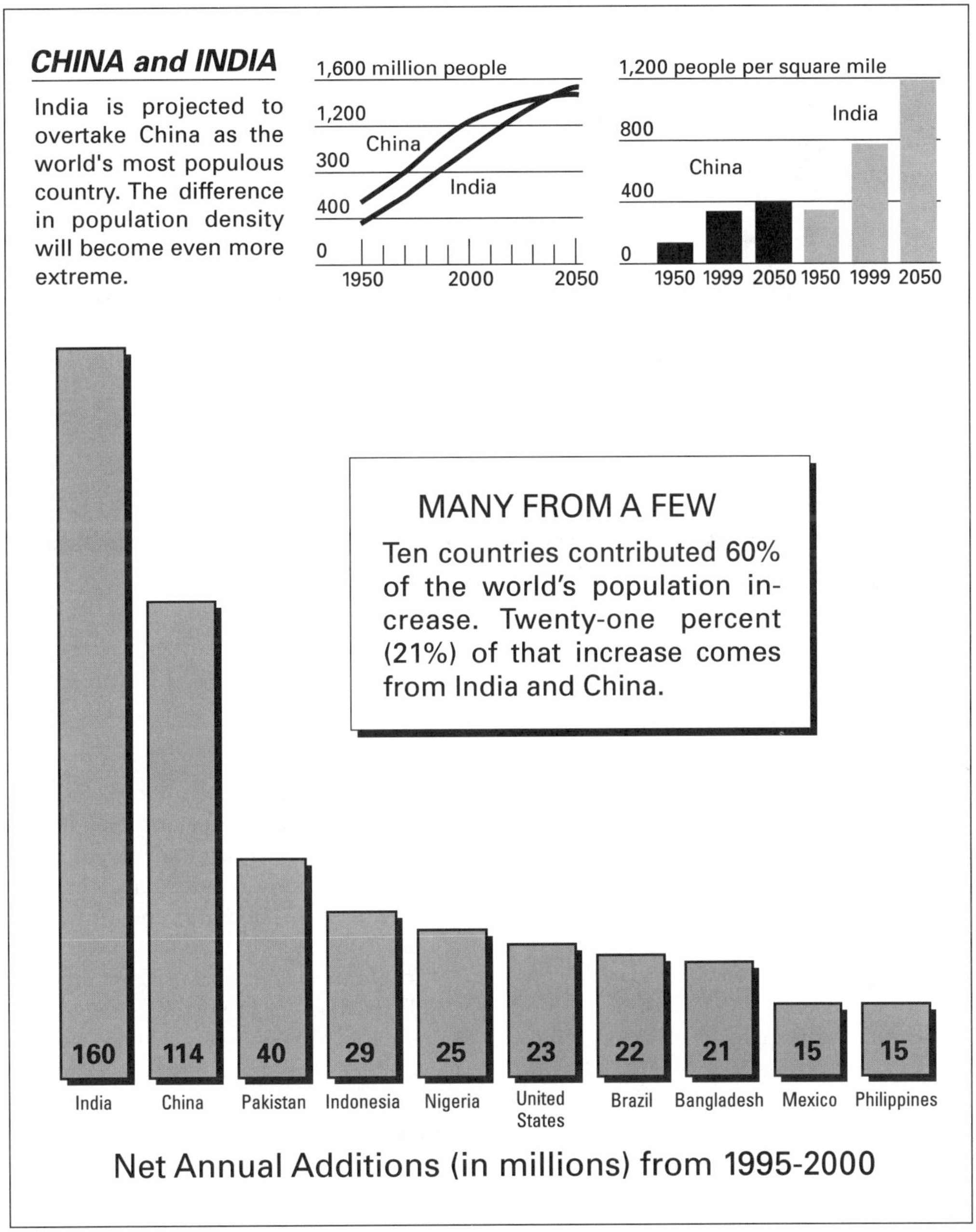

Reference: U.N. Population Division; U.S. Census Bureau

FIGURE 17-3
World population by billions.

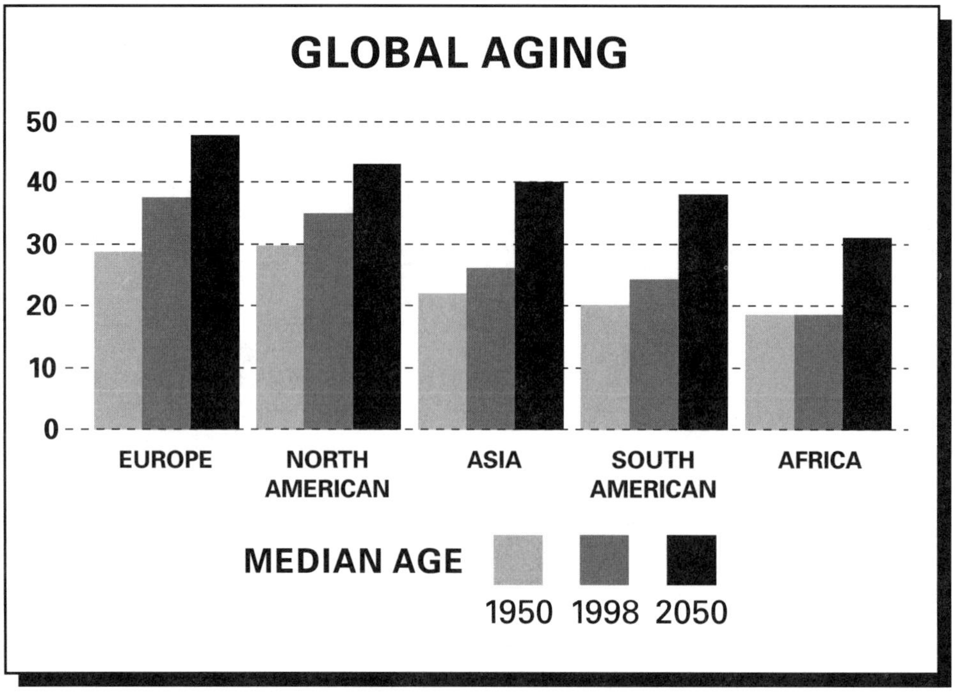

Reference: United Nations Population Division

FIGURE 17-4
Global aging.

double from 39 to 69 million and elderly persons will constitute 20 percent of the population. This aging trend brings up all kinds of resource and ethical issues for counties around the world.

Future of Family Nursing: Theory, Practice, Research, Education and Social Policy

First, what is the future of family nursing theory, practice, research, education, and social policy? *Family nursing theory* is an emerging area of study within the nursing profession. As mentioned in Chapter 2, family nursing theory has drawn from family social sciences theories, family therapy theories, and nursing models and theories. The trend will continue to use integrated (eclectic) models and further develop ideas that are unique to nursing as a discipline.

Family nursing practice is an evolving specialty area within nursing (Kirschling et al, 1994) and will continue to significantly impact health care in the future, especially with the current focus on health care reform in the United States. The barriers discussed in Chapter 1 that confront the practice of family nursing need to be addressed in the new health care delivery systems. As health care is moved into family homes in the community, nurses will be called upon to serve families as the unit-of-care.

Most *family nursing research* has traditionally focused on individuals rather than families as a whole. Research pertaining to families and mental health is further advanced than that concerning families and physical health. Recently nursing has awakened to the connection between family dynamics and health and illness. More family-centered nursing research needs to be conducted by scholars in family nursing.

Family nursing education will continue to include more family-focused study in the nursing curricula. Recent studies in family nursing education (Hanson & Heims, 1992; Hanson et al, 1992; Wright & Bell, 1989) reported that (1) more family content is being included in undergraduate and graduate nursing curricula but the content could be made more explicit, (2) an eclectic approach to family assessment is taught rather than using specific models, and (3) many clinical practicums are still focused on individuals rather than families as a unit. For family nursing to be practiced in community-based settings, more nurses need to be educated in family nursing.

The implications of these nursing education trends and predictions have many ramifications for development of *family social policy*. As professionals, nurses participate in the development of legislation and governmental policy. Legislative and legal actions that have a direct or indirect impact on families are called family policy. All governmental laws, whether at the local, county, state or national level, affect families either directly or indirectly. The range of social policy decisions that affects families is vast, including health care access and coverage, low income housing, social security, taxes, welfare, food stamps, pension plans, affirmative action, and education. Despite this fact, Zimmerman (1992) wrote "Although all governmental policies affect families, in both negative and positive ways, the United States has little overall, official explicit family policy" (p. 4).

Healthy People was the first program initiated by the federal government in 1979 that resulted in national health targets (*Healthy People: The Surgeon General's Report on Health Promotion and Disease Prevention*). The five challenging goals were to reduce mortality among various age groups: infants, children, adolescents, young adults, and adults. Through the combined efforts of the nation's public health agencies, most of the goals were accomplished by 1990. *Healthy People 2000* (U.S. Dept of Health and Human Services, 1990) developed objectives for the next 10 years built on the lessons of the first Surgeon General's report and was the product of unprecedented collaboration among government, voluntary and professional organizations, businesses, and individuals. The framework of *Healthy People 2000* consisted of three broad goals: increase the span of healthy life for Americans, reduce health disparities among Americans, and achieve access to preventive services for all Americans. This broad approach to health promotion, health protection, and prevention services provided direction for individuals to change personal behaviors and for organizations and communities to support good health through health promotion policies. Recently, the U.S. Department of Health and Human Services (1998) developed another proposal entitled *Healthy People 2010 Objectives,* which is a draft of proposed programs for the first decade of the new century (2000 to 2010). The context in which this new proposal was developed differed from the earlier program because of advancement in preventive therapies, vaccines and pharmaceuticals, assistive technologies, and computerized systems, which have changed the face of health care and how it is practiced. New relationships will be defined between public health departments and health care delivery organizations. With demographic changes in the United States reflecting an older and more racially diverse population, these new facts will create new demands on public health and overall health care systems. Global forces, including food supplies, emerging infectious diseases, and environmental interdependence, will also present new public health challenges. The two major goals of this latest mandate are to: (1) increase quality and years of healthy life and (2) eliminate health disparities. Each goal contains numerous objectives and explains how they can be reached (Box 17–1). More information about this program can be reached on the "Healthy People 2010 Home Page" at http://health.gov/healthypeople under Stakeholders' Report. *Healthy People 2010* is the United States' contribution to the World Health Organization's (WHO) "Health for All" strategy. The United States hopes to provide models for world policy and strategies for health improvement. The final document was released to the public in January 2000 at the Healthy People 2010 consortium meeting in Washington, DC.

Other Factors Influencing Family Nursing

Religion

Religious institutions have a major impact on families and their health practices. Many of the traditions of family life are closely tied to religious ceremonies, including weddings, births, initiations into adulthood, and healing rituals. Families have passed these practices from generation to generation. Also, many families find it helpful to use spiritual sources for strength, meaning, and assistance when they are experiencing hardship, using such strategies as prayer, becoming more involved in religious activities, and developing greater faith (Burr et al, 1993). Furthermore, religion has been recognized as playing an important role in the mental health of individuals and families, in their outlook on life and lifestyle (Fong & Sandhu, 1993). Family nurses need to be aware of families' cultural and religious beliefs and practices. Because of the diversity of religious practices within even small communities today, nurses will encounter various spiritual customs that may influence families' responses to health care practices.

Box 17–1

HEALTHY PEOPLE 2010

Goals

1. Increase quality and years of healthy life
2. Eliminate health disparities

Objectives

I. Promote Healthy Behaviors

1. Physical activity and fitness
2. Nutrition
3. Tobacco use

II. Promote Healthy and Safe Communities

4. Educational and community-based programs
5. Environmental health
6. Food safety
7. Injury/violence prevention
    a. Injuries that cut across intent
    b. Unintentional injuries
    c. Violence and abuse
8. Occupational safety and health
9. Oral health

III. Improve Systems for Personal and Public Health

10. Access to quality health services
    a. Preventive care
    b. Primary care
    c. Emergency services
    d. Long-term care and rehabilitative services
11. Family planning
12. Maternal, infant, and child health
13. Medical product safety
14. Public health infrastructure
15. Health communication

IV. Prevent and Reduce Diseases and Disorders

16. Arthritis, osteoporosis, and chronic back conditions
17. Cancer
18. Diabetes
19. Disability and secondary conditions
20. Heart disease and stroke
21. HIV
22. Immunization and infectious diseases
23. Mental health and mental disorders
24. Respiratory diseases
25. Sexually transmitted diseases
26. Substance abuse

Source: U.S. Department of Health and Human Services. Office of Public Health and Science. (1998). *Healthy People 2010 Objectives*. Washington, DC: U.S. Government Printing Office.

Sexuality

Sexuality is another element affecting families today. With the sexual revolution of the late 1960s and 1970s, brought about by the development of the birth control pill, premarital sexual behavior became more common and cohabitation became an accepted form of family life. Births to unmarried women have increased over the past decade. For example, the percentage of births to unmarried women between the ages of 15 and 44 increased from 18.4 percent to 24.5 percent between 1980 and 1987 and is now approximately 33 percent (U.S. Bureau of the Census, 1990). Today, the threat of AIDS has heightened awareness of the danger of random sexual activity. However, it is too early to analyze the effects of AIDS on the sexuality of Americans or to say whether the sexual revolution is truly over.

Health Care Technology

The complexity of health care practices has increased significantly in the past two decades as a result of advances in technology. With ongoing technological development, health care will continue to see rapid changes. It will be a challenge for family nurses to continue providing personalized care with high-touch delivery to family members as a balance to the dehumanization that can occur with highly technical patient care.

Changes in technology have not only increased the complexity of health care but have also changed the nature of nursing practice in acute care settings and in the home. Patients today stay in the hospital for much shorter periods of time and return to their homes while still requiring care. Thus, the family must either provide the care or ensure that appropriate providers come into the home for follow-up care. In addition, the use of computers is changing practice. For example, minimum data sets have been created to track delivery of care with the result that data on assessments, interventions, referrals, follow-up, and other parameters are now providing ongoing information that can be used in planning effective health care for families.

The use of video technology and satellite telecommunication systems is relatively new. One of the major uses today is for health education, both basic education and continuing education. Nurses in rural areas receive continuing education and are able to pursue advanced degrees via educational video networks. Patient care via telecommunications systems is becoming more common, primarily through consultation with experts via interactive video.

GENETICS

Genetics is the central science for health care in the future. In a guest editorial for the *Journal of Family Nursing,* Feetham (1999, p. 3–9) summarized some statements pertaining to nurses' need for a paradigm shift in regard to their understanding of human genetics in their practice. The burgeoning genetic knowledge as a result of the Human Genome Project makes identification of individuals at risk for disease and the diagnosis and treatment of disease possible in ways that were inconceivable until quite recently. These findings result in unique challenges for families and require health professionals to understand how discoveries in chromosomal genetics will increase their ability to interpret the clinical symptoms of patients and inform their clinical management. Nurses must understand the trajectory of these genetic discoveries and that the knowledge of risk may change over time.

The Human Genome Project began in the mid-1980s and is an international research program led in the U.S. by the Department of Energy and the National Institutes of Health. This project results in information that affects our understanding of the mechanisms for the diagnosis and treatment of disease to promote health and to prevent or delay the onset of disease. This knowledge has major implications for all health professionals working with individuals and their families. Genetic discoveries help health scientists to treat primary dysfunction or disease progression rather than treatment symptoms.

Nurses need to be aware of the research and to stay current in their areas of specialization. Genetics is an area where family nurses can provide significant leadership. The paucity of attention to family systems and family relationships in the collection and dissemination of genetic information places family members and families at increased risk. Most health professionals do not practice within the context of the family. Nurses need to assist families and know that family relationships may be affected as a result of the process of risk identification. Families expect nurses to interpret public, clinical, and scientific literature, and that includes new cutting-edge genetic research. Nurses can help by encouraging individuals to consider how genetic testing results may affect family relationships. Nurses need to be aware that genetic discoveries have significant ethical, legal, and social implications. The National Coalition for Health Professional Education in Genetics (HCHPEG) promotes professional education and access to information about human genetic advances (www.nchpeg.org). Nursing should provide leadership to the genetic revolution, and family nursing has a specific role in this revolution (see Appendix A for other Internet contacts).

Health Care Reform

Health care reform is a major issue in America today. Some of the questions being asked include: Does every person have the right to health care? What does universal access really mean? How will individuals pay for their health insurance? If not individuals, who should pay for health care? Should there be a standard benefit health insurance package to which individuals have a right? The rising costs of health care have made it impossible to ignore these issues any longer. Nearly all the states, as well as the federal government, are examining health care. We see the emergence of managed care as a primary mode of organizing health care delivery. In a managed care system, insurance companies contract with selected health care providers to furnish a comprehensive set of health care services to individuals who are enrolled in an insurance program with a predetermined monthly premium (Iglehart, 1992). Participants in managed care systems generally have a primary care provider who manages their care, and there are financial incentives for patients to use the providers and facilities associated with the managed care plans in which they are enrolled. As managed care plans are emerging, variations in the mode of operation are also emerging, including which health care providers are to be included and what services will be covered.

The role of public health departments, which have been the primary providers of health care to poor families in many areas of the country, are also changing. In some instances, public clinics are becoming part of managed-care health plans. Many of these decisions are being made at the community level. It is critical that nurses participate in the decision making and advocate the role of nursing in future health care systems.

Nurses who receive third-party reimbursement must continue to be visionary in guiding their practice to ensure their being included in managed-care plans. As a primary care provider, nurses who practice from a family nursing perspective will have an advantage in managing health care of their patients. Understanding the dynamics of families and involving all family members in health care will be an advantage. Although the numbers of nurses graduating with advanced degrees has increased markedly during the past 20 years, there are still insufficient numbers of primary care nurses and nurses with a sound foundation in family nursing practice.

To have an impact on health care delivery, nurses need to become active at every level of the political system and advocate for family issues. Voting is no longer enough. Nurses must get to know the political candidates and elected officials in their cities, districts, and states; attend campaign events; write letters on health care issues from a nursing perspective; offer assistance in analyzing issues related to health care reform; and volunteer to serve on local or state commissions or boards related to health. The challenge today is to establish health care systems in which nurses are provided opportunities to work with families as well as individuals. With the rising cost of health care and attempts to get these costs under control, budgets are under constant scrutiny. It is essential that family nurses demonstrate through practice and research the benefits of family health care.

Vosburgh and Simpson (1993) reported that families respond positively to nurses practicing with a family nurse perspective. Additional studies are needed to examine the effectiveness of family nursing practice. Nurses must help families meet the developmental and situational transitions in life. One aim for the future must be to develop "family hardiness," or the ability to internalize a sense of control, a sense of meaningfulness to life, and a commitment to explore new challenges (McCubbin & McCubbin, 1993). Nurses must not only provide the physical care that individual family members need but also incorporate counseling and health promotion and prevention at every contact with the client. In the twenty-first century, we can no longer afford to overlook the family's role in health protection and promotion. The health care system must view families as a significant influence on health care outcomes.

The changes in health care that are on the horizon mean that families must become better educated consumers of health care services. Families need to understand their rights and the options available to them. More than ever, families will need to become adept at participating in the decisions that will affect their health. Nurses need to acquire the knowledge and skills to empower families through participating in community organizing, coalition building, and other political activities.

SUMMARY

This century has been characterized by an increasingly technological and global transnational society, transcending the boundaries of the traditional nuclear family and demanding increasing instrumental and emotional investment in the work sphere (Dreman, 1997a). Changing gender roles, decreased marriage and fertility rates, increased divorce rates, ambiguity in parental roles, "high-tech" reproductive methods, family violence, and other evolving phenomena have resulted in a breakdown in the traditional family infrastructure, which once served as a basis for the education, nurturance, and identity of its members. Individualism, autonomy, and the pursuit of career-related status may usurp traditional family values, such as community, belonging, and family-related status, as society "progresses" along the inevitable pathways of increasing modernization. Families *can* provide the stability, belonging, and sense of community necessary to a society characterized by flux, alienation, and individualism. The prevailing theme seems to be that a sense of family roots and belonging may complement rather than undermine a person's search for autonomy by diminishing the existential anxiety precipitated by a changing and sometimes incomprehensible world. Family stability promotes flexibility in the face of change, family and communal belonging promotes healthy autonomy, and interpersonal nurturance and connectedness contribute to individuality and achievement. Work and domestic realms are complementary, rather than antagonistic spheres of influence, and cross-fertilize and contribute to optimal performance in each domain.

Survival in the future depends not so much on what a person knows, but how a person learns (Pesut, 1997). To some degree, all nurses are futurists. A good futurist characterizes society or situations being studied and accounts for present situations, generates a coherent image of the future, and provides a road map or description of how to get there. A continuum of time defines the past, present, and future. No facts exist about the future; rather, we have historical facts, present options, and projected possibilities for the future. The future represents freedom, power, and hope.

The movement of family health care nursing requires nurses to expand beyond the traditional family-as-context approach. A more comprehensive and integrated approach allows family nurses to practice incorporating the family as context, the family as client, the family as system, and the family as a component of society. Family health care nursing is challenging and rewarding and represents the future practice of all nurses. Join us in defining the future of family nursing in the new millenium!

Study Questions

1. Match the cultural periods of American families (a to c) with their typical characteristics (I to V).
   a. Traditional family
   b. Individualism
   c. New familism
      I. Leveling off of divorce rates
      II. High birth rates
      III. High degree of marital stability
      IV. Decline in birth rates
      V. Increased flexibility
2. What are the specific family demographic trends in the U.S.?
3. What other trends have you noticed in your country?
4. Name some world demographic changes that you are aware of.
5. What other observations have you made about the world?
6. Why and how is family nursing theory, practice, research, education, and social policy important for the future of family health care nursing?

Discussion Questions

1. What do you see as the future for families in the U.S. and around the world? Describe the rationale for your response.
2. Pretend you could look into a crystal ball, and name one prediction for the future of families and one for family nursing.
3. What role will you play in the future of family health care nursing?
4. Discuss the implications that religion, sexuality, and health care technology have for the future of family health care nursing. What are some other factors that will affect family health care nursing that are not listed in this chapter?

References

Burr, W.A., et al. (1993). *Family Science*. Pacific Grove, CA: Brooks/Cole.

Burton, L.M., et al. (1995). Context and surrogate parenting among contemporary grandparents. In S.M.H Hanson, et al. *Single Parent Families: Diversity, Myths and Reality*. New York: Haworth Press.

Calhoun, A.W. (1960). *A Social History of the American Family*. New York: Barnes & Noble.

Children's Defense Fund. (1990). Children MO: A report card, briefing book and action primer. Washington, DC: Children's Defense Fund.

Coontz, S. (1992). *The Way We Never Were: American Families And The Nostalgia Trap*. New York: Basic Books.

Doherty, W.J. (1992). Private lives, public values: The new pluralism. *Psychology Today, 25*(3):32–37, 82.

Dreman, S. (1997a). Is the family viable? Some thoughts and implications for the third millennium. In S. Dreman (Ed.) *The Family On The Threshold Of The Twenty-first Century: Trends And Implications*. Mahwah, NJ: Lawrence Erlbaum.

Dreman, S. (1997b). On the threshold of a new era: An introduction. In S. Dreman (Ed.) *The Family On The Threshold Of The twenty-first Century: Trends And Implications*. Mahwah, NJ: Lawrence Erlbaum.

Feetham, S. (1999). The future in family nursing is genetics and it is now. *Journal of Family Nursing, 5*(1):3–9.

Fong, L., & Sandhu, D. (1993). Religion and the family in a global context. In K. Altergott, (Ed.), *One World: Many Families*. Minneapolis: National Council on Family Relations.

Gelles, R.J. (1995). *Contemporary Families: A Sociological View*. Thousand Oaks: Sage.

Hammond, A. (1998). *Which World? Scenarios For The twenty-first Century*. Washington, DC: Island Press/ Shearwater Books.

Hanson, S.M.H., & Heims, M.L. (1992). Family nursing curricula in U.W. schools of nursing. *Journal of Nursing Education, 31*(7):305–308.

Hanson, S.M.H., et al. (1992). Education for family health care professionals: Nursing as a paradigm. *Family Relations, 41*:49–53.

Iglehart, J.K. (1992). The American health care system, managed care. *The New England Journal of Medicine, 327*:742–747.

Kaakinen, J. (1999). An ecological view of elders and their families: Needs for the twenty-first century. In Dempsey, C. & Butkus, R. (Eds.). *All Creation is Groaning*. Collegeville, Minn: Liturgical Press.

Kinsella, K. (1996). Aging and the family: Present and future demographic issues. In Blieszner, T., & Bedford, V. (Eds.). *Aging and the Family: Theory and Research*. Westport, CT: Praeger.

Kirschling, J. M., et al. (1994). "Success" in family nursing: Experts describe phenomena. *Nursing and Health Care, 15*:186–189.

McCubbin, M.A., & McCubbin, H.I. (1993) Families coping with illness: The resiliency model of family stress adjustment, and adaptation. In C.B. Danielson, et al. *Families, Health & Illness: Perspectives on Coping in Intervention* (pp. 21–65). St. Louis: Mosby.

Riche, M.F. (1998). *From Pyramids to Pillars: The New Demographic Reality*. Washington DC: Communications Consortium Media Center.

Pesut, D.J. (1997). Facilitating futures thinking. *Nursing Outlook, 45*:155.

Popenoe, D. (1993). American family decline, 1960–1990: A review and appraisal. *Journal of Marriage and the Family, 55*:527–555.

Spanier, G.B. (1989). Bequeathing family continuity. *Journal of Marriage and the Family, 51*:313.

U.S. Bureau of the Census. (1990). Statistical Abstracts of the United States, 1990. Washington, DC: U.S. Government Printing Office.

U.S. Bureau of the Census. (1991a). Current population reports, Series P-60, No. 173. Child support and alimony: 1989. Washington, DC: U.S. Government Printing Office.

U.S. Bureau of the Census. (1991b). Current population reports, Series P-20, No. 461. Marital status and living arrangements: March 1991. Washington, DC: U.S. Government Printing Office.

U.S. Bureau of the Census. (1992a). Current population reports, Series P-20, No. 458, Household and family characteristics: 1991. Washington, DC: U.S. Government Printing Office.

U.S. Bureau of the Census. (1992b). Current population reports, P23–180. Marriage, divorce, and remarriage in the 1990s. Washington, DC: U.S. Government Printing Office.

U.S. Bureau of the Census. (1992c). Current population reports, P20, No. 468. Marital status and living arrangements: March 1992. Washington, DC: U.S. Government Printing Office.

U.S. Bureau of the Census. (1992d). Current population reports, P23–181. Households, families and children: A 30-year perspective. Washington, DC: U.S. Government Printing Office.

U.S. Bureau of the Census. (1994a). The Earnings Ladder. Washington DC: US Department of Commerce.

U.S. Bureau of the Census. (1994b). Current Population Reports, P20, No. 477 and P20, No. 478.Washington DC: U.S. Government Printing Office.

U.S. Bureau of the Census. (1994c). Current Population Reports Series P20, No. 483. S. W. Rawlings and A. Saluter, Household and Family Characteristics: March

1994. Washington, DC: U.S. Government Printing Office. Table A, p. vii.

U.S. Bureau of the Census. (1995a). Current Population Reports. P60, No. 184. Statistical Abstract of the United States, 1995. Washington, DC: U.S. Government Printing Office.

U.S. Bureau of the Census. (1995b). Marital Status and Living Arrangements, March 1995. Washington, DC: U.S. Government Printing Office.

U.S. Bureau of the Census. (1995c). Statistical Abstract of the United States. Washington, DC: U.S. Government Printing Office.

U.S. Department of Health and Human Services, Office of Public Health and Science. (1998). Healthy People 2010 Objectives: Draft for public comment. Washington, DC: U.S. Goverment Printing Office. ISBN 0-16-049722-1.

U.S. Public Health Service, U.S. Department of Health and Human Services. (1990). Healthy People 2000: National Health Promotion and Disease Prevention Objectives. Washington, DC: Government Printing Office (017-001-00473-1).

Vosburgh, D., & Simpson, P. (1993). Linking family theory and practice: A family nursing program. *Image: Journal of Nursing Scholarship*, *25*(3):231–235.

Whitehead, B.D.(1992). A new familism? *Family Affairs*, *5*(1–2).

Wilcox, B.L. (1997). Genetic technology: The brave new world? *Family Futures*, *1*(4):4–5.

Wisensale, S. K. (1992). Toward the twenty-first century: Family change and public policy. *Family Relations*, *41*:417–422.

Wright, L., & Bell, J. (1989). A survey of family nursing education in Canadian universities. *The Canadian Journal of Nursing Research*, *21*(3):59–74.

Zimmerman, S.L. (1992). Family trends: What implications for family policy? *Family Relations*, *423*:429.

Bibliography

Altergott, K. (Ed.). *One World. Many Families.* Minneapolis: National Council of Family Relations.

American Nurses' Association. Cabinet on Nursing Research. (1985). *Directions For Nursing Research: Toward The Twenty-First Century*. St. Louis: American Nurses Association.

Aydelotte, M.K. (1987). Nursing's preferred future. *Nursing Outlook*, *11*:4–120.

Barnum, B. (Ed.). (1989). Trends in the nineties. *Nursing & Health Care*, *10*:1–50.

Bender, D.L. & Leone, B. (Eds.). *The Family in America: Opposing Viewpoints*. San Diego: Greenhaven Press.

Cherlin, A., & Furstenberg, F. F. (1982, Fall). The shape of the American family in the year 2000. Washington, DC: American Council of Life Insurance.

Chilman, C. S. (1986). Some critical issues facing the United States in the 1990s and (if we're lucky) beyond. In R. H. Jewson & P. W. Dail (Eds.), *In Praise of 50 Years: The Groves Conference on the Conservation of Marriage and the Family*. Lake Mills, IA: Graphic Publishing.

Dilworth-Anderson, P., et al. (1993). The importance of values in the study of culturally diverse families. *Family Relations*, *42*:238–242.

Family Service America. (1984). *The State of Families 1984–85*. Milwaukee, WI: Family Service America.

Family Service America. (1987). *The State of Families*. 2: *Work and family* (pp. 1–95). Milwaukee, WI: Family Service America.

Feetham, S.L. (1999). Families and the genetic revolution: Implications for primary healthcare, education, and research. *Families, Systems & Health*, *17*(1):27–43.

Ferketich, S.L., & Mercer, R.T. (1992). Focus on psychometrics: Aggregating family data. *Research in Nursing and Health*, vol *15*(4):313–317.

Fine, M.A. (1993). Current approaches to understanding family diversity. *Family Relations*, *42*:235–237.

Glenn, N. (1997). *Closed Hearts, Closed Minds: The Textbook Story of Marriage*. New York, NY: Institute for American Values.

Glick, P. C. (1988). Fifty years of family demography: A record of social change. *Journal of Marriage and the Family*, *50*:861–873.

Hareven, T. (1982). American families in transition: Historical perspectives on change. In F. Walsh (Ed.), *Normal Family Process*. (pp. 446–465). New York: Guilford.

Institute Council on Families in America. (1995). *Marriage in America: A Report to the Nation*. New York: Institute for American Values.

Kirkendall, L. A., & Gravatt, A. E. (Eds.). (1984). *Marriage and the Family in the Year 2020*. New York: Prometheus Books.

Levine, M.O., et al. (1983). Traditional and alternative family life styles. In M.O. Levine, et al. (Eds.) *Developmental Behavioral Pediatrics*, pp. 193–208. Philadelphia: W.B. Saunders.

McCubbin, H., et al. (1987). FHI: The Family Hardiness Index. In H. McCubbin and A. Thompson (Eds.) *Family Assessment Inventories For Research And Practice*. Madison: University of Wisconsin.

Norton, A. J., & Moorman, J. E. (1987). Current trends in marriage and divorce among American Women. *Journal of Marriage and the Family*, *49*:483–497.

Olson, D.G., & Hanson, M.K. (Eds). (1990). *2001: Preparing Families for the Future*. Minneapolis: National Council on Family Relations.

Orthner, D. (1991). The family in transition. In D. Blankenhorn, et al. (Eds.) *Rebuilding The Nest: A New Commitment To The American Family*. Milwaukee, WI: Family Service America.

Popenoe, D. (1988). *Disturbing The Nest: Family Change And Decline In Modern Societies*. New York: Aldine de Gruyter.

Popenoe, D. (1989). The family transformed. *Family Affairs*, *2*(2 3):1–15.

Popenoe, D., & Whitehead, B.D. (1999). Should we live together? What young adults need to know about cohabitation before marriage. The National Marriage Project, Rutgers University, 25 Bishop Place, New Brunswick, New Jersey. 08901-1181. 732-932-2722. E-mail: marriage@rci.rutgers.edu

Price, S., & Elliott, B. (1993). *Vision 2010: Famlies & health care*. Minneapolis: National Council on Family Relations, 3989 Central Avenue, Suite 550, Minneapolis, MN 55421. ISBN #0-916174-39-5.

Public Health Service, U.S. Department of Health and Human Services. (1990). Healthy people 2000: National health promotion. and disease prevention objectives. Washington, DC: Government Printing Office (#17-001-00473-1).

Riche, M.F. (1998). *From Pyramids To Pillars: The New Demographic Reality*. Manuscript presented at the United Nations Population Fund Technical Meeting on Population Aging, Brussels, Belgium, Oct 6–9, 1999. (Brochure developed by Communications Consortium Media Center at 1200 New York Ave. NW, Suite 300, Washington, DC 20005-1754.)

Scanzoni, J. (1983). *Shaping Tomorrow's Family: Theory And Policy For The Twenty-first Century*. Beverly Hills, CA: Sage.

Schneider, J.A. (1986). Rewriting the SES: Demographic patterns and divorcing families. *Social Science and Medicine*, *23*:211–222.

Spanier, G. B. (1986). The changing American family: Demographic trends and prospects. In P. W. Dail & R. H. Jewson (Eds.) *In Pause Of Fifty Years: The Groves Conference On The Conservation Of Marriage & Family*, Lake Hills, IA: Graphic Publications.

Sprey, J. (1988). Current theorizing on the family: An appraisal. *Journal of Marriage and the Family*. *50*:875–890.

Williams, D.M. (1989) Political theory and individualistic health promotion. *Advances in Nursing Science*, *12*:1425.

Zigler, E., & Black, K.B. (1989). America's family support movement: Strengths and limitations. *American Journal of Orthopsychiatry*, *I*:6–19.

Appendix A

RESOURCE LIST FOR FAMILY NURSING

COMMUNITY AND NATIONAL RESOURCES

Administration for Children and Families (ACF)
200 Independence Ave SW
Washington, DC 20201
HYPERLINK: http://www.acf.dhhs.gov/index.htm

Administration on Aging
U.S. Department of Health and Human Services
Executive Office Center
2101 East Jefferson St
Rockville, MD 20852
(800) 358-9295
http://www.aoa.dhhs.gov

Administration on Children and Families
Switzer Building, Room 330
C Street SW
Washington, DC 20201
(202) 205-8347
FAX: (202) 205-9721

Agency for Health Care Policy and Research (AHCPR)
Public Health Service
Executive Office Center, Suite 501
2101 E. Jefferson St
Rockville, MD 28052
http://www.ahcpr.gov

AIDS Caregivers Support Network
2536 Alki Avenue SW, #138
Seattle, WA 98116
(206) 937-3368
http://www.wolfenet.com

AIDS Healthcare Foundation
6255 W. Sunset Boulevard, 21st Floor
Los Angeles, CA 90028
(323) 860-5200
http://www.aidshealth.org

Alzheimer's Disease and Related Disorders Association (ADRDA)
919 N. Michigan Ave, Suite 1000
Chicago, IL 60611-1676
(800) 272-3900
http://www.alzheimers.org

American Association for Marriage and Family Therapy
1133 15th Street NW, Suite 300
Washington, DC 20005-2710
(202) 452-0109
FAX: (202) 223-2329
http://www.aamft.org

American Association of Homes for the Aging
901 E. Street NW, Suite 500
Washington, DC 20036
(202) 233-4000

American Association of Retired Persons (AARP)
601 E. Street NW
Washington, DC 20049
(202) 434-2777
ElderWeb
http://www.elderweb.com

American Cancer Society
1599 Clifton Road
Atlanta, GA 30329-4251
(800) ACS-2345
http://www.cancer.org

American Diabetes Association
1660 Duke St
Alexandria, VA 22314
(800) 342-2383
http://www.diabetes.org

American Family Society
P.O. Box 80
Rockville, MD 20851

American Health Care Association
1200 15th Street NW
Washington, DC 20005
(202) 833-2050

American Heart Association
7272 Greenville Avenue
Dallas, TX 75231
(214) 373-6300
http://www.americanheart.org

American Lung Association
1740 Broadway
New York, NY 10019-1740
(212) 315-8700
http://www.lungusa.org

American Pain Society
4700 W. Lake Avenue
Glenview, IL 60025
(847) 375-4714
http://www.ampainsoc.org

American Parkinson Disease Association
1250 Hylan Blvd
Staten Island, NY 10305
(800) 223-2732

Arthritis Foundation
3400 Peachtree Road, Suite 1101
Atlanta, GA 30326
(404) 266-795

Arthritis Foundation
1330 West Peachtree Street
Atlanta, GA 30309
(404) 872-7100
http://www.arthritis.org

Association of African American People's Legal Council
PO Box 20053
Detroit, MI 48220

Association of Critical Care Nurses
101 Columbia
Aliso Viejo, CA 92656
(949) 362-2000
http://www.aacn.org

Center for Family Resources
384 Clinton Street
Hempstead, NY 10550

Center for Food Safety and Applied Nutrition
Food and Drug Administration (FDA)
200 C Street SW
Washington, DC 20204
(202) 205-5615
FAX: (202) 205-5532

Center for Mental Health Services
Substance Abuse and Mental Health Services Administration (SAMHSA)
Parklawn Building, Room 18C-07
5600 Fishers Lane
Rockville, MD 20857
(301) 443-7790
FAX: (301) 443-7912

Center for Practice and Technology
Agency for Health Care Policy and Research
6010 Executive Boulevard, Suite 300
Rockville, MD 20852
(301) 594-4015
FAX: (301) 594-4027

Center for Substance Abuse Prevention
Substance Abuse and Mental Health Services Administration
Rockwall II Building, Room 950
5600 Fishers Lane
Rockville, MD 20857
(301) 443-9931
FAX: (301) 443-6394

Center for Substance Abuse Treatment
Substance Abuse and Mental Health Services Administration (SAMHSA)
Rockwall II Building, Room 800
5600 Fishers Lane
Rockville, MD 20857
(301) 443-7924
FAX: (301) 480-6077

Centers for Disease Control and Prevention
1600 Clifton Rd
Atlanta, GA 30333
(404) 639-3311
http://www.cdc.gov/

Centers for Disease Control and Prevention
Office of Program Planning and Evaluation
Building 16, Room 5145, MS D23
1600 Clifton Road NE
Atlanta, GA 30333
(404) 639-7070
FAX: (404) 639-7171

Child Abuse and Neglect Programs
200 Independence Ave SW
Washington, DC 20201
http://www.acf.dhhs.gov/index.htm

Child Care and Development Fund
200 Independence Ave SW
Washington, DC 20201
http://www.acf.dhhs.gov/index.htm

Child Support Enforcement Program
200 Independence Ave SW
Washington, DC 20201
http://www.acf.dhhs.gov/index.htm

Child Welfare Services
200 Independence Ave SW
Washington, DC 20201
http://www.acf.dhhs.gov/index.htm

Children's Health Insurance Program (CHIP)
Health Care Financing Administration
7500 Security Boulevard
Baltimore, MD 21244
(410) 786-3000
http://www.hcfa.gov/init/children.htm

Department of Health and Human Services
200 Independence Ave SW
Washington, DC 20201
http://www.os.dhhs.gov/

Division of Adolescent and School Health
National Center for Chronic Disease Prevention and Health Promotion
Centers for Disease Control and Prevention
4770 Buford Highway NE, Mailstop K-29
Atlanta, GA 30341-3724
(770) 488-3254
FAX: (770) 488-3110

Division of Health Promotion Statistics
National Center for Health Statistics
Centers for Disease Control and Prevention
6525 Belcrest Road, Room 770
Hyattsville, MD 20782
(301) 436-3548
FAX: (301) 436-8459

Division of Prevention Research and Analytic Methods Epidemiology Program Office
Centers for Disease Control and Prevention
Mailstop D01
Atlanta, GA 30333
(404) 639-4455
FAX: (404) 639-4463

Division of Public Health
Public Health Program Practice Office
Centers for Disease Control and Prevention
4770 Buford Highway NE, Mailstop K-29
Atlanta, GA 30341-3742
(770) 488-2469
FAX: (770) 488-2489

Emergency Nurses Association
915 Lee Street
Des Plaines, IL 60016-6569
(800) 900-9659
http://www.ena.org

Family Preservation and Family Support
200 Independence Ave SW
Washington, DC 20201
http://www.acf.dhhs.gov/index.htm

Family Resources Coalition
200 South Michigan Avenue, Suite 1520
Chicago, IL 60604

Food and Drug Administration
Parklawn Building, Room 15A-08
5600 Fishers Lane, MS HFY-40
Rockville, MD 20857
(301) 443-5470
FAX: (301) 443-2446

Foster Care/Adoption Assistance/Independent Living
200 Independence Ave SW
Washington, DC 20201
http://www.acf.dhhs.gov/index.htm

Head Start
200 Independence Ave SW
Washington, DC 20201
http://www.acf.dhhs.gov/index.htm

Health Resources and Services Administration
Parklawn Building, Room 14–33
5600 Fishers Lane
Rockville, MD 20852
(301) 443-2460
FAX: (301) 443-9270

Housing and Urban Development
451 Seventh St SW
Washington DC 20410
http://www.hud.gov/index.html

Indian Health Service
12300 Twinbrook Parkway, Suite 610
Rockville, MD 20852
(301) 443-1054
FAX: (301) 443-7538

Institution for American Values
1841 Broadway, Suite 211
New York, NY 10023
(212) 246-3942
FAX: (212) 541-6665
E-mail: HYPERLINK mail to:iav@worldnet.att.net iav@worldnet.att.net

International Childbirth Education Association (ICEA)
PO Box 20048
Minneapolis, MN 55420
http://www.icea.org

La Leche League International
1400 N. Meacham Road
Schaumburg, IL 60173-4048
http://www.lalecheleague.org

Maternal and Child Health Bureau
Health Resources and Services Administration
5600 Fishers Lane
Rockville, MD 20857

Medicaid
Health Care Financing Administration
7500 Security Boulevard
Baltimore, MD 21244
(410) 786-3000
http://www.hcfa.gov/medicaid/medicaid.htm

Medicare
Health Care Financing Administration
7500 Security Boulevard
Baltimore, MD 21244
(410) 786-3000
http://www.hcfa.gov/medicare/medicare.htm

Mended Hearts
7320 Greenville Avenue
Dallas, TX 75231
(800) 242-8721
http://www.mendedhearts.org

National Asian Pacific Center on Aging
1511 Third Ave, Suite 914
Seattle, WA 98101
(206) 624-1221
www.ncoa.org/lcao/members/napca.htm

National Association for Hispanic Elderly
234 East Colorado Blvd, Suite 300
Pasadena, CA 91101
(626) 564-1988
www.nih.gov/nia/related/aoaresrc/dir/127.htm

National Association of Adult Day Care
180 East 4050 South
Murray, UT 84107
(801) 262-9167

National Association of Area Agencies on Aging
(202) 296-8130

National Association of Home Health Agencies
426 C Street NE, Suite 200
Washington, DC 20002
(202) 547-1717

National Cancer Institute
National Institutes of Health
Building 31, Room 10A49
31 Center Drive, MSC 2580
Bethesda, MD 20892-2580
(301) 496-9569
FAX: (301) 496-9931

National Caucus for the Black Aged
1424 K Street NW, Suite 500
Washington, DC 20006
(202) 797-8227

National Center for Chronic Disease Prevention and Health Promotion
Centers for Disease Control and Prevention
4770 Buford Highway NE, Mailstop K10
Atlanta, GA 30341-3724
(770) 488-5000
FAX: (770) 488-5966

National Center for Health Statistics
6525 Belcrest Road
Hyattsville, MD 20782-2003
http://www.cdc.gov/nchswww

National Center for HIV, STD, and TB Prevention
Centers for Disease Control and Prevention
1600 Clifton Road NE, Mailstop E-07
Atlanta, GA 30333
(404) 639-8008
FAX: (404) 639-8600

National Center for Infectious Diseases
Centers for Disease Control and Prevention
1600 Clifton Road NE, Mailstop C-12
Atlanta, GA 30333
(404) 639-3401
FAX: (404) 639-3039

National Center for Injury Prevention and Control
Division of Unintentional Injury
Centers for Disease Control and Prevention
4770 Buford Highway NE, Mailstop K59
Atlanta, GA 30341-3724
(770) 488-4652
FAX: (404) 488-4338

National Center for Injury Prevention and Control
Division of Violence Prevention
Centers for Disease Control and Prevention
4770 Buford Highway NE, Mailstop K60
Atlanta, GA 30341-3724
(770) 488-4276
FAX: (404) 488-4349

National Centers for Chronic Disease Prevention and Health Promotion
Centers for Disease Control and Prevention
4770 Buford Highway NE, Mailstop K40
Atlanta, GA 30341-3724
(770) 488-5403
FAX: (770) 488-5971

National Coalition of Hispanic Health Human Services Organizations
1501 Sixteenth St, NW
Washington, DC 20036
(202) 387-5000

National Council on Family Relations
3989 Central Ave NE, Suite 550
Minneapolis, MN 55421
(888) 781-9331
(612) 781-9331
FAX: (612) 781-9348
http://www.ncfr.org

National Council on the Aging
409 Third Street SW, Suite 202
Washington, DC 20024

National Gay and Lesbian Task Force
1700 Kalorama Road NW
Washington, DC 20009-2624
(202) 332-6483
FAX: (202) 332-0207
TTY: (202) 332-6219
http://www.ngltf.org/

National Gerontological Nursing Association
7250 Parkway Drive, Suite 510
Hanover, MD 21706

National Heart, Lung and Blood Institute
National Institutes of Health
31 Center Drive, MSC 2486
Bethesda, MD 20892-2486
(301) 496-5437
FAX: (301) 480-4907

National Hispanic Prenatal Hotline
(800) 504-7081

National Hospice Organization
301 Maple Avenue W, Suite 506
Vienna, VA 22180
(703) 938-4449

National Immunization Program
Centers for Disease Control and Prevention
1600 Clifton Road NE, Mailstop E-05
Atlanta, GA 30333
(404) 639-8200
FAX: (404) 639-8626

National Indian Council on Aging
10501 Montgomery Blvd NE, Suite 210
Albuquerque, NM 87110
(505) 292-2001
www.omhrc.gov/mhr2/orgs/88O0655.htm

National Institute of Arthritis and Musculoskeletal and Skin Diseases
National Institutes of Health
Natcher Building
45 Center Drive
Bethesda, MD 20892-6600
(301) 594-5014
FAX: (301) 402-2406

National Institute of Dental Research
National Institutes of health
Building 45, Room 3 AN-44B
45 Center Drive, Mailstop 6401
Bethesda, MD 20892-6401 (301) 594-5391
FAX: (301) 480-8254

National Institute of Diabetes and Digestive and Kidney Diseases
National Institutes of Health
Building 45, Room 6AN38J
9000 Rockville Pike
Bethesda, MD 20892
(301) 594-8867
FAX: (301) 480-4237

National Institute of Mental Health
National Institutes of Health
Parklawn Building, Room 9C25
5600 Fishers Lane
Rockville, MD 20857
(301) 443-3533
FAX: (301) 443-8022

National Institute of Occupational Safety and Health
Centers for Disease Control and Prevention
200 Independence Ave SW, Room 733G
Washington, DC 20201
(202) 401-0721
FAX: (202) 260-4464

National Institute on Aging
P.O. Box 8057
Gaithersburg, MD 20892-8057
(301) 496-1752
http://www.nia.gov

National Institutes of Health (NIH)
Building 1, Room 260
9000 Rockville Pike
Bethesda, MD 20892
(301) 496-1508
FAX: (301) 402-2517
(301) 496-6614
FAX: (301) 480-9654
http://www.nih.gov/

National Kidney Foundation
30 East 33rd Street
New York, NY 10016
(800) 622-9010
http://www.kidney.org

National Multiple Sclerosis Society
205 East 42nd Street
New York, NY 10017
(212) 986-3240

Office of Clinical Standards and Quality Health Care
Health Care Financing Administration
S1-13-23 South Building
C3-24-07 South Building
&500 Security Boulevard
Baltimore, MD 21244-1850

Office of Disease Prevention and Health Promotion
200 Independence Avenue, SW, Room 738G
Washington, DC 20201
(202) 260-2652
FAX: (202) 205-0463

Office of Disease Prevention and Health Promotion
738-G Humphrey Building
200 Independence Ave, SW
Washington, DC 20201
FAX: (202) 205-9478

Office of Minority Health (OMH)
Rockwall II Building, Suite 1000
5515 Security Lane
Rockville, MD 20857
(301) 443-5084
FAX: (301) 594-0767

Office of Minority Health
Resource Center
Box 37337
Washington, DC 20013-7337
(800) 444-6472
FAX: (301) 589-0884

Office of Policy and External Affairs
Agency for Toxic Substances and Disease Registry
1600 Clifton Road, NE, Mailstop E60
Atlanta, GA 30333
(404) 639-0500
FAX: (404) 639-0522

Office of Policy, Planning, and Evaluation
National Institute of Environmental Health Sciences
National Institutes of Health
Building 101, Room B250
PO Box 12233, Mail Drop B2-08
111 Alexander Drive
Research Triangle Park, NC 27709
(919) 541-3484
FAX: (919) 541-4737

Office of Population Affairs
Suite 200 West
4350 East West Highway
Bethesda, MD 20814
(301) 594-7608
FAX: (301) 594-5980

Office of Women's Health
712E HHH Building
200 Independence Avenue SW
Washington, DC 20201
(202) 690-7650

Office on Disability and Health
National Center for Environmental Health
Centers for Disease Control and Prevention
4770 Buford Highway NE, Mailstop F029
Atlanta, GA 30341-3724
(770) 488-7094
FAX: (770) 488-7075

Office on Smoking and Health
National Center for Chronic Disease Prevention and Health Promotion
Centers for Disease Control and Prevention
4770 Buford Highway NE, Mailstop K50
Atlanta, GA 30341-3724
(770) 488-5797
FAX: (770) 488-5767

Older Women's League
1325 G Street NW
Lower Level B
Washington, DC 20005

Parents, Friends, and Families of Lesbians and Gays (PFLAG)
1101 14th Street NW, Suite 1030
Washington, DC 20005
(202) 638-4200
FAX: (202) 638-0243
http://www.pflag.org/pflag.html

Physical Activity and Health Branch
Division of Nutrition and Physical Activity
National Center for Chronic Disease Prevention and Health Promotion
4770 Buford Highway NE, Mailstop K-47
Atlanta, GA 30341-3724
(770) 488-5513
FAX: (770) 488-5486

President's Council on Physical Fitness and Sports
731-H Hubert Humphrey Building
200 Independence Avenue, SW
Washington, DC 20201
(202) 690-5148
FAX: (202) 690-5211

Public Health Program Practice Office
Centers for Disease Control and Prevention
4770 Buford Highway NE, Mailstop K-36
Atlanta, GA 30341-3724
(770) 488-2402
FAX: (770) 488-2428

Sigma Theta Tau International
Virginia Henderson Library
550 West North Street
Indianapolis, IN 46202
(317) 634-8171
(888) 634-7575
(800) 634-7575
FAX: (317) 634-8188
E-mail: HYPERLINK: mailto:education@stti-sun.iupui.edu
education@stti-sun.iupui.edu
www.nursing.society.org

Substance Abuse and Mental Health Services Administration
Parklawn Building, Room 12C-26
5600 Fishers Lane
Rockville, MD 20857
(301) 443-6067
FAX: (301) 594-6159

Temporary Assistance for Needy Families
200 Independence Ave SW
Washington, D.C. 20201
http://www.acf.dhhs.gov/index.htm

The Association of Women's Health, Obstetric, and Neonatal Nurses (AWHONN)
700 14th Street NW, Suite 600
Washington, DC 20005-2019
http://www.awhonn.org

The Child Welfare League of America
440 First Street NW, Third Floor
Washington, DC 20001-2085
(202) 638-2952
FAX: (202) 638-4004
http://www.cwla.org/cwla/index.html

The Human Rights Campaign
919 18th Street, NW
Washington, DC 20006
(202) 628-4160
FAX: (202) 347-5323
http://www.hrc.org/

The International Lactation Consultant Association (ILCA)
4101 Lake Boone Trail, Suite 201
Raleigh, NC 27607
http://www.ilca.org

The National Clearinghouse on Child Abuse and Neglect
330 C Street SW
Washington, DC 20447
(800) 394-3366 or (703) 385-7565
FAX: (703) 385-3206
http://www.calib.com/nccanch/index.htm

The National Health Information Center (NHIC)
P.O. Box 1133
Washington, DC 20013-1133
(800) 336-4797 or (301) 565-4167
FAX: (301) 984-4256
http://nhic-nt.health.org/

The National Organization for Women
1000 16th Street NW, Suite 700
Washington, DC 20036
(202) 331-0066
FAX: (202) 785-8576
TTY: (202) 331-9002
http://www.now.org/

U. S. Bureau of the Census
U. S. Department of Commerce
Washington, DC 20233
URL: HYPERLINK: http://www.census.gov
http://www.census.gov

United Ostomy Association
2001 West Beverly Blvd
Los Angeles, CA 90057
(213) 413-5510

Veterans Administration
810 Vermont Avenue, NW
Washington, DC 20420
(202) 233-4000

Visiting Nurses Association of America
3801 East Florida Avenue, Suite 900
Denver, CO 80210
(800) 426-2547

Welfare to Work Challenge
200 Independence Ave SW
Washington, DC 20201
http://www.acf.dhhs.gov/index.htm

Work and Family Information Center
The Conference Board
845 Third Avenue
New York, NY 10022

World Future Society (WFS)
7910 Woodmont Ave, Suite 450
Bethesda, MD 20814
(800) 989-8274

Youth Programs
200 Independence Ave SW
Washington, DC 20201
(301) 443-2170
FAX: (301) 443-1797
http://www.acf.dhhs.gov/index.htm

WEB SITES

A network of online therapists with various specialties
$80 per session
http://www.concernedcounseling.com

Alliance of Genetic Support Groups
http://www.medhelp.org/geneticalliance

American Association of Therapeutic Humor
http://www.aath.org/

American Heart Association
Physical Activity and Cardiovascular Health: Fact Sheet, 1999
http://www.americanheart.org

American Nurses Association
http://www.nursingworld.org/

American Nurses Foundation
http://www.nursingworld.org/anf
E-mail: HYPERLINK mailto:ANF@ana.org ANF@ana.org

At a cost of $850, a 16 week program for eating disorders
http://www.edrecovery.com

Bandaides and Blackboards
http://funrsc.fairfield.edu/jfleitas/contents.html

Brownson's guide to nursing organizations
http://members.tripod.com/DianneBrownson/organizations.html

Commission on Family and Medical Leave Act
http://www.dol.gov/dol/esa/public/regs/compliance/whd/fmla/family.htm

Contact for medical information
www.webmd.com

Current licensing requirements for marriage and family therapy for each state in the US
http://www.enol.com/shrman/MFT/professional/mftstates

Diversity Rx is a clearinghouse of information on the World Wide Web on how to meet the language and cultural needs of minorities, immigrants, refugees and other diverse populations seeking health care. "Diversity Rx is sponsored by The National Conference of State Legislatures, Resources for Cross Cultural Health Care, and the Henry J. Kaiser Family Foundation."
http://www.diversityrx.org

Dogpile Search Engine
http://www.dogpile.com/

Down Syndrome WWW Page
http://www.nas.com/downsyn

Family Trends
http://www.infoplease.lycos.com/ipa/A0001548.html
For $30, a series of questionnaires aimed at helping people deal with stress.
http://www.masteringstress.com

Futuristic Book Store
www.wfs.org/wfs

General Accounting Office
http://www.gao.gov

Genetics Education Center
http://www.kumc.edu/instruction/medicine/genetics/homepage.html

GeroWeb
http://www.iog.wayne.edu/GeroWebd/GeroWeb.html

Global RN discussion list
School of Nursing
University of California
San Francisco
http://nurseweb.ucsf.edu/www/globalrn.htm

Great Plains Genetics
http://www.unmc.edu/mrimedia/gpgsn/genetics.html

HealthGate
http://www.healthgate.com

Human Development and Family Life Bulletin
http://www.hec.ohio-state.edu/famlife/bulletin/bullmain.htm

Human Genome Project Information
http://www.ornl.gov/TechResources/Human_Genome/home.html

Institute for Family-Centered Care
http://www.familycenteredcare.org

International Society of Nurses in Genetics
http://nursing,creighton.edu/isong/index.html

Internet Sites of Interest to Aging Research
http://www.rand.org:/centers/aging/related.html

Maps & Driving Directions (start and end destinations)
http://maps.yahoo.com/

National Center for Health Statistics
Centers for Disease Control
www.cdc.gov/nchs

National Coalition for Health Professional Education in Genetics (NCHPEG)
www.nchpeg.org

National Down Syndrome Society
http://www.ndss.org

National Heart, Lung and Blood Institute (NHLBI)
Simple Lifestyle Changes
http://www.nhlbi.nih.gov

National Institute of Nursing Research
http://www.nih.gov/ninr/

National Institutes of Health
http://www.nih.gov

National Student Nurses Association
http://www.nsna.org/

Office of Minority Health Resource Center
http://www.omhrc.gov

Online therapists with tips on how to pick and what to expect
http://www.metaoia.org/imhs

Pharmacy information
http://www.drugstore.com

Phone Directory searches (by city, type of business, name)
http://www.teldir.com/us/bn/

Real Education
web-based educational instruction
http://www.realeducation.com/

Resources for Nurses and Families
http://pegasus.cc.ucf.edu/~wink

See video: "Shattering the Silences"
http://www.pbs.org/shattering

Sigma Theta Tau
E-mail: HYPERLINK mailto:research@stti.iupui.edu research@stti.iupui.edu

Time Conversions
http://www.globalmetric.com/time/

US Census Bureau information
http://www.census2000.org

Whole Nurse
http://www.wholenurse.com/nursing.htm

World Future Society (WFS)
www.wfs.org/wfs

ZipCode Look Up
http://www.zipinfo.com/

JOURNALS*

AWHONN Lifelines
J B Lippincott Company
12107 Insurance Way
Hagerstown, MD 21740

Birth
110 El Camino Real
Berkeley, CA 94705

Family Relations
NCFR
3989 Central Avenue NE, Suite 550
Minneapolis, MN 55421

Journal of Obstetric, Gynecologic, and Neonatal Nursing (JOGNN)
J B Lippincott Company
12107 Insurance Way
Hagerstown, MD 21740

Journal of Perinatal and Neonatal Nursing
Aspen Publishers, Inc.
7201 McKinney Circle
Frederick, MD 21701

MCN: The American Journal of Maternal Child Nursing
555 West 57th Street
New York, NY 10019

*See also community and national resources for their organizations official journals. For example, the National Council on Family Relations publishes the journals *Family Relations* and the *Journal of Marriage and the Family*. Also see chapter 1 for a list of journals pertaining to families.

Appendix B

GLOSSARY

Ableism: prejudice against those without full physical capabilities.

Acculturation: a process in which gradual changes are produced by the influence of one culture on another so that the two cultures become more like each other.

Acute illness pattern: the temporary alteration of daily routines to deal with the crisis of acute diseases and injuries, such as communicable diseases, bone fractures, and appendicitis. After disease treatment, families usually return to predisease family routines.

Adaptive family health model: in this model, families are adaptive if they have the ability to change and grow and possess the capacity to rebound quickly after crisis.

Advance directive: a written agreement established between a patient and a care provider to withhold heroic measures or life-sustaining treatment if their condition becomes irreversible. These agreements are usually written at a time when the individual is healthy or able to make conscious decisions about their welfare.

Advocate: a person who speaks or acts on behalf of those who cannot protect or speak for themselves.

Affirming communication: family communication characterized by taking care not to hurt other members emotionally or physically, taking time to hear what others have to say, conveying respect for others' feelings, and ending conflicts on a positive note.

Aggregate of people: a group of people with similar characteristics, such as all people infected with HIV, all those diagnosed with juvenile onset diabetes, or all homeless families.

Alienation: feeling separate from larger social groups to the extent that the individual suffers emotional pain.

Analysis: critical review of collected data to identify and remedy gaps and inconsistencies and compilation of that data in an organized manner, so as to determine those concerns or problems with which the client needs assistance or guidance. The analysis phase ends with the identification of the pertinent nursing diagnosis.

Analysis: the organization, reduction, categorization, and summarization of data to obtain answers to research questions.

Assessment: (1) a continuously evolving process of data collection in which the nurse, drawing on the past and the present, is able to predict or plan the future. Typically it is the initial phase of the nursing process that progresses into diagnosis, planning, intervention, and evaluation; (2) the first step of the nursing process, which involves the gathering of data through reviewing the human situation and the physical, emotional, and social status of the client to obtain complete and accurate data for the purpose of determining needs for care.

Assimilationist: to assimilate means to lose individual identity (cultural, racial, sexual traits) to align more closely with social norms. A common example of assimilation is the experience of immigrants who do not pass their native language on to their children.

Attachment: an enduring emotional tie between persons that develops and grows over time and that is not transient or easily abandoned. Attachment is specific and unique to the involved individuals and implies love, tenderness, and affection. Involved individuals seek proximity to each other and yearn to be in each other's presence. Attachment relationships can withstand anger, frustration, and periods of separation.

Biological family: family relationships defined by genetic connection.

Bisexual: this term is often used to describe people whose sexual objects of choice include both men and women.

Blaming the victim: instead of considering greater social structures and their impact on the world, those who suffer are blamed. For example, low-income housing projects are required to have removed all lead-based paints. However, many have not; so many children still suffer from poisoning, which comes from eating paint chips (which are sweet). Families are then targeted by public health officials with public service campaigns to alert them to the danger. If the kids get sick, the parents are blamed, not the tardy landlord.

Childbearing cycle: The period of time, beginning with the pre-conceptual period, when a parent considers getting pregnant, the prenatal period of pregnancy, the labor and birth, and the postpartum period, during which the woman's body returns to the normal pre-pregnancy physiologic state and family adapts to a new member.

Chosen family: family relationships defined by anything besides genetics, e.g., love, sex, affection, money, housing.

Chronic illness pattern: the "long haul" in which families permanently reorganize their daily routines to accommodate long-term diseases and conditions.

Clinical family health model: examined from this perspective, a family is healthy if its members are free of physical, mental, and social dysfunction.

Coming out: the informal process gay people go through in revealing their sexual preference to their family, friends, and coworkers.

Community as client: a broad interpretation of the unit of service that addresses the entire community's needs.

Concepts: building blocks of theory that represent the main ideas expressed by the theory; sometimes termed variables. They exist on a continuum from empirical (concrete) to abstract. Examples of concrete concepts are gender and age; abstract concepts, family and health.

Conceptual model or framework: the terms "model" and "framework" are sometimes used interchangeably to mean a set of interrelated concepts that symbolically represent and convey a mental image of a phenomenon. They are less predictive than a theory and only symbolize that there is a relationship among the concepts in the framework. For example, nursing models are not considered stringent enough to be theories because they are not predictive.

Confluence: the process of combining two or more activities at the same time. In families, this may promote togetherness.

Contingency contract: a contract with a health professional or other support person that includes the process of setting a goal and identifying costs and rewards of goal attainment. The purpose of the contingency contract is to reinforce behaviors needed to reach a goal.

Contract: a binding agreement between two or more parties.

Creative thinking: the ability to produce work that is both novel and appropriate. A novel product is one that is original and not predictable. An appropriate product satisfies problem constraints, fulfills a need, is sensible, and useful.

Critical thinking: purposeful, self-regulatory judgment, which results in interpretation, analysis, evaluation, and inference, as well as the explanation of the evidential, conceptual, methodological, criteriological, or contextual considerations on which that judgment was based; a statement of expert consensus for purposes of educational assessment and instruction.

Culture: sets of shared world views and adaptive behaviors derived from simultaneous membership in a variety of contexts, such as ecological setting (rural, urban, suburban), religious background, nationality and ethnicity, social class, gender-related experiences, minority status, occupation, political leanings, migratory patterns, and stage of acculturation, or values derived from belonging to the same generation, partaking of a single historical moment, or upholding a particular ideology.

Data: pieces of information collected in a study to answer research questions.

Developmental or normative transitions: predictable family changes related to the oldest child's development that occur in an expected time line congruent with movement through the eight family stages. Even though families have children in more than one developmental stage, it is assumed that parents have some experience with the earlier stages of family development because of the parenting of the first child.

Developmental task: psychological and social tasks associated with growth and change or transition. Specifically, the developmental tasks of pregnancy are those associated with transition to parenthood and the psychosocial assimilation of the expected baby into the life of the mother and father.

Deviant: those people or things that do not fit social norms are "deviant." The term "deviation" was originally from the field of statistics, describing the data that lay outside of the bell curve.

Disease prevention: activities that protect the population from actual or potential diseases and disabilities and their consequences.

DNR orders: Do not resuscitate orders are explicit instructions that are written by a physician directing care providers not to revive or sustain the vital functions of persons in respiratory or cardiac arrest.

Durable power of attorney: a document that names a person who would make treatment decisions for a patient if they were not able to make them for themselves. Generally it is a person who knows the patient and his or her values well and is in a good position to represent their wishes to the patient's physician.

Empowerment: the process of providing information and resources to help others to reach a goal.

Energized family: a family unit that responds to the needs and interests of all members, while coping effectively with life transitions and problems. An energized family is flexible, has an equal distribution of power, and has a health-promoting lifestyle.

Epidemiology: the science that is concerned with health events in human populations.

Essentialism: reducing the cause of a characteristic or behavior to one cause. Biologic essentialism explains everything as a product of genes or blood.

Ethclass: the intersection of social class and ethnicity. This intersection produces identifiable dispositions and behavioral patterns in families.

Ethical principles: general action guides specifying moral actions that are prohibited, required, or permitted in certain circumstances.

Ethics: the enterprise of disciplined reflection on the moral intuitions and moral choices that people make.

Ethnicity: different from racial groups, ethnic groups are those people who share cultural practices and characteristics, such as a food, clothing, religion, music, and the like, in any combination. A group's sense of "peoplehood" based on a combination of race, religion, ancestral history, and nationality.

Ethnography: a qualitative research methodology primarily used to study cultures.

Eudiamonistic family health model: professionals who use this model as their philosophy of practice focus on efforts to maximize the family's well-being and to support the entire family and individual members in reaching their highest potential.

Evaluation: the fifth step of the nursing process, evaluation is the appraisal of the changes experienced by the client in relation to goal achievement and realization of expected behavioral outcomes as a result of the actions of the nurse. (Yura, H. and Walsh, M. B. (1988). *The Nursing Process: Assessing, Planning, Implementing and Evaluating,* p. 163. Norwalk, Appleton & Lange.)

Expressive behaviors: actions designed to provide affective support.

Family appraisal of the illness: the way the family sees the illness.

Family as a component of society: focus of assessment and intervention is on the family as an institution in society. The family as a whole interacts with other institutions (educational, religious, economic, health) to receive, exchange, or give communication and services.

Family as a system: focus of assessment and intervention is on the interactions between family members. The family is viewed as an interactional system, in which the whole is more than the sum of its parts. The focus is on the individual and family simultaneously.

Family as the client: focus of assessment and intervention is on all individual family members. The family is in the foreground and the individuals are in the background. The family is the sum of individual family members.

Family as the context: focus of assessment and intervention is on the individual client. The individual is in the foreground and the family is in the background. The family is the context for the individual as either a resource or a stressor to their health and illness.

Family career: the dynamic process of change that occurs during the life span of the unique group called the family. American families are diverse and are created through marriage, remarriage, adoption, and partnerships. Family careers include family stages and transitions that can occur in a nonlinear fashion.

Family-centered care: (or family-centered maternity/newborn care or family-centered childbearing care): the delivery of safe, quality health care while recognizing, focusing on, and adapting to both the physical and psychosocial needs of the client-patient, the family, and the newly born. The emphasis is on the provision of maternity/newborn health care, which fosters family unity while maintaining physical safety.

Family child health nursing: focuses on the relationships, family tasks, and nursing care related to children's health.

Family coping: family strategies, patterns, and behaviors designed to maintain or strengthen the family as a whole, maintain the emotional stability and well-being of its members, obtain or use family and community resources to manage the situation, and initiate efforts to resolve family hardships created by a stressor. The family's efforts to strengthen the family as a unit, maintain the well-being of its members, and use family and community resources to manage stress and hardship.

Family function: The purpose that the family serves for: (1) its members and (2) for the society in which it exists.

Family health: a dynamic, changing relative state of well-being that includes theological, psychological, spiritual, sociological, and cultural factors of the family system. A holistic term referring to functional and dysfunctional families. The term further encompasses the biologic and spiritual aspects of family life.

Family health care nursing: the process of providing for the health care needs of families that are within the scope of nursing practice. Family health care nursing can be aimed at the family as context, the family as a whole, the family as a system, or the family as a component of society.

Family health promotion: behaviors of the family that are undertaken to increase the family's well-being or quality of life.

Family Leave Act: on February 5, 1993, President Clinton signed the 1993 Family Leave Act, which required employers with more than 50 workers to provide up to 12 weeks of unpaid leave to employees at a child's birth or adoption or to care for members of their families who are ill.

Family life cycle theory: a descriptive developmental theory about the tasks and processes for families. Stages are based on the age of the oldest child of a nuclear family. The most common family life cycle theory by Duvall has been criticized for not being applicable to nontraditional families. Similar theories for divorced and blended families have been proposed.

Family process: the ongoing interaction between the family members through which they accomplish their instrumental and affective tasks.

Family resources: attributes and supports that are available for use by the family

Family stages: refers to Duvall's eight stages of family development, based on the oldest child, and described as the expected changes in childrearing families. These are marriage without children, childbearing, preschool children, school children, adolescents, launching of young adults (first child gone to last child leaving home), middle age of parents (empty nest to retirement), and aging of family members (retirement to death of both parents).

Family structure: the ordered set of relationships among the parts of the family and between the family and other social systems.

Family transitions: family developmental and situational events that signal a reorganization of family roles and tasks during family careers.

Family types: predictable and discernible patterns of family functioning.

Family values: a family's system of ideas, attitudes, and beliefs about the worth or priority of entities, or ideas that bind together the members of a family in a common culture.

Family: refers to two or more individuals who depend on one another for emotional, physical, or economical support. The members of the family are self-defined.

Family-centered care: an approach to child health care based on the assumption that the family is the child's primary source of strength and support.

Fetal personhood: arising out of abortion debates, fertilization debates, and fetal surgery technology, the concept of fetal personhood indicates that a fetus has legal and ethical rights outside of its mother's.

Fictive kin: a concept from anthropology along the lines of chosen family but carrying the implication that the fictive kin isn't "real."

Functional kin: when fictive kin become fully integrated as a family.

Gay: equivalent to "homosexual," gay is a preferred term for those people whose sexual object of choice is of the same sex. This may be used to refer to women or men.

Gender: the way in which different sexes behave. Femininity encompasses long hair, makeup, and soft speech; masculinity includes athletic prowess, aggressiveness, and never wearing dresses. Femininity is usually associated with females and masculinity with males. However none of these behaviors is biologically driven; there is no gene in women telling them to curl their hair. Females and males in practice combine many masculine and feminine traits in their daily lives.

Genome project: Originally begun in 1990, the U. S. Human Genome Project is coordinated by the U. S. Department of Energy and the National Institutes of Health. The project is expected to be completed by the year 2003. Project goals are to: (a) identify all of the estimated 80,000 to 100,000 genes in human DNA, (b) determine the sequences of the 3 billion chemical bases that make up human DNA, (c) store this information in databases, (d) develop tools for data analysis, and (e) address the ethical, legal, and social issues that may arise from the project. (*http://www.ornl.gov/TechResources/Human Genome/ home.html)*

GLBT: "Gay, Lesbian, Bisexual, and Transgendered"

Grounded theory: a qualitative methodology used to collect and analyze data with the goal of developing theories and theoretical propositions that are closely connected (or "grounded") in real-world observations.

Head Start: A national program that provides comprehensive developmental services for low-income, pre-school children, ages 3 to 5, as well as social services for their families. Education, social and emotional development, physical and mental health, and nutrition are all components.

Health patterns: the daily activities and behaviors families and their members perform to promote and protect optimal physical, mental, and social well-being, not merely to ensure the absence of disease and incapacitation.

Health promotion: activities that improve or maintain the well-being of people.

Heterosexism: prejudice against people who are not heterosexual or straight.

Homelessness: a state of losing one's possessions, doubling up with relatives during hard times, or simply having no home.

Homophobia: fear of homosexuals and GLBT folks.

Homosexual: this term was invented at the beginning of the twentieth century by psychoanalysts studying people who found themselves attracted to their own sex. Because of the term's use as a disease category, it is generally not used within the communities to which it refers. See Gay, Lesbian, Bisexual and Queer.

Hypothesis: a statement that postulates some sort of relationship between concepts and propositions that is crucial to a theory. It is a way of stating an expected relationship between concepts. For example, children who are raised in healthy families are more likely to be healthy themselves.

Ideological code: words and beliefs that seek to guide how members of society perceive the world.

Illness patterns: the processes and phases of illness that families go through to manage a disease and the medical treatments that become a part of their daily lives. Families usually respond differently to acute, chronic, and life-threatening phases of illness.

Implementation: the fourth step of the nursing process; it involves carrying out or putting into effect the care plan developed during the planning phase.

Incendiary communication: communication characterized by bringing up old unresolved issues, failing to calmly talk things through to reach a solution, yelling and screaming at other family members, and walking away from conflicts without much resolution.

Individual development: the expected changes in each family member associated with growth and development.

Individuation: the time provided for each family member to be alone to develop a sense of self and spirituality.

Instrumental behaviors: actions designed to complete a task.

Integrated model: the result of combined concepts from several theories to formulate or provide direction for interventions when working with families. For example, the family assessment intervention model, the structural/functional model, and the Calgary family model are examples of integrated approaches. See Chapters 2 and 8 in this textbook.

Interracial: families or people of more than one race.

In vitro fertilization (IVF): embryos are generated outside of the body and transferred (at least two) after successful fertilization with sperm.

Labeling: labeling theory suggests that we give people labels (loser, woman, black, Latino, cop, addict) to categorize them and so know how to interact with them. If someone is simply a woman, she loses the complexity of her humanity.

Lesbian: Equivalent to "homosexual," lesbian is a preferred term for women whose sexual objects of choice are other women.

Life-threatening illness pattern: the family's responses to caring and preparing for the death of a member at the end of life, as well as the grieving, mourning, and healing after the death.

Living will: a legal document stating what medical treatment a patient chooses to omit or refuse in the event that he or she is terminally ill and is unable to make those decisions for himself or herself.

Macrolevel: a level of analysis that focuses on the larger forms of social behavior; for example, social systems, social institutions, or the relationship between social institutions.

Meals on Wheels: community program that delivers food to homebound people.

Measurement: the assignment of numbers to individuals, objects, events, or situations according to specified rules; the process of using an instrument to measure a particular attribute, assigning numbers to the attributes, and using the data for statistical analysis. Measurement can be a part of the assessment process.

Medicaid: a jointly funded, federal and state health insurance program for certain low-income and needy people.

Medicare: the nation's largest health insurance program, covering 37 million people who are age 65 and over and those who have permanent kidney failure and people with certain disabilities.

Methods: the steps, procedures, and strategies for gathering and analyzing data in a study.

Microlevel: a level of analysis that focuses on the smaller forms of social behavior; for example, everyday interaction within the family.

Nonnormative event: describes stressful events that occur unexpectedly, leaving little or no time to prepare for them.

Norm: culturally expected behavior, appearance, or structure.

Normative event: term usually used to describe events that may be perceived as stressful but can be anticipated and planned for to reduce the effects of the stress. For example, the birth of a baby can be a stressful event for families, but they have several months to prepare for the new member's arrival.

Normative events: those forces that structure members of society to fit norms.

Nuclear family: a stereotypical structure of one mother, one father, and two children.

Nurse-client contract: an agreement between the health professional and client (family) to work together to attain goals that are determined by the client.

Nursing diagnosis: a clinical judgment about individual family or a community response to actual and potential health problems or life processes. Nursing diagnoses provide the basis for selection of nursing interventions to achieve outcomes for which the nurse is accountable.

Nursing process: an orderly, systematic manner of determining the client's problems, making plans to solve them, initiating the plan or assigning others to implement it, and evaluating the extent to which the plan was effective in resolving the problems identified.

Parish nurse: a nurse who works with a faith community and combines the activities of spiritual counseling with health promotion, disease prevention, and health maintenance for parishioners and families.

Partner: an alternative to the terms girlfriend, boyfriend, or spouse. Often used within GLBT communities.

Pedophilia: adult sex with children.

Permeability of family boundaries: the status of a family boundary that selectively allows access or admittance to some influences but not others. Family boundaries are permeable to the extent that some influences are allowed admittance while others are excluded. Totally closed boundaries do not allow outside forces to influence the family system, but totally open boundaries allow all influences to affect the family. Boundaries of the family are healthy to the extent that their permeability allows needed influences to be admitted while destructive influences are prohibited or screened out.

Phenomenology: the holistic study of human experience that emphasizes its complexity and stresses the need to study experience as it is lived.

Planning: the third step of the nursing diagnosis. It involves the selection or design of nursing interventions in consultation and collaboration with the client, which facilitates the achievement of the desired objectives. It is the process by which objectives are determined, interventions chosen, and the care plan is written.

Population: the entire set of individuals, objects, events, or situations that meet sample criteria for inclusion in a study.

Postpartum period: defined medically as the 6 weeks during which the mother's body returns to the prepregnant physiological state. Psychological changes may take longer.

Power: the net ability or capability of actors (A) to produce or cause (intended) outcomes or effects, particularly on the behavior of others (O) or others' outcomes.

Prevention: (1) primary: focuses on preventing the occurrence of health problems; (2) secondary: designed to identify and treat health problems early; (3) tertiary: aimed at correcting health problems and preventing further deterioration.

Propositions: statements about the relationship between two or more concepts. An example is that the family unit interacts with the health of the individual members of the family.

PSDA: the Patient Self-Determination Act that was passed by the U.S. Congress in 1991. The PSDA is a federal law that requires hospitals and nursing homes to provide patients with information about their rights as a patient. Patients must be informed of their rights under state law to make their own medical care decisions.

Public health nursing: the practice of promoting and protecting the health of populations using knowledge from the nursing, social, and public health sciences.

Qualitative data: derived from family assessment and describes family's characteristics or qualities. The characteristics or attributes of a family are usually derived from open-ended questions and summarized in narrative form.

Qualitative research: the systematic collection, organization, and interpretation of nonnumerical data.

Quantitative data: derived from family assessment and measures, counts, or compares properties or aspects of the family. This information is usually derived from closed-ended questions that assign a value to the answers that are then submitted for analysis through descriptive or inferential statistics.

Quantitative research: the systematic collection, organization, manipulation, and interpretation of numerical data.

Queer: at one time a slur against GLBT people, queer has been reclaimed as a term to describe sexual orientation, to reflect the continuum of sexual practices and tastes.

Race: apparently straightforward, the concept of race has a complicated history. When examining census records over this century, the categories have expanded from Irish, Italian, Northern European, Negro, and octoroon to white, nonwhite Hispanic, Asian, Pacific Islander, Native American (sometimes by tribe), African American, Caribbean American, and so on. All of these people have been in this country throughout the century but their racial category recognition has changed. Sociologists now define race as a group of people with shared physical characteristics.

Religion: an organized system of beliefs, practices, and forms of worship.

Religiosity: a continuum with intrinsic religious motivation on one end and extrinsic religious motivation on the other end.

Religiousness: adherence to the beliefs and practices of an organized church or religious institution.

Research design: the overall plan for collecting and analyzing data.

Risk: the probability that individuals in the community will be affected by a health problem.

Role delineation: the identification of the behavioral expectations associated with a role.

Role enactment: behavior demonstrated by a person in the performance of a role.

Role strain: difficulty in the delineation and enactment of a role.

Role: The behavioral expectations attached to a position.

Role-performance family health model: This view of family health is based on the view that family health is the ability of family members to perform their routine roles and achieve developmental tasks.

Sample: subset of a population selected to participate in a research study.

Sampling plan: process of selecting a portion of the population to represent the entire population.

Secondary data: collected for one study and later reanalyzed for another study, usually to test new research hypotheses.

Selective reduction: the procedure of removing (aborting) unwanted fetuses in multiple pregnancies.

Self-care contract: contract developed independent of a health professional. The contract is between two individuals for the purpose of improving a health behavior.

Sex: the reproductive structure of human bodies. Although generally thought to include only males (penis, testes, scrotum, chest hair) and females (vagina, ovaries, uterus, breasts), one in every 2,000 live births is "intersexed." These infants are born with a mixture of female and male traits. Most are then surgically "assigned" to one sex. This term describes only biology, not behavior.

Sexism: prejudice against a person because of their sex. Generally applied to expectation that women are not as qualified or competent as men.

Sexual orientation: the object (person) towards which sexual desire is directed, the object one wants to explore sexually.

Sexuality: sexual acts that give an individual pleasure.

Situational or nonnormative transitions: unpredictable events such as changes in personal relationships, roles, and status; the environment, physical and mental capabilities, and possessions. These may occur at any time or during any family developmental stage.

Social class: a large group of people with relatively similar incomes, amount of wealth, life conditions, life chances, and lifestyles. Synonymous terms are "socioeconomic status" and "social status."

Social support: the amount of help actually received, satisfaction with that help, and the person's network providing that help. Help received may be in the form of instrumental or physical aid, information, emotional support, or the appraisal of one's role performance.

Solidarity: strong shared group identity that leads to promotion of that group and its causes. Class solidarity would include working for unions to secure or better the life of those within the working class.

Spiritual well-being: a sense of inner peace, compassion for others, reverence for life, gratitude, and appreciation of both unity and diversity; it includes the conviction that there is a purpose and meaning in life, a relationship with God, and realistic views of adversity and loss.

Spirituality: generally encompasses a sense of relation or connectedness within oneself, others, nature, and God, or a higher power, that draws one beyond oneself.

Stereotype: exaggerated, often extreme, expectations of certain people, which keep people from recognizing difference and humanity. For example, the stereotypical nurse is a white woman, when in truth many men of color work in the field: denying them recognition makes their successful functioning difficult.

Stigma: derived from the Christian tradition, stigmata refers to the blood on the palms and feet of Christ when nailed to the cross. A stigma is a social marker that labels people negatively as a deviant. Stigma may be about race, physical disability, sex, sexual orientation, clothing, tattoos, and religion.

Straight: a colloquial term for heterosexual people.

Stressor: a demand placed on the family that produces, or has the potential of producing, changes in the family system.

Theory: a set of statements that tentatively describe, explain, or predict relationships between concepts. They are selected and organized as abstract representations of phenomenon. Examples of theories are family systems theory and family development theory.

Transgender: different than transsexual, transgendered people feel more comfortable displaying or living in the gender that is different than their sex. For example, a woman who binds her breasts and wears men's suits or a man who wears makeup and dresses. Transgendered people are not necessarily gay: a transgendered man may still desire women. However, as a result of social and historical forces, they are included with others who have suffered opp424ression for expressing themselves "differently," such as gays, lesbians, and bisexuals.

Transsexuals: people who have undergone some form of physical change (hormones, surgery, or both) to achieve a body to suit the gender they prefer. For example, a transsexual biological female who feels more "real" as a man will take on masculine attributes as well as male hormones, a radical mastectomy, and construction of male genitalia. There is as continuum of options.

Unacculturated families: families that have not integrated dominant American core values and practices into their lives.

Underclass: the poorest families, those who live in persistent poverty.

Vertical diffusion: A dynamic that occurs when one family member initiates a health behavior change and thereby influences another family member to make a similar change.

Welfare reform: Personal Responsibility and Work Opportunity Reconciliation Act (1996); an effort to "reform" welfare and its purported abuses.

Xenophobia: fear of outsiders (from country, community, town, social group).

Appendix C

FAMILY SYSTEMS STRESSOR-STRENGTH INVENTORY (FS^3I)

Shirley May Harmon Hanson • Karen B. Mischke

INSTRUCTIONS FOR ADMINISTRATION

The Family Systems Stressor-Strength Inventory (FS^3I) is an assessment and measurement instrument intended for use with families (see Chapter 8). It focuses on identifying stressful situations occurring in families and the strengths families use to maintain healthy family functioning. Each family member is asked to complete the instrument on an individual form before an interview with the clinician. Questions can be read to members unable to read.

After completion of the instrument, the clinician evaluates the family on each of the stressful situations (general and specific) and the strengths they possess. This evaluation is recorded on the family member form.

The clinician records the individual family member's score and the clinician perception score on the Quantitative Summary. A different color code is used for each family member. The clinician also completes the Qualitative Summary, synthesizing the information gleaned from all participants. Clinicians can use the Family Care Plan to prioritize diagnoses, set goals, develop prevention and intervention activities, and evaluate outcomes.

Family Name ______________________________ Date __________
Family Member(s) Completing Assessment ______________________________
Ethnic Background(s) ______________________________
Religious Background(s) ______________________________
Referral Source ______________________________
Interviewer ______________________________

	Family Members	Relationship in Family	Age	Marital Status	Education (highest degree)	Occupation
1.						
2.						
3.						
4.						
5.						
6.						

Family's current reasons for seeking assistance:

____

____

____

Source: Mischke-Berkey, K. & Hanson, S. M. H. (1991). *Pocket Guide to Family Assessment and Intervention.* St. Louis: Mosby; Hanson, S. M. H. (1996). *Familiy Nursing Assessment and Intervention.* In *Family Health Care Nursing: Theory, Practice and Research.* Ed. 1. S. M. H. Hanson & S. T. Boyds (eds). Philadelphia: F. A. Davis.

PART I: FAMILY SYSTEMS STRESSORS (GENERAL)

DIRECTIONS: Each of the 25 situations/stressors listed here deals with some aspect of normal family life. They have the potential for creating stress within families or between families and the world in which they live. We are interested in your overall impression of how these situations affect your family life. Please circle a number (0 through 5) that best describes the amount of stress or tension they create for you.

	Family Perception Score						Clinician Perception
Stressors:	**Not Apply**	**Little Stress**		**Medium Stress**		**High Stress**	**Score**
1. Family member(s) feel unappreciated	0	1	2	3	4	5	________
2. Guilt for not accomplishing more	0	1	2	3	4	5	________
3. Insufficient "me" time	0	1	2	3	4	5	________
4. Self-image/self-esteem/ feelings of unattractiveness	0	1	2	3	4	5	________
5. Perfectionism	0	1	2	3	4	5	________
6. Dieting	0	1	2	3	4	5	________
7. Health/Illness	0	1	2	3	4	5	________
8. Communication with children	0	1	2	3	4	5	________
9. Housekeeping standards	0	1	2	3	4	5	________
10. Insufficient couple time	0	1	2	3	4	5	________
11. Insufficient family playtime	0	1	2	3	4	5	________
12. Children's behavior/ discipline/sibling fighting	0	1	2	3	4	5	________
13. Television	0	1	2	3	4	5	________
14. Overscheduled family calendar	0	1	2	3	4	5	________
15. Lack of shared responsibility in the family	0	1	2	3	4	5	________
16. Moving	0	1	2	3	4	5	________
17. Spousal relationship (communication, friendship, sex)	0	1	2	3	4	5	________
18. Holidays	0	1	2	3	4	5	________
19. In-laws	0	1	2	3	4	5	________
20. Teen behaviors (communication, music, friends, school)	0	1	2	3	4	5	________
21. New baby	0	1	2	3	4	5	________
22. Economics/finances/ budgets	0	1	2	3	4	5	________
23. Unhappiness with work situation	0	1	2	3	4	5	________
24. Overvolunteerism	0	1	2	3	4	5	________
25. Neighbors	0	1	2	3	4	5	________

Additional Stressors: ______________________________

Family Remarks: ______________________________

Clinician: Clarification of stressful situations/concerns with family members.

Prioritize in order of importance to family members: ______________________________

PART II: FAMILY SYSTEMS STRESSORS (SPECIFIC)

DIRECTIONS: The following 12 questions are designed to provide information about your specific stress-producing situation/problem, or area of concern influencing your family's health. Please circle a number (1 through 5) that best describes the influence this situation has on your family's life and how well you perceive your family's overall functioning.

The specific stress-producing situation/problem or area of concern at this time is: ______________________________

	Family Perception Score					Clinician Perception
Stressors:	**Little**		**Medium**		**High**	**Score**
1. To what extent is your family bothered by this problem or stressful situation? (e.g., effects on family interactions, communication among members, emotional and social relationships)	1	2	3	4	5	______
Family Remarks: ______________________________						
Clinician Remarks: ______________________________						
2. How much of an effect does this stressful situation have on your family's usual patterning of living? (e.g., effects on lifestyle patterns and family developmental task)	1	2	3	4	5	______
Family Remarks: ______________________________						
Clinician Remarks: ______________________________						
3. How much has this situation affected your family's ability to work together as a family unit? (e.g., alteration in family roles, completion of family tasks, following through with responsibilities)	1	2	3	4	5	______
Family Remarks: ______________________________						
Clinician Remarks: ______________________________						

Has your family ever experienced a similar concern in the past?

1. YES — If YES, complete question 4
2. NO — If NO, complete question 5

Stressors:	Little		Medium		High	Clinician Perception Score
	Family Perception Score					
4. How successful was your family in dealing with this situation/problem/concern in the past? (e.g., workable coping strategies developed, adaptive measures useful, situation improved) Family Remarks: ______ Clinician Remarks: ______	1	2	3	4	5	______
5. How strongly do you feel this current situation/problem/concern will affect your family's future? (e.g., anticipated consequences) Family Remarks: ______ Clinician Remarks: ______	1	2	3	4	5	______
6. To what extent are family members able to help themselves in this present situation/problem/concern? (e.g., self-assistive efforts, family expectations, spiritual influence, & family resources) Family Remarks: ______ Clinician Remarks: ______	1	2	3	4	5	______
7. To what extent do you expect others to help your family with this situation/problem/concern? (e.g., what roles would helpers play; how available are extra-family resources) Family Remarks: ______ Clinician Remarks: ______	1	2	3	4	5	______

Stressors:	Poor		Satisfactory		Excellent	Score
8. How would you rate the way your family functions overall? (e.g., how your family members relate to each other and to larger family and community) Family Remarks: ______ Clinician Remarks: ______	1	2	3	4	5	______

	Family Perception Score					Clinician Perception
Stressors:	**Poor**		**Satisfactory**		**Excellent**	**Score**
9. How would you rate the overall physical health status of each family member by name? (Include yourself as a family member; record additional names on back.)						
a. ________	1	2	3	4	5	______
b. ________	1	2	3	4	5	______
c. ________	1	2	3	4	5	______
d. ________	1	2	3	4	5	______
e. ________	1	2	3	4	5	______
10. How would you rate the overall physical health status of your family as a whole?	1	2	3	4	5	______
Family Remarks: ________						
Clinician Remarks: ________						
11. How would you rate the overall mental health status of each family member by name? (Include yourself as a family member; record additional names on back.)						
a. ________	1	2	3	4	5	______
b. ________	1	2	3	4	5	______
c. ________	1	2	3	4	5	______
d. ________	1	2	3	4	5	______
e. ________	1	2	3	4	5	______
12. How would you rate the overall mental health status of your family as a whole?	1	2	3	4	5	______
Family Remarks: ________						
Clinician Remarks: ________						

PART III: FAMILY SYSTEMS STRENGTHS

DIRECTIONS: Each of the 16 traits/attributes listed below deals with some aspect of family life and its overall functioning. Each one contributes to the health and well-being of family members as individuals and to the family as a whole. Please circle a number (0 through 5) that best describes the extent that the trait applies to your family.

		Family Perception Score					Clinician Perception
My Family:	**Not Apply**	**Seldom**		**Usually**		**Always**	**Score**
1. Communicates and listens to one another	0	1	2	3	4	5	______
Family Remarks: ______							
Clinician Remarks: ______							
2. Affirms and supports one another	0	1	2	3	4	5	______
Family Remarks: ______							
Clinician Remarks: ______							
3. Teaches respect for others	0	1	2	3	4	5	______
Family Remarks: ______							
Clinician Remarks: ______							
4. Develops a sense of trust in members	0	1	2	3	4	5	______
Family Remarks: ______							
Clinician Remarks: ______							
5. Displays a sense of play and humor	0	1	2	3	4	5	______
Family Remarks: ______							
Clinician Remarks: ______							
6. Exhibits a sense of shared responsibility	0	1	2	3	4	5	______
Family Remarks: ______							
Clinician Remarks: ______							
7. Teaches a sense of right and wrong	0	1	2	3	4	5	______
Family Remarks: ______							
Clinician Remarks: ______							
8. Has a strong sense of family in which rituals and traditions abound	0	1	2	3	4	5	______
Family Remarks: ______							
Clinician Remarks: ______							

		Family Perception Score					Clinician Perception
My Family:	**Not Apply**	**Seldom**		**Usually**		**Always**	**Score**
9. Has a balance of interaction among members	0	1	2	3	4	5	______
Family Remarks: ______							
Clinician Remarks: ______							
10. Has a shared religious core	0	1	2	3	4	5	______
Family Remarks: ______							
Clinician Remarks: ______							
11. Respects the privacy of one another	0	1	2	3	4	5	______
Family Remarks: ______							
Clinician Remarks: ______							
12. Values service to others	0	1	2	3	4	5	______
Family Remarks: ______							
Clinician Remarks: ______							
13. Fosters family table time and conversation	0	1	2	3	4	5	______
Family Remarks: ______							
Clinician Remarks: ______							
14. Shares leisure time	0	1	2	3	4	5	______
Family Remarks: ______							
Clinician Remarks: ______							
15. Admits to and seeks help with problems	0	1	2	3	4	5	______
Family Remarks: ______							
Clinician Remarks: ______							
16a. How would you rate the overall strengths that exist in your family?	0	1	2	3	4	5	______
Family Remarks: ______							
Clinician Remarks: ______							

16b. Additional Family Strengths: ______

16c. Clinician: Clarification of family strengths with individual members: ______

FAMILY SYSTEMS STRESSOR-STRENGTH INVENTORY (FS^3I)
SCORING SUMMARY
SECTION 1: FAMILY PERCEPTION SCORE

INSTRUCTIONS FOR ADMINISTRATION

The Family Systems Stressor-Strength Inventory (FS^3I) Scoring Summary is divided into two sections: Section 1, Family Perception Scores and Section 2, Clinician Perception Scores. These two sections are further divided into three parts: Part I, Family Systems Stressors: General; Part II, Family Systems Stressors: Specific; and, Part III, Family Systems Strengths. Each part contains a Quantitative Summary and a Qualitative Summary.

Quantifiable family and clinician perception scores are both graphed on the Quantitative Summary. Each family member has a designated color code. Family and clinician remarks are both recorded on the Qualitative Summary. Quantitative summary scores, when graphed, suggest a level for initiation of prevention/intervention modes: Primary, Secondary, and Tertiary. Qualitative summary information, when synthesized, contributes to the development and channeling of the Family Care Plan.

Part I Family Systems Stressors (General)

Add scores from questions 1 to 25 and calculate an overall numerical score for Family System Stressors (General). Ratings are from 1 (most positive) to 5 (most negative). The Not Apply (0) responses are omitted from the calculations. Total scores range from 25 to 125.

Family Systems Stressor Score: General

$\frac{(\quad)}{25} \times 1 =$

Graph score on Quantitative Summary, Family Systems Stressors: General, Family Member Perception. Color code to differentiate family members

Record additional stressors and family remarks in Part I, Qualitative Summary: Family and Clinician Remarks.

Part II Family Systems Stressors: Specific

Add scores from questions 1–8, 10, and 12 and calculate a numerical score for Family Systems through Stressors: Specific. Ratings are from 1 (most positive) to 5 (most negative). Questions 4, 6, 7, 8, 10, and 12 are reverse scored.* Total scores range from 10–50.

Family Systems Stressor Score: Specific

$\frac{(\quad)}{10} \times 1 =$

Graph score on Quantitative Summary: Family Systems Stressor: Specific (Family Member Perceptions). Color code to differentiate family members.

Summarize data from questions 9 and 11 (reverse scored) and record family remarks in Part II, Qualitative Summary: Family and Clinician Remarks

Part III Family Systems Strengths

Add scores from questions 1 to 16 and calculate a numerical score for Family Systems Strengths. Ratings are from 1 (seldom) to 5 (always). The Not Apply (0) responses are omitted from the calculations. Total scores range from 16 to 80.

$\frac{(\quad)}{16} \times 1 =$

Graph score on Quantitative Summary: Family Systems Strengths (Family Member Perception).

Record Additional Family Strengths and Family Remarks in Part III, Qualitative Summary: Family and Clinician Remarks.

Source: Mischke-Berkey, K. & Hanson, S. M. H. (1991). Pocket guide to family assessment and intervention. St. Louis: Mosby.

*Reverse Scoring:
Question answered as (1) is scored 5 points
Question answered as (2) is scored 4 points
Question answered as (3) is scored 3 points
Question answered as (4) is scored 2 points
Question answered as (5) is scored 1 point

SECTION 2: CLINICIAN PERCEPTION SCORES

Part I Family Systems Stressors (General)*

Add scores from questions 1 to 25 and calculate an overall numerical score for Family System Stressors (General). Ratings are from 1 (most positive) to 5 (most negative). The Not Apply (0) responses are omitted from the calculations. Total scores range from 25 to 125.

Family Systems Stressor Score: General

$\frac{(\ \ )}{25} \times 1 =$

Graph score on Quantitative Summary, Family Systems Stressors: General (Clinician Perception).

Record Clinicians' clarification of general stressors in Part I, Qualitative Summary: Family and Clinician Remarks

Part II Family Systems Stressors: Specific

Add scores from questions 1–8, 10, & 12 and calculate a numerical score for Family Systems Stressors: Specific. Ratings are from 1 (most positive) to 5 (most negative). Questions 4, 6, 7, 8, 10, & 12 are reverse scored.* Total scores range from 10–50.

Family Systems Stressor Score: Specific

$\frac{(\ \ )}{10} \times 1 =$

Graph score on Quantitative Summary: Family Systems Stressor: Specific (Clinician Perception).

Summarize data from questions 9 & 11 (reverse order) and record Clinician Remarks in Part II, Qualitative Summary: Family and Clinician Remarks.

Part III Family Systems Strengths

Add scores from questions 1 to 16 and calculate a numerical score for Family Systems Strengths. Ratings are from 1 (seldom) to 5 (always).

The Not Apply (0) responses are omitted form the calculations. Total scores range from 16 to 80.

$\frac{(\ \ )}{16} \times 1 =$

Graph score on Quantitative Summary: Family Systems Strengths (Clinician Perception).

Record Clinicians' clarification of family strengths in Part III, Qualitative Summary: Family and Clinician Remarks.

---

*Reverse Scoring:
Question answered as (1) is scored 5 points
Question answered as (2) is scored 4 points
Question answered as (3) is scored 3 points
Question answered as (4) is scored 2 points
Question answered as (5) is scored 1 points

QUANTITATIVE SUMMARY FAMILY SYSTEMS STRESSORS: GENERAL AND SPECIFIC FAMILY AND CLINICIAN PERCEPTION SCORES

DIRECTIONS: Graph the scores from each family member inventory by placing an "X" at the appropriate location. (Use first name initial for each different entry and different color code for each family member.)

	Family Systems Stressors: General			Family Systems Stressors: Specific	
Scores for Wellness and Stability	**Family Member Perception Score**	**Clinician Perception Score**	**Scores for Wellness and Stability**	**Family Member Perception Score**	**Clinician Perception Score**
5.0			5.0		
4.8			4.8		
4.6			4.6		
4.4			4.4		
4.2			4.2		
4.0			4.0		
3.8			3.8		
3.6			3.6		
3.4			3.4		
3.2			3.2		
3.0			3.0		
2.8			2.8		
2.6			2.6		
2.4			2.4		
2.2			2.2		
2.0			2.0		
1.8			1.8		
1.6			1.6		
1.4			1.4		
1.2			1.2		
1.0			1.0		

*PRIMARY Prevention/Intervention Mode: Flexible Line	1.0–2.3
*SECONDARY Prevention/Intervention Mode: Normal Line	2.4–3.6
*TERTIARY Prevention/Intervention Mode: Resistance Lines	3.7–5.0

*Breakdowns of numerical scores for stressor penetration are suggested values

FAMILY SYSTEMS STRENGTHS
FAMILY AND CLINICIAN PERCEPTION SCORES

DIRECTIONS: Graph the scores from the inventory by placing an "X" at the appropriate location and connect with a line. (Use first name initial for each different entry and different color code for each family member.)

Sum of strengths available for prevention/ intervention mode	Family Systems Strengths	
	Family Member Perception Score	Clinician Perception Score
5.0		
4.8		
4.6		
4.4		
4.2		
4.0		
3.8		
3.6		
3.4		
3.2		
3.0		
2.8		
2.6		
2.4		
2.2		
2.0		
1.8		
1.6		
1.4		
1.2		
1.0		

*PRIMARY Prevention/Intervention Mode: Flexible Line	1.0–2.3
*SECONDARY Prevention/Intervention Mode: Normal Line	2.4–3.6
*TERTIARY Prevention/Intervention Mode: Resistance Lines	3.7–5.0

*Breakdowns of numerical scores for stressor penetration are suggested values

QUALITATIVE SUMMARY
FAMILY AND CLINICIAN REMARKS

PART I: FAMILY SYSTEMS STRESSORS: GENERAL

Summarize general stressors and remarks of family and clinician. Prioritize stressors according to importance to family members.

____
____
____

PART II: FAMILY SYSTEMS STRESSORS: SPECIFIC

A. Summarize specific stressor and remarks of family and clinician.

____
____
____

B. Summarize differences (if discrepancies exist) between how family members and clinician view effects of stressful situation on family.

____
____
____

C. Summarize overall family functioning.

____
____
____

D. Summarize overall significant physical health status for family members.

____
____
____

E. Summarize overall significant mental health status for family members.

____
____
____

PART III: FAMILY SYSTEMS STRENGTHS

Summarize family systems strengths and family and clinician remarks that facilitate family health and stability.

____
____
____

FAMILY CARE PLAN*

Diagnosis General & Specific Family System Stressors	Family Systems Strengths Supporting Family Care Plan	Goals Family & Physician	Prevention/Intervention Mode		Outcomes Evaluation and Replanning
			Primary, Secondary, or Tertiary	Prevention/Intervention Activities	

*Prioritize the three most significant diagnoses.

Appendix D

THE FRIEDMAN FAMILY ASSESSMENT MODEL (SHORT FORM)

There are two forms of the Friedman Family Assessment Model: short and long. Only the short form is presented here.

Before using the following guidelines in completing family assessments, two words of caution: First, not all areas included below will be germane for each of the families visited. The guidelines are comprehensive and allow depth when probing is necessary. The student should not feel that every subarea needs be covered when the broad area of inquiry poses no problems to the family or concern to the health worker. Second, by virtue of the interdependence of the family system, one will find unavoidable redundancy. For the sake of efficiency, the assessor should try not to repeat data, but refer the reader back to sections where this information has already been described.

IDENTIFYING DATA

1. **Family Name**
2. **Address and Phone**
3. **Family Composition**
   See Form D–1.
4. **Type of Family Form**
5. **Cultural (Ethnic) Background**
6. **Religious Identification**
7. **Social Class Status**
8. **Family's Recreational or Leisure-time Activities**

DEVELOPMENTAL STAGE AND HISTORY OF FAMILY

9. **Family's Present Developmental Stage**
10. **Extent of Family Developmental Tasks Fulfillment**
11. **Nuclear Family History**
12. **History of Family of Origin of Both Parents**

ENVIRONMENTAL DATA

13. **Characteristics of Home**
14. **Characteristics of Neighborhood and Larger Community**
15. **Family's Geographical Mobility**
16. **Family's Associations and Transactions With Community**
17. **Family's Social Support System or Network**

FAMILY STRUCTURE

18. **Communication Patterns**
    Extent of Functional and Dysfunctional Communication (types of recurring patterns)
    Extent of Emotional (Affective) Messages and How Expressed
    Characteristics of Communication Within Family Subsystems
    Extent of Congruent and Incongruent Messages
    Types of Dysfunctional Communication Processes Seen in Family
    Areas of Open and Closed Communication
    Familial and Contextual Variables Affecting Communication

Source: Friedman, M.M., (1998). *Family Nursing: Research, Theory and Practice,* 4th Edition, pp. 579–581. Stamford, Conn: Appleton & Lange.

19. **Power Structure**
    Power Outcomes
    Decision-making Process
    Power Bases
    Variables Affecting Family Power
    Overall Family System and Subsystem Power
    (Family Power Continuum Placement)
20. **Role Structure**
    Formal Role Structure
    Informal Role Structure
    Analysis of Role Models (optional)
    Variables Affecting Role Structures
21. **Family Values**
    Compare the family to American or family's reference group values and/or identify important family values and their importance (priority) in family.
    Congruence Between the Family's Values and the Family's Reference Group or Wider Community
    Congruence Between the Family's Values and Family Member's Values
    Variables Influencing Family Values
    Values Consciously or Unconsciously Held
    Presence of Value Conflicts in Family
    Effect of the Above Values and Value Conflicts on Health Status of Family

FAMILY FUNCTIONS

22. **Affective Function**
    Family's Need-Response Patterns
    Mutual Nurturance, Closeness, and Identification
    Separateness and Connectedness
23. **Socialization Function**
    Family Child-rearing Practices
    Adaptability of Child-rearing Practices for Family Form and Family's Situation
    Who Is (Are) Socializing Agent(s) for Child(ren)?
    Value of Children in Family
    Cultural Beliefs That Influence Family's Child-rearing Patterns
    Social Class Influence on Child-Rearing Patterns
    Estimation About Whether Family Is at Risk for Child-rearing Problems and If So, Indication of High Risk Factors
    Adequacy of Home Environment for Children's Needs to Play
24. **Health Care Function**
    Family's Health Beliefs, Values, and Behavior
    Family's Definitions of Health: Illness and Their Level of Knowledge
    Family's Perceived Health Status and Illness Susceptibility
    Family's Dietary Practices
    Adequacy of family diet (recommended 3-day food history record).
    Function of mealtimes and attitudes toward food and mealtimes.
    Shopping (and its planning) practices.
    Person(s) responsible for planning, shopping, and preparation of meals.
    Sleep and Rest Habits
    Physical Activity and Recreation Practices (not covered earlier)
    Family's Drug Habits
    Family's Role in Self-care Practices
    Medically Based Prevention Measures (physicals, eye and hearing tests, and immunizations)
    Dental Health Practices
    Family Health History (both general and specific diseases—environmentally and genetically related)
    Health Care Services Received
    Feelings and Perceptions Regarding Health Services
    Emergency Health Services
    Source of Payments for Health and Other Services
    Logistics of Receiving Care

FAMILY STRESS AND COPING

25. **Short- and Long-term Familial Stressors and Strengths**
26. **Extent of Family's Ability to Respond, Based on Objective Appraisal of Stress-producing Situations**
27. **Coping Strategies Used** (present/past)
    Differences in family members' ways of coping
    Family's inner coping strategies
    Family's external coping strategies
28. **Dysfunctional Adaptive Strategies Used** (present/past; extent of usage)

FORM D–1
Family Composition Form

Name (Last, First)	Gender	Relationship	Date/Place Of Birth	Occupation	Education
1. (Father)					
2. (Mother)					
3. (Oldest child)					
4.					
5.					
6.					
7.					
8.					

Appendix E

STUDY QUESTIONS AND ANSWERS

CHAPTER 1

1. Define family.

As a starting point students are asked to think about whom they consider their own family to be. Nurses working with families should ask people whom they consider to be their family and include those members in health care planning. In this chapter, Hanson defined family as "two or more individuals who depend on one another for emotional, physical, and economical support. The members of the family are self-defined."

2. Define family health.

There are many ways to define what is meant by family health. Hanson defined family health as "a dynamic, changing relative state of well-being, which includes the biological, psychological, spiritual, sociological, and cultural factors of the family system."

3. List five traits that are common in healthy families.

Any of the following answers: communicates and listens to one another, affirms and supports one another, teaches respect for others, develops a sense of trust in members, displays a sense of play and humor, exhibits a sense of shared responsibility, teaches a sense of right and wrong, has a strong sense of family in which rituals and traditions abound, has a balance of interaction among members, has a shared religious core, respects the privacy of one another, values service to others, fosters family table time and conversation, shares leisure time, admits to and seeks help with problem.

4. Define family health care nursing.

Definitions may be tailored by the individual nurse to fit their practice. Hanson defined family health care nursing as "the process of providing for the health care needs of families that are within the scope of nursing practice. Family health care nursing can be aimed at the family as context, the family as a whole, the family as a system, or the family as a component of society."

5. Which of the following statements are true about family nursing practice?

a. Family care is concerned with the experience of the family over time.
b. Family nursing is directed at families whose members are both healthy and ill.
c. The family nurse is responsible along with the family itself for defining who is the family.
d. If family nursing practice is successful, the family members will simultaneously achieve maximum health.

Answer: All the above statements (a, b, c, d) are true about family nursing practice.

6. Describe the difference between family as a client and family as a system.

The family as a client centers on the assessment of all individual family members where the family is in the foreground and individuals are in the background. The family is the sum of individual family members with a focus on each and every individual such as one may see in a family medical practice office. The family as system views the family as an interactional system whereby the interactions between family members become the target for nursing interventions. The nurse focuses on the individual and family simultaneously.

7. Name and describe three of the many roles that nurses can assume with families.

Any of the following three roles are identified and discussed.

Health teacher. The family nurse teaches about family wellness, family illness.

Coordinator/collaborator/liaison. The family nurse coordinates the care that families may receive, collaborating with the family in the planning of this care.

Deliverer/supervisor of technical care. The family nurse delivers or supervises the actual physical/mental care that families receive in various settings.

Family advocate. The family nurse advocates for families by speaking out for them or by empowering families to speak for themselves.

Consultant. The family nurse consults and advises families or agencies to facilitate family-centered care.

Counselor. The family nurse plays a mental health therapeutic role by helping families solve problems or change behavior in coping with health and illness issues.

Case finder/epidemiologist. The family nurse is involved in case finding or is a tracker of disease/problems.

Environmental modifier. The family nurse consults with families or other professionals to modify the larger or small environment that impacts family health.

Clarifier-interpreter. The family nurse clarifies and interprets data to family members pertaining to diagnosis, treatment, and prognosis of health and illness conditions.

Surrogate. The family nurse may substitute for another person in the family system.

Researcher. The family nurse identifies practice problems and through the process of scientific investigation, finds solutions.

Role model. The family nurse serves as a role model to other people through her activities.

Case manager. The family nurse provides coordination and collaboration between a group of families and the health care system.

8. The primary mode of supervising students studying family nursing is through:

a. Audio tapes of interactions between students and families
b. Video tapes of interactions between students and families
c. Process recordings developed by the student
d. Direct supervision of student and family interactions

Answer: All of the answers are true: a, b, c, d

9. Which of the following nursing specialties have historically focused on the quality of family health?

a. Maternity nursing
b. Pediatric nursing
c. Public health nursing
d. All of the above

Answer: The correct response is: d

10. Family health care nursing is a specialty that started near the end of the twentieth century.

Answer: False. Family nursing has roots in society from prehistoric times. Most notable of the earlier writings came from Florence Nightingale.

11. Discuss three traditional functions performed by families over history that still exist today. What are two functions that have become more meaningful in modern times?

Families existed to achieve economic survival.
Families existed to reproduce the species.
Families existed to provide protection from hostile forces.
Families passed along the religious faith (culture).
Families educated their children (socialization).
Families conferred social status on their children.
In modern times, the relationship and health function of families have received more attention.

CHAPTER 2

1. Which of the following statements about theories is accurate?

a. Theories are subject to rules of organization.
b. Theories are statements about how some part of the world works.
c. Theories represent logical and intelligible patterns that make sense of observations.
d. All of the above.

Answer: d

2. The conceptual and theoretical frameworks that provide the foundation for family nursing have evolved from the following three major traditions and disciplines: ______________, ______________, and ______________.

Answer: Family social science, family therapy and nursing

3. Discuss why it is important for nurses to integrate conceptual and theoretical frameworks when working with families.

Families are complex small groups in which multiple processes and dynamics occur simultaneously. Families do not function in one way alone. Today, no one theory or conceptual framework from family social science, family therapy theory, or nursing fully describes the dynamics of family life. Nurses who use only one theoretical approach to working with families are limiting the possibilities for families. Integrating theories allows nurses to view the family from a variety of perspectives, which increases the probability the interventions selected will be implemented by the family, as they "fit" their structure, processes, and style of functioning. Instead of fragmented knowledge and piecemeal interventions, nursing practice is then based on an organized, realistic conceptualization of families. Nurses who use an integrated theoretical approach build on the strength of families in creative ways.

Discussion Question

Select a research article that investigates a question or describes family function. Review it to determine the conceptual framework or theoretical approach(s) used to support the study and the findings. Was the article approached from any of the three disciplines and traditions discussed in the chapter? Did the researchers use an integrated approach to make sense out of the concept studied? How did the theoretical concepts they studied contribute or limit the findings about families? How will this knowledge assist nurses in caring for families?

CHAPTER 3

1. How does the unit of analysis in family nursing research influence the nature of the research?

The unit of analysis influences who is included in the study and how the data is collected and analyzed. How does it influence the type of research questions addressed? The unit of analysis influences what is foreground and what is background (e.g., individual/family member, individual/family subgroup, family system, individual/family system); that is, what phenomena are the focus of study and what is context? The unit of analysis influences not only how the question is framed but also influences the nature of the information we will obtain. How does it influence the data received? Give an example of each. The unit of analysis determines who is the source for information about the family and, consequently, how it is obtained. For example, the individual family member can report individual perceptions via interview or self-report on questionnaires; research about battered women's experiences or parenting experiences are examples. Relational data include information from two or more related persons about an individual or family subsystem (e.g., marital or sibling); research on parent-child relationships is an example. Family-level information depends on transactional data that may be obtained by an interview with the whole family, an observational method, or by combining self-report responses in some way; research questions about family adaptation to a chronic illness or loss are an example. All of the aforementioned strategies are used to study research questions that involve the individual family member(s) and the family system; for example, research about spouses who care for persons with Alzheimer's disease or parents of children with a chronic condition can address: (a) individual characteristics, especially those embedded in the family member role (spouse, mother, father), (b) relational characteristics, such as marital quality, and (c) family as system, such as family coping.

2. Why is it important for family nurse researchers to define "family" explicitly in a study?

To build the science of family nursing, researchers have to be sure that who is included in the study and the data collected are consistent with how the findings are used.

3. Choose one of the research designs used in family research and give an example of a family research question that would be appropriate for that design.

Exploratory: "What is the experience of substance-abusing mothers as they progress through recovery" or "What is the family experience when a child has ADHD?"

Descriptive: "What types of stressors do families with adolescents experience and what are their usual coping strategies?" (e.g., purpose to describe stressors and coping strategies using quantitative measures). "What are the health concerns among rural families of school-aged children?"

Correlational: "What is the relationship between parents' expectations for their children's development and their style of discipline?" "Are social support and communication quality related to the well-being of parents of chronically ill children?"

Experimental: "Does a nurse coaching intervention improve the coping strategies used by families in which the mother has been treated for breast cancer?" "Does a nursing support intervention improve family functioning after a member's cardiac surgery?"

Longitudinal: "What is the impact on the family during the first year after a cancer diagnosis?" "How do prenatal interventions influence mother-infant interaction during the first year of the infant's life?"

4. Briefly discuss two challenges associated with sampling in family research.

I: Whether the families who actually participate represent the population or groups to whom findings and conclusion are to be generalized; representativeness and applicability of findings are concerns for socioeconomic status, health condition, developmental age/status, ethnicity, and culture. II: Attrition is a concern (by illness, death, relocation, and refusal to continue) and whether or not there is a bias because of attrition that would influence interpretation of the findings.

5. How questions are asked can make a significant difference in the quality of data when self-report methods are used in family research. Describe three strategies to improve the quality of the data collected.

The questions should be clear and not ambiguous; examples of items or questions or possible ways of evaluating what the question is about can help. The vocabulary that fits the education and experience of the participants should be used. Questions should focus on a single idea and provide a clear frame of reference. Questions should ask for information the participant has and avoid speculation about how others might think or feel. Closed-ended questions with fixed responses help for objective scoring; open-ended questions allow for clarification and elaboration. Both types have strengths and limitations.

6. Distinguish between reliability and validity of measurement in family research.

Reliability ensures the dependability and consistency of a measure, whereas validity refers to the appropriateness of the specific use of a measure. Both are crucial to meaningful data.

7. Why is quantitative family research multivariate in nature?

In family nursing research, we are usually interested in multiple concepts and multiple variables, hence the term "multivariate."

8. Give two reasons why a family nurse researcher might choose qualitative methods to answer a research question.

I: Qualitative methods are valuable for obtaining in-depth information about why people behave, think, and make meaning as they do: very useful, therefore, for many of the questions nurse researchers have about how families experience and/or respond to various health and illness experiences. II. In addition, qualitative methods allow for the discovery or uncovering of perceptions, understandings, meanings, and psychosocial context that pre-existing measures do not address or ask about; in other words, there is emphasis on discovery or uncovering rather than assessing along existing dimensions.

9. Briefly discuss three ethical considerations in family nursing research.

I: Personal disclosure carries risks to participants, from unpleasant feelings to adverse responses. II. Involvement of children and adolescents requires their assent. III: Use of videotapes requires attention to storage, duration of storage, how used, and how destroyed. IV: Privacy and confidentiality of individuals, especially children or other dependents, and couples must be maintained. V: Intrusion on family's private living space can influence conclusions. VI. Reporting requirements and legal mandates for maltreatment of children, elders, and disabled persons. VII. Guidelines for responding to "clinically urgent" situations or clinically relevant information that are collected.

10. List six issues that should be evaluated in family and family nursing research.

- Whether an explicit family conceptual or theoretical framework is used; basic assumptions should be clear.
- Concept of the family should be explicit and consistent with the theoretical framework.
- A clear definition of the family must be included, specifying who is included in data collection.
- There must be logical consistency in the methods of the research, from unit of analysis, question, design, modes of data collection, measures, and/or data analysis.
- Actual or potential ethical considerations should be addressed.
- The findings need to add to the knowledge base about families and have relevance to nursing practice.

11. The authors list areas for future work in family nursing research. Which area do you believe should be addressed first if the goal is improvement of family nursing practice? Why?

Student should select one of the following and provide their own rationale:

- Family intervention studies
- Studies of families representing diversity in structure, ethnicity and living situation
- Studies that focus on relationships between families and other social systems
- Attention to unit of analysis
- Theory development and theoretical consistency
- Biosocial research and genetics

CHAPTER 4

1. Analyses of family structure, function, and process are limited because the majority of family studies focus on

a. Extended, multigenerational families.
b. Nontraditional family structures.
c. Poor, black, single-parent families.
d. White, middle-class, two-parent families.

Answer: d

2. Which of the following family types is most likely to have the fewest resources to cope with stress?

a. Blended families
b. Cohabiting families
c. Extended families
d. Single-parent families

Answer: d

3. Married men are healthier than single men because they

a. Are less readily sanctioned.
b. Engage in more healthy activities.
c. Experience fewer stressors.
d. Tend to be much happier.

Answer: b

4. Which of the following is a functional prerequisite for the family system?

a. Adaptation
b. Determination
c. Recreation
d. Socialization

Answer: a

5. Which of the following familial roles has undergone the most change in the last two decades?

a. Housekeeper
b. Provider
c. Recreational
d. Therapeutic

Answer: b

6. What is the most common source of role strain in young women with children under 6 years of age?

a. Definition of the situation
b. Lack of role consensus
c. Lack of role knowledge
d. Role overload

Answer: d

7. The woman is most likely to influence the outcome of familial decision making when she is

a. Educated

b. Rich
c. Pregnant
d. White

Answer: b

8. In a healthy family, power

a. Is equally divided among family members.
b. Is the purview of the husband.
c. Resides in the parental coalition.
d. Is an outmoded notion.

Answer: c

9. A healthy family system is characterized by

a. Absence of disease.
b. Parent-child coalitions.
c. Open communication.
d. Stereotyped interactions.

Answer: c

CHAPTER 5

1. The growing significance of cultural diversity in the United States is emphasized by the fact that more than one in four residents is non-white or of Hispanic origin. Which ethnic group experienced the highest increase in growth between 1980 and 1990?

a. Hispanic origin
b. Asian/Pacific Islander
c. Native American
d. African-American

Answer: b

2. The country of origin of an individual is primarily related to his or her:

a. Racial classification
b. Social class
c. Ethnic classification
d. Cultural classification

Answer: c

3. Factors that contribute to differences in health status in various cultural groups and social classes include all of the following except:

a. Inadequate access to preventive and basic health-care resources
b. Family and personal lifestyle differences
c. Exposure to environmental hazards
d. Personality differences
e. Income inequality and rising unemployment

Answer: d

4. Which of the following types of families are more likely to experience poor health within their family?

a. Lower-class families
b. Middle-class families
c. Upper middle-class families
d. Economically affluent families

Answer: a

5. Ethnic families that have integrated dominant American core values and practices in their lives are considered to be:

a. Ethnocentric
b. Unacculturated
c. Culturally competent
d. Acculturated

Answer: d

6. Culturally derived family values influence family health by setting priorities with respect to making family decisions. "Familism" in the Latino culture is an example of which cultural orientation?

a. Time orientation
b. Family versus self-interest
c. Active versus passive orientation
d. Past versus present

Answer: b

7. Which of the following three philosophical/religious beliefs and value systems are more likely to influence the majority of Asian Americans?

a. Judeo-Christian beliefs, Muslim, and Confucianism
b. Taoism, Buddhism, and Confucianism
c. Buddhism, Hinduism, and Shintoism
d. Hinduism, Taoism, and Muslim

Answer: b

8. Women's participation in the labor force has contributed to all of the following changes in family roles, power relationships, and communication patterns except:

a. More open communication
b. Greater sharing of child care roles in family
c. Less sharing of power in marital relationships
d. Sharing of breadwinner role between husband and wife

Answer: c

9. Ethnic differences in family coping patterns are seen among traditional or unaccculturated families. Which of the following coping strategies would commonly be used by Chinese families? (You may choose one or more answers).

a. Family group reliance
b. Role flexibility
c. Spiritual support
d. Maintaining family cohesiveness

Answer: a and d

10. Families who live below the poverty line are at greater risk of experiencing which of the following?

a. Homelessness
b. Poorer health status
c. Lack of access to health services
d. Higher mortality rates
e. All of the above

Answer: e

CHAPTER 6

1. Match the following characteristics with family type:

a. Flexibility is a strength	1. Regenerative family
b. Values family time	2. Resilient family
c. Family hardiness	3. Rhythmic family
d. Emotional closeness within the family	
e. Views illness as a challenge	
f. Routines provide sense of security	

Answers a. 2, b. 3, c. 1, d. 2, e. 1, f. 3

2. What are the five characteristics of an illness according to John Rolland, the author of *Families, Illness, & Disability*?

Onset, course, outcome, type and degree of incapacitation, and degree of uncertainty

3. List three characteristics of a family that indicate a shared religious core.

A faith in God. Family support system that encourages nurturing and affirming relationship. Parental responsibility for passing on religious faith.

4. Identify a family policy currently being debated with the state where you reside.

Will vary by state

5. The United States Constitution provides a guideline for establishing the rights of the family within society. True or False

Answer: False

6. Legal definitions of the family have been challenged as family structures have changed over the past two decades. True or False

Answer: True

7. The principle of beneficence supports the decision to ignore signs of neglect until physical abuse has occurred. True or False

Answer: False

CHAPTER 7

1. In what way is the use of the nursing process unique in providing care for the family as client?

The family must be visualized in terms of its functions and needs. The family as a unit, and each of its members, must be assessed in terms of the ability to meet the collective needs of the family as well as those of each member. The nurse is dealing with many individuals rather than a single person and with the multiple relationships that exist between and among the persons involved. Each step of the nursing process is applied to the unit of care, the family, as well as to particular family members.

2. Describe two diagnostic classification systems that might be used in interpreting data and identifying the specific health care needs of families.

The NANDA system is currently being used by some nurses to describe the health care concerns of the family. Nursing diagnoses are defined as clinical judgments about responses of the individual, family, or community to actual or potential health problems and/or life processes. NANDA includes the statement that the nurse independently selects the interventions appropriate to the identified problem and is accountable for the outcomes of interventions. A taxonomy of diagnostic labels has been developed for the use of professional nurses in defining client problems.

3. What are the limitations of the NANDA system in the defining of family health care needs?

The NANDA system is seen by many as having limited usefulness in family health care because the system has only seven diagnosis labels approved for testing that specifically address family health care concerns. Also, it is seen by some as a system that does not address health promotion needs. Only one diagnosis title specifically deals with this area. There is an effort at this time to increase the emphasis on the development and incorporation of heath promotion nursing diagnosis labels into the NANDA taxonomy.

4. What is an ecomap?

An ecomap is a diagram of a particular family's relationships, including those between and among its members, and with the environment. Extended family are included, and strengths, weaknesses, and social support systems are shown.

5. Discuss how family health care might be evaluated.

Family nursing care is evaluated by monitoring the progress of the family as a unit, and each of its members as specified, in the achievement of the objectives mutually agreed. Specific criteria that will indicate success are identified in consultation and collaboration with the family during the planning process. The achievement of the stated outcome indicates that the desired level of functioning has been achieved. Inability to function at the defined level, complete the designated tasks, or demonstrate the particular behaviors indicates satisfactory progress has not been made.

CHAPTER 8

1. Family assessment and family measurement mean the same thing. True or False

Answer: False

2. Once the nurse assesses the family, they have all the information needed to develop a comprehensive care plan. True or False

Answer: False

3. Match the following terms:

a. Measurement	i. Systematic collection of data
b. Assessment	ii. Assigning numbers to an attribute
c. Qualitative	iii. Data that describe family characteristics
d. Quantitative	iv. Data that compare, measure, or count family properties

Answers: a. ii, b. i, c. iii, d. iv

4. The Family Systems Stressor-Strength Inventory is a measurement instrument that evolved out of the model of the nursing theorist:

a. Sister Callista Roy
b. Dorthea Orem
c. Madelaine Leininger
d. Betty Neuman

Answer: d

5. Family stability is the goal of which model?

a. Friedman's family assessment model
b. Calgary family assessment model
c. Family assessment and intervention model

Answer: c

6. Friedman's model and the CFAM model yield substantially different kinds of information. True or False

Answer: False

7. Friedman's model is based on which of the following theoretical frameworks?

a. Structural–functional theory
b. Systems theory
c. Developmental theory
d. All of the above

Answer: d

8. Wright and Leahey's model is based on which of the following theoretical frameworks?

a. Structural theory
b. Systems theory
c. Developmental theory

d. Communications theory
e. Functional theory

Answer: e

9. Genograms and ecomaps should only be used with families if you are working with the whole group. True or False

Answer: False

10. Nursing instrumentation is at an early stage of development. True or False

Answer: True

11. How does family assessment fit into what we call nursing process?

Assessment is the first step in the family nursing process and it yields descriptive information on the family. Chapter 7 of this book describes five steps of the nursing process, e.g., assessment, analysis, planning, implementation and evaluation, and how to apply this to family situations.

12. How is family assessment different from individual assessment?

Individual assessment focuses on one person. Family assessment focuses on the family as content, the family as client, the family as a system, and the family as a component of society. Family assessment is much more comprehensive than individual assessment. This approach from individual to whole family assessment requires a paradigm shift from who we think of family as our client.

13. Give some examples of how qualitative measurement is used in your daily life. Do the same with quantitative measurement.

Quantitative and qualitative information are obtained during assessment of individuals or families. Quantitative measurement is often called measurement and can be assigned numbers that represent the amount and kind of specified attribute. The data can be nominal or ordinal or interval in nature. Examples are: blood pressure, temperature, numbers of family members, gender, weight. Qualitative data is what we obtain through assessment and interviewing clients. This information is descriptive in nature and not amenable to being assigned numbers. The data is usually nominal in nature. Examples are: history of disease process, family genogram, and patient's reactions to condition. Can you think of other qualitative and qualitative information that we use in nursing practice?

14. Compare measurement and assessment.

Quantitative data is used synonymously with the word measurement. Measurement gives us data to which numbers can be assigned. Assessment usually yields qualitative data, which is descriptive in nature and is not assigned numbers. See answer to Question 13.

15. Discuss the current status of the development of family measurement.

Family assessment guidelines have appeared in several nursing textbooks in the past decade. However, the development of family measurement instruments has only recently received major attention. There is a paucity of materials that can be used for family nursing measurement. Much more theoretical and psychometric work pertaining to family measurement needs to be done by future family nursing and family social science scholars.

16. Summarize the key parts of each family assessment model and discuss how they are different or overlap.

There are three family assessment models presented in this chapter. Each is unique, creating a different data base on which to plan interventions. The family assessment and intervention model and the FS^3I (Berkey & Hanson) are used to measure specific family dimensions such as family stressors and strengths. The FS^3I yields both qualitative and quantitative data. The family assessment model and short form (Friedman) is broader and more general and is particularly useful for viewing families in the context of their community. This approach yields assessment/qualitative data by using an interview guide consisting of specific categories. The Calgary family assessment model (Wright & Leahey) is broad in perspective, focusing on internal relationships (interactions) within the family rather than the interface between the family and community or specific family qualities. All three approaches can be used alone or in combination.

CHAPTER 9

1. Many factors help determine whether a family is involved in health promotion. Which of the following factors may influence promotion of a family's health?

a. Type of family
b. Quality of family interaction
c. Developmental level of family
d. Quality of family housing
e. All of the above

Answer: a

Questions 2 through 6 are based on the following vignette:

The Jones family has four members: Tyrone, the father, age 39; Marcia, the mother, age 30; Barbara, age 8; and James, age 15. James has hemophilia, and he has AIDS, which he contracted from a blood transfusion about 3 years ago. He began to show symptoms a year ago, was prescribed an experimental drug, and is currently asymptomatic. He attends high school daily but tires easily. The parents come in to the HIV clinic with James for a routine checkup. They say that he does not have much to say and stays in his room a lot after school; in fact, all the family members stay in their own rooms most of the time. Meals are usually eaten separately. James says he eats dinner in his room most evenings and complains about feeling lonely and avoided. The parents, in turn, feel that James is avoiding them at meals.

2. What stage of the family health and illness cycle is this family experiencing?

a. The vulnerability and symptom-experiencing cycle
b. The health phase
c. Chronic adjustment/adaptation phase
d. Rehabilitation

Answer: c

3. Family process influences how a person adapts to a family health issue. Which of the following processes would be most helpful in improving the quality of this family's life?

a. Insist that James eat with family.
b. Ignore the problem, it will take care of itself.
c. Schedule a family meeting where each family member talks about how he or she feels about James' health.
d. Schedule a family meeting and explain that the family is grieving and decide not to worry about it.

Answer: c

4. Which of the following best describes key traits of a healthy family that this family does not appear to have?

a. Resiliency, spending time together, and positive communication
b. Resiliency, spending time together, and adaptability
c. Happiness, financial security, shared vacations
d. Flexibility, sense of humor, positive communication

Answer: b

5. Internal family factor that is influencing the level of this family's well-being is:

a. James' disease
b. Reaction of peers to AIDS
c. Community fear of the family of AIDS
d. Poor family communication

Answer: d

6. To empower this family to resolve the crisis so that James does not feel alone and the rest of the family does not feel avoided, the nurse would:

a. Teach them exactly what to do to resolve the problem.
b. Encourage James to eat once a week with the family.
c. Teach them family communication and problem solving.
d. Allow them to work the issue out by themselves.

Answer: c

CHAPTER 10

1. Early predecessors of childbearing family nurses were

a. Childbirth educators.
b. Nurse midwives.
c. Nursery nurses.
d. Public health nurses.

Answer: d

2. Currently the best theory to guide childbearing family nursing is

a. Family systems.
b. Structural-functional.
c. Change theory.
d. None of the above.

Answer: d

3. Families with closed boundaries are often not accessible to nursing interventions because

a. These families do not have children.
b. These are unstable families.
c. Family members do not interact with each other.
d. These families reject influences from the outside environment.

Answer: d

4. Childbearing family nurses may ask about a family's space arrangement for an expected baby to assess if the family

a. Is meeting its basic needs.
b. Is accepting the reality of the expected baby.
c. Has fears about the survival of the baby.
d. All the above.

Answer: d

5. Priority for research related to childbearing family is

a. The effectiveness of family nursing interventions.
b. Development of theories that describe childbearing families.
c. The importance of immediate contact between newborn babies and their parents.
d. How the "Baby Boom" of the 1950s influenced present-day childbearing family nursing.

Answer: a

6. Write a care plan to help the Johnson family develop a relationship with Jason while he is in the special care nursery.

Discuss his expectations about being a father

Encourage him to discuss his expectations with his partner

Educate both mothers and fathers about the realities of being parents

Encourage women to regard their partners as parents instead of helpmates, supports, and bystanders

Encourage couples to share the enjoyable and not-so-enjoyable tasks of child care

Explore ways fathers can share in infant feeding when mothers are breastfeeding

Encourage her mother to attend a grandparents class that includes current recommendations about newborn care

Provide up-to-date reading materials for both women

Teach the client nonthreatening ways to communicate with her mother, such as the use of "I" messages

Encourage the client to ask her mother to tell her about how she dealt with crying and how she learned about it. Also encourage client to share what she is learning with her mother.

Do not "take sides" in this discussion. It is important for nurses not to feel disappointed when their clients do not take their advice. Enhancing the mother-daughter relationship is more important than determining who is right.

Postpartum depression affects how mothers interact with their babies. This can interfere with nurturing babies and role learning. Other family members experience stress and change in relationships that affect family members' motivation and morale.

A care plan for a family with an infant in a special care nursery should include interventions to promote attachment such as encouraging frequent contact between the family and the infant, having the family take over as much of the care of the baby as possible, and pointing out the characteristics and behaviors of baby so the family know the baby as a unique individual.

Nurses need to make the special care nursery a welcoming environment for families through open-door policies, comfortable and home-like furnishing, pleasant staff, and consideration of women's postpartum physical and emotional needs. Providing privacy for the family with the baby can enhance family-infant interaction. Encouraging the family to establish rituals with Jason can foster family development.

The expectations of a family such as the Johnson's usually are not met with a preterm birth. All nurses in contact with the family should encourage the Johnson's to discuss their expectations and disappointments. Nurses can help the family form realistic expectations about the baby in special care.

Mary is showing signs of postpartum depression which can interfere with her interactions with Jason. She should be referred for appropriate treatment. Preterm babies often do not have clear cues. Mary should be aware of this. Nurses can coach her on interpreting Jason's cues.

Mary Johnson planned to breastfeed Jason. Nurses in both the special care nursery and her community should support her in maintaining lactation and initiating breastfeeding.

The Johnson family is new to the community. Nurses can refer the family to support systems to help alleviate stress. Stressed families often have difficulty in maintaining and developing positive relationships.

CHAPTER 11

1. The family child health nurse determines the most *appropriate* health promotion activities with a family with young children through analysis of:

a. Children's health practices
b. Patterns of parenting, and family and child developmental tasks
c. Parents' and grandparents' health beliefs
d. Patterns of disease and illness reorganization task management

Answer: b. Through analysis of the individual family and the family career, i.e., their stages of family development, family transitions, individual development, and patterns of health disease and illness.

2. Family child health nurses practice family-centered health care, which is most accurately characterized as:

a. Fostering partnerships between members of different families
b. Providing consistently high-quality care for all families
c. Forming partnerships between families and nurses
d. Viewing the nurse as the constant in family and child health

Answer: c. Family centered care is collaborative. Partnerships include viewing the family as one important constant in the child's life.

3. The family interaction model has three major concepts. Which one of the following is not one of these major concepts?

a. Task development cycles
b. Individual development
c. Family career
d. Patterns of health, disease, and illness

Answer: a. Tasks may have development cycles, but this activity is not one of the major concepts of the family interaction model.

4. Which of these principles should family nurses incorporate in their care in order to help a family with a child who has diabetes?

a. Patterns of illness are usually predictable in families
b. Protection is paramount in each interaction
c. Patterns of illness and disease differ in different families
d. Reorganization of family routines is discouraged

Answer: c. Family patterns of health, disease, and illness vary widely. Family responses, which become the substance of the family transitions, also vary.

5. Using the family interaction model, the family child health nurse knows that one of the more important assessments of families experiencing a chronic illness of their child is:

a. Definition of the disease with which the child has been diagnosed
b. How the family's past crises have altered their growth
c. Definition of the limitations that the family is experiencing
d. How the family's past experience with the illness affects the current situation.

Answer: d. Using concepts of family career, individual development, and patterns of health, disease and illness, the nurse inquires about the particular family's experiences and responses.

6. Why is it important for family child health nurses to explore a family's developmental tasks when analyzing the family's response to an illness event?

Understanding the family's present developmental stage, the extent to which the family is fulfilling its family developmental tasks, and the family's history, as well as both parents' families of origin, gives insight into the family's challenges at the current stage. The nurse can assess the age of the oldest child and other children to learn what developmental stages the family is now passing through. Knowing the past family experiences helps the nurse build on the family's strengths and define what areas may need teaching and support.

7. What principles of family-centered care would family child health nurses use with a hospitalized infant and family?

Answer: The principles of family-centered care include:

(a) Recognizing families as "the constants" in children's lives, while the personnel in the health care system fluctuate

(b) Openly sharing information about alternative treatments, ethical concerns, and uncertainties about health care treatments

(c) Forming partnerships between families and health professionals to decide what is important for families

(d) Respecting the racial, ethnic, cultural, and socioeconomic diversity of families and their ways of coping

(e) Supporting and strengthening families' abilities to grow and develop.

Discussion Questions

1. Discuss with your classmates your experiences with families. Compare your expectations as you think about the behaviors of types of children and families with whom you are familiar and those with whom you are less familiar.
2. Compare how you, a family child health nurse, would discuss health outcomes with a family in the following situations: a family with a chronically ill child, a family with an acutely ill child, a family with a child with a life-threatening illness. Consider families with multiple children in which one has an illness or disease and the others do not.
3. Obtain a child or family health policy in your city, state, or county. Discuss the implications of that policy for families with a chronically ill child and for a family who has few or limited financial resources or has no health insurance.

CHAPTER 12

1. Which of the following factors has led to the growth of family nursing in medical-surgical settings:

a. Consumer demands for unfragmented and holistic care
b. Early hospital discharge
c. Empirical evidence that families influence patient recovery
d. All of the above

Answer: d

2. All of the following characteristics are likely to increase the degree of family stress associated with hospitalization *except*:

a. Sudden illness onset with no time to prepare
b. Repeated family experience with the illness
c. Few sources of guidance for the family
d. Significant disruption of family functioning as a result of the hospitalization

Answer: b

3. Nurses caring for families in medical-surgical settings need to consider the following factors of the "therapeutic quadrangle":

a. Illness, family, doctor, patient
b. Illness, doctor, nurse, patient
c. Illness, family, health care team, patient
d. Family, health care team, social work services, chaplain services

Answer: c

4. Helping families maintain healthy lifestyles is a major aim for nurses during the:

a. Pre-illness phase
b. Acute illness phase
c. Chronic illness phase
d. Terminal illness phase

Answer: a

5. Establishing a calm and relaxed atmosphere that will support a trusting and empathetic relationship describes which of the following family nursing interventions:

a. Proximity enhancement
b. Information management
c. Assurance provision
d. Comfort facilitation

Answer: c

6. Minimization of family disruption effects describes which category of family nursing interventions?

a. Family support
b. Family process management
c. Promotion of family integrity
d. Family involvement

Answer: b

7. Which of the following family behaviors is rarely displayed during the chronic phase of illness?

a. Accepting the imminence of death
b. Carrying out prescribed treatment regimens
c. Finding the necessary money and resources to facilitate care
d. Preventing the social isolation caused by lessened contact with others

Answer: a

8. Relationships between the family and the health care team move through stages. The stage characterized by family renegotiation of trust with health care professionals is called the stage of:

a. Naive trust
b. Disenchantment
c. Guarded alliance
d. None of the above

Answer: c

9. What factors should be considered when determining hospital visiting policies?

a. Patient preferences
b. Family preferences
c. Nursing care needs
d. All of the above

Answer: d

10. Which of the following is not an advantage to having families present when nurses and physicians carry out resuscitative efforts?

a. Assurance that the patient is dying
b. Less nursing staff time is needed for giving explanations, since the family has witnessed activities firsthand.
c. It helps the family accept the reality of death.
d. It provides the family with an opportunity to say what they need to say while there is still a chance the patient can hear.

Answer: b

11. Families of patients with AIDS may experience:

a. Social stigmatization
b. Guilt
c. Economic hardship
d. All of the above

Answer: d

CHAPTER 13

1. Which of the following recent trends have influenced both the client's treatment needs and the system of care delivery in family mental health nursing?

a. Freudian psychoanalytic movement, deinstitutionalization
b. Downward turn in the economic market, consumer advocacy
c. Health care reform, shortened length of hospital stay, more manageable medication protocols
d. Freudian psychoanalytic movement, the medical model

Answer: c

2. Family mental health nurses who are using structural family theory to guide their practice would assess which of the following areas in families?

a. Differentiation of self, anxiety, and triangulation
b. Power, subsystems, and boundaries
c. Multigenerational trust, multigenerational loyalty, and other multigenerational family processes
d. Disconfirmation, disqualification, and double-bind messages

Answer: b

3. Family mental health nurses who are using Bowen's family theory to guide their practice would assess which of the following areas in families?

a. Differentiation of self, anxiety, and triangulation

b. Power, subsystems, and boundaries
c. Multigenerational trust, multigenerational loyalty, and other multigenerational family processes
d. Disconfirmation, disqualification, and double-bind messages

Answer: a

4. Family mental health nurses who are using contextual family theory to guide their practice would assess which of the following areas in families?

a. Differentiation of self, anxiety, and triangulation
b. Power, subsystems, and boundaries
c. Multigenerational trust, multigenerational loyalty, and other multigenerational family processes
e. Disconfirmation, disqualification, and double-bind messages

Answer: c

5. Family mental health nurses who are using communication theory to guide their practice would assess which of the following areas in families?

a. Differentiation of self, anxiety, and triangulation
b. Power, subsystems, and boundaries
c. Multigenerational trust, multigenerational loyalty, and other multigenerational family processes
d. Disconfirmation, disqualification, and double-bind messages

Answer: d

6. Family mental health nurses who are using a multiple systems view to guide their practice would assess which of the following areas in families?

a. Family interactional patterns
b. Biological factors
c. Psychological factors
d. Cultural, environmental, and spiritual factors
e. All of the above

Answer: e

7. Nancy is an advanced practice nurse practicing family nursing in a community mental health center. She is developing a health promotion program for the community. Health promotion seeks to:

a. Increase positive coping abilities and counteract harmful conditions that may produce disability
b. Provide early diagnosis and treatment and prompt referral as necessary
c. Assist the client and the family to resume the highest level of productivity in all aspects of daily living
d. Assist the client and the family to cope with residual disability that warrants continued assistance

Answer: a

8. After a potentially lethal suicide attempt by drinking rat poison, 33-year-old Maria was admitted to the intensive care unit for stabilization of her physical condition. The nurses sought a consultation from the mental health consultation liaison nurse. The role of the consultation liaison nurse in a medical treatment setting is to:

a. Refer the client for inpatient psychiatric treatment
b. Help the client and the family begin to understand the crisis that has just occurred and options for family treatment
c. Provide intensive psychotherapy
d. Focus on assisting the client and the family to open lines of direct communication

Answer: b

9. John has been suffering from the debilitating effects of schizophrenia for the past 10 years. Following his most recent discharge from the hospital, he was admitted to a psychoeducational program. A psychoeducational program might include all of the following elements *except*:

a. Information about the availability of specific community services
b. Helping the family to understand how they caused John's illness
c. Detailed information about the illness, treatment plans, and medications
d. Home visits by a mental health nurse specialist

Answer: b

10. Melissa is a 19-year-old who has recently been diagnosed with bipolar disorder. She was admitted to an in-patient treatment setting that

emphasizes family-focused treatment. Family-focused treatment is likely to include:

a. Use of therapeutic leave of absences to provide a break from the demands of treatment
b. Custodial care and companionship from the nurses
c. Regular scheduled conferences that include the family in setting treatment goals
d. The use of psychopharmocological interventions only

Answer: c

CHAPTER 14

1. Which of the following statements are true?

a. Adult children should be discouraged from talking to their elderly parents about their benefits and finances.
b. Older families, like older people, seem more alike than different.
c. Families provide the bulk of health care to older people.
d. Sons and daughters share the care of elderly parents equally.

Answer: c

2. List and describe three common, normative events that can trigger significant transitions in older families.

Answer: Retirement, death of a spouse, change in health status

3. Social support outside the family is important in helping older individuals remain independent and functioning in the community. Name four factors or conditions that may hinder or limit the availability of social support.

Answer: Finances, transportation, lack of knowledge, isolation related to cultural or ethnic differences

4. A major goal of gerontological family nursing is:

a. To help the family system restore and maintain the functioning and health of its older members.
b. To assist the family in making health care placement decisions for its older members.
c. To set appropriate caregiving goals for the family.
d. To help the family avoid the need for institutionalization of elderly members.

Answer: a

5. List and discuss three potential stressors that are commonly experienced by the "sandwich generation." How might these affect their coping and adaptation to a decline in health of aging parents?

Multiple competing demands (i.e., care of children, parent care, job responsibilities), one-parent families, financial demands

6. Which of the following is (are) true statement(s)?

a. Most older persons tend to rely heavily on the formal health care system to meet their needs.
b. The formal health care system is set up to meet the needs of the family.
c. Older people tend to rely on family assistance and "make do" until a crisis occurs.
d. Families caring for an elderly member with a dementing illness are at greater risk for poor health and/or elder mistreatment.

Answer: c

7. Which of the following is (are) true statement(s)?

a. Chapters and articles that describe the unique characteristics of various cultural and ethnic groups provide universally accurate information about individuals and families.
b. Variability within cultural groups may be as great as variability between cultural groups.
c. The inclusion of diversity content in the nursing curriculum eliminates the problems of stereotyping and bias in nursing assessments.

Answer: b

CHAPTER 15

1. Describe the target of care for community public health nursing.

Answer: The target of care is the community: the community is the client receiving care. Individuals, families, and groups are subunits of the community. Nurses working in community settings direct care toward individuals, families, and groups, and the community serves as the context within which care is given.

2. Identify nursing's historical roots in caring for families in community settings.

Visiting nurses were described as early as the pre-Christian era in India, Egypt, Greece, and Rome. In the mid-1800s, the role was expanded to include health education, not just care of the sick. The role of visiting nurse expanded to include all family members. In 1893, Lillian Wald established a home visiting service in New York City to serve the sick poor. In the early 1900s, subspecialties in community health nursing developed. Some nurses cared for mothers/infants and others worked in areas like mental health. Community health nurses did not fully direct their practice to the family as a unit until the 1950s and this remained their perspective until the 1970s.

3. Analyze how the practices of family and community public health nursing interface.

The trend in the delivery of health care has been to move health care to community settings: thus family nursing is very pertinent to public and community health nurses. Some community health nurses have redirected their care toward the community as client, with the family as an important subunit: others have continued to emphasize the family as the central unit service. Community health nurses contribute to the growth and health of the community and society through the assistance given to family groups.

4. Define the following: epidemiology, public health nursing, community as client, aggregate of people, health promotion, disease prevention, and primary, secondary, and tertiary prevention.

Epidemiology: the study of the distribution of states of health and the causes of deviations from health in populations, and the application of this study to control the health problems.

Public health nursing: the synthesis of nursing knowledge and practice and the science and practice of public health, implemented via systematic use of the nursing process and other processes, designed to promote health and prevent illness in population groups. The focus of care is the aggregate. The goal of care is the promotion of health and the prevention of illness.

Community as client: target of service (i.e., the population group for whom healthful change is sought).

Aggregate of people: groups of people with some common characteristics.

Health promotion: "the process of enabling people to increase control over, and to improve their health" (Ottawa Charter, 1986, p. 1).

Disease prevention: activities that have as their goal the protection of people from the ill-effects of actual or potential health threats.

Primary prevention: actions designed to prevent a disease from occurring; reduces the probability of a specific illness occurring and includes active protection against unnecessary stressors or threats.

Secondary prevention: early diagnosis and prompt treatment: includes activities such as screening for diseases.

Tertiary prevention: activities aimed at correcting health problems and preventing further deterioration. It also focuses on preventing recurrences of the problem.

5. List at least one example of a public health intervention for each level of prevention.

An example of primary is provision of and training in the use of barrier contraceptives.

An example of secondary prevention is obtaining a Pap smear to detect cervical dysplasia.

An example of tertiary prevention is rehabilitation of an injured worker to return to work.

Discussion Question

1. Identify a policy that affects families in your community.

Answer: Will vary

CHAPTER 16

1. Identify two examples of "family" that are outside of and contradict the stereotypical "nuclear family."

Answer: Divorced families, step families, chosen families, foster families.

2. Describe at least one policy shift in access or cost of personal health services that has an impact on the health of families.

Increased insurance coverage, increasing likelihood of routine care; loss of coverage, decreasing likelihood of dental or other care services; parental work requirements, making it difficult to get children to care; additional coverage of prescription drugs could reduce hospitalization of those with chronic illnesses

3. Describe social discrimination as it affects family experiences.

Insistence on "family" defined as a father/mother dyad can limit child-rearing options for GLBT families; rules on family foster care or adoption can limit range of choices for child placement; expectation that mothers will provide care can impoverish a family

4. List at least three services available to families because of public policies.

Family medical leave, aid to needy families, Head Start, Medicaid, day care for low income families, foster care for children at risk, home care for the elderly under Medicare

5. Why is it important that a nurse never presume to define "family" for a patient?

A patient with a nontraditional family configuration may assume that the nurse will discriminate and will withhold information that could make a significant difference in planning for and giving care.

6. Discuss areas in which advocacy by nurses could be significant for family social policy.

The nurse's insight into family structure and health can inform public debates on income, welfare, health, child care or environmental policy.

CHAPTER 17

1. Match the cultural periods of American families with their typical characteristics.

a. Traditional family	_____	I. Leveling off of divorce
b. Individualism	_____	II. High birth rates
c. New familism	_____	III. High degree of marital stability
	_____	IV. Decline in birth rates
	_____	V. Increased flexibility

Answer: 1. c, 2. a, 3, a, 4. b, 5. c

2. What are the specific family demographic trends in the U.S.?

Examples are: marriage rates remain high, divorce rates remain high, increasing numbers of single parent families, birth rates are down, birth rates to never-married women are high, couples delay first marriage, women represent an increasing percentage of the work force, people are living longer, a larger percentage of the U.S. population are old.

3. What other trends have you noticed in your country?

4. Name some world demographic changes that you are aware of.

Examples are: Increasing world population particularly in underdeveloped countries, increased aging populations occurring throughout the world, increased technology bringing the world community closer to one another, health issues around the world are similar, and what affects one country affects all other countries

5. What other observations have you made about the world?

6. Why and how is family nursing theory, practice, research, education, and social policy important for the future of family health care nursing?

Family nursing theory, practice, and research are essential components of the nursing profession. Theory provides a foundation for us to understand our observations and to practice nursing. Nursing practice informs nursing research on the issues that need to be investigated. The outcome of nursing research is to inform better practice. Nursing theory, practice and research (TPR) needs to be taught to upcoming generations of nurses in our educational institutions. Nursing theory, practice, and research provide information for family health and social policy. Changes in one part of these intertwined components affect other components. This book has addressed all of these important components of family health care nursing.

Discussion Questions

1. What do you see as the future for families in the U.S. and around the world? Describe the rationale for your response.

2. Pretend you could look into a crystal ball, and name one prediction for the future of families and one for family nursing.
3. What role will you play in the future of family health care nursing?
4. Discuss the implications that religion, sexuality, and health care technology have for the future of family health care nursing. What are some other factors that will affect family health care nursing that are not listed in this chapter?

INDEX

An *f* following a page number indicates a figure; a *t* indicates a table.